TEXTBOOK OF
MEDICAL PHYSIOLOGY

VOLUME 1:
CELLULAR MECHANISMS, NEURAL INTEGRATION, AND SYSTEMIC REGULATION

Dr. Shipra Chandra

ALLIED
HEALTH
PRESS

Textbook of Medical Physiology

Volume 1: Cellular Mechanisms, Neural Integration, and Systemic Regulation

Author: **Dr. Shipra Chandra**

Allied Health Press
4164 Lakeshore Road
Burlington ON L7L 1A4
Canada
www.alliedhealthpress.com
Email: orders@arclereducation.com

ISBN: 978-1-77956-778-9

ABOUT THE AUTHOR

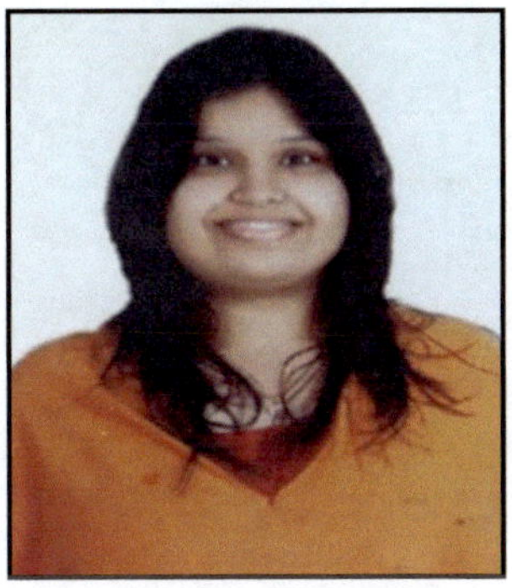

Dr. Shipra Chandra born in Delhi in 1983, completed school from a government school in Delhi in 2001 with First division. Being a science student , took admission in Chemistry Honors at Kirori Mal College, Delhi University. But the wonders of Human Body always fascinated me and I continued preparing for Pre Medical Test (PMT) despite being in a reputed college and course.

By the Grace of God and blessings of my family I secured 5th rank in CPMT 2002 along-with being waitlisted at DPMT and securing rank in AIEEE exam. Joined MBBS on 14/11/2002 at the most prestigious King George Medical College, Lucknow, U.P. Completed MBBS in First division in 2008 and joined AIIMS, New Delhi Department of Emergency Medicine for work experience in 2009 but continued the preparation for Post Graduation Entrance Test and cracked the UP-PGME in 2010 and was allotted MD Physiology from King George Medical University.

After completing the MD in 2013, I again cleared AIIMS, New Delhi entrance test for Senior Residency. Learned a lot during my 3 year tenure from 2013 to 2016 at AIIMS. Following which I joined Fortis Hospital Shalimar Bagh and continued search for a Government Job. Gave the interview at U.P. Public Service Commission in 2017, cracked it and joined as Assistant Professor at Sarojini Naidu Medical College, Agra in 2017. I have 7 research publications , one book chapter and guided 3 MD students during my tenure. Promoted to the post of Associate Professor in 2022 and currently working in the same capacity.

Brief Table of Contents

Getting Started with This Book

Chapter Openers

A list of Chapter Outline is presented providing a brief Introduction to what will be covered in the chapter.

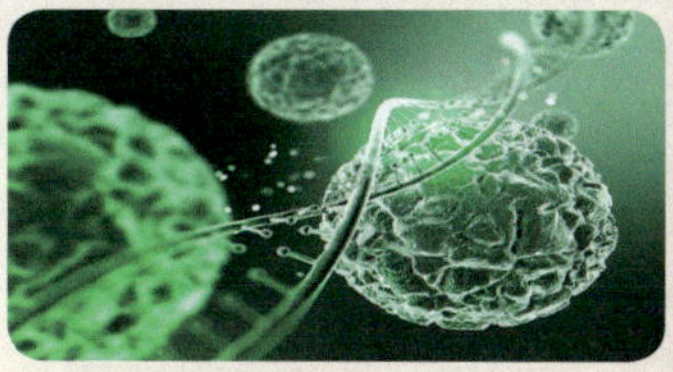

LEARNING OBJECTIVES

After studying this chapter, you will be able to:

1. Discuss the scientific method in biology;
2. Explain the cell theory;
3. Discuss the genetics and heredity;
4. Evolution and natural selection;
5. Focus on ecology and ecosystems;
6. Learn about human biology;
7. Evaluate the plant biology;
8. Explain the microbiology;
9. Focus on current trends in biology.

Introduction

Often referred to as the science of life, biology is a broad field of study aimed at comprehending the several kinds of life on Earth, from tiny creatures to sophisticated multicellular entities. Comprising several subfields, including molecular biology, ecology, and evolutionary biology, each of which advances our knowledge of living systems, this field clarifies the mechanisms controlling life events, including development, reproduction, and interaction with the surroundings, which is the central goal of biology. Moreover, biology fills in the void between the natural sciences and medicine by offering a necessary understanding of health, illness, and the interactions between organisms and their environments. Dealing with urgent global issues such as climate change, biodiversity loss, and new diseases depends on an awareness of these complex biological interactions, therefore highlighting the critical part biology plays in modern civilization. Fundamentally, biology explores and tests ideas about the living world using the scientific method. Through methodical observation and experimentation,

1.1. The Scientific Method in Biology

Learning Outcome

1. Describe the steps of the scientific method;
2. Focus on hypothesis formation;
3. Learn about experimental design.

Learning Outcomes

The beginning of each section of every chapter contains a set of Learning Outcomes that inform students of concepts they should understand. These outcomes help students understand what they should be able to do if they have mastered the material in that section.

Test Your Knowledge

Throughout each chapter, Test Your Knowledge cues you to note which topics have been covered and to self-test your understanding of the material presented.

Test Your Knowledge

1. Explain why correlation does not imply causation in scientific experiments.
2. How does the scientific method help reduce the influence of personal opinions in research?

Chapter Summary

The Summary Section appear at the end of each chapter and summarize main concepts covered throughout the chapter. These points provide key concepts in an engaging and meaningful way.

Summary

The investigation of biological principles highlights the importance of a comprehensive view of life by reflecting the intricate interactions that occur within living systems. The complexity of biology goes beyond individual species or systems, as this essay highlights; it also includes the interactions that mold ecosystems and affect biodiversity. Researchers can conduct in-depth analyses of metabolomic data using sophisticated technologies like MetaboAnalyst, which offer insights into the molecular mechanisms underlying these interactions. As demonstrated by the developments in MetaboAnalyst, for example, the integration of diverse omics data promotes a thorough understanding of metabolic pathways and helps identify important biological markers necessary for research on development and disease (Chong et al., 2018). Additionally, the phenomenon of ecological invasions is a key component of biological research and a vital field of study. The introduction of non-native species into unfamiliar habitats has significant ramifications and calls for multidisciplinary management strategies. Examining the origins and effects of these biological incursions, invasion science has become a crucial field that highlights the need to comprehend ecological dynamics and community interactions. As interest in biological invasions increases, new findings are emerging that put conventional ecological theories and practices to the test. The importance of incorporating various scientific viewpoints is shown by this developing discipline, which also highlights how invasive species shape ecosystems and advances our knowledge of ecological resilience (David et al., 2013). When taken as a whole, these discoveries from invasion science and metabolomics highlight the value of multidisciplinary biology research. Fostering cross-disciplinary collaboration and utilizing technological breakthroughs to improve our comprehension of intricate biological interactions are crucial as we look to the future of biological research. In addition to deepening our understanding of the complexities of life, this method lays the groundwork for tackling urgent environmental issues. Future studies can ensure the continued relevance of biology in a world that is constantly changing by acknowledging the interconnection of biological systems and opening the door to creative solutions that support sustainability and biodiversity conservation. We might imagine a thorough comprehension of life that serves both academia and society at large through ongoing investigation and integration of scientific knowledge.

Knowledge Assessment

The chapter includes material designed to review and reinforce each content. It includes Critical Thinking Questions to help test of your understanding of information presented in the chapter and Short answer Questions to review your understanding of the key concepts presented in the chapter.

Critical Thinking Questions

1. **Who is known as the "Father of Modern Biology"?**
   a. Aristotle
   b. Charles Darwin
   c. Gregor Mendel
   d. Louis Pasteur
2. **What is the basic unit of life?**
   a. Atom
   b. Molecule
   c. Cell
   d. Organism
3. **Which branch of biology studies the interaction of organisms with their environment?**
   a. Genetics
   b. Ecology
   c. Physiology
   d. Botany
4. **Which macromolecule is the main source of energy for living organisms?**
   a. Proteins
   b. Lipids
   c. Carbohydrates
   d. Nucleic acids
5. **DNA is primarily responsible for which function in living organisms?**
   a. Energy production
   b. Protein synthesis
   c. Storing genetic information
   d. Regulating body temperature

Short Answer Questions

1. What is biology, and why is it important to study biology?
2. What are the three main domains of life, and how are they different from one another?
3. Define homeostasis and give an example of how it works in living organisms.
4. What is the cell theory, and why is it fundamental to biology?
5. How do autotrophs and heterotrophs differ in the way they obtain energy?
6. What is the scientific method, and how is it applied in biological research?
7. Discuss how biology helps address global challenges such as climate change, disease, and food security.
8. Explain the levels of biological organization from the smallest unit to the largest. Provide examples at each level.
9. Describe the relationship between structure and function in biology, giving specific examples from cells or organs.
10. How has the discovery of genetics shaped our understanding of inheritance and variation among organisms?

Supplementary Materials

Key Terms: A list of key terms is given for quick reference

KEY TERMS FROM THIS CHAPTER

Annotation enrichment analysis	Biological structure	Cell
Cell theory	Cellular structure	Ecology
Ecosystems	Genetics	Human biology
Microbiology	Natural selection	Organism
Plant biology		

Further Resources: Recommendations for additional readings, websites, and multimedia resources.

References

1. Argelaguet, R., Velten, B., Arnol, D., Dietrich, S., Zenz, T., Marioni, J. C., Buettner, F., et al. (2018). Multi-omics factor analysis—A framework for unsupervised integration of multi-omics data sets. *Molecular Systems Biology, 14*. https://doi.org/10.15252/msb.20178124.
2. Bacher, S., Blackburn, T. M., Essl, F., & Genovesi, P. (2017). *Socio-Economic Impact Classification of Alien Taxa (SEICAT)*. https://core.ac.uk/download/286567949.pdf (accessed on 8th March 2025).
3. Barnett, R., Brace, S., Cucchi, T., & Dobney, K. (2013). *Divergent Evolutionary Processes Associated with Colonization of Offshore Islands*. https://core.ac.uk/download/20664364.pdf (accessed on 8th March 2025).

Detailed Table of Contents

CHAPTER 12

Renal Physiology: Structure and Filtration 403

Index 437

LIST OF FIGURES

PREFACE

Physiology gives the foundation for the medical sciences by outlining the functional mechanisms of the human body. It combines molecular biology, anatomy, and clinical medicine, enabling one to understand how cells, tissues, and systems interact to maintain life. By focusing on mechanisms of function—rather than just anatomical shape—physiology educates students and practitioners to comprehend normal function and derangement in disease.

The field advances with ongoing discoveries on ion channels, neurotransmitters, hormonal feedback, and feedback mechanisms, thereby further elucidating the relationships between health and disease. Physiological functions are no longer researched in stationary models but now encompass systems biology, integrated data, and bioengineering methods. In this regard, accurate and available knowledge of physiology remains crucial to students, teachers, clinicians, and scientists.

This book, *Textbook of Medical Physiology, Volume 1: Cellular Mechanisms, Neural Integration, and Systemic Regulation,* provides a step-by-step account of the fundamental principles of human physiology. A combination of clear exposition with related clinical data, the book is intended to be helpful both for educational purposes and daily use. The volume is suitable for medical students, students in allied health sciences, and those in biological sciences, offering a comprehensive coverage of the fundamental systems that maintain human life, from traditional principles to the latest knowledge.

- Chapter 1 introduces physiology and the law of homeostasis as the unifying concept that governs the operation of every function in the body. It accounts for the birth of physiological science in the past and gives definitions of key terms, feedback loops, and control systems. The importance of stabilizing the internal environment and why stability within the internal environment is regulated between systems is also introduced, making readers appreciate physiological interdependence.
- Chapter 2 characterizes cell membrane physiology, emphasizing membrane structure, ion channels, transport mechanisms, and electrochemical gradients. The chapter includes discussions of passive and active transport, membrane potential, osmosis, and the role of cellular compartments. The chapter lays the groundwork for understanding how individual cell function is responsible for tissue and organ behavior.
- Chapter 3 examines the physiological processes of muscle function, , such as skeletal, cardiac, and smooth muscle. Topics covered are excitation-contraction coupling,

sliding filament theory, energy sources for contraction, and muscle tension control. Clinical applications of conditions like myasthenia gravis and muscular dystrophy are integrated to enhance applied learning.

- Chapter 4 describes nerve physiology in terms of action potential generation and conduction, synaptic transmission, and the action of neurotransmitters. Neuronal structural and functional classification, myelination functions, and synaptic plasticity are described. This chapter facilitates sensory input and motor output of the body.
- Chapter 5 is focused on the autonomic nervous system (ANS), presenting the sympathetic and parasympathetic divisions and their control of involuntary processes. Neurotransmitter circuits, autonomic reflexes, and various types of receptors are addressed, along with their physiological effects on the cardiovascular, respiratory, gastrointestinal, and urogenital systems. Pharmacological considerations are introduced.
- Chapter 6 covers the central nervous system, , such as the organization of the brain and spinal cord, sensory and motor tracts, and functional areas of the cerebral cortex. The brainstem and hypothalamus, key control centers, are covered, in addition to higher functions , such as consciousness, sleep, memory, and language. An introduction to cerebrospinal fluid dynamics and the blood-brain barrier is also covered in the chapter.
- Chapter 7 covers the physiology of the special senses of vision, hearing, taste, smell, and equilibrium. The chapter covers sensory receptor types, transduction pathways, and neural processing in the sensory cortices. Clinical conditions, , such as hearing loss, anosmia, and visual field defects, are referenced to relate theoretical constructs to actual presentations.
- Chapter 8 discusses blood physiology, outlining the parts and functions of plasma, red blood cells, white blood cells, and platelets. Hematopoiesis, blood types, immunity, and hemostasis are discussed together with regulatory factors. Anemia, leukopenia, and disorders of coagulation present a clinical picture of blood function.
- Chapter 9 covers cardiac physiology in the context of the examination of heart structure and electrical function. Topics addressed are the cardiac cycle, heart sounds, myocardial conduction, and cardiac output. Autonomic regulation of heart rate and contractility, as well as concepts in electrocardiography (ECG), are covered to provide students with an in-depth understanding of heart function and rhythm interpretation.
- Chapter 10 deals with the topic of vascular physiology, , such as the regulation of blood pressure, vascular resistance, microcirculation, and venous return. The chapter outlines how baroreceptors, chemoreceptors, and hormonal control mechanisms maintain vascular stability. Pathophysiologic considerations, , such as hypertension and shock, are discussed for their clinical significance.
- Chapter 11 discusses pulmonary physiology, dealing with the mechanics of breathing, gas exchange, lung volumes, and control of breathing. Ventilation-perfusion matching, oxygen transport, and carbon dioxide elimination are also discussed, along with conditions , such as hypoxia and respiratory acidosis. The impact of environmental and pathological factors on lung function is also highlighted.
- Chapter 12 covers renal physiology, specifically the structure of the kidneys and glomerular filtration. Nephron anatomy, filtration pressures, and selective membrane permeability in urine formation are described in detail. Regulation of water, electrolytes, and waste excretion is outlined, paving the way for more advanced renal considerations in subsequent volumes.

This textbook is written for undergraduate students in medical, nursing, dental, allied health, and biomedical sciences. It is also valuable for residents and practitioners to re-examine basic physiology in the clinical environment. The organized approach and clinical correlations make it a perfect one for instructors, while extensive diagrams and overview summaries aid independent study.

INTRODUCTION TO PHYSIOLOGY AND HOMEOSTASIS

1

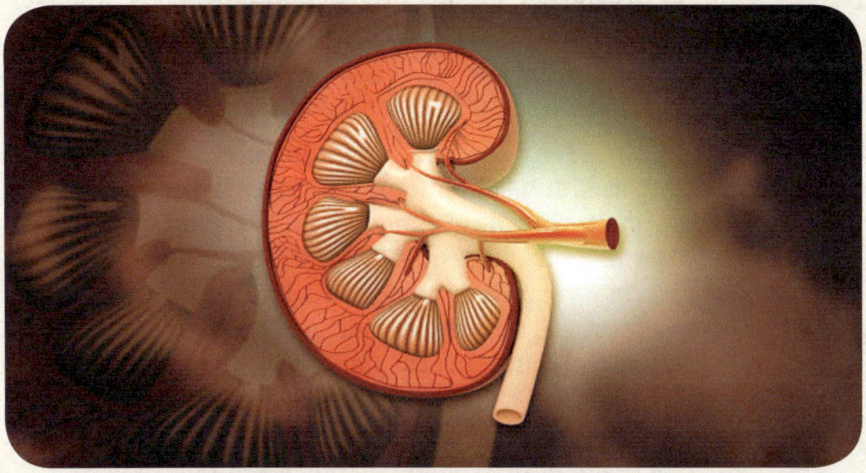

Introduction

Physiology, as a significant branch of biological science, examines the intricate functions and processes that define living organisms. In examining the biochemical activities that define life, physiology seeks to understand how these processes bring about growth, reproduction, and homeostasis. Physiology is studied at different levels of organization, ranging from cell processes to complex systems in multicellular organisms. For instance, the basic biochemical processes of life, which are common to all forms of life, illustrate the universality of bodily functions on this planet, as noted by Smith and Morowitz (2004). Investigating these processes not only enhances our understanding of life itself but also provides clues to the mechanisms of health and disease that are critical to the development of medical science and medicine. One of the key characteristics of physiology is the focus on homeostasis, the dynamic equilibration of internal environments essential for survival. Homeostasis encompasses various mechanisms that enable organisms to maintain a stable internal environment, even

LEARNING OBJECTIVES

After studying this chapter, you will be able to:

1. Discuss the key concepts in physiology;
2. Describe the homeostasis: the concept;
3. Discuss the physiological systems involved in homeostasis;
4. Highlight mechanisms of homeostatic regulation;
5. Learn about major organ systems involved in homeostasis;
6. Evaluate the impact of environmental factors on homeostasis.

when external conditions fluctuate. Physiological systems, , such as the thermoregulation of endothermic animals or the osmoregulation of aquatic animals, demonstrate how organisms modulate their environment while maintaining optimal function. These regulatory processes are crucial for sustaining life, highlighting the interface between physiological function and environmental interaction.

Additionally, a comparative study of homeostatic mechanisms in different species helps portray the evolutionary adjustments that define these vital processes, thereby enabling us to gain a deeper understanding of biological diversity and ecological equilibrium. Physiology also bridges boundaries with other fields, providing an integrated description of life phenomena. As demonstrated by cross-disciplinary approaches that dissect emotions using robotic models, the depth of physiological response is beyond the reach of any single approach.

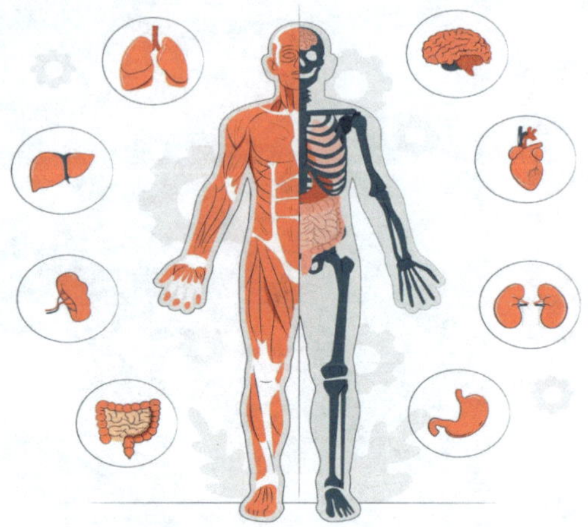

Figure 1.1 Physiology and Homeostasis.

Source: https://static.toiimg.com/thumb/msid-100620098,imgsize-33518,width-400,resizemode-4/100620098.jpg.

The intersection of information from psychology, neuroscience, and robotics captures the multidimensionality of physiology and its meanings for broader scientific inquiries. Physiological research, in this sense, extends beyond biological function and explores the emotional and cognitive aspects of living organisms. This overall systematization of the physiological processes not only maximizes their significance within individual organisms but also emphasizes their functions as components of ecosystems, hence fostering an increased appreciation of the interdependencies of life forms (Figure 1.1).

Overview of Physiological Processes

In physiology, an understanding of the complex interrelations of biological processes is vital for appreciating how homeostasis is maintained in the body. Physiological processes involve a wide variety of processes like metabolism, respiration, and homeostasis. These processes work in tandem to maintain the interior environment stable, irrespective of changes in the exterior environment. At the hub of such an endeavor is systems biology, which integrates models and data across varying biological scales from molecular interactions through complete organ systems. Recent advances in Computational Aided Process Engineering (CAPE) have facilitated examining these interactions more intensively, enabling analysis and design of biological systems on the basis of a multi-scale strategy. Notably, research studies have begun to simulate the dynamics of such systems as blood flow in endothelial cells and demonstrated how the mechanical forces are involved in cellular regulatory processes and emphasizing the complexity of physiological interactions (Allen et al., 2009). One fundamental feature of physiological functions is the regulation of nutrient uptake, specifically in the gastrointestinal tract. The complicated dynamics of digestion and nutrient absorption serve as a model of how physiologic systems are involved in homeostasis. Zinc, a trace element that is essential, has a tightly controlled mechanism of absorption in the small intestine. Multiple dietary and intrinsic factors affect zinc bioavailability, ultimately on systemic levels. Current research more and more employs *in vitro* cell models for studying zinc transport across the intestinal epithelium, particularly with human intestinal cell lines , such as Caco-2. The models assist in closing the loophole between laboratory findings and human physiology and confirm the significance of exploring background mechanisms in an effort to ensure nutrient homeostasis is achieved effectively (Haase et al., 2020). Along with this, the physiological processes maintaining fluid and electrolyte balance also illustrate the body's sophisticated homeostatic mechanisms. The kidneys play a key role in filtering blood, removing waste products, and regulating fluid content. Through nephron units, the kidneys regulate the reabsorption of water and electrolytes according to systemic changes like dehydration or excess intake of fluids, maintaining osmotic balance and blood pressure. In addition, homeostatic regulation is also determined by hormonal stimulation, , such as aldosterone and antidiuretic hormone (ADH), which regulate the kidneys' reaction to various physiological demands. The dynamic interaction between renal function and hormonal regulation demonstrates the complexity of homeostasis and the need for integrative physiology in order to fully understand the complexity of these processes acting together in maintaining life. By such investigations, researchers try not only to account for normal body functions but also for the treatment of pathological states caused by homeostatic imbalances.

Importance of Studying Physiology

Physiology is most significant in the comprehension of complicated processes of living organisms, particularly in the context of homeostasis, the process by which physiologic phenomena remain stable despite environmental variation. By examining the mechanisms of physiological processes, scientists gain profound insight into how organisms respond and adapt to their environment and react to various stimuli. These insights are not only essential in basic biological research but also in applied medicine. For instance, the understanding of neurophysiology and sensory systems is used in determining therapy for neurological ailments and sensory loss, illustrating the applied relevance of physiological research to enhancing human health and well-being (Lange et al., 2025). The relevance of physiology further goes beyond immediate health implications; it includes comprehension of biological continuity and adaptation as a whole. When organisms travel through an altering environment, the principles of homeostasis are not static but dynamic, transgenerational processes. By investigating developmental physiology, researchers discover how homeostatic processes evolve with the passage of time and influence structure and function transgenerationally. These perceptions test conventional views of biological stability and emphasize the need for a systems view of biology, taking into account the interaction of multiple physiological processes in adaptation and evolution (Torday, 2015). This view not only enhances our understanding of life itself but also guides the preservation of different species and ecosystems. Furthermore, a firm understanding of physiology provides a fundamental foundation for advancing medical science, engineering, and ecology. As physicians strive to address complex issues, , such as metabolic disease and chronic disease, knowledge of physiology underlies the development of targeted therapeutic strategies. Furthermore, applying physiological principles to biotechnological innovation, , such as regenerative medicine and artificial organs, is the multidisciplinary aspect of the subject. Thus, the application of physiology to learn is not merely for educational needs; it is a basic input to develop future advances beyond the normal parameters, eventually resulting in survival and improvement of life on Earth (Figure 1.2).

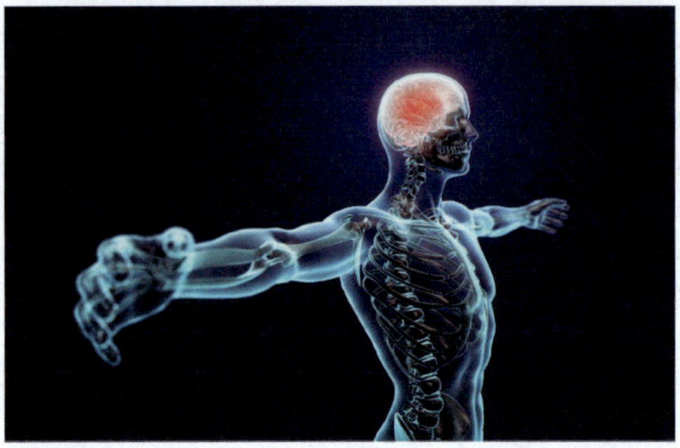

Figure 1.2. Anatomy And Physiology.

Source: https://static.physoc.org/app/uploads/2019/03/22194355/human.jpg.

Relationship Between Physiology and Other Biological Sciences

The association of physiology with other biological sciences is automatically related to the entire knowledge of homeostasis. Homeostasis is the mechanism whereby organisms maintain constant internal conditions despite the changing situations in the outside environment. It is a survival mechanism and a connection between physiology and molecular biology and ecology. For instance, molecular mechanisms explain how proteins and hormones induce change in physiological processes and therefore an organism's health and robustness. In this respect, the role of physiological parameters is complemented by molecular data, enabling scientists to develop targeted interventions and therapies that cure a plethora of diseases. Understanding of homeostasis in this integrative perspective ultimately refines our comprehension of biological systems, demonstrating how physiology remains a key in the interlocking system of biological sciences. As physiological processes react to environmental fluctuation, it is easier to see the relationship between ecology and physiology. How life exists with respect to its surroundings must be examined through physiological adaptations that ensure survival. For instance, in assessing the impact of changing salinity conditions on organisms , such as the delta smelt in estuarine habitats, physiological inquiry focuses on osmoregulation mechanisms essential for internal balance across varied conditions. Through the integration of ecological and physiological insights, scientists are able to demystify intricate relationships and forecast how organisms react to environmental stressors. These multidisciplinary approaches not only teach us about individual species but also tell us about broader ecological patterns and how knowing physiology is integral to addressing issues that result from environmental change, as detailed in the research regarding delta smelt and how they adjust their behavior to changing salinity levels (Connon et al., 2016).

Moreover, merging physiological studies with the other fields of biology further improves the understanding of evolutionary processes. Evolutionary biology examines the processes through which species change over a period of time, and physiology provides the functional basis for such evolution. By studying the physiological traits, , such as metabolic rate or mode of reproduction, scientists are in a position to find out the selective pressures driving the evolutionary processes of organisms. For example, the theory of feedback loops in endocrine control illustrates how physiological functions influence and are influenced by evolutionary forces. Such phenomena create a dynamic framework where physiological changes across generations produce adaptations that optimize an organism's fitness in its setting (Bich et al., 2020). Therefore, the interaction between physiology and the other life sciences, especially evolutionary biology, highlights the significance of a holistic perspective on the processes of life, which leads to an appreciation of the intricacies in biological systems and their continued evolution.

1.1. Key Concepts in Physiology

Learning Outcome

1. Explain homeostasis and its importance;
2. Emphasize feedback mechanisms in physiological control;
3. Learn about organization levels in biological systems.

Key ideas of physiology form the foundation of understanding how living organisms are capable of being successful at homeostasis and responding to their surroundings. Physiology includes an essential component of studying organ systems and the integrative functions of organ systems. Each organ system operates through complex interactions, allowing survival and adaptability. For instance, the cardiovascular, respiratory, and renal systems coordinate to regulate blood pressure, oxygenation, and the removal of waste products, illustrating the homeostatic principles that regulate physiological processes. Such synergistic interaction among many systems not only ensures internal stability but also allows for the organism to react well to changes from outside. Hence, knowledge of these interfaces is the key to understanding how organisms perform optimally under varying conditions. Moreover, the concept of pleiotropy shows the complexity of physiological adaptation and response across time. Pleiotropic activities take place when one gene regulates multiple phenotypic traits, demonstrating a deterministic correspondence between genetic evolution and physiological complexity. This principle depicts how multicellular organisms developed advanced responses to demands in the environment through evolutionary mechanisms that entwine gene expression with physiology. By observing how pleiotropic characters develop, we gain insight into the adaptive processes that have enabled organisms to thrive under conditions of immense ecological stress. Investigations have shown this intricate interaction between genes and complex characters to be a cornerstone in the endeavor to gain insight into health and disease in various organisms (Torday, 2015). Along with this, progress in physiological modeling, as seen through the HD Physiology Project, illustrates that it is possible to integrate knowledge on different levels of biological context. The project indicates the creation of holistic models that simulate physiological and pathological states and thus further develop understanding of dynamic biological processes. By means of multilevel functional simulations, the models facilitate an understanding of how different variables can influence homeostasis in real-time. The implications of these models extend far beyond mere simulation; they also bring the possibility for imaginative drug efficacy determinations and therapeutic strategies. With advancing research, these integrated viewpoints emphasize the value of a wide-ranging understanding of physiology and cement the idea of homeostasis as a complex interconnection of interacting biological systems (for HD physiology project investigators et al., 2017) (Figure 1.3).

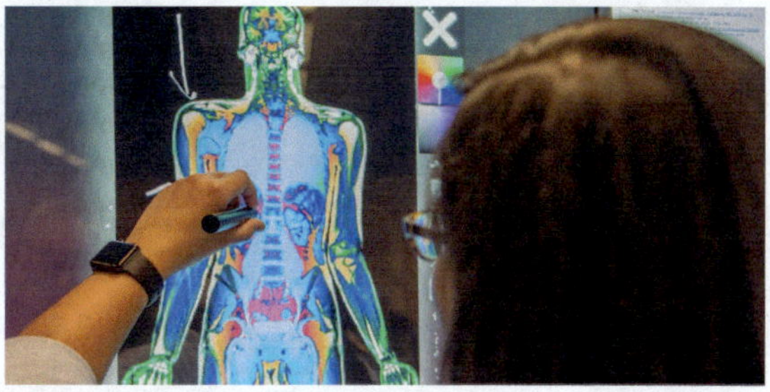

Figure 1.3. Medical physiology.

*Source:*https://www.unmc.edu/gradstudies/_images/programs/masters-physiology-large.jpg.

1.1.1. Homeostasis and Its Significance

The concept of homeostasis is at the core of appreciating physiological function in living organisms. Homeostasis refers to the ability of biological systems to maintain internal stability regardless of fluctuating external conditions. The adaptation processes on various levels, from cellular to organismal, that maintain crucial parameters, e.g., temperature, pH, and levels of electrolytes, within a narrow range for optimal function. By way of constant monitoring and adjustment of physiological states, homeostasis enables organisms to respond to alterations effectively, highlighting its significance in survival and health. Aside from short-term survival, the significance of homeostasis also stems from its capacity for long-term species evolutionary adaptation to ensure they survive in altered environments and conditions. A more sophisticated view of homeostasis describes it as dynamic, converting the existing belief that homeostasis is a mere maintenance process to history. Instead, as elaborated in developmental physiology, homeostasis can be viewed as a vigorous, intergenerational process that sustains the maintenance, continuity, and alteration of physiological structures and functions over time (Torday, 2015). This perspective highlights the dynamic aspect of homeostatic control, with a focus on the fact that it is not a state of equilibrium but rather a dynamic process with intricate signaling pathways and cellular cooperation. The recognition of homeostasis as a diachronic process highlights the importance of viewing physiological processes based on systems biology to shed more light on the underlying principles of life, adaptation, and overall biological organization. Furthermore, homeostatic theory illustrates significant regulatory processes , such as feedback loops, particularly in endocrinology. The philosophy is centered on the maintenance of vital levels of substances , such as glucose within the plasma through interdependent systems of feedback. However, an organicist perception of endocrine regulation upholds that living structures consist of interdependent structural constraints that regulate glycemia by their mutual interaction (Bich et al., 2020). This paradigm gives a more accurate description of homeostatic functioning past the mere feedback loop, exposing the complexities involved in sustaining metabolic equilibrium. Scientists may employ such paradigms to create new mathematical models that yield a better understanding of endocrine dynamics as well as advance our general understanding of homeostasis in physiological contexts (Figure 1.4).

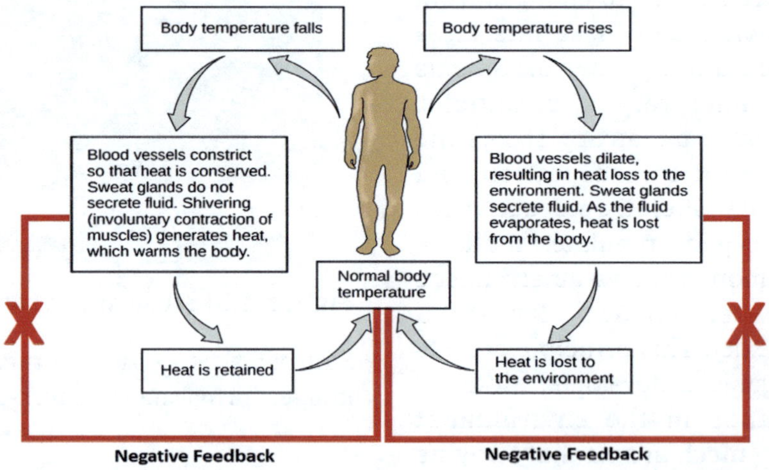

Figure 1.4. Temperature-regulation-in-homeostasis-with-feedback.

*Source:*https://cdn.wou.edu/chemistry/files/2019/01/Temperature-regulation-in-homeostasis-with-feedback.png.

1.1.2. Feedback Mechanisms in Physiological Regulation

The feedback mechanism principle underlines the concept of physiological regulation and homeostasis. Feedback loops are essential control mechanisms in biological systems that enable organisms to respond dynamically to internal and external stimuli. Feedback loops can either be negative or positive. Negative feedback mechanisms operate to correct departures from a set point to restore balance and maintain homeostasis. For instance, maintaining body temperature is a quintessential example of this, in which thermoreceptors detect temperature changes, causing processes that release heat through vasodilation or conserve heat through vasoconstriction. Positive feedback mechanisms, however, amplify the initial stimulus, with the process normally being in childbirth, as the release of oxytocin intensifies the uterine contractions. The interplay of these feedback systems ensures that the physiological processes are accurately balanced, thereby ensuring overall functionality and stability of the organism. The relevance of redox homeostasis even goes to demonstrate how fragile feedback mechanisms of physiological regulation are. The maintenance of redox balance, specifically the dynamic equilibrium between oxidants and antioxidants, is vital for cellular function. The new understanding of electrophiles as signaling molecules has reoriented our perception of redox signaling during homeostasis. Contrasting with the traditionally held assumptions of antioxidants as a general defense, recent studies argue that a balanced physiological state is established through the subtle balance between nucleophile and oxidant signaling. Alternatively, feedback loops swiftly reverse redox dysbalances, allowing constant modulation to adapt to cellular requirements. In accordance with recent literature, oxidant-nucleophile balance is established during redox homeostasis in which persistent feedback retains the balance, ultimately ensuring cellular strength and adaptive responses to physiological stress (Forman et al., 2016). In the same manner, feedback regulatory loops are also of crucial significance in the metabolism of basic amino acids, , such as arginine. Arginine not only serves as a building block of proteins but also as a biosynthetic precursor of various secondary metabolites and signaling molecules. Feedback inhibition plays a significant role in controlling enzymes during the arginine biosynthesis pathway in plants, as the concentration of arginine influences the activity of vital metabolic enzymes like ornithine transcarbamoylase and argininosuccinate synthetase. The studies demonstrate that arginine level fluctuations are responsible for initiating feedback mechanisms to ensure proper homeostasis of the amino acid, thereby harmonizing metabolic processes with physiological requirements of plants. Evidence from studies corroborates that regulatory mechanisms have evolved in sync with the higher demand of arginine in seed plants and underscore the intricate coordination involved in maintaining metabolic homeostasis in response to environmental challenges (Canovas-Ramos et al., 2019).

1.1.3. Levels of Organization in Biological Systems

An understanding of organization levels within biological systems is critical to the apprehension of physiology and homeostasis complexities. The cellular organization constitutes the most basic level, whereby individual cells are the functional units of life. Every cell type possesses specialized functions that feed into tissue functional operation, which is made up of populations of identical cells functioning in collaboration. As the hierarchy ascends, tissues develop into organs, and organs aggregate to organ systems, yielding elaborate networks with emergent properties unavailable at lower levels. This structured format allows complex interactions that coordinate vital physiological processes , such as the uptake of nutrients and the disposal of wastes, which are critical in sustaining homeostasis and life. In homeostasis, the concept of feedback mechanisms comes into play as it illustrates how biological systems regulate themselves. Feedback loops are similar to control circuits in which the output of a process influences its continued operation. A classic example of the system is the control of blood glucose: when the concentration of glucose rises, insulin is released to lower its concentration, and its decrease introduces glucagon into the scene in a bid to regain equilibrium. This dynamic relationship is equivalent to a profound relationship of functional structures as constraints within the organism, with a focus on organizational closure in physiological processes. Organizational closure can be more clearly understood in the regulation of metabolism, defining the complex relationships between different physiological systems, particularly when controlling complex activities , such as glucose metabolism (Bich et al., 2020). Moreover, homeostasis is not only an issue of momentary physiology, but also a diachronic model traversing an organism's development and evolutionary history. Homeostasis may be seen as a dynamic model constantly reacting to both internal signals and external environmental factors. Throughout the life of a person, physiological functions, all facilitated by cooperation between various levels of organization, aim towards attaining stability despite variability. This plasticity involves intricate cell-cell communication at critical development stages, explaining how the organism develops and changes over the course of time. By applying these principles together in a systems biology approach, researchers can develop an enhanced understanding of homeostasis through the integration of developmental science with traditional physiological research, effectively moving away from reductionist perspectives in biology (Torday, 2015).

Test Your Knowledge

1. What is the difference between negative and positive feedback mechanisms, and how do they help maintain homeostasis?
2. How does the body use a negative feedback loop to regulate blood glucose levels following a meal?

1.2. Homeostasis: The Concept

Learning Outcome

1. Explain the definition and examples of homeostasis;
2. Define the role of homeostatic mechanisms within the body;
3. Understand the effects of homeostatic imbalance.

An appreciation of homeostasis requires a deep understanding of its role in maintaining the constancy of biological processes. The concept itself stems from the fact that organisms need to regulate their internal states as a response to changes outside. It is a matter of life and death and comprises complex feedback mechanisms that keep physiological parameters, e.g., temperature, pH, and ionic concentration within narrow ranges. The dynamic nature of homeostasis means that even though the systems are in a state of continuous striving for equilibrium, they also exhibit remarkable sensitivity to change, which points towards the fine balance between flexibility and stability. This view encourages further investigation of the philosophical constructs in connection with the organism itself and its interactions within ecological systems. Instead of looking at an organism as a machine, there is scope for investigating it as a networked entity functioning within an overarching biological system, thereby deepening the knowledge of homeostasis and its relevance. Besides that, the latest research has also touched on the technological developments that facilitate homeostasis to be studied at different scales. One such initiative of this trend towards the use of computational frameworks simulating physiological and disease processes is the HD Physiology Project. This initiative emphasizes the importance of high-level definitions in understanding how the systems interact in order to sustain life. By way of generating multilevel functional simulations, the project not only contributes to knowing about homeostatic function but also addresses therapeutic implications, , such as the evaluation of drug effects on cardiac stability. Such revelations are an enlarging interface between biology and technology where quantitative models help enhance the interpretation of physiological data, ultimately leading to better therapeutic modalities and a broader understanding of homeostasis. Thus, the evolution of these approaches makes it possible to explore homeostatic mechanisms more widely by bridging gaps between traditional biology and modern computational approaches. The philosophical underpinnings of the definition of organism make it more difficult for us to understand homeostasis.

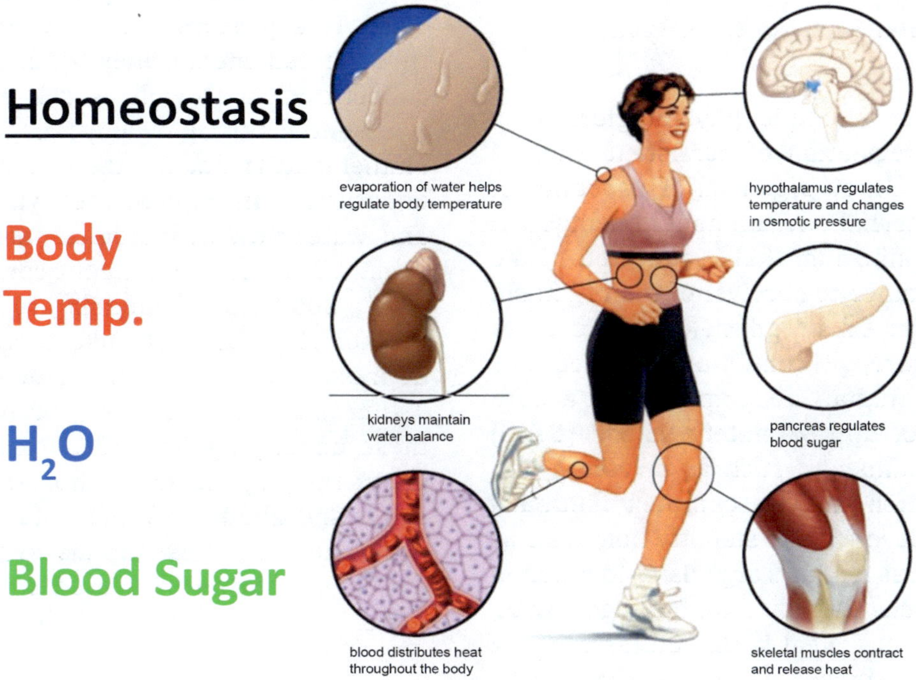

Figure 1.5. Homeostasis and response.

*Source:*https://sciencetallis.weebly.com/uploads/9/9/6/6/99666290/homeostasis-body-temp-h2o-blood-sugar_orig.jpg.

The controversy that remains on the classification of organisms has implications in comprehending homeostatic processes. Reductionist critics argue that a strictly mechanistic conception of organisms deprives them of their richness and complexity. Instead, an emergent philosophy of organisms, based on various philosophical arguments, positions them as adaptive systems that can interact with their environment dynamically. This perspective questions the question of how homeostasis works not merely a static equilibrium but as a responsive process that alters with the organism. By looking at the organism in a philosophical context, we may be uncovering levels of knowledge that enhance our knowledge of homeostasis and its critical functions in life. By embracing the complexity of organisms, we can use it to enhance the more integrated study of physiological control, disrupting the conventional thought that has dominated biological thinking for so long (Figure 1.5).

1.2.1. Definition and Examples of Homeostasis

Homeostasis is a simple physiological term meaning the regulation of persistent internal conditions within an organism, irrespective of fluctuating external environmental changes. It is dynamic equilibrium that is reflected in the critical importance to survival of the organism and it incorporates many physiological processes like temperature, pH, and fluid balance. For instance, the human body maintains a core temperature of approximately 98.6°F (37°C) through mechanisms , such as sweating and shivering, which involve complex feedback mechanisms. Beyond mere stability, homeostasis is crucial because it allows organisms to function at optimal levels, thereby maintaining growth, reproduction, and health. An understanding of homeostatic mechanisms is enlightening regarding the complexity of biological systems and the pathologic effects of dysregulation, producing numerous disorders. One traditional illustration of homeostasis is in the regulation of blood glucose levels, which is a key aspect of metabolic homeostasis. When blood glucose rises after a meal, pancreatic beta cells secrete insulin, enabling cells to absorb glucose and lowering blood sugar. During low blood glucose, alpha cells of the pancreas secrete glucagon, triggering the release of glucose from liver stores. This intricate interplay of hormones is a prototype for a negative feedback loop, a primary mechanism in homeostasis. Furthermore, the study of systems-level behavior at the tissue level, , such as the integration of the metabolic networks, shows the intricate process of maintaining homeostasis. An illustration is the recent work in Computer Aided Process Engineering (CAPE), aiming at integrating various biological models in order to better understand these regulation mechanisms and enhance our knowledge of their clinical relevance and potential therapeutic intervention (Allen et al., 2009). Moreover, ionic electrodiffusion and osmosis water flow demonstrate another aspect of homeostasis in cells. This process occurs when ions diffuse through cell membranes, both regulating ion concentration as well as cell volume, which is essential for many physiological functions. Mathematical modeling, under partial differential equations, can explain the dynamics of ionic and water flow in biological tissue, under the constraint of thermodynamic consistency (Mori et al., 2014). Such models are also required in exploring disorders like cortical spreading depression, a derangement of ionic and cell volume homeostasis in the brain. By studying these underlying processes, researchers learn about the ways in which homeostasis may be upset and about how the potential effects on health develop, thus emphasizing the necessity for balance to be preserved within biological systems.

1.2.2. Role of Homeostatic Mechanisms in the Body

The homeostatic mechanisms form the cornerstone of physiological stability within the human organism. They work through a complex system of feedback mechanisms, enabling organisms to achieve balance in spite of external and internal fluctuations.

For instance, the body's thermoregulation shows us this process; as temperature in the environment rises, physiological responses , such as sweating and vasodilation are initiated to enable the removal of excess heat. Conversely, in a cold setting, shivering and vasoconstriction are stimulated. This continuous interaction not only guards against extreme deviations from baseline physiologic values but also shows us the body's high adaptability to respond to various stressors. This adaptive flexibility points to a broader perspective of homeostasis, illustrating its essential role not as a state but as a process dynamically adjusting physiological functions in real-time, making it fundamental to survival and health. Beyond investigation, the concept of homeostasis extends beyond direct physiological response and enters into developmental physiology. Homeostatic processes play a critical role in the control of cellular activities in growth, repair, and adaptation to alterations in the external environment. An example is the complex network of signaling pathways mediating cell proliferation and differentiation for ensuring tissue structural and functional integrity. It becomes relevant in an organizational context when appreciating how organisms react to stressors that disrupt their internal physiological norm. The dynamic interplay between homeostasis and cellular repair systems highlights how, in addition to conserving current states, homeostatic function aids the adaptation and evolution of organisms through time. From a diachronic perspective, homeostasis is not a static destination but an open system that makes stability and adaptability possible as one moves through a constantly changing world (Torday, 2015). Besides, the role of stem cells within tissue homeostasis is proof of the complexity and significance of homeostatic control in maintaining cellular integrity. Such specialized cells play a critical role in replacing dying or old cells, so that tissues can keep on functioning throughout the life of an organism. The regenerative ability of certain tissues, , such as the intestinal epithelium, is a case in point, where stem cells actively participate in such self-renewal. Research in model systems, e.g., Drosophila melanogaster, has provided insight into the regulatory mechanisms governing such homeostatic processes. How disruptions, e.g., trauma or degeneration with age, impact stem cell function and hence tissue homeostasis underscores the delicate balance of biological systems. Thus, the ongoing activity of stem cells in homeostatic systems emphasizes that it is not merely a response process to be in a state of physiological balance but an active survival and health mechanism (Carroll et al., 2015) (Figure 1.6).

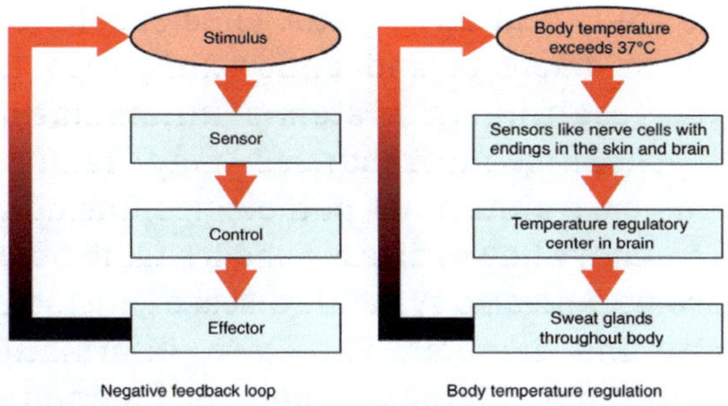

Figure 1.6. Homeostasis feedback.

Source: https://cdn.kastatic.org/ka-perseus-images/8528b0149aa08e36c0305fb9f259949d5984950d.png.

1.2.3. Consequences of Homeostatic Imbalance

Homeostasis is a crucial aspect of physiological processes, maintaining internal conditions stable despite outside fluctuations. When homeostatic functions fail, resulting imbalances may cascade and produce unwanted health effects. A heart-wrenching example is the process of aging, which is marked by a progressive decline in homeostatic regulation. The failure occurs in the form of cellular senescence, when cells lose their capability to reproduce and carry out their functions. Therefore, physiological processes are disrupted, exposing people to infections and chronic diseases, like cardiovascular diseases and cancer. Such consequences underscore the importance of homeostasis, not only for health but also for longevity, illustrating the intricate interaction between age-related changes and homeostatic collapse (Rodrigues et al., 2021). Another significant consequence of homeostatic imbalance is found in the gastrointestinal tract, or the gut microbiota. The gut harbors a dense microbial community that plays an essential role in maintaining immune function as well as metabolic homeostasis. In the event of imbalance in this microbiota, or what is referred to as dysbiosis, gut barrier function could be compromised. This dysfunction leads to the translocation of pathogenic substances, , such as bacteria and endotoxins, into the blood, resulting in systemic inflammation. Such chronic disturbances may lead to various gastrointestinal pathologies, including inflammatory bowel disease and irritable bowel syndrome, and also systemic diseases, including obesity and diabetes. Therefore, information regarding gut microbiota and its function in homeostatic maintenance is crucial for the prevention and management of disease (Ghosh et al., 2021). The effect of homeostatic imbalance extends beyond individual systems and into multiple physiological realms. For instance, the immunosenescent immune system, a process known as immunosenescence, illustrates that homeostasis breakdown can impact immunity and overall health. As the immune system ages, it becomes weaker at combating infection, not just raising susceptibility to various pathogens but also to chronic inflammatory diseases, or inflammaging. This coordination between immunosenescence and other bodily systems is part of a bigger pattern of dysfunction that develops as a consequence of the initial loss of homeostasis. Lastly, these interdependent outcomes emphasize the imperative need to give precedence to homeostatic maintenance in all physiological processes towards augmenting resilience against health problems caused by age and lifestyle (Rodrigues et al., 2021) (Figure 1.7).

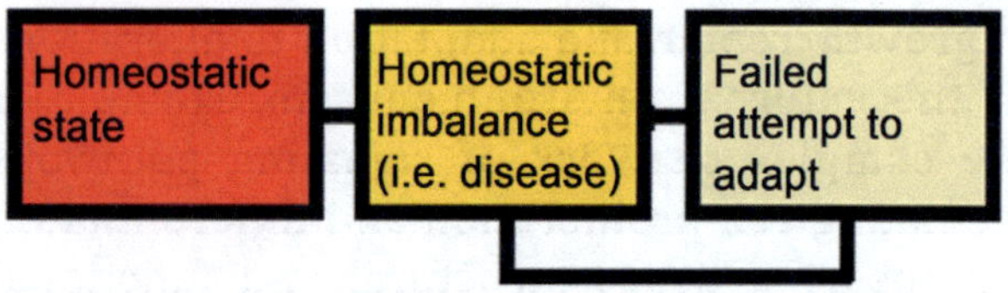

Figure 1.7. Homeostatic imbalance.

Source: https://study.com/cimages/multimages/16/homeostasis.png..

Test Your Knowledge

1. What is homeostasis, and why is it important for normal body function in living organisms?
2. How do receptors, control centers, and effectors work together to establish homeostasis in the body?

1.3. Physiological Systems Involved in Homeostasis

Learning Outcome

1. Explain the function of the nervous system in homeostasis;
2. Define the endocrine system's contribution;
3. Explain how physiological systems communicate with one another.

Homeostasis is a natural aspect of physiology, encompassing a variety of systems functioning in concert to achieve internal stability in the face of external change. One of the most important systems employed in this process is the endocrine system, which employs hormones to regulate a range of functions, including metabolism, growth, and stress response. Feedback mechanisms are crucial in this regulation, so that levels , such as glucose can be kept within a very narrow range required for cellular function. Under an organicist strategy, such a complex interaction could be viewed in terms of closure of constraints that define the interdependence of the functional structures in charge of metabolic processes.

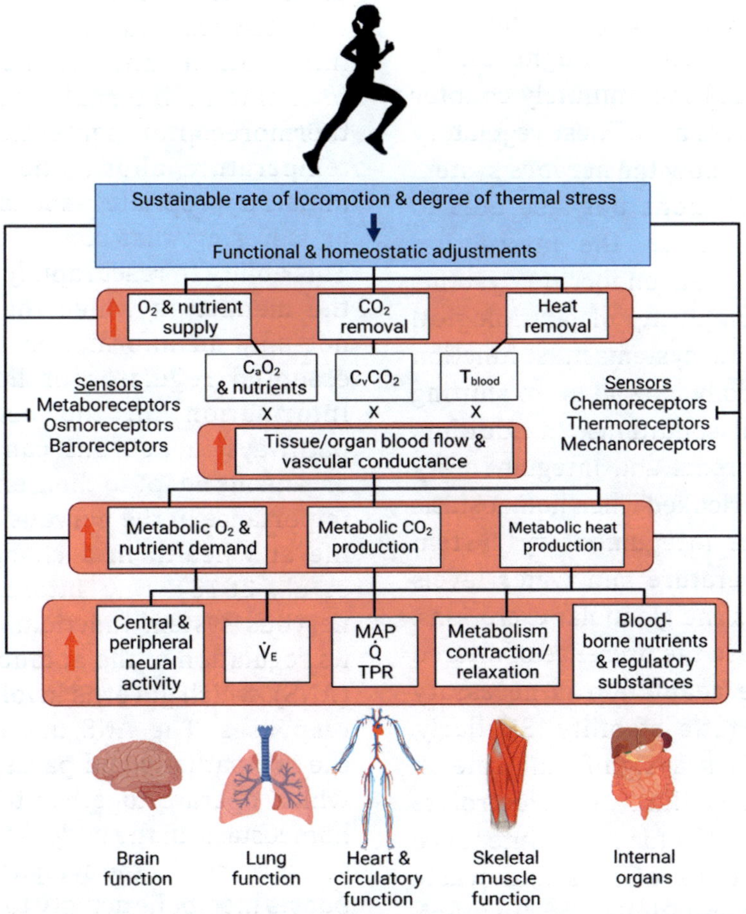

Figure 1.8. Integrative view of physiological systems during exercise and thermal stress.

*Source:*https://pub.mdpi-res.com/cells/cells-11-00383/article_deploy/html/images/cells-11-00383-g006.png?1643085627.

Such a strategy changes our perspective of the endocrine system from the simple feedback model to one that highlights subtle interactions that must be incorporated for homeostasis to be achieved, hence presenting a richer perspective of physiological regulation (Bich et al., 2020). The nervous system is also part of homeostatic mechanisms, managing rapid physiological responses to environmental changes. It consists of a collection of neurons transmitting signals within the body to bring about instant responses to a stimulus, , such as changes in temperature or the perception of danger. The system operates through reflex arcs for the ability to react quickly to maintain equilibrium. For instance, thermoregulation is ensured by mechanisms like sweating or shivering brought on by hypothalamic responses that minutely counter the production and loss of heat. These regulatory pathways demonstrate how the nervous system not only detects alterations but also acts to restore homeostasis. Thus, the interaction between the nervous and endocrine systems is reflective of the complexity of physiological regulation, wherein both systems must function together so that the body may adapt to shifting internal and external conditions. In addition, the operation of the renal and integumentary systems cannot be overlooked when homeostasis is under review. The integumentary system regulates body temperature and water levels through skin functions and glandular excretions. This is especially true in the presence of altered environments, where adaptation is necessary to preserve homeostatic stability. Similarly, the renal system plays a significant role in the regulation of body fluid and electrolyte balance, clearing the blood for the maintenance of proper concentrations of ions and waste products. Salinity fluctuations, for instance, have a significant influence on the internal regulation of compositions by organisms, , such as in some fish, which vary their osmoregulation processes to accommodate fluctuating salinity in the environment. The integration of the two views from both the integumentary and the renal systems creates a more complete understanding of how homeostasis is created and maintained under various physiological states (Connon et al., 2016) (Figure 1.8).

1.3.1. The Nervous System's Role in Homeostasis

The nervous system plays a central role in homeostasis, orchestrating a dynamic and intricate interplay between various physiological systems. It achieves this through a network of neurons that constantly communicate with tissues and organs, processing sensory information and coordinating responses to maintain internal stability. For instance, thermoreceptor perception of alterations in temperature allows the nervous system to initiate appropriate responses, , such as sweating or shivering, that conserve body temperature. This ability to react rapidly to stimuli illustrates the manner in which the nervous system is not only an information conduit but also an essential regulator of homeostatic activity. Information on the complexity of these pathways in neurons can inform us on how organisms adapt to their environments, and the importance of the nervous system in sustaining life and health in a changing world (Alcedo et al., 2013). One interesting aspect of the nervous system functioning in homeostasis is its regulation of the autonomic nervous system (ANS), which governs involuntary physiological responses. The ANS has two main branches: the sympathetic and parasympathetic systems, which operate together to produce a state of homeostasis in the body. As an instance, during a stress response, the sympathetic nervous system boosts metabolic activity to prepare the body for fight or flight, and the parasympathetic system promotes relaxation and energy conservation once the danger has passed. This homeostasis is vital for ensuring the stability of the internal environment of the body in the presence of external stressors. The nervous capacity for fine-tuning physiological mechanisms through sophisticated feedback systems is best exemplified by these systems (Gopika et al., 2024). Moreover, the process of the enteric nervous system (ENS) is a testament to the connection between the nervous system and digestive homeostasis. The ENS, or second brain, oversees gut function and is charged with homeostatic regulation of the gastrointestinal processes of digestion and absorption. By coordinating signaling pathways that govern the release of digestive enzymes and the passage of food through the gastrointestinal tract, the ENS allows for proper assimilation of nutrients and removal of waste. This complex interaction underscores the central role not just in short-term response, but also in long-term physiological homeostasis. Interaction between the ENS and overall homeostasis demonstrates how the nervous system regulates essential bodily functions while responding to environmental and internal changes (Alcedo et al., 2013) (Figure 1.9).

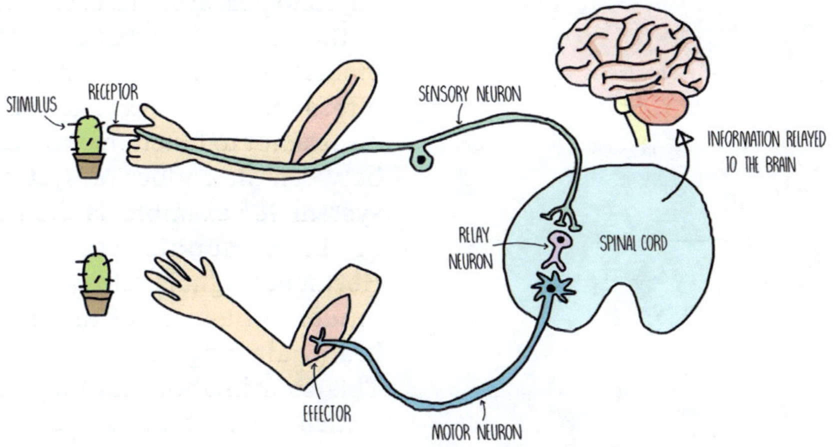

Figure 1.9. Homeostasis and the nervous system.

Source: https://images.squarespace-cdn.com/content/v1/5c5aed8434c4e20e953d6011/1609170858693-EY2P548Y7X1BGBXZ0UKK/nervous+system+reflex+action.jpg.

1.3.2. The Endocrine System's Contribution

The endocrine system is essential in the regulation of homeostasis by managing physiological processes through the release of hormones into the bloodstream. Hormones, being chemical messengers, allow an organ or tissue to talk to another organ or tissue, allowing the body to respond appropriately to internal and external stimuli. For example, when the body is under stress, the hypothalamus tells the adrenal glands to release cortisol, a hormone that is involved in the stress response. This activity not only affects metabolic function but also is implicated in emotional well-being and total resistance to stressors. Proper functioning of the endocrine system, thus, is required in order to ensure that various body systems function together in harmony, thereby ensuring the intricate processes of homeostasis required to sustain life. The interaction of the endocrine system with other systems of the body is also complex and critical. The endocrine system itself is not autonomous, but instead is in a dialog state with the nervous and immune systems to regulate a wide range of body processes. For instance, the hypothalamic-pituitary axis is a critical brain-endocrine interface that oversees responses to changing physiological states. Hormones , such as insulin, which regulate glucose metabolism, demonstrate how this system affects energy balance and, thus, general well-being. The controlling mechanisms of the systems become unbalanced and create pathology, , such as diabetes mellitus or thyroid disease, highlighting the significance of the role of the endocrine systems in homeostasis and the prevention of long-term illness. The ability of the endocrine systems to adapt to changes over time is also critical to long-term health and well-being.

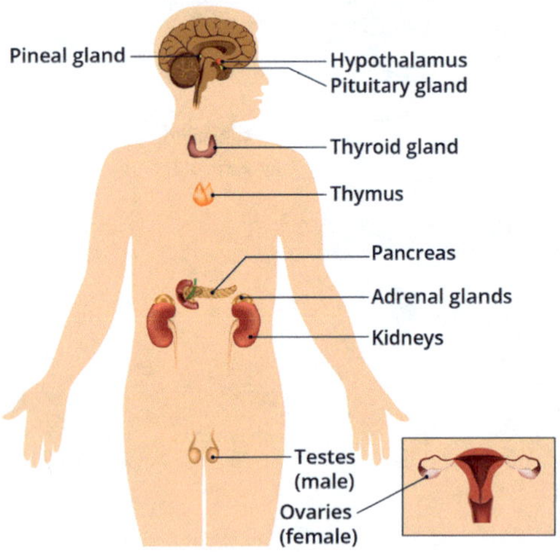

Figure 1.10. Endocrine glands and their hormones.

*Source:*https://media.healthdirect.org.au/images/inline/original/endocrine-glands-and-their-hormones-85e01a.png.

As individuals age, for instance, the body experiences alterations in hormone secretion that can influence muscle mass, fat distribution, and metabolic function. Conditions , such as sarcopenia, characterized by loss of muscle mass and quality, illustrate the systemic alterations of aging and their impact on homeostasis. The redistribution of body fat, especially when it invades skeletal muscle, may have the ability to alter muscle function and the overall metabolic efficiency, further underscoring the need for endocrine balance (Carter et al., 2019). Awareness of these changes and their effects on physiology is necessary to create interventions that would reverse the pathophysiology of aging and facilitate healthy aging processes by sustaining homeostasis in the endocrine system (Figure 1.10).

1.3.3. Interaction Between Different Physiological Systems

The delicate interaction between various physiological systems is essential to homeostasis in the human body. Each system—whether the endocrine, nervous, or immune system—is interdependent and functions harmoniously in an attempt to function optimally. The interaction between the endocrine system and the nervous system, for example, is the best representation of such sophisticated interdependence. Hormonal signals released by endocrine glands influence neurotransmitter actions within the brain, altering responses to outside stimuli. This coordination not only regulates functions , such as metabolism and growth but also intentionally synchronizes body responses in stress or physical activity. This understanding is crucial to ongoing study in physiological well-being as well as in the treatment of illnesses arising when homeostasis is disrupted. Other than the endocrine and nervous systems, the gastrointestinal and immune systems also present widespread interactions that affect overall well-being. For example, gut microbiota presents very intricate communication with intestinal epithelial cells (IECs) concerning local and systemic immunity. Dysbiosis in the gut may weaken this interaction, resulting in compromised immunity and conditions , such as Irritable Bowel Syndrome (IBS-D). In this case, diet therapy may be a therapeutic intervention used to restore homeostasis by exerting a positive influence on gut flora balance. Effective management calls for a comprehensive understanding of how gastrointestinal alterations may have physiological effects across different systems to ultimately inform the creation of correct nutrition recommendations required for health (Wu et al., 2024). Also, physiological interactions contribute to bone metabolism and health, which suggests a broader focus on systems biology. An exploration of interactions between numerous hormone receptors and bone cells is a complicated network that is crucial for bone integrity. For instance, receptor activator of nuclear factor kappa B (RANK) and RANK ligand (RANKL) are key regulators of bone remodeling, but their function is subject to modulation by systemic factors , such as hormone and inflammatory cytokine levels. This highlights a general principle of physiological exploration: that to appreciate the dynamic interaction between the various components of biological systems, it is crucial to view them from a systems perspective. Mathematical modeling and successive simulations may also assist in clarifying these relationships further, providing insights into perturbations' effects on different physiological systems and their roles in health issues and emphasizing the inter-system interaction in homeostasis preservation (Kariya, 2024).

Test Your Knowledge

1. What function does the nervous system play in rapid homeostatic control, and how do reflex arcs serve in this function?
2. How does the endocrine system establish long-term homeostasis through the release of hormones and feedback control?

1.4. Mechanisms of Homeostatic Regulation

Learning Outcome

1. Describe the negative feedback loops;
2. Define the positive feedback mechanisms;
3. Describe the examples of homeostatic regulation in action.

Homeostatic regulation is a sophisticated process that maintains the physiological stability of organisms over a period of time. Historically viewed as a servo-mechanism that maintains physiological balance, homeostasis is a more inclusive, dynamic model when viewed in terms of developmental physiology. Such a perspective portrays the dynamic relationship of various biological systems in which homeostasis is not merely maintaining the status quo but also adapting and evolving based on shifting environmental needs. As highlighted by the literature, cellular signaling during embryogenesis and subsequent physiology supports a meaningful comprehension of homeostasis as a dynamic, intergenerational process. This kind of information contradicts classical views of homeostasis and promotes a Systems model of Biology where interconnectedness and plasticity of life processes are focal (Torday, 2015).

One of the most important aspects of this homeostatic regulation is tissue fidelity, especially in mature organisms where there is a delicate balance to be achieved between cellular turnover and regeneration. The mechanisms that contribute to tissue homeostasis involve the elimination of senescent or damaged cells in an efficient manner and the activation of stem cells to generate new cells. Tissue areas like the intestinal epithelium are particularly well known for their ability to regenerate and are therefore excellent systems to study stem cell-mediated homeostasis. The identification of stem cell niches in single tissues, including the midgut of Drosophila melanogaster, revolutionized our understanding of how cellular dynamics contribute to maintaining homeostasis. Not only do such specialized sites promote the optimal physiological function, but they also facilitate adaptation when stress, damage, or aging exists and, as a result, elucidate the complex interactions that contribute to homeostatic integrity (Carroll et al., 2015). Moreover, the study of homeostatic control also encompasses understanding the effects of disruption in such processes. Either resulting from acute trauma or chronic pathologies , such as aging, homeostatic disruption may lead to pathological states.

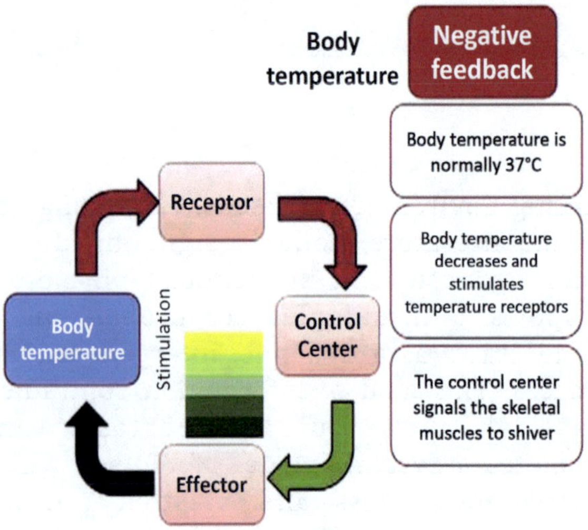

Figure 1.11. Homeostatic control mechanisms.

Source: https://i.ytimg.com/vi/kCWCuztw1kk/sddefault.jpg?sqp=-oaymwEmCIAFEOAD8quKqQMa8AEB-AH-BIAC4AOKAgwIABABGH8gOChBMA8=&rs=AOn4CLAHrUkfnH2lCbFax3_5w0Nhmz2abg.

Regeneration after injury is a very significant reaction that asserts the robustness of homeostatic mechanisms; however, chronic disruption accelerates tissue function degeneration. Determining how homeostatic processes are disturbed and the resulting cellular response can inform therapeutic intervention to restore balance. As scientists delve into the complex planes of interaction between stem cells and their niches, they can learn about the processes of healing as well as potential weaknesses within the homeostatic system and thus enhance our general understanding of physiological health and disease (Carroll et al., 2015) (Figure 1.11).

1.4.1. Negative Feedback Loops

The negative feedback loop theory is crucial in describing how homeostasis occurs in biological systems. Negative feedback loops are mechanisms whereby a change in a physiological variable triggers responses that are in opposition to the change, leading to stability. For instance, in the case of thermoregulation, when the body temperature is above the set point, body processes like sweating and vasodilation increase to lose heat and return the body temperature to normal. Conversely, when body temperature falls too low, responses , such as shivering and vasoconstriction are elicited to generate and preserve heat. Through this process, it is demonstrated how negative feedback mechanisms play a vital role in keeping physiological parameters within their optimal levels to facilitate survival and performance in various living organisms. Other than thermoregulation, blood glucose maintenance is another fine example of negative feedback in metabolism. When blood glucose rises following a meal, the pancreatic β-cells secrete insulin, causing cellular absorption of glucose and promoting its storage as glycogen. During a decrease in blood glucose, insulin secretion is inhibited, preventing an over-decrease in the glucose level. Furthermore, glucagon secreted by pancreatic α-cells during low blood sugar levels causes the breakdown of glycogen into glucose, maintaining the balance. This interaction demonstrates the manner in which negative feedback loops are pivotal in regulating metabolism, demonstrating the significance of ongoing adaptation and precise signaling in energy homeostasis as well as metabolic health. Negative feedback loops are not limited to the maintenance of immediate homeostatic conditions but also play a dominant role in long-term physiological reactions. Regulation of such hormones as cortisol is an example. When stressed, cortisol is released to stimulate energy stores; chronic increases in cortisol trigger feedback inhibition of the pituitary and hypothalamus to shut off its further release. This mechanistic process prevents levels of the hormones from reaching toxic proportions and provides a protective defense against hypercortisolism and other diseases. Therefore, the physiology of negative feedback loops demonstrates their intrinsic significance not only in short-term response but also in long-term health and stability, underscoring their role in physiological regulation and prevention of disease (Galicia-García et al., 2020; Onishi et al., 2021) (Figure 1.12).

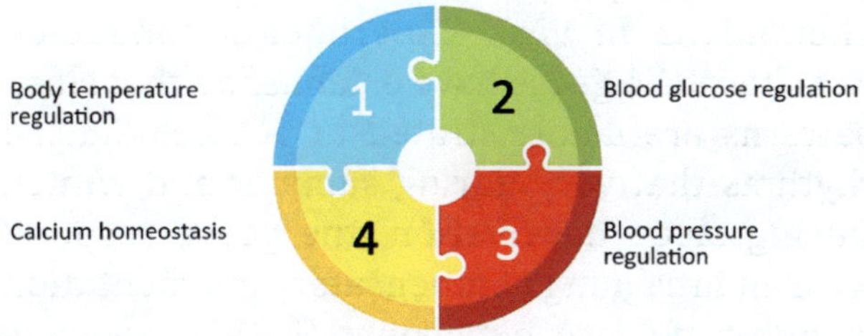

Figure 1.12. Homeostasis with negative-feedback-loops.

*Source:*https://fastercapital.co/i/Homeostasis--Maintaining-Homeostasis-with-Negative-Feedback-Loops--Examples-of-Negative-Feedback-Loops-in-Action.webp.

1.4.2. Positive Feedback Mechanisms

In physiology, positive feedback processes play an essential role in amplifying some physiological processes, generally giving rise to dynamic and, at times, rapid changes in an organism. Unlike negative feedback loops, which are designed for the restoration of balance and homeostasis, positive feedback enhances physiological responses, driving processes to completion. This is best illustrated with childbirth, where the release of oxytocin makes the uterine contractions progressively stronger until delivery. This is a case of positive feedback establishing a definitive endpoint. These systems, while part of the biological process in some instances, also illustrate the balance between homeostasis and system disruption required to produce a significant impact, which demonstrates the intricacy of physiological interaction within living systems. The role of positive feedback is not confined to immediate physiological processes but can also affect the larger biological systems in the long run. As an example, the concept of homeostasis originates from the interaction between various feedback processes that maintain an organism in balance. However, from the point of view of developmental physiology, homeostasis is not just a stable state but a process that is influenced by intergenerational factors. According to recent evidence, such feedback loops may generate robust relationships at cellular and systemic levels and enable processes , such as embryogenesis and tissue regeneration. This perspective allows for a conceptualization of adaptation and survival of organisms in a deeper manner, , such as an appreciation for the function of positive feedback during evolutionary biology and ongoing refinement of physiological structure and function. This systems-level complexity necessitates a systems biology approach, integrating both forms of feedback for total comprehension of life. Furthermore, the environmental setting of positive feedback systems cannot be overstressed, especially in ecosystems and global stability. The planet Earth is such a complex system in which abiotic and biotic components engage in a feedback loop responsible for homeostasis. The stability of such a system, as marked by its changing biological entities, suggests the role of positive feedback in maintaining balance in ecosystems. It is suggested by research that enhancing biological diversity enhances ecosystem resilience, illustrating how positive feedback stabilizes systems with changing conditions of the environment.

This dynamic mechanism is important in understanding the Earth's capacity for self-organization to homeostatic states, demonstrating that life and its environment's relationship has its foundation in a delicate harmony of feedback systems. Thus, recognition of the role of positive feedback supports an understanding of how complex systems can robustly adapt to changed circumstances, a fundamental element within the broader context of homeostasis and physiology (Dyke et al., 2013; Torday, 2015) (Figure 1.13).

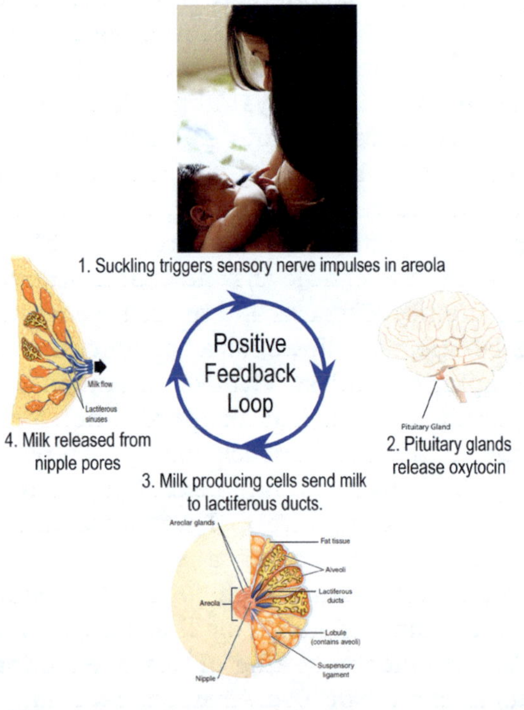

Figure 1.13. Positive feedback mechanisms.

*Source:*https://cdn.storymd.com/optimized/kAvL03ied1/original.png.

1.4.3. Examples of Homeostatic Regulation in Action

Homeostatic regulation is a central part of the physiological process by which organisms maintain internal stability despite external change. A very obvious example can be observed in thermoregulation, whereby the human body attempts to maintain its core temperature around 37 degrees Celsius. When the body temperature rises because of environmental heat or exertion, mechanisms , such as vasodilation and sweating are activated. Vasodilation increases blood flow to the skin to facilitate heat loss, and sweat glands excrete water, which reduces the temperature of the body as it evaporates. Conversely, during cold weather, there is vasoconstriction, which preserves heat. The interaction of these processes emphasizes the dynamic nature of homeostasis, demonstrating how the body's reactions are tightly tuned to achieve balance, as evidenced by the physiological processes maintaining the internal environment essential for survival and health (Prasad et al., 2024). Sleep regulation is another example par excellence of homeostatic phenomena *in vivo*. Experiments conducted with barnacle geese have established that sleep patterns are demonstrated to possess diurnal rhythms that vary during summer and winter. During sleep deprivation, the geese respond with an intriguing compensatory augmentation of non-rapid eye movement (NREM) sleep in summer but not in winter, indicating a faint homeostatic response. This seasonality of adaptability suggests that these birds possess a plastic homeostatic regulatory system of sleep such that they are able to alter their sleep needs in response to environmental changes and pressures (van Hasselt et al., 2020). Such types of results are significant in identifying how organisms control habits and physiological processes to optimize health, emphasizing the importance of homeostasis in the preservation of life processes. Lastly, the hormone cortisol demonstrates homeostatic regulation in its involvement in the stress response. If the body perceives a stressor, the hypothalamus will trigger the adrenal glands to release cortisol, which in turn will aid in mobilizing energy reserves and controlling immune function. This action is required to preserve homeostasis in cases of acute stress. However, chronic levels of cortisol will lead to dysregulation, which in turn negatively affects numerous body systems and results in disease states , such as anxiety or metabolic disease. Thus, while cortisol is essential in enabling immediate homeostatic response, chronic elevationhighlights the balance the body must achieve between effectively responding to stressors and avoiding long-term adverse effects (Prasad et al., 2024). These comments account for the complexities of homeostatic processes and their association with general health.

Test Your Knowledge

1. What are the three main components of a homeostatic control system and what is each one's role?
2. How does negative feedback sustain constant states throughout the body and in what way is it dissimilar from positive feedback?

1.5. Major Organ Systems Involved in Homeostasis

Learning Outcome

1. Describe the endocrine system and regulation via hormones;
2. Explain the nervous system and how it maintains homeostasis;
3. Explain the immune system's role in homeostasis.

Homeostasis is a complex interaction of various systems of organs that work synergistically to maintain internal conditions in the face of changing conditions outside. Of these, the endocrine system plays a key role by secreting hormones that regulate metabolism, growth, and fluid balance. For instance, hormones , such as insulin and glucagon by the pancreas control blood sugar levels, and the adrenal glands produce corticosteroids that control stress responses. The interactive nature of such hormonal responses illustrates the body's ability to restore balance through feedback. In addition, homeostatic functions of the endocrine system are also intertwined with other systems, i.e., the nervous system, to bring about immediate responses to changes in the external environment, thereby affirming the integration of body systems in homeostatic regulation (Torday, 2015).

Another critical organ system responsible for homeostasis is the renal system, which is responsible for maintaining the body's fluid and electrolyte balance and blood pressure. The kidneys eliminate waste products and excess salts from the bloodstream and conserve essential constituents. Through mechanisms , such as glomerular filtration and tubular reabsorption, the renal system achieves homeostasis by regulating the composition and volume of body fluids. Sodium intake, for example, influences the blood's volume and pressure, necessitating strict control mechanisms for responding to sodium changes. Recent studies describe how brain signaling cascades interact with renal physiology to manage blood pressure, detailing the highly regulated feedback relationships between the renal system and larger physiological systems

(Neal et al., 2016). Shining light on these interactions further explains how the body is able to maintain stable internal environments when faced with external disruption.

The nervous system also plays a role in homeostatic regulation via the coordination of the processes of different systems of organs and the induction of reflex physiological responses. The ANS, once again divided into sympathetic and parasympathetic branches, directly regulates heart rate, digestion, and respiratory rate, among many others. For example, in stress, the sympathetic branch initiates the fight-or-flight mechanism, increasing heart rate and shunting blood to essential muscles. The parasympathetic branch, on the other hand, causes relaxation and digestion, attempting to restore balance after stressors have been dissipated. Interestingly, the integration of sensory input enables the nervous system to detect changes in the internal environment and react in turn to them, thus reflecting its vital role in maintaining homeostasis. By examining the cross-talk between the major organ systems, we are able to appreciate the subtle physiological nuances behind human health and homeostasis (Figure 1.14).

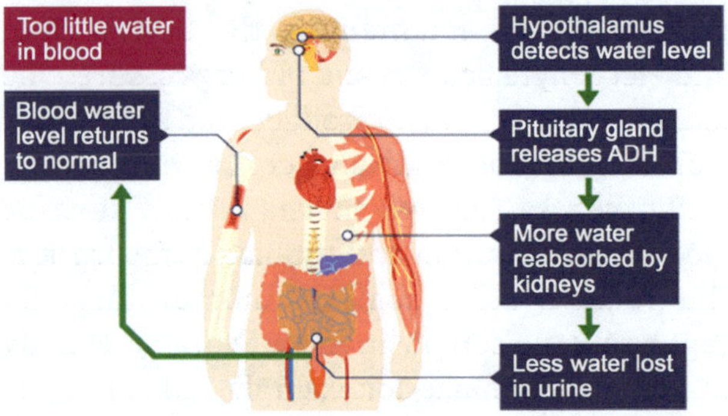

Figure 1.14. Organ systems involved in homeostasis.

*Source:*https://bam.files.bbci.co.uk/bam/live/content/zvf8mp3/medium.

1.5.1. The Endocrine System and Hormone Regulation

The endocrine system is very crucial in maintaining homeostasis in the human body by regulating hormones. Hormones, which are chemical messengers secreted into the blood by endocrine glands, influence numerous physiological processes , such as growth, metabolism, and reactions to stress. Unlike the nervous system, which provides quick and temporary responses to stimulation, the endocrine system takes time and its action lasts longer. One of the most important problems the endocrine system solves is the control of plasma blood glucose, a process in which feedback mechanisms play a predominant role. Feedback mechanisms work by sampling hormone levels and correcting by changing hormone release, thus keeping plasma glucose levels within a tight, optimal range. This subtle balance illustrates how the endocrine system works tirelessly to uphold physiological stability, a feature of health in human beings. In the study of endocrine regulation, it helps to see the organizational closure idea, which proposes that biological systems consist of interdependent functional structures that act as constraints. This explanation supplements our understanding of endocrine regulation beyond the reductionist feedback loop idea. For instance, aspects of glucose metabolism contain several hormones and feedback pathways that inter-relate mutually to create a complex set of influences. Using principles of closure of constraints, each of the entities within this process possesses a tiered set of interactions to feed into the overall stability of glycaemia. Such organizational frameworks can allow for the development of sophisticated mathematical models, enabling scientists to explore the intricate dynamics of hormone regulation in a systematic fashion. An organicist approach allows for a better, more integrated understanding of the endocrine system and makes it possible to better understand diseases , such as diabetes and metabolic disease. In addition, the action of some of these hormones, , such as nesfatin-1, suggests the chemical diversity and complexity in endocrine regulation. Nesfatin-1 is a peptide that has implications for metabolic control as well as homeostasis and affects hunger- and energy-dependent behaviors. Chronic administration of nesfatin-1 has been shown to completely alter blood pressure regulation, with special focus on stress factors. The modulation of hormones , such as angiotensin and cortisol, and the plasma concentration of nesfatin-1, is indicative of the complex interplay of a number of regulatory processes in the body. These findings place forth nesfatin-1 as not only a player in energy homeostasis but also as a key regulator in responding to physiological stressors. The identification of these mechanisms reveals the intricate means by which the endocrine system encourages homeostasis, thus illustrating the vital relationship between hormonal regulation and the health of man (Figure 1.15).

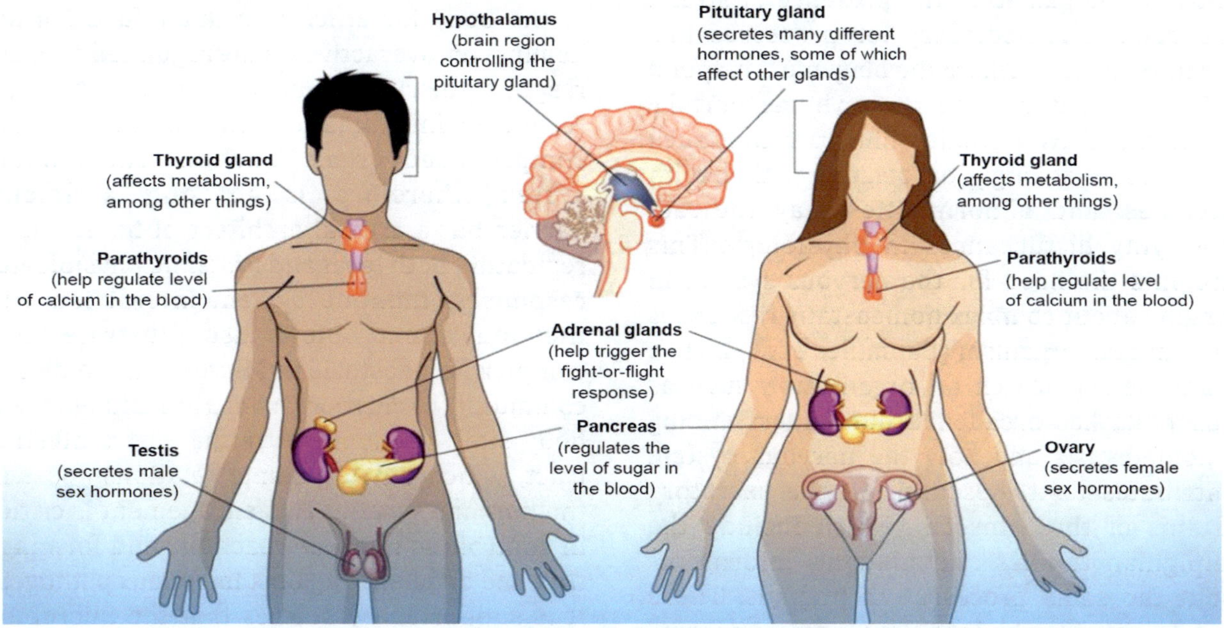

Figure 1.15. Endocrine system.

*Source:*https://www.sakethospital.in/wp-content/uploads/2023/12/Add-a-heading.jpg..

1.5.2. The Nervous System and Its Role in Homeostasis

The nervous system plays a central role in maintaining homeostasis in the human body by processing sensory data and coordinating a response to internal and external changes. Comprised of the peripheral nervous system (PNS) and central nervous system (CNS), it serves to transmit information among various body systems to provide rapid adaptations for survival. The nervous system is kept informed of such measures as hydration status, temperature, and pH levels through specialized receptors, which detect ranges that fall outside of normal. When a deviation has been observed, the CNS deciphers the data and controls responses , such as altered heart rate, respiratory rate, and endocrine secretion. The interaction enables physiological processes to adjust dynamically, thereby allowing an organism to stay in equilibrium even with environmental changes. In these ways, the nervous system illustrates its significance in the maintenance of homeostasis and overall health. Aside from its role as a regulator, the nervous system is also involved in homeostasis through complex feedback mechanisms that focus on communication between different physiological systems. For instance, ANS regulates unconscious functions , such as digestion, heart rate, and respiratory rhythm so that energy allocation and metabolic processes adapt to changing requirements. The parasympathetic and sympathetic branches of the ANS create a delicate balance between inhibition and stimulation, enabling strong homeostatic control to be gained in the presence of stress. This balance is necessary for processes like thermoregulation, where the body must respond rapidly to avoid hypothermia or hyperthermia. Furthermore, HRV studies illustrate that such a balance is strongly associated with health outcomes, and abnormalities may indicate underlying disturbances in physiology. This pinpoints the need for the nervous system in bringing about complex homeostatic responses in the human organism (Bahmiller et al., 2014). In addition, research on organisms , such as Drosophila has broadened our understanding of homeostasis and how the nervous system contributes to it. Research on the excretory systems of these insects, which include the Malpighian tubules and hindgut, informs us about the same processes in humans. These models give insight into how neuroendocrine signals influence renal function, fluid transport, and cellular communication within the gut, all of which are critical for maintaining electrolyte balance and osmotic homeostasis. By studying these more basic systems, scientists can uncover principles that have wide relevance in human physiology, which highlight common mechanisms for governing homeostatic regulation. In addition, the flexibility of such models allows for exploring many of the disease processes of man, illustrating the interrelated nature of the nervous system with other physiologic systems and its absolute center in acquiring and sustaining homeostasis (Cohen et al., 2020).

1.5.3. The Role of the Immune System in Maintaining Homeostasis

The immune system plays the essential role of maintaining homeostasis by protecting the body against dangerous invaders, but also moderating its response so as not to harm the tissues. This control keeps the immune system from overreacting to such foreign invaders as bacteria, viruses, and fungi without triggering autoimmune diseases. While a well-regulated immune response plays a role in the maintenance of homeostasis within the internal environment of the body for efficient cellular function and healing, an overactive or dysregulated immune response disrupts homeostatic regulation and results in inflammation, chronic disease, and compromised organ function. The immune system, therefore, is not only a defense barrier but a critical architect of homeostasis, regulating both local and systemic physiological responses. Immune system interaction with the body's microbiota also illustrates how complex homeostasis is. Microbiota is a diverse community of microorganisms inhabiting various body sites, predominantly the gastrointestinal tract, which have dynamic relationships with the immune system. This engagement is critical in controlling immune reactions and forming a first line of defense against infectious pathogens. It is supported by studies that the microbiota can program both the innate and adaptive branches of the immune response, rendering the body proficient at distinguishing between perilous pathogens and non-detrimental entities. Through maintenance of an ideal balance of microbiota, the immune system helps suppress inflammatory responses that can disrupt homeostasis and instead maintain a balance critical for wellbeing and health (Brown et al., 2016). Thus, therapeutic strategies focused on interrupting gut microbiota might be pivotal to restoring homeostasis disrupted by immune dysfunction. The immune system also maintains homeostasis through tissue repair and regeneration following damage. When tissue injury occurs, the immune system initiates processes that enhance wound healing, which can involve mechanisms , such as inflammation followed by resolution. Immune cells, , such as macrophages, secrete signal molecules triggering tissue repair through the induction of cell proliferation and migration necessary for regeneration. The role of heat shock proteins, , such as HSP27 and HSP72, has also been highlighted in the mediation of protective responses, particularly through their interaction with intestinal microbiota and involvement in cellular stress responses (Liu et al., 2013). Here, the immune system is responsible for restoring tissue integrity and functional homeostasis, illustrating its multifunctional role not only in protection but in mechanisms of repair and recovery necessary to sustain life (Figure 1.16).

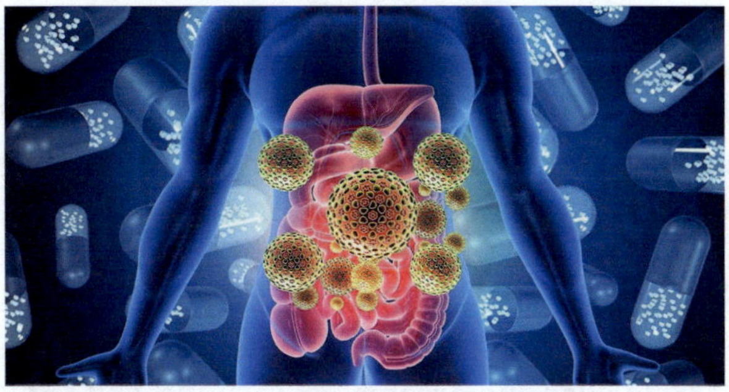

Figure 1.16. Maintaining immune system homeostasis.

Source: https://www.chiroeco.com/wp-content/uploads/2023/05/AdobeStock_312008058.jpeg.

Test Your Knowledge

1. How does the nervous system sense changes in the internal environment and coordinate responses to maintain homeostasis?
2. What is the function of the endocrine system in long-term homeostatic regulation through hormone signaling?

1.6. Impact of Environmental Factors on Homeostasis

Learning Outcome

1. Describe the control of temperature and thermoregulation;
2. Describe the influence of hydration and osmotic balance;
3. Describe the influence of altitude and pressure on physiological processes.

Homeostasis, the internal stability that is achieved by organisms in response to fluctuating external conditions, is influenced by a number of environmental factors. These are temperature, salinity, and availability of nutrients, and they have the potential to exert considerable influence on physiological processes. For instance, an increase in temperature can potentially elevate metabolic rates, thus impacting the organism's energy requirement and overall health. In aquatic environments, for instance, estuaries, changes in salinity can trigger osmoregulation problems that compel species to re-establish their physiological processes. The delta smelt (*Hypomesus transpacificus*), an endangered fish from the San Francisco Estuary, is a classic illustration of how changes in salinity impact homeostasis. These organisms must utilize conserved molecular processes in order to change their osmoregulatory physiology upon being challenged with salinity change, illustrating the intricate relationship between environmental drivers and physiological homeostasis (Connon et al., 2016).

Additionally, the interaction between environmental drivers and homeostasis is further illustrated through the role of metal ions in biological processes. Essential metallic elements , such as sodium and potassium are required for ion gradient maintenance across membranes within cells and osmoregulation. The ions facilitate essential transport physiology, particularly during stress phases of the environment. The functions of these metals extend beyond physiological processes only; an example is calcium ions, which serve as second messengers, relaying signals from the outside world and mediating back to it, and transport structural roles within cells. Excessive levels of some metals are capable of inducing oxidative stress and thus leading to cell damage and compromising homeostatic equilibrium. Thus, recognizing the dual role of metal ions as normal functioning of essential nutrient activities and potential toxicity is important in appreciating how environmental conditions influence homeostatic control in organisms (Dow et al., 2017). As global climate change continues to redefine environmental conditions, the stresses of homeostasis will increase for the vast majority of species. The interplay of molecular and organismal responses in sublethal response and physiological adaptation research is central to understanding these effects. For example, delta smelt demonstrates that even with a robust physiological capacity to survive fluctuating salinity, the energetic expense of possessing such adaptations might limit their habitat utilization and survival. Applying mechanistic approaches with causal links among physiological responses and environmental variation allows researchers to enhance the prediction of species resilience and distribution patterns in climate change conditions. This understanding not only enhances the field of physiology but also has global implications for conservation and ecosystem management, prioritizing the importance of developing an integrative knowledge base around the dynamic interaction of environmental factors and homeostasis (Connon et al., 2016) (Figure 1.17).

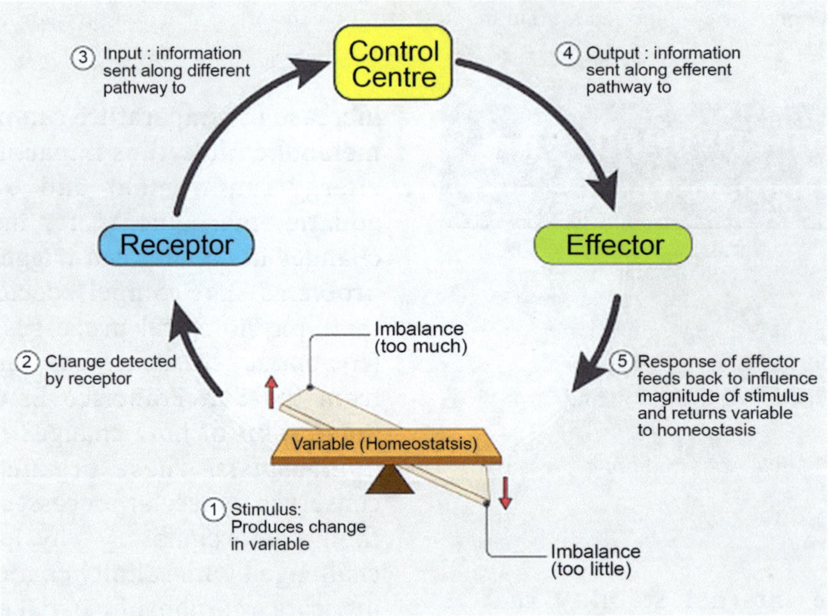

Figure 1.17. Homeostasis in the ecosystem.

Source: https://cdn-images.prepp.in/public/image/92bbaa32b8eee5500849abe4e4bc21dd.png?tr=w-510,h-454,c-force.

1.6.1. Temperature Regulation and Thermoregulation

The human body maintains a consistent internal environment, a process highly important for ideal physiological function referred to as homeostasis. Temperature control is an essential aspect of this homeostatic equilibrium, since the body can coordinate the numerous responses it generates to keep a core temperature of approximately 37°C (98.6°F). The thermoregulatory response entails a complex interplay of various physiological and behavioral mechanisms, controlled largely by the hypothalamus. This central processing unit integrates sensory information regarding ambient temperatures and elicits appropriate responses, , such as stimulating sweat glands or controlling blood flow to the skin. Further, this system also takes into account thermoregulatory needs in states of illness, where fever response may be reflective of intrinsic pathophysiological changes that need further investigation and understanding, highlighting the importance of precise temperature control in clinical practice (Tawfik, 2020). The neural control of thermoregulation has a central network that incorporates the body's response to alterations in temperature.

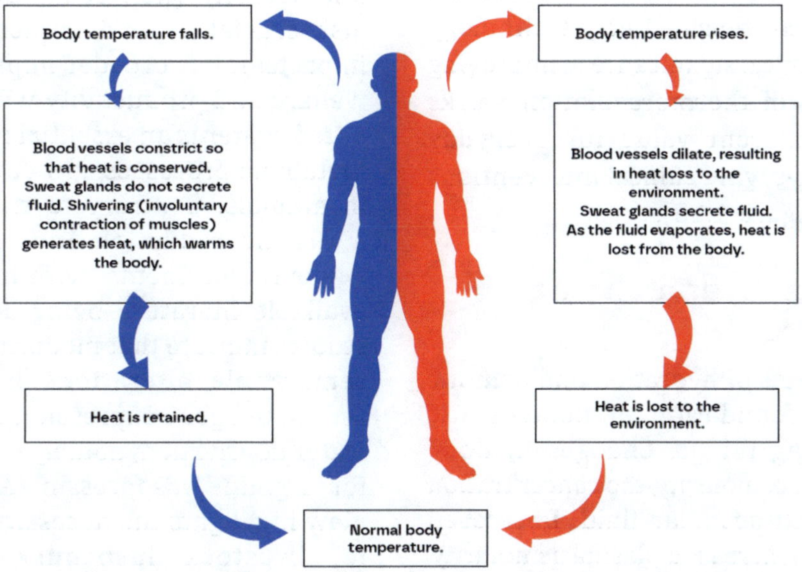

Figure 1.18. Thermoregulation-human-body.

Source: https://news.six2.com/content/uploads/SIXS-thermoregulation-Human-Body-1024x756.jpg.

This network utilizes a chain of neurotransmitters and neural pathways to regulate aspects , such as cutaneous vasoconstriction, shivering, and the stimulation of the brown adipose tissue to generate heat. Since the body experiences environmental temperature changes, it triggers these thermoeffectors to retain or lose heat to ensure normal function and prevent thermal stress. The efferent branches of this thermoregulatory circuit demonstrate a remarkable degree of organization, which demonstrates how discrete yet interconnected systems work together for a common purpose, thermohomeostasis. This fundamental understanding of the neural process of thermoregulation is important to advance the therapeutic techniques that adjust body temperature in various clinical settings (Morrison et al., 2018). In seeking the meaning of thermoregulation, it is important to appreciate its role in immune responses and overall energy homeostasis. The body's temperature-regulating systems not only serve the purpose of insulating against exterior temperature extremes but also are centrally involved in infectious disease processes. Fever, for instance, is an immediate response to infection, raising the body's temperature as a mechanism against pathogen reproduction. Comprehension of fever's physiologic and immunologic underpinnings, as exhaustively explored in books , such as Understanding Fever and Body Temperature: A Cross-disciplinary Approach to Clinical Practice, provides helpful clinicosophy for clinicians. The intersection of historical context, thermometry technology innovations, and clinical significance in improving an understanding of thermoregulation works to support its inherent value for everyday physiology and life-saving clinical interventions (Tawfik, 2020) (Figure 1.18).

1.6.2. Effects of Hydration and Osmotic Balance

The combined effects of hydration and osmotic balance are the foundation of homeostatic regulation in living things. Changes in body hydration influence osmolarity, the concentration of solute in the extracellular fluid. Decreased hydration results in increased plasma osmolarity, with mechanisms that work to correct the imbalance. The kidneys play a central role in this process by altering urine concentration through the regulation of water reabsorption. By stimulating antidiuretic hormone (ADH) pathways, the body holds water and reduces osmolarity, maintaining hemostatic stability. These physiological responses illustrate the direct role of hydration in regulating osmotic balance, validating the necessity of fluid intake to maintain ideal health and function. Research has shown that acute and chronic hydration states can profoundly affect homeostatic control. In dehydration, particularly where there are high environmental stresses , such as space travel, researchers noticed a considerable headward fluid shift leading to disturbances typical of impaired osmotic balance, like headache and vestibular disturbance. Such complications point to the adaptation mechanisms of the body and how it can include the modulation of hormone secretion to regulate cardiovascular and fluid status in response to stress. Neural and hormonal mechanisms converging to prove the complexity of osmotic balance demonstrate that even a small perturbation can result in significant health implications, supporting the absolute necessity of hydration regulation in various settings, including extreme ones like microgravity (Keil et al., 2025). Hydration is also crucial beyond immediate physiological impacts; it has broader implications for animal welfare and productivity within agriculture. As noted, water is an essential nutrient to facilitate metabolic processes, growth, and reproduction in animals. Contrary to this, there has been a drastic reduction in studies of livestock water requirements, with most of the existing available literature being decades old. Recent studies indicate that modern beef cattle develop remarkable alterations in osmoregulation-associated gene expression under conditions of water deprivation, notably concerning pathways for arginine vasopressin (AVP). This genomic view highlights the necessity of new regulation for livestock husbandry, emphasizing the importance of hydration in ensuring sustained productivity under increasingly uncertain climatic patterns. In the end, an extensive understanding of how hydration affects osmotic balance is crucial to human health as well as farm efficiency (Arachchilage et al., 2023).

1.6.3. Influence of Altitude and Pressure on Physiological Processes

The interaction of altitude, atmospheric pressure, and body function is key to the understanding of how organisms preserve homeostasis under different surroundings. With an elevation increase, atmospheric pressure decreases, resulting in diminished oxygen availability. This hypoxia condition plays a significant role in respiration and circulation, as the body must undergo adaptations to provide sufficient oxygenation to tissues. For instance, above altitudes of 3,000 meters, individuals develop physiological challenges , such as shortness of breath and fatigue due to decreased oxygen partial pressure, which can drop to as low as 26% of sea-level levels. The human body responds by activating compensatory mechanisms, including increased respiratory rate and cardiac output, to optimize oxygen utilization and maintain vital functions. Therefore, the physiological reactions to altitude illustrate the subtle balance required to achieve homeostasis under challenging environmental conditions. The adaptations expressed in high-altitude flying birds also illustrate the powerful effect of lowered air pressure on physiological function. In migration, resident as well as migratory species of birds are confronted with hypoxic conditions, demanding a specialized reaction. Birds exhibit numerous physiological adaptations, including increases to their cardiovascular and pulmonary systems, to mitigate the impact of lowered oxygen levels. For example, larger hearts and greater capillary densities ensure improved oxygen transport to tissues. Additionally, adaptations , such as increased wing size and altered flight mechanics enable birds like the hummingbird to hover in hypodense air environments effectively. These morphological changes ensure that there is a balance between aerodynamics and energy efficiency, emphasizing the importance of evolutionary adaptations toward maintaining performance and survival across varying altitudinal zones. In general, the impact of altitude and pressure on physiological processes emphasizes the complexity of homeostatic mechanisms across various species. With organisms approaching higher altitudes, adaptation potential becomes critical to maintain sustained function and survival. Studies have highlighted a variety of strategies adopted by various taxa, particularly in conditions that are harsh as well as where the costs of physiology are higher. Not only does it inform us about animal physiology, but also about what can be achieved in human physiological responses to altitude exposure, say in altitude training or mountain climbing considerations. Finally, an understanding of these physiological adaptations deepens our knowledge of homeostasis, showing the incredible resilience of life against environmental stresses and challenges (Altshuler & Dudley, 2006).

Test Your Knowledge

1. How is exposure to extreme temperatures (heat or cold) influenced by the body's capacity to maintain thermal homeostasis?
2. How is dehydration or excessive water intake able to upset homeostatic fluid balance, and how does the body react?

SUMMARY

In conclusion, physiological interdependence and the law of homeostasis ensure the complexity of biological systems. The mechanisms ensure the maintenance of internal stability against external change, demonstrating the body's extremely resilient nature. Understanding mechanisms of homeostasis is crucial for the appreciation of how living organisms respond to environmental change, emphasizing the evolutionary significance of such physiological responses. Function of the sympathetic nervous system, further in survival processes , such as fight or flight, emphasizes the active interaction between organ systems and the central nervous system. Multi-faceted coordination is reflective of the reason behind the ongoing importance of physiological psychology research to demonstrate these complex relationships, particularly of gender differences during responding to stressors (Miara et al., 2013). Moreover, research into homeostatic processes continues in the disease and health context. Because physiological processes can be tested by pharmacological approaches or pathologic insults, understanding these disruptions is crucial in formulating effective treatment regimens. For instance, heart failure represents a significant clinical syndrome, defined by mitochondrial dysfunction and altered patterns of gene expression, as found in recent investigations. The persistence characteristics of agents like melatonin exhibit mechanistic intervention approaches that can circumvent drug-induced cardiac dysfunction, as a refinement of our knowledge of homeostasis under pathological stress (Ganeshan, 2019). This knowledge not only informs clinical application but also facilitates an integrated understanding of physiological resilience and susceptibility to stressors. In conclusion, harmonization of physiology and homeostasis underscores the complexity of the biological system and its inherent capacity to change. Continued research here continues to reveal complex relationships among the organ systems, the environment, and therapeutic maneuvers. As researchers discover more about the breakdown and repair of homeostasis, new challenges for developing innovative treatment approaches arise. Ultimately, a proper understanding of these principles equips upcoming healthcare professionals and researchers with the knowledge necessary to address health priorities. Through continued inquiry into the multifaceted nature of physiology and homeostasis, we can encourage innovation that enhances individual health as well as aggregate health outcomes.

The homeostatic principle is the core of a physiological understanding and the maintenance of life. Homeostasis refers to the dynamic equilibrium that biological systems strive to achieve for maximum operation regardless of changes in the external environment. The intricate balance is created by various feedback mechanisms through which organisms can perceive and counteract alterations within and outside their immediate surroundings. For instance, physiological mechanisms , such as temperature regulation and fluid balance are necessary for the maintenance of cellular function and general health. In exploring these core principles, it is evident that homeostasis is not merely a static condition but rather a continuously regulated state, essential for survival across diverse organisms, from simple single-celled organisms to complex multicellular life forms. The relationship between biological systems and their environments is exemplified by the Earth's complex ecological systems, which reflect homeostatic principles on a planetary scale. According to current evidence, abiotic and biotic organisms interact such that the Earth becomes stable and allows for the presence of other ecosystems. Gaia homeostasis theory addresses the mechanisms by which life and its physical environment interact in their mutual effect in order to generate states of equilibrium with the ability to resist perturbations from the external environment. This synergy confirms the merit of feedback loops in supplying resilience, further evidence of the premise that biological diversity is essential to ecosystems' stability. Experimental results derived from conceptual models have verified that greater biological diversity is correlated with greater stability, highlighting a key element of homeostasis beyond specific species and geographic locales (Dyke et al., 2013). A closer examination of human physiological processes reveals that homeostasis mechanisms are similarly evidenced in scientific investigations of human health, particularly in the description of illnesses , such as cystic kidney diseases (CKDs). CKDs illustrate the pathological disruption of homeostasis, in which the development of cysts interferes with normal renal function through defective cellular mechanisms. Studies have shown significant conservation of mechanisms between species, which suggests a common evolutionary origin of excretory systems, and which can be used to explain the complex human health issues. By using invertebrate models , such as planarians, scientists have been able to study the underlying biology of fundamental biological processes underpinning CKDs, and thus validate basic homeostatic principles relevant in clinical practice. These investigations not only enhance our knowledge of physiology but also provide new insights into therapeutic intervention, reminding us of the overriding significance of homeostasis to health (Vu et al., 2015).

KEY TERMS FROM THIS CHAPTER

- Blood Glucose Regulation
- Blood Pressure
- Body Temperature
- Cellular Respiration
- Control Center
- Effector
- Electrolyte Balance
- Endocrine System
- Feedback Loop
- Homeostasis
- Hormones
- Internal Environment
- Metabolism
- Negative Feedback
- Nervous System
- Osmoregulation

CRITICAL THINKING QUESTIONS

1. **What is the main role of homeostasis in the human body?**
   a. To encourage rapid changes in the internal conditions
   b. To maintain a constant internal environment
   c. To resist all the changes in the body
   d. To speed up all the metabolic processes
2. **What is an example of a negative feedback mechanism?**
   a. Blood clotting
   b. Childbirth contractions
   c. Regulation of body temperature
   d. Lactation during breastfeeding
3. **What organ is significantly responsible for maintaining blood glucose levels?**
   a. Heart
   b. Liver
   c. Pancreas
   d. Kidney
4. **Which region of the brain regulates most of the homeostatic processes like temperature and thirst?**
   a. Cerebellum
   b. Medulla oblongata
   c. Hypothalamus
   d. Cerebrum
5. **Which hormone is secreted when the blood sugar is too high?**
   a. Glucagon
   b. Insulin
   c. Adrenaline
   d. Cortisol

Short Answer Questions

1. Define homeostasis.
2. What is a negative feedback mechanism?
3. Name the two significant systems that are involved in maintaining homeostasis in the body.
4. What is the normal range of human body temperature?
5. Describe how the body maintains temperature homeostasis in hot and cold environments.
6. Explain the role of the endocrine system in homeostasis with examples of particular hormones.
7. Explain negative feedback control of blood glucose levels using insulin and glucagon.
8. Explain the differences and similarities between negative and positive feedback mechanisms using physiology examples.

Answers to Critical Thinking Questions

1. (b); 2. (c); 3. (c); 4. (c); 5. (b)

REFERENCES

1. Alcedo, J., Flatt, T., & Pasyukova, E. G. (2013). Neuronal inputs and outputs of aging and longevity. *Frontiers in genetics, 4*, 71. https://doi.org/10.3389/fgene.2013.00071(accessed on 16th June 2025).
2. Thi-Kim Vu, H., Rink, J. C., McKinney, S. A., McClain, M., Lakshmanaperumal, N., Alexander, R., & Sánchez Alvarado, A. (2015). Stem cells and fluid flow drive cyst formation in an invertebrate excretory organ. *eLife, 4*, e07405. https://doi.org/10.7554/eLife.07405Allen, R., Bogle, I. D. L., & Sumner, T. (2009). The role of Computer Aided Process Engineering in physiology and clinical medicine. https://core.ac.uk/download/1674037.pdf (accessed on 16th June 2025).
3. Douglas L. Altshuler, Robert Dudley, The physiology and biomechanics of avian flight at high altitude, Integrative and Comparative Biology, Volume 46, Issue 1, February 2006, Pages 62–71, https://doi.org/10.1093/icb/icj008(accessed on 16th June 2025).
4. Bich, L., Mossio, M., & Soto, A. M. (2020). Glycemia regulation: From feedback loops to organizational closure. https://core.ac.uk/download/287611700.pdf (accessed on 16th June 2025).
5. Cañamero, L. (2019). Embodied robot models for interdisciplinary emotion research. https://core.ac.uk/download/287581878.pdf (accessed on 16th June 2025).
6. Canovas-Ramos, F. M., De la Torre, F., El-Azaz, J., et al. (2019). Biochemical regulation of arginine biosynthesis in plants. https://core.ac.uk/download/223069350.pdf (accessed on 16th June 2025).
7. Carroll, L., Cordero, J., & Naszai, M. (2015). Intestinal stem cell proliferation and epithelial homeostasis in the adult *Drosophila* midgut. https://core.ac.uk/download/42368228.pdf (accessed on 16th June 2025).
8. Carter, C. S., Justice, J. N., & Thompson, L. (2019). Lipotoxicity, aging, and muscle contractility: Does fiber type matter? https://open.bu.edu/bitstream/2144/40625/7/carter_justice_thompson_Lipotoxicity_paper_04302019.pdf (accessed on 16th June 2025).
9. Connon, R. E., Dexter, J., Fangue, N. A., et al. (2016). Sublethal salinity stress contributes to habitat limitation in an endangered estuarine fish. https://core.ac.uk/download/323068737.pdf (accessed on 16th June 2025).
10. Quintana, D., & Guastella, A. J. (2020). An allostatic theory of oxytocin. *Trends in Cognitive Sciences, 24*, 515–528. https://doi.org/10.1016/j.tics.2020.03.008 (accessed on 16th June 2025).
11. Zheng, D., Liwinski, T., & Elinav, E. (2020). Interaction between microbiota and immunity in health and disease. *Cell Research, 30*, 492–506. https://doi.org/10.1038/s41422-020-0332-7
12. Delafield-Butt, J. (2009). Containment and reciprocity in biological systems: A putative psychophysical organizing principle. https://core.ac.uk/download/9040029.pdf (accessed on 16th June 2025).
13. Dow, J. A. T. (2017). The essential roles of metal ions in insect homeostasis and physiology. https://core.ac.uk/download/96881956.pdf (accessed on 16th June 2025).
14. Dyke, J. G., & Weaver, I. S. (2013). The emergence of environmental homeostasis in complex ecosystems. https://core.ac.uk/download/18935006.pdf (accessed on 16th June 2025).

15. Forman, H. J., Maiorino, M., & Ursini, F. (2016). Redox homeostasis: The golden mean of healthy living. https://core.ac.uk/download/84920832.pdf (accessed on 16th June 2025).

16. Gopika, S., & Kulkarni, P. V. (2024). Critical review on physiological aspects of *Samana Vata*. https://core.ac.uk/download/617190090.pdf (accessed on 16th June 2025).

17. Haase, H., & Maares, M. (2020). A guide to human zinc absorption: General overview and recent advances of *in vitro* intestinal models. https://core.ac.uk/download/322792238.pdf (accessed on 16th June 2025).

18. Jackson, R., & Williams, D. L. (2016). Availability of information on reptile health and welfare from stores selling reptiles. https://core.ac.uk/download/77412350.pdf (accessed on 16th June 2025).

19. Ganeshan, T. K. (2019). Investigating the protective role of the natural hormone melatonin, in reducing drug-induced cardiotoxicity in the therapy of chronic diseases. https://core.ac.uk/download/287605215.pdf (accessed on 16th June 2025).

20. Keil, L. C., & Severs, W. B. (2025). Effects of CSF hormones and ionic composition on salt/water metabolism. https://core.ac.uk/download/pdf/42811529.pdf (accessed on 16th June 2025).

21. Lange, K. A. (2025). *Physiology of Man and Animals in the Tenth Five-Year Plan: Proceedings of the Thirteenth Congress of the I. P. Pavlov All-Union Physiological Society*. https://core.ac.uk/download/pdf/42860886.pdf (accessed on 16th June 2025).

22. Rodrigues, L. P., Teixeira, V. R., Alencar-Silva, T., Simonassi-Paiva, B., Pereira, R. W., Pogue, R., & Carvalho, J. L. (2021). Hallmarks of aging and immunosenescence: Connecting the dots. *Cytokine & Growth Factor Reviews, 59*, 9–21. https://doi.org/10.1016/j.cytogfr.2021.01.006 (accessed on 16th June 2025).

23. Onishi, M., Yamano, K., Sato, M., Matsuda, N., & Okamoto, K. (2021). Molecular mechanisms and physiological functions of mitophagy. *The EMBO Journal, 40*. https://doi.org/10.15252/embj.2020104705 (accessed on 16th June 2025).

24. Miara, A. (2013). Differences in sympathetic nervous response due to gender. https://open.bu.edu/bitstream/2144/12160/6/Miara_Amy_2013_nosig_nocv.pdf (accessed on 16th June 2025).

25. Tawfik, M. M. (2020). Understanding fever and body temperature: A cross-disciplinary approach to clinical practice. *Anesthesia & Analgesia, 130*, e174–e174. https://doi.org/10.1213/ane.0000000000004777 (accessed on 16th June 2025).

26. Mori, Y. (2014). A multidomain model for ionic electro diffusion and osmosis with an application to cortical spreading depression. http://arxiv.org/abs/1410.8391 (accessed on 16th June 2025).

27. Neal, C. M. (2016). Evaluating techniques in tissue clarification using CLARITY imaging and investigating where sodium is sensed in the body. https://core.ac.uk/download/142066226.pdf (accessed on 16th June 2025).

28. van Hasselt, S. J., Mekenkamp, G. J., Komdeur, J., Allocca, G., Vyssotski, A., Piersma, T., Rattenborg, N., et al. (2020). Seasonal variation in sleep homeostasis in migratory geese: A rebound of NREM sleep following sleep deprivation in summer but not in winter. *Sleep, 44*. https://www.semanticscholar.org/paper/e9448f23542ee58570c6818105e7e6f293187d55 (accessed on 16th June 2025).

29. Morrison, S. F., & Nakamura, K. (2018). Central mechanisms for thermoregulation. *Annual Review of Physiology, 81*, 285–308. https://doi.org/10.1146/annurev-physiol-020518-114546 (accessed on 16th June 2025).

30. Prasad, H. M. S., Bhuvana, C. S., & Kamath, N. (2024). Critical appraisal of homeostasis with its interpretation in Ayurveda. *Global Journal for Research Analysis*. https://www.semanticscholar.org/paper/76559efa2b91283a85d4c55e21258e48015c22b8 (accessed on 16th June 2025).

31. Ghosh, S., Whitley, C. S., Haribabu, B., & Jala, V. R. (2021). Regulation of intestinal barrier function by microbial metabolites. *Cellular and Molecular Gastroenterology and Hepatology, 11*, 1463–1482. https://doi.org/10.1016/j.jcmgh.2021.02.007 (accessed on 16th June 2025).

32. Torday J. S. (2015). Homeostasis as the Mechanism of Evolution. *Biology*, *4*(3), 573–590. https://doi.org/10.3390/biology4030573(accessed on 16th June 2025).

33. Torday, J. S. (2015). Pleiotropy as the mechanism for evolving novelty: Same signal, different result. https://core.ac.uk/download/323075977.pdf (accessed on 16th June 2025).

34. Galicia-García, U., Benito-Vicente, A., Jebari, S., Larrea-Sebal, A., Siddiqi, H., Uribe, K. B., Ostolaza, H., et al. (2020). Pathophysiology of type 2 diabetes mellitus. *International Journal of Molecular Sciences, 21*, 6275–6275. https://doi.org/10.3390/ijms21176275 (accessed on 16th June 2025).

35. Wickramasinghe Vithana Arachchilage, H. C. (2023). Identification of genes expressed in the anterior pituitary associated with water restriction in beef cattle. https://core.ac.uk/download/588707434.pdf (accessed on 16th June 2025).

36. Wolfe, C. T. (2010). Do organisms have an ontological status? https://core.ac.uk/download/11922649.pdf (accessed on 16th June 2025).

37. Wu, X., Cao, Y., Liu, Y., & Zheng, J. (2024). A new strategy for dietary nutrition to improve intestinal homeostasis in diarrheal irritable bowel syndrome: A perspective on intestinal flora and intestinal epithelial interaction. *Nutrients, 16*. https://www.semanticscholar.org/paper/21de59f6dfd2d3c90f880dff31a3156e45f1c2dd (accessed on 16th June 2025).

38. Kariya, Y. (2024). [Challenges in understanding the biological and pharmacological responses based on emergent complexity in biological systems: From bone metabolism to general physiology]. *Yakugaku Zasshi: Journal of the Pharmaceutical Society of Japan, 144*(9), 865–870. https://www.semanticscholar.org/paper/3b9c4e0fe557db73aa62c87bbc54404c6b6a7e1c (accessed on 16th June 2025).

CELL MEMBRANE PHYSIOLOGY

2

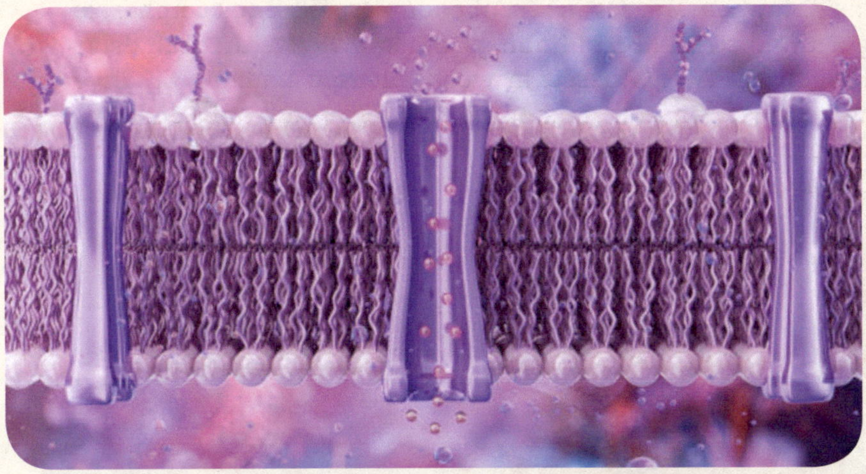

LEARNING OBJECTIVES

After studying this chapter, you will be able to:

1. Describe the structure of the cell membrane;
2. Describe the functions of the cell membrane;
3. Describe the transport mechanisms;
4. Describe the membrane potential;
5. Describe the cell membrane and homeostasis;
6. Assess the pathological conditions regarding the cell membrane.

Introduction

Cell membrane physiology is a fundamental branch of the biological sciences that focuses on the structure, function, and dynamics of cellular membranes. Being the interface between the cell and its extracellular environment, the cell membrane is a vital component of homeostasis, communication, and the regulation of the transport of materials in and out of the cell. The selective permeability of the membrane is the result of the conformation of the lipid bilayer, which is mostly composed of phospholipids and proteins. Through various mechanisms , such as passive and active transport, cells regulate the internal composition, which is essential for such processes as nutrient uptake, waste expulsion, and signal transduction. Understanding the processes of cell membranes not only describes basic cellular processes but also opens the door to additional medical and biotechnological investigations. Cell membrane physiology is explored in diverse applications, particularly in pharmacology and disease treatment. For instance, a study highlighted by Sanjaya et al. indicates that cell membrane interruptions can impact physiological functions radically, producing deleterious effects , such as decreased nutrient uptake and tissue injury, as in the case of infection of Spodoptera litura larvae with SlNPV. This demonstrates how a viral infection can interrupt cell membrane integrity, causing catastrophic histological damage. By understanding these interactions, researchers are able to design special therapies that reinforce membrane stability or reverse deleterious effects elicited by pathogens. Cell membrane physiology is thus not a speculative science; it is at the core of developing novel treatments to reverse cellular dysfunctions. The applicability of cell membrane physiology is also not restricted to the physiology of single cells but has more global implications for multicellular organisms. Membrane dynamics form the basis of basic processes , such as cell signaling, immune function, and overall tissue homeostasis. The ability of cells to communicate and cooperate with one another is based on their ability to interpret and respond to extracellular signals using membrane proteins, receptors, and related signaling pathways. Moreover, recent open-access trends emphasize the public nature of this field, enabling wider distribution of findings and knowledge that can drive forward advances in cell biology and medicine. As discussed in work released under a Creative Commons Attribution license, ongoing research on cell membrane dynamics not only enriches academic debate but also enhances the potential for practical real-world application, verifying cell membranes at the focal point of biological process and human wellbeing (Figure 2.1).

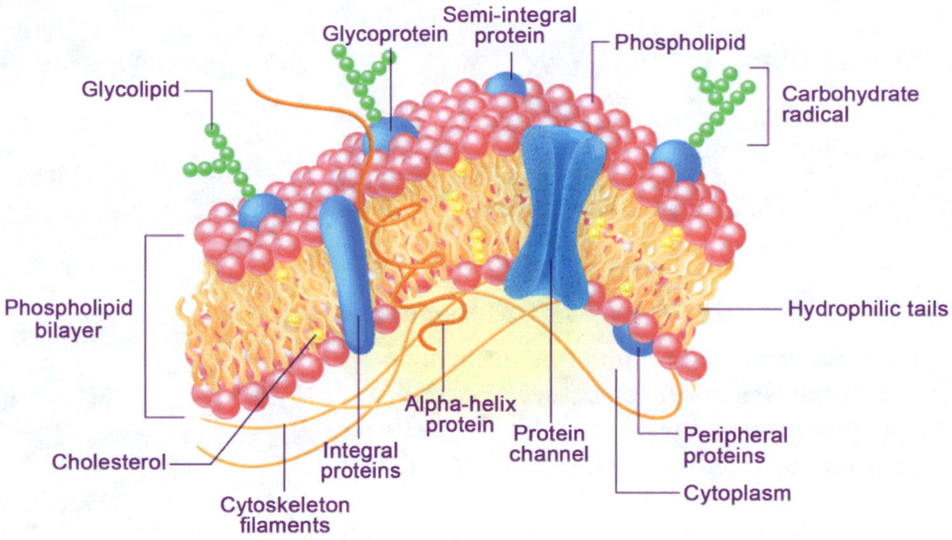

Figure 2.1. Cell membrane physiology.

Source: https://cdn1.byjus.com/wp-content/uploads/2022/12/Plasma-Membrane.png.

Definition of Cell Membrane

The cell membrane, or simply referred to as the plasma membrane, is a dynamic and vital component of all living cells and functions as a barrier that maintains the peculiar inner environment of the cell. The cell membrane is primarily composed of a phospholipid bilayer and is studded with proteins, cholesterol, and carbohydrates, which are the determinants of its fluidity and function. These hydrophilic heads face outwards towards the aqueous environments, both intra- and extracellular, while the hydrophobic tails face inwards, creating a semi-permeable barrier. The cell membrane's selective permeability plays a critical role in managing the movement of ions, nutrients, and waste products, which is crucial in maintaining homeostasis and facilitating communication between cells. One of the fundamental roles of the cell membrane is the control of material transport. The membrane employs various methods, , such as passive and active transport, to control the flow of molecules. For instance, passive transport is felt in diffusion, where material moves from an area of high concentration to a low concentration without the consumption of energy. By contrast, active transport is energy-dependent, frequently in the form of ATP, to transport substances against their concentration gradient. Such transport functions are important for several physiological processes, , such as the uptake of nutrients and the elimination of waste, and the upkeep of ionic gradients vital for cellular processes like signaling and the contraction of muscles. The interaction of these transport mechanisms highlights the importance of the cell membrane to cell physiology and organism health. More recent work has investigated more advanced models of cell membrane behavior, particularly in terms of fluid dynamics and electrolyte balance. For example, ionic electrodiffusion and osmotic water flow models describe cell volume and intracellular electrolyte regulation, a process that is at the core of homeostasis and physiological function. These types of balance between ion flow across the membrane, as described in established pump-leak models, regulate cell volume, and their loss has significant effects on cellular stability and operation. These models give a clearer picture of the physiological function of cell membranes, revealing their inherent function to sustain life and their responsiveness to various external and internal stimuli, , such as changes in ion concentration and availability of energy (Eisenberg et al., 2011; Mori et al., 2011).

Significance of the Cell Membrane in Cellular Processes

The cell membrane is a critical barrier that divides the interior of the cell from the exterior world and therefore, bears the responsibility of cellular function. The lipid bilayer not only offers structural strength but also selective permeability, such that essential nutrients are allowed in and harmful compounds are excluded. The unique molecular composition of phospholipids and proteins in the membrane results in a dynamic system that is capable of responding to cellular needs that are ever-changing. The capacity to respond enables cells to maintain homeostasis, manage chemical gradients, and respond to extracellular stimuli, all of which are critical to function and survival. In addition, the fluid mosaic model explains this structure, emphasizing that the mobile nature of components in the membrane provides for successful communication and interaction with other cells and the surroundings, further emphasizing the role of the cell membrane in cellular physiology. Also, the cell membrane plays a fundamental role in signal transduction, which is essential for the maintenance of communication channels that regulate cellular functions. Membrane proteins, , such as receptors, are responsible for detecting environmental signals and transmitting the signal into the cell. The receptors have the capability to bind several ligands, initiating intricate intracellular cascades of signaling, which eventually lead to physiological responses, , such as cell growth, differentiation, and metabolism. For instance, the role of caveolae, cholesterol-rich membrane domains that have been extensively studied; these are signaling hubs that govern the reaction to extracellular signals and control essential processes, including regulation of oxygen diffusion (Zuniga-Hertz & Patel, 2019). This high-level communicative ability shows not just how cellular identity is determined by the cell membrane but also how adaptive reactions to modifications of the cellular environment are facilitated. Moreover, the cell membrane-extracellular matrix (ECM) interaction illustrates how the membrane integrates outside mechanical signals into cellular processes. Fibroblasts, for example, are adhered to the ECM and utilize membrane-bound receptors to respond to mechanical cues, which regulate activities , such as collagen alignment during wound healing. The fibroblast-ECM interactions, as evidenced by dynamic collagen fiber orientation, facilitate profound cellular responses that further the tissue regeneration process (Maini et al., 2005). The mechanisms demonstrate the interconnectedness of cellular function and the cell membrane's structural components, commenting on its ability to coordinate complex biological processes and on its important contribution to wound healing and tissue repair. These functions highlight the requirement of the cell membrane in ensuring cellular health and effectively responding to environmental stresses (Figure 2.2).

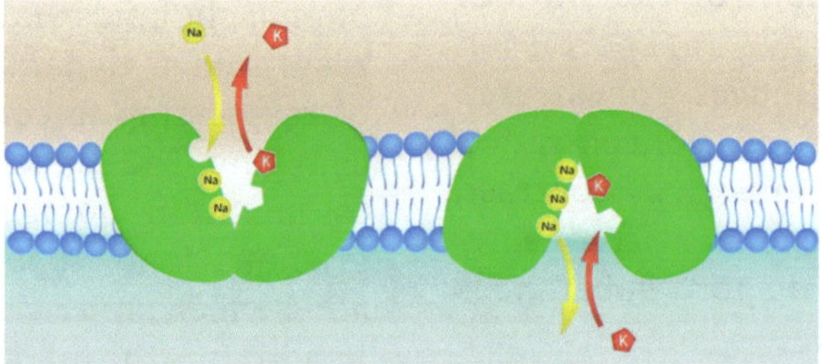

Figure 2.2. Cell membrane functions and importance.

Source: https://study.com/cimages/videopreview/videopreview-full/0q247j9umd.jpg.

2.1. Structure of the Cell Membrane

Learning Outcome

1. Describe the composition of the phospholipid bilayer;
2. Highlight the role of proteins in the structure of the membrane;
3. Understand the fluid mosaic model explanation.

The structure of the cell membrane is important in maintaining cellular integrity and regulating the movement of materials in and out of the cell. Composed largely of a phospholipid bilayer, the membrane contains a fluid mosaic model that allows the dynamic movement of lipids and proteins. This structure not only facilitates selective permeability, a basic process that regulates what enters and leaves the cell, but also provides a platform for membrane proteins. These proteins carry out many essential functions, including serving as receptors for signaling molecules, enzymes for chemical processes, and transport channels. Membrane structure also facilitates cellular signaling and communication so that the cell can respond appropriately to environmental stimuli. Most fundamental to understanding the cell membrane's purpose is its interaction with the cytoskeleton, which assists in maintaining cellular form and supporting membrane structure. The cell membrane has been shown to exhibit viscoelastic properties that are controlled by the supporting cytoskeletal matrix, indicative of profound interdependence between the cell's structures. By applying techniques , such as passive particle tracking microrheology, researchers have demonstrated that cellular viscoelastic moduli are highly related to the cytoskeleton architecture (Carlsson et al., 2013). This provides additional understanding of how modifications in the cytoskeleton can direct membrane dynamics and consequently have an impact on everything from the mobility of cells to the cell's reaction to stress. Moreover, the cell membrane structure is not rigid; it can change depending on various physiological stimuli. Like fibroblasts, which exhibit coordinated movements influencing the extracellular matrix, affecting both cell membrane structure as well as function during processes like wound healing. When collagen becomes aligned due to fibroblast movement, changes in membrane properties and behaviors can be anticipated (Maini et al., 2005). These interactions improves the comprehension of cellular reactions to the external world, illustrating the significance of membrane structure to cell physiology in general. The dynamic nature of the cell membrane emphasizes its intrinsic capacity to integrate structural stability with functional versatility, which is required for the maintenance of cellular homeostasis (Figure 2.3).

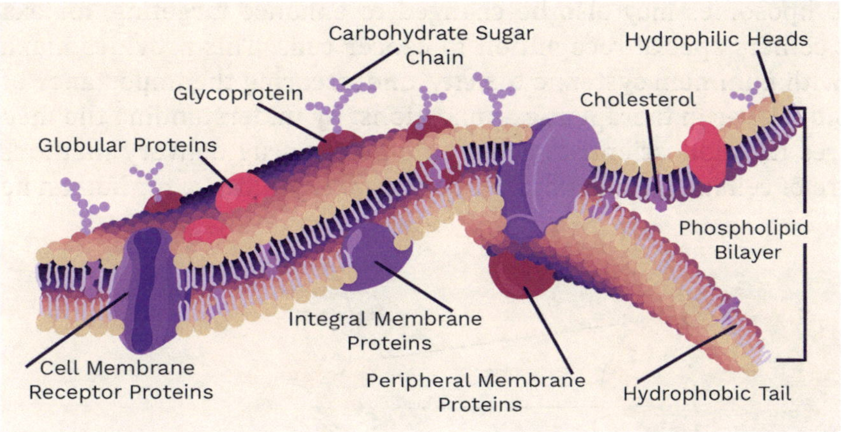

Figure 2.3. Cell membrane structure.

Source: https://www.thoughtco.com/thmb/gEjN01_wm9QX5NAVyHSEBNVBNLs=/1500x0/filters:no_upscale():max_bytes(150000):strip_icc()/cell-membrane-373364_final-5b5f300546e0fb008271ce52.png.

2.1.1. Phospholipid Bilayer Composition

The phospholipid bilayer is the simple structural component of the cell membrane and is responsible for the properties and function of the membranes. It is composed of two phospholipid layers and forms a hydrophobic center within which the phospholipid bilayer acts as a barrier to most water-soluble molecules. The amphipathic nature of the phospholipids, whereby their hydrophilic heads are directed outwards towards the aqueous environment and their hydrophobic tails inward, forms this fundamental barrier. This structure not only protects cellular content but also provides a platform for membrane proteins to perform best. Additionally, composition adjustments in bilayers, including phospholipid variations and the addition of cholesterol, further modulate fluidity and permeability, which play a significant role in the facilitation of homeostasis within the cell. Recognition of such compositional nuances is pivotal in the comprehension of how cells respond to environmental signals and stimuli. Cholesterol is a structural component of the phospholipid bilayer and contributes significantly to the stability and fluidity of the membrane. It intercalates between the phospholipids and reduces the solute and ion permeability of the membrane, thereby enhancing the membrane's integrity under most physiological conditions. Increased levels of cholesterol have been implicated in the formation of particular membrane regions known as lipid rafts, which act as platforms for protein sorting and signaling (Zuniga-Hertz & Patel, 2019). Lipid rafts play a role in a wide range of cell processes, including receptor-mediated signaling and endocytosis. In addition, the encounter of cholesterol and phospholipids is central to the formation of caveolae, membrane structures with invaginations that are implicated in signal transduction and cellular responses to mechanical stress or changes in oxygen levels. The assembly of the phospholipid bilayer is thus fundamental not only to structural integrity but also to facilitating refined cellular interactions. Advances in understanding phospholipid bilayer properties have been employed to develop targeted drug delivery systems, particularly for the treatment of diseases like cancer. For instance, temperature-sensitive liposomes encapsulating chemotherapeutic drugs , such as doxorubicin use the properties of phospholipid bilayers to deliver drugs under controlled release at high temperatures (Alawak et al., 2019). The structure of these liposomes may also be changed to enhance targeting, for example, by surface modification that confers special recognition to cancer cells. This provides maximum therapeutic activity of drugs with minimum systemic toxicity, underscoring the importance of the composition of the phospholipid bilayer in therapeutic applications. By understanding the mechanism by which these lipid mixtures function, scientists can create better drug delivery methods, and this shows the dynamic nature of cell membrane physiology and its significance for human health (Figure 2.4).

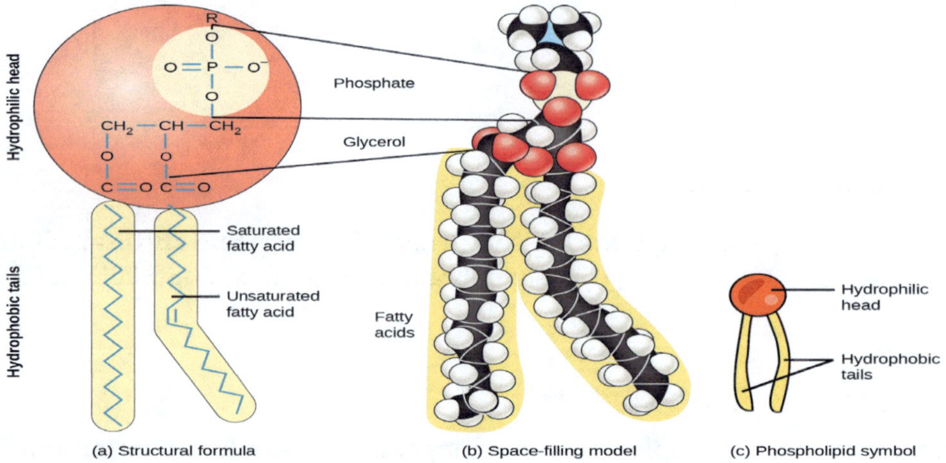

Figure 2.4. Phospholipid-bilayer.

Source: https://microbenotes.com/wp-content/uploads/2022/09/Phospholipid-Bilayer.jpg.

2.1.2. Role of Proteins in Membrane Structure

Proteins play a key role in the structural stability and function of cell membranes, which have significant functions in varied physiological activities. These membrane proteins, which are integrated into the lipid bilayer, have varied functions like transport, signaling, and structural support. These proteins either have the capability of spanning through the membrane multiple times or might be localized on one surface, a characteristic which accounts for the selective permeability of the membrane. While assisting ions and molecules to cross the cell barrier, these proteins not only regulate the osmotic balance of the cells but also participate in intercellular communication.

Their spatial organization within the membrane can not only influence individual cell behavior but also tissue structure as a whole, and hence, membrane proteins play a vital role in cellular homeostasis. The dynamic function of membrane proteins is also evidenced by their involvement in membrane remodeling, e.g., under conditions of cellular stress or during the cell cycle. For instance, DP1 and reticulons are primary proteins of the assembly of the endoplasmic reticulum (ER) that participate in membrane and secretory protein synthesis. Its organization has a direct bearing on its ability to correctly fold proteins and manage intracellular calcium levels necessary for most signaling processes. Maintaining the ER structure by these ER-associated proteins has a direct causal relation to intracellular function, demonstrating how specialized proteins ensure cellular membrane integrity and function. Abnormalities in these proteins have also been found to result in defective cell function and have been linked to numerous diseases, indicative of their physiological role as well. In addition, membrane protein-membrane lipid bilayer interactions are complex and sophisticated since membrane proteins can alter membrane properties and dynamics. For example, in Gram-negative bacteria, the TolC protein is an outer membrane efflux pump that plays a critical role in toxin efflux and in the preservation of membrane integrity upon stress. This multifaceted role of TolC thus not only illustrates the importance of TolC in enterobacterial physiology but also the more general significance of membrane proteins for adaptive cellular responses. Experiments indicate that the phenotypic consequences of tolC mutations are often interdependent, reaffirming that membrane proteins can have effects on a variety of physiological pathways via their interaction with lipid bilayers and other cellular entities. As ongoing studies increasingly unveil the intricacies of membrane protein functions, their essential functions in cellular physiology are becoming more and more increasingly apparent, and their role in disease mechanisms and therapeutic strategies continues to expand (Figure 2.5).

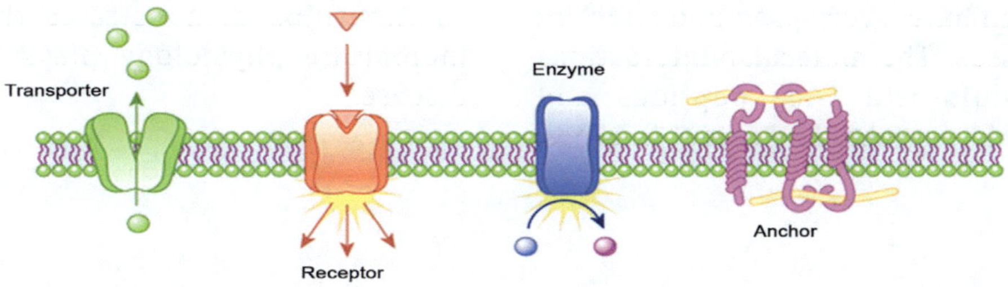

Figure 2.5. Role of proteins in membrane structure.

Source: https://www.nature.com/scitable/content/ne0000/ne0000/ne0000/ne0000/14706234/U3CP1-4_MemProteinFunction_ksm.jpg.

2.1.3. Fluid Mosaic Model Explanation

The fluid mosaic model is a key concept in the study of the structure and function of biological membranes, particularly cellular integrity and communication and transport across the cell membrane. The fluid mosaic model presents the cell membrane as a dynamic and fluid structure composed of a phospholipid bilayer with proteins, cholesterol, and carbohydrates dispersed throughout. The phospholipids are arranged in such a manner that their hydrophilic heads face towards the external aqueous medium and their hydrophobic tails are drawn back inside, creating a semi-permeable membrane. The membrane fluidity is crucial, which enables lateral movement of proteins and lipids, and this opens the way to a heterogeneous distribution of membrane constituents. This fluidity is also important for processes , such as cell signaling, endocytosis, and exocytosis, as it enables the membrane to rapidly reorganize as a reaction to environmental change or as a demand by the cell. One component of the fluid mosaic model is the existence of lipid rafts, which are enriched microdomains within the membrane that facilitate some cellular processes. Here in lipid-ordered areas, with a high concentration of saturated lipids and cholesterol, some proteins aggregate to optimize signaling mechanisms and membrane interactions. Cholesterol distribution has a significant function in the modulation of membrane fluidity and stability, particularly in the functionality of proteins. Furthermore, lipid asymmetry in the bilayer is significant in maintaining both structural integrity and signaling ability. As these lipid microdomains have been associated with disease states, , such as Alzheimer's disease, changes in the lipid composition can have a very profound effect on cellular processes. The molecular interactions between amyloid-beta (Aβ) peptides and membrane lipids, suggested by recent findings, emphasize the intricate relationship between lipid dynamics and pathogenesis, further validating the importance of the fluid mosaic model of cell membrane physiology. Besides its role in structural integrity and signaling, the fluid mosaic model guides our understanding of pathologies related to membranes. Changes in lipid composition, , such as increased cholesterol or altered lipid saturation, could lead to changes in membrane characteristics, favoring diseases like Alzheimer's. The positioning of cholesterol in membrane microdomains has been shown to influence amyloid precursor protein processing and Aβ deposition, events that are central to Alzheimer's pathogenesis. Such interactions are the traditional means by which membrane biophysics changes can trigger or exacerbate disease processes, a demonstration of the model's applicability in the clinic. By exploring the fluid mosaic model, researchers can read the mechanisms behind many diseases and propose potential therapeutic approaches that appeal to membrane dynamics, designing new interventions and treatment strategies in neurological diseases. Mastering these intricate relationships demonstrates the pivotal role membrane physiology plays in health and disease.

Test Your Knowledge

1. What is the fluid mosaic model, and how does it describe the structure and dynamic state of the cell membrane?
2. How is the phospholipid bilayer organized, and why is this type of structure important to membrane fluidity and permeability?

2.2. Functions of the Cell Membrane

Learning Outcome

1. Explain the selective permeability to cell membrane physiology;
2. Define cell membrane communication and signaling;
3. Learn cellular homeostasis transport mechanisms.

The cell membrane serves as a critical interface that divides the interior of the cell from its exterior environment, thus maintaining cellular integrity and homeostasis. Composed largely of a bilayer phospholipid with inserted proteins, the membrane carries out various significant functions. It also acts as a selective barrier, regulating the passage of ions and molecules in and out of the cell, and is necessary to uphold the appropriate internal environment for metabolic processes. Membrane proteins also permit communication with the external milieu so that cells may be informed to generate an array of physiological responses, , such as the secretion of hormones or changes in cell behavior. This cell membrane signaling and chemical exchange potential highlights the importance of the cell membrane in controlling cellular function and responding to stimuli from the environment, marking it as a sophisticated part of cellular physiology (Chowdhury et al., 2017). In addition to its selectively permeable barrier role, the cell membrane is also essential for the processes of endocytosis and exocytosis, routes through which cells ingest substances and expel materials, respectively. Through these processes, the membrane plays an active role in taking in nutrients, removing waste, and recycling membrane proteins, all of which are vital to cellular existence. Of notable interest is the recycling of proteins , such as the Cystic Fibrosis Transmembrane Conductance Regulator (CFTR), which is facilitated through specific molecular pathways that ensure appropriate localization and density of these proteins within the membrane. These are controlled to maintain physiological functions , such as transepithelial anion secretion. Through these pathways, particularly intracellular trafficking proteins like the Rab GTPases, scientists have a better understanding of both healthy physiology and the pathophysiology of numerous illnesses (Silvis et al., 2009). Furthermore, the sensitivity of the cell membrane to and response against mechanical stimulation is crucial for the growth, function, and repair of tissue. Mechanotransduction, the process by which cells convert mechanical stimuli into biochemical responses, is controlled by various receptors that are incorporated into the membrane.

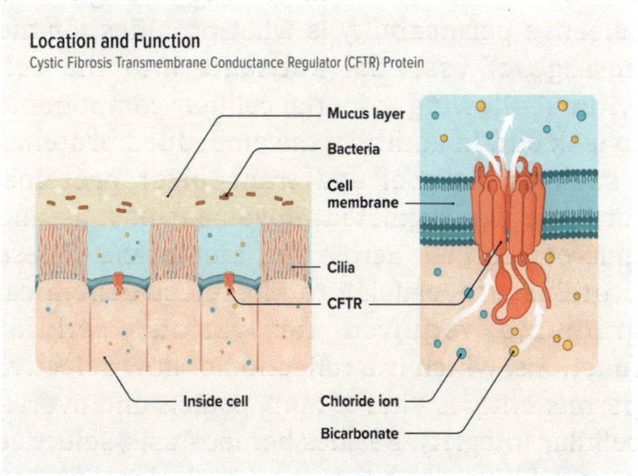

Figure 2.6. Cystic fibrosis transmembrane conductance regulator (CFTR).

Source: https://post.healthline.com/wp-content/uploads/2023/04/2852947-Location-and-Function-of-Cystic-Fibrosis-Transmembrane-Conductance-Regulator-CFTR-Protein-1296x919.png.

The receptors can perceive a change in the stiffness of the extracellular matrix or the imposition of an external force, leading to alterations in cellular behavior. These responses are central to physiological processes like wound repair, where cells have to move and divide based on mechanical stimuli. The intricate interplay between the mechanical properties of the membrane and its biological nature underscores the significance of membrane physiology in health and disease, providing increased insight into cellular movement vital to the development of therapeutic approaches (Chowdhury et al., 2017) (Figure 2.6).

2.2.1. Selective Permeability

Selective permeability is a basic concept in cell membrane physiology, summarizing the capability of membranes to regulate the transport of substances into and out of the cell. This owes primarily to the phospholipid bilayer, which is hydrophobic and rejects polar molecules and ions from passing through. This selective permeability is what provides for the passage of essential nutrients into the cell without allowing essential cellular components to leak out. In addition, the embedded proteins, , such as channel and transporter proteins, facilitate the regulated movement of ions and macromolecules across the membrane. These proteins are crucial to the electrochemical gradients required for various cellular functions, which is a reflection of how selective permeability is vital to homeostasis and overall cellular integrity. Besides homeostasis, selective permeability is also essential in cell signaling and communication. The operation of some pathways heavily relies on the accurate modulation of ion concentrations inside and outside the cell membrane. For instance, extracellular ATP release through Cx43 hemichannels has been linked to intercellular communication and the discovery of how selective permeability influences broader physiological processes. The heightened actin/myosin contractility may counteract the opening of such hemichannels, highlighting a highly developed regulatory mechanism governing cellular signaling pathways. The ability to selectively allow or restrict particular ions or molecules can have a dramatic effect on cellular response, promoting complicated physiological responses and adaptations important for health and disease management. Moreover, implications of selective permeability extend into cellular energy metabolism, particularly involving mitochondrial function. Mitochondria are the key organelles for ATP synthesis, and their selective permeability to calcium ions ($Ca2^{+}$) shows the intricate relationship between membrane dynamics and metabolic function. Uptake of $Ca2^{+}$ into the mitochondria is highly regulated, with an impact on a wide variety of cellular processes, including energy production, signaling pathways, and cell survival. A disturbance of calcium homeostasis—usually by dysregulation of selective permeability—may result in harmful effects like cell death. Understanding these mechanisms not only provides greater insight into cell physiology but also points to the criticality of maintaining selective permeability to avoid pathophysiological conditions, thereby contributing to ongoing research in cellular disease and disease management (Bultynck et al., 2014; Quintana et al., 2017) (Figure 2.7).

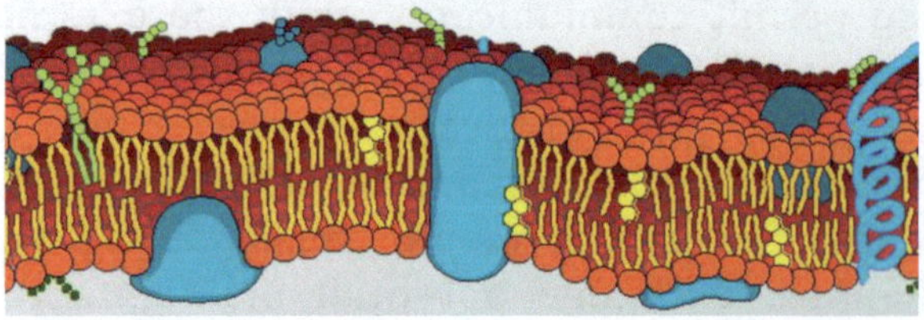

Figure 2.7. Selective permeability.

Source: https://study.com/cimages/videopreview/videopreview-full/humdygb8k3.jpg.

2.2.2. Communication and Signaling

The intricate signaling and communication processes underlie cell membrane function to facilitate crucial interactions among and between cells. Through various mechanisms, cells communicate information to enable timely and appropriate physiological responses. Gap junctions, particularly those made up of proteins called connexins, represent one such dynamic form of intercellular communication. In primary bovine corneal endothelial cells, for instance, the communication is primarily established by the release of extracellular ATP via Cx43 hemichannels. The mechanism is implicated in the propagation of calcium ($Ca2^+$) waves, a crucial component of signaling that coordinates cellular responses to external stimuli and internal changes in tissues. Besides, through regulation of the operation of such channels, researchers are discovering new drugs for diseases linked to abnormal signaling pathways, pointing toward the significance of how the membrane system of communication is comprehended and regulated in a physiological context (Bultynck et al., 2014).

The interpolated structure of the intercellular space lies at the core of mediating communication and signaling pathways. In multicellular systems, organization in space among cells influences their ability for effective communicate biochemical messages effectively. This is observable when looking at how cells communicate to form functional entities and thus gain metabolic self-production as well as self-preservation. The coordination of signaling via the extracellular matrix demonstrates the relevance of spatial organization among cell-cell interactions. In contrast to focusing on cell differentiation or cell dimensions, it becomes increasingly evident that the functional hierarchy of intercellular space is an important factor. Researching these spatial relationships helps scientists uncover how multicellular systems maintain coherence and integrity and reveal the complexities of physiological processes and interactions that underlie cell functions (Bich et al., 2019). With growing complexity in cell signaling pathways, so does the need to research the pathological significance of their dysregulation. Signaling dysregulation can lead to a broad variety of health disorders, including cancer and senescence-like degeneration, which are typically associated with failures of the organizational structure of the intercellular environment. An understanding of how intercellular communication is disrupted illuminates the pathogenesis of such diseases. Considering cell signaling from the organismic perspective highlights the importance of maintaining the integrity of tissue communication networks. Also, novel approaches targeting precise channel functionalities can have the potential to mitigate effects of pathologies resulting from cellular signaling loss of function. Hence, study of the variability of communication and signaling in the field of cell membrane physiology is essential in formulating theoretical comprehension as well as practical innovations in medical research (Bultynck et al., 2014; Bich et al., 2019) (Figure 2.8).

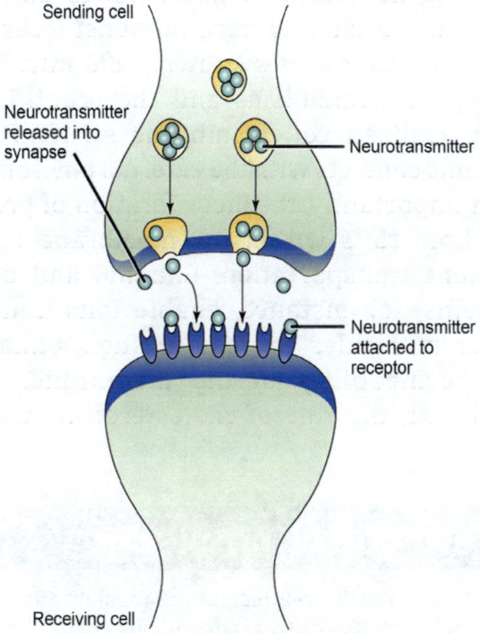

Figure 2.8. Communication and signaling to the functionality of cell membranes.

Source: https://cdn.kastatic.org/ka-perseus-images/a034cb7 d0abe5fce1a8682 a8ba5dd32fe5e1617c.png.

2.2.3. Transport Mechanisms

Transport mechanisms form the foundation of cell membrane physiology and regulation of cellular homeostasis. They are categorized into two broad categories: passive and active transport, and each of them has a distinct function in the cell. Molecules moving against their concentration gradient without the utilization of energy are seen in passive transport, a process that is exhibited by diffusion and facilitated diffusion. Water and small neutral molecules prefer to move through these channels across the lipid bilayer, maintaining the cell's interior environment undisturbed. Active transport, however, requires energy to move materials against the concentration gradient, thereby allowing cells to acquire necessary nutrients or remove waste products. Such processes emphasize the importance of the cell membrane's position as a selective barrier, allowing necessary components to enter the cell while excluding harmful substances from entry. It also involves knowing the intricacy of transport mechanisms and the identification of specialized cell membrane structures for dynamic contacts with the external environment. Most importantly, the incorporation of proteins and lipid rafts within the membrane enables efficient transportation. Channel and carrier proteins, for instance, enable ions and even larger molecules to pass through, enhancing the permeability of the membrane. Apart from that, the role of cholesterol in structure cannot be overstressed as it controls fluidity and stability that are mandatory for the efficient functioning of transport proteins. The discovery of caveolae, which are cholesterol-rich regions of membranes, has also boosted cell signaling and transport knowledge. These areas are involved in regulatory functions when responding to environmental stimuli, meaning membrane architecture has a significant impact on transport mechanisms and cellular response (Zuniga-Hertz & Patel, 2019). Experimental understanding of transport mechanisms contributes to cell membrane physiology. Recent studies have used mathematical modeling and fluorescence techniques to explain the dynamics of ion transport through membranes, providing measurable parameters for permeability and reflection coefficients in different cell types, , such as nephron segments of the kidney (Fushimi et al., 1991). Empirical research has explained the nuances of salt and water transport and the delicate balance maintained within cells under shifting physiological conditions. The understanding of transport processes is thus central to cellular biology as well as critical for biomedicine applications. By explaining how cells regulate the influx and efflux of substances, the work helps to inform advances in therapeutic interventions aimed at fixing dysfunctional transport functions in disease pathology. The study of the mechanisms remains to provide fascinating new information about cellular life and adaptive processes with respect to signals from the environment.

Test Your Knowledge

1. How does the cell membrane regulate the movement of materials into and out of the cell, and what are the major modes of transport employed?
2. How is the cell membrane involved in cell signaling and communication with the external world?

2.3. Transport Mechanisms

Learning Outcome

1. Explain the processes of passive transport;
2. Define the active transport processes;
3. Explain the bulk transport (vesicular transport).

Transport mechanisms are key in the upkeep of cellular homeostasis through facilitating the movement of substances across the cell membrane. Passive and active transport procedures are the general categories of transport mechanisms. Passive transport includes osmosis and diffusion, which allow molecules to move against or in their concentration gradients without utilizing energy. For instance, low-molecular-weight nonpolar molecules like oxygen and carbon dioxide pass freely through the lipid bilayer, important for vital physiological functions , such as respiration. Active transport, however, uses energy, normally in the form of ATP, to move substances against their concentration gradient, thus enabling the cell to control some internal environments to sustain its existence and activity. This dynamic relationship between passive and active processes is indicative of the complexity and effectiveness of cell membrane physiology such that essential molecules are permitted to enter or exit the cell according to necessity. In the field of transport processes, vesicular traffic is an important one, particularly in terms of cellular signaling and material exchange. The small GTPase RAB11 family proteins are key regulators of this process, coordinating the transport of vesicles that contain important cargo , such as hormones, neurotransmitters, and even waste products. Control of RAB11 pathways can have a considerable impact on normal cell physiology since these proteins not only coordinate the delivery of essential molecules but also function in forming autophagic precursors relevant for maintaining cellular health. These alterations can lead to pathological conditions, including cancer, where the ability to properly regulate vesicular transport can determine cell survival and growth. This knowledge of the role of RAB11 in vesicular traffic illustrates how transportation mechanisms are finely integrated with bigger cellular processes and disease states and also how crucial they are in cell membrane physiology research (Bosia et al., 2021). Besides, transport processes are not limited to ionic and molecular movement but also include the organization of the extracellular matrix (ECM), which plays a crucial role in tissue repair and regeneration. For example, dermal wound healing is significantly influenced by collagen alignment and fibroblast function and interaction with the ECM. A multiscale model has been developed to simulate the dynamics of collagen deposition and alignment to account for how fibroblasts transport and reorganize themselves in collagen and fibrin networks. The transport phenomena are then used to predict how alterations in fibroblast velocity or variations in growth factor levels, e.g., TGF-β, can impact the healing process as well as the development of a scar. This link between transport mechanisms and tissue morphogenesis serves to underscore the importance of the research on transport dynamics not only in cellular physiology but also in tissue engineering and regenerative medicine (Maini et al., 2005) (Figure 2.9).

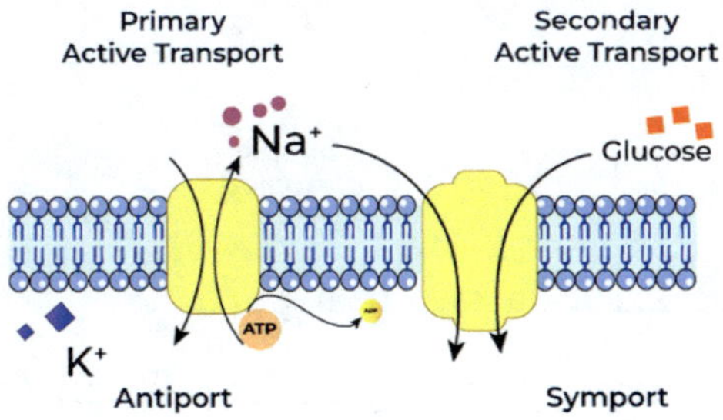

Figure 2.9. Transport mechanisms.

Source: https://media.geeksforgeeks.org/wp-content/uploads/20231231181024/Primary-and-Secondary-Active-transport.png.

2.3.1. Passive Transport Processes

Passive transport processes are very important mechanisms through which substances pass across cellular membranes without the necessity for energy expenditure. This type of transport relies on natural concentration gradients existing across cell membranes; materials will move from areas of greater concentration to areas of lesser concentration. Simple diffusion, facilitated diffusion, and osmosis are included in these processes. Simple diffusion is the movement of small, nonpolar molecules, , such as oxygen or carbon dioxide, directly through the lipid bilayer. On the other hand, facilitated diffusion uses selective transport proteins to allow larger or polar molecules, like glucose or ions, to pass through the membrane. Selective permeability of cell membranes is central to the homeostasis of the cell and constitutes a hallmark demonstration of the significance of passive transport in cell membrane physiology. Osmosis, which is a type of special passive transport, is the movement of water molecules across semi-permeable membranes. Water will move from hypotonic solutions, in which it is higher concentration, into hypertonic solutions, where it is lower concentration, until equilibrium is established. This is important for cell function because the process of managing osmotic pressure affects cell size and shape and, therefore, many physiological processes. For instance, plant cells use osmotic pressure to support turgor and thereby produce structural strength. In cells of animals, the regulation of water movement by osmosis is crucial in maintaining cellular volume and preventing lysis or crenation under fluctuating conditions of the environment. Osmosis dynamics are directly related to the fluid balance in biological systems, and therefore, this conveys the complexity of passive transport processes. The relevance of passive transport extends beyond the confines of simple cell functions and into broader biological situations. For instance, the regulation of ionized potassium in the extracellular space relies on passive transport mechanisms in order to prevent conditions that bring about pathological states , such as neural excitability. Secondly, the novel Kirchoff-Nernst-Planck (KNP) model has significant findings with regard to ion dynamics in astrocytes because it elucidates how spatial potassium buffering operates to provide optimal conditions for neuronal signaling.

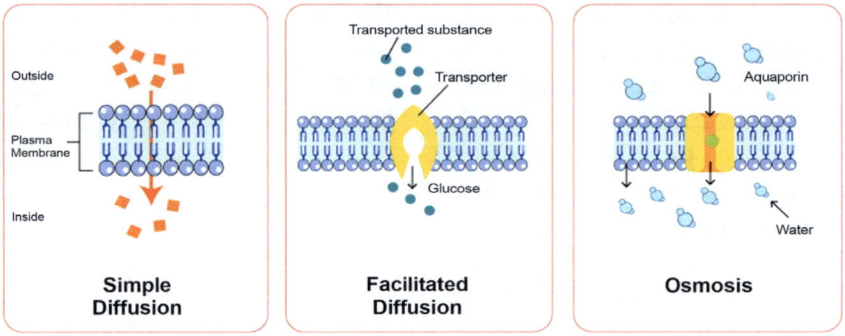

Figure 2.10. Passive transport.

Source: https://media.geeksforgeeks.org/wp-content/uploads/20240103161614/Passive-Transport.png.

The process of passive transport thus not only aids cellular homeostasis but also affects intercellular communication and tissue health in general. Furthermore, understanding the principles of passive transport informs us better about many physiological occurrences in all forms of life, from unicellular organisms to multicellular organisms of even greater complexity like mammals and fungi, as in studies in organismal physiology (Boswell et al., 2017; Destexhe et al., 2019) (Figure 2.10).

2.3.2. Active Transport Processes

Active transport processes are the foundation of cellular physiology because they enable the transport of ions and molecules in opposition to their concentration gradients. This is required for cell homeostasis, for the intake of required nutrients, and for waste substance elimination. Unlike passive transport processes, which rely on diffusion and spontaneous movement of materials from areas of high concentration to low concentration areas, active transport entails energy input, usually in the form of adenosine triphosphate (ATP). This energy investment is critical in mechanisms , such as the sodium-potassium pump, which helps regulate cellular volume and membrane potential, thus highlighting the crucial role of active transport in cellular health and function. Second, the mechanism of active transport differs across different cells or organisms.

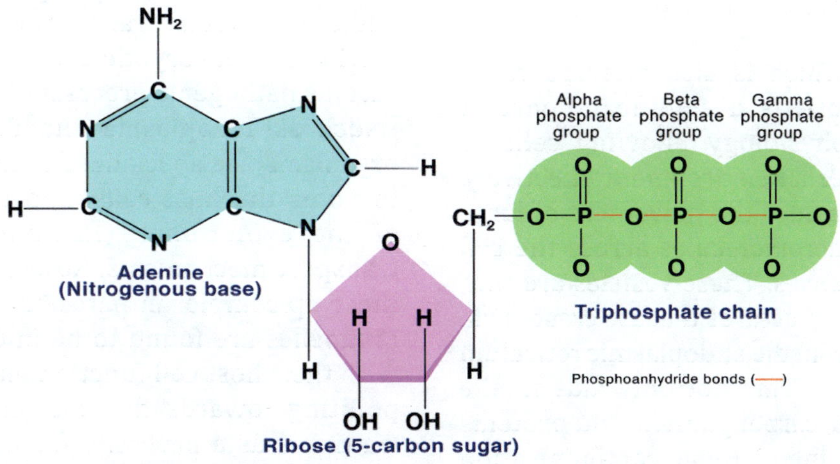

Figure 2.11. Adenosine triphosphate (ATP).

Source: https://www.sciencefacts.net/wp-content/uploads/2021/12/Adenosine-Triphosphate-ATP-Structure.jpg.

Various types of active transport systems have evolved in order to satisfy specific physiological needs, i.e., primary. Primary active transport uses ATP itself to move substances, whereas secondary active transport relies on the electrochemical gradients created by primary transporters. The complexity of the systems is a sign of their versatility to facilitate cells to survive in diverse environments. For example, in bacteria, active transport is essential in the nutrient uptake and protection against harmful substances so that certain species can outcompete others in their environmental niches, as demonstrated by the action of the proton motive force under protonophores' influence. This reflects the worldwide implications of active transport in cellular adaptation and survival processes (Kim et al., 2021). Lastly, regulation of active transport phenomena involves critical importance in various physiological conditions, influencing cellular function as well as greater biological structures." For instance, in the human body, interference with active transport can lead to grave illnesses like diabetes and hypertension. It has been theorized that the normal functioning of active transport contributes to effective healing and repair of tissues and wounds, primarily by controlling the ion balance and cell responses (Maini et al., 2005). Furthermore, knowledge of the processes allows therapeutic intervention approaches to alter active transport systems for enhanced recovery from injury or mitigation of the effects of diseases with characteristics of cellular deregulation. Hence, it is important to research active transport mechanisms both from the aspect of basic biological information and development in clinical applications (Figure 2.11).

2.3.3. Bulk Transport (Vesicular Transport)

Bulk transport, which is also referred to as vesicular transport, is a significant part of cell membrane physiology, allowing cells to regulate their internal environment effectively. Bulk transport includes the movement of large molecules and macromolecules across the cell membrane via vesicles. These vesicles are tiny, membrane-bound structures that are created via budding, usually from the endoplasmic reticulum or Golgi apparatus. This not only aids in the transport of lipids, carbohydrates, and proteins but also helps in intercellular communication and nutrient assimilation. It is the understanding of vesicular transport that is responsible for explaining many cellular functions and can provide insights into pathological conditions in which these functions are disrupted, thereby highlighting its role in the regulation of cellular homeostasis. The Golgi apparatus plays a crucial role in the vesicular transport of lipids and proteins as a processing and sorting plant of the cell. Research work on this organelle has been enhanced significantly, thus clarifying the structure and function in the formation of vesicles and transport. In reaching the Golgi, proteins that have been synthesized in the endoplasmic reticulum undergo glycosylation as well as modification in numerous other aspects, ultimately regulating their destinations in the cell or their expulsion outside the cell. Continued studies of the Golgi have generated controversies over its dynamism and debates of its whole range of functions. For instance, research examining the role of the Golgi apparatus in both normal physiology and disease states, , such as cancer, emphasizes additional studies of its complex processes and functions in the vesicular transport mechanisms (Farquhar et al., 1998). In addition, vesicular transport is not only the sole privilege of eukaryotic cells but is also vital in various pathogenic processes in some parasites, , such as Toxoplasma and Plasmodium. The organisms use specialized secretory organelles to enter the host cells, and this is indicative of the evolutionary flexibility of vesicular transport mechanisms. Research indicates that these apicomplexan parasites' apical secretory organelles are found to be in close correlation with their host cell function manipulation, thus pointing towards the dual character of bulk transport as a necessity for pathogen survival as well as a vital element of host cell biology. Recent research has revealed that such a parasite has optimized its endosomal processes to ensure maximum delivery of proteins that are crucial for its survival, illustrating a remarkable level of synergy between vesicular transport and host-pathogen interactions (Fomovska et al., 2013). Not only does knowledge of the process enhance our understanding of cell membrane physiology, but it also raises implications of therapeutic interventions against these diseases.

Test Your Knowledge

1. What is bulk (vesicular) transport and how does it differ from mechanisms of passive and active transport?
2. Describe the process of endocytosis and distinguish phagocytosis, pinocytosis, and receptor-mediated endocytosis.

2.4. Membrane Potential

Learning Outcome

1. Identify the membrane potential;
2. Define the function of ion channels and pumps;
3. Describe its significance in nerve impulse transmission.

Membrane potential is important to understand if one wants to grasp cell function and communication. The membrane potential is the voltage across a cell's plasma membrane, and the main driving force behind this is the distribution of ions , such as sodium, potassium, and chloride. When a cell is at rest, it will typically have a negative membrane potential of approximately -70 mV due to differential membrane permeability to various ions and the action of ion pumps, specifically the sodium-potassium pump. This resting potential determines a threshold for excitability so that neurons and muscle cells will respond to stimuli. The slight imbalance of ion concentration across the membrane is an electrochemical gradient that drives the passive transport of ions and thereby influences cellular activity , such as neurotransmission, muscle contraction, and overall metabolism. Membrane potential can alter to have significant physiological impacts. For instance, depolarization occurs when the membrane potential becomes less negative, typically triggered by action potentials in neurons. In such circumstances, voltage-gated sodium channels are opened, allowing sodium ions to flood the cell and cause an action potential. This abrupt change in membrane potential is responsible for the transmission of the nerve impulse and muscle contraction. Repolarization to recharge the membrane potential comes after depolarization through the opening of potassium channels, allowing potassium ions to leave the cell. This dynamic interplay between repolarization and depolarization is essential to the conduction of electrical impulses and is an important component of cellular communication. As such, understanding the nuances of membrane potential dynamics is important for comprehending many physiological and pathologic states. The physiological significance of membrane potential escalates from individual cells to entire biological systems, influencing the secretion of hormones and the release of neurotransmitters, among others. Membrane potential is not static, but dynamic, and responds to stimulation by changing, which allows cells to initiate varied responses. And neither should the role of lipid composition in the membrane be ruled out, as some lipids possess biophysical properties that affect membrane curvature and potential.

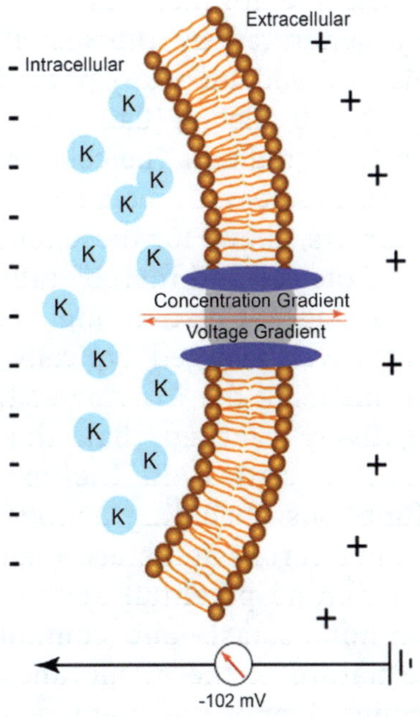

Figure 2.12. Membrane potential.

Source: https://ars.els-cdn.com/content/image/3-s2.0-B9780121486600500068-f05-03-9780121486600.jpg.

Experiments illustrate that the characteristics of some lipid subclasses, , such as cardiolipin in mitochondrial membranes, have the potential to influence overall cellular function and health, pointing to a complex relationship between cell physiology and membrane potential deserving of examination. Better understanding of these interactions will enhance our current knowledge of cellular dysfunction in diseases, highlighting the importance of investigating membrane potential within the broader subject area of cell membrane physiology (Maini et al., 2005; Budin et al., 2024) (Figure 2.12).

2.4.1. Definition of Membrane Potential

The membrane potential theory is key to understanding the physiology of cells because it describes the electrical potential difference across a cell membrane. This potential is principally generated by the distribution of ions, in this case, sodium (Na+), potassium (K+), chloride (Cl-), and calcium (Ca2+), which create a concentration gradient. The cell membrane's selective permeability, facilitated by ion channels and transporters, allows for these ions to move in and out of the cell and thereby influence the membrane voltage. At rest, normal mammalian cells are negatively charged, typically at a level of -70 mV, meaning the interior of the cell is more negatively charged than the outside. Polarization is critical in the majority of cellular functions, including action potential generation in neurons and muscle contraction, putting membrane potential at the forefront of cellular homeostasis and communication. The labile nature of the membrane potential is also accounted for by the interaction between active and passive transport processes, which maintain ionic gradients that are essential for cellular function. The sodium-potassium pump (Na+/K+ ATPase) is a primary contributor by actively transporting three sodium ions out of the cell and two potassium ions into the cell, thus contributing to the negative intracellular environment. As ions migrate based on their chemical gradients, they trigger electrical changes that mirror the physiological state. For epithelial cells, research has established how pump-leak models can beautifully explain ion and water balance through cell membranes, thus controlling cell volume and ionic composition under various physiological states (Mori et al., 2011). This equilibrium between membrane potentials and ionic flows is the foundation of understanding complex physiological processes. Embrane potential is not an unchanging property but a vital parameter that responds to various cellular stimuli. Membrane depolarization or hyperpolarization can be caused by changes in stimulation, thus influencing excitability and signal transmission in excitable tissues. The synergy of osmotic and electrodiffusion processes demonstrates the manner in which cellular milieus modulate membrane potential fluctuations. Existing models have enlightened the energy dynamics of such processes and how entropic, elastic, and electrostatic forces collaborate to influence membrane behavior (Eisenberg et al., 2011). Therefore, an understanding of membrane potential involves inherent concepts of ion transport, electrical signaling, and cellular homeostasis, which serve to be a cornerstone for studying the physiology of the cell membrane and its applications to overall biological systems.

2.4.2. Role of Ion Channels and Pumps

Another important part of cell membrane physiology is the role played by ion channels and pumps in cellular homeostasis and intercellular communications. Ion channels are transmembrane proteins that form pores for selective ion movement, , such as sodium, potassium, calcium, and chloride. They are often voltage-gated, ligand-gated, or mechanically gated, causing the cell to react to stimuli of any sort. For instance, transmission at the neuronal level relies on the efflux and influx of sodium and potassium ions through voltage-gated channels to create action potentials used in the transmission of signals along nerves. Regulation of these channels directly influences neuronal excitability and synaptic transmission and illustrates their versatility in processes ranging from muscle contraction, hormone release, and sensation. In contrast to ion channels, ion pumps actively move ions across the membrane against their concentration gradient and utilize energy derived from the hydrolysis of ATP. The sodium-potassium pump (Na+/K+ ATPase) is one of the most well-characterized ion pumps and is responsible for maintaining the electrochemical gradient across the plasma membrane. Through the expulsion of three sodium ions in exchange for two potassium ions, this pump sustains the negative resting membrane potential required for cell function. Such interference can lead to cell dysfunction and has been implicated in various pathologies, from neurodegenerative diseases and cardiac arrhythmias to cancer. Information about the influence of these pumps on ion homeostasis not only provides insight into fundamental physiology but also indicates where therapeutic targets for the treatment of associated diseases might be located. In addition, the coordination between ion channels and pumps regulates the overall ionic cellular environment, which influences intracellular signaling pathways. Dendritic spines, however, are small bumps on neurons responsible for synaptic plasticity and transmission. Modern mathematical models have shown us that the volume and shape of these spines can help control calcium dynamics necessary for neurotransmitter release (Bartol et al., 2019). The models suggest that the volume-to-surface area ratio of dendritic spines dictates the efficiency of ion channels and pumps in controlling calcium influx and efflux. Accordingly, the physical anatomy of a spine can impose a gigantic impact on synaptic activity, vindicating the fact that ion pumps and channels are crucial in fine-tuning cellular processes accountable for cognition and the encoding of memories (Figure 2.13).

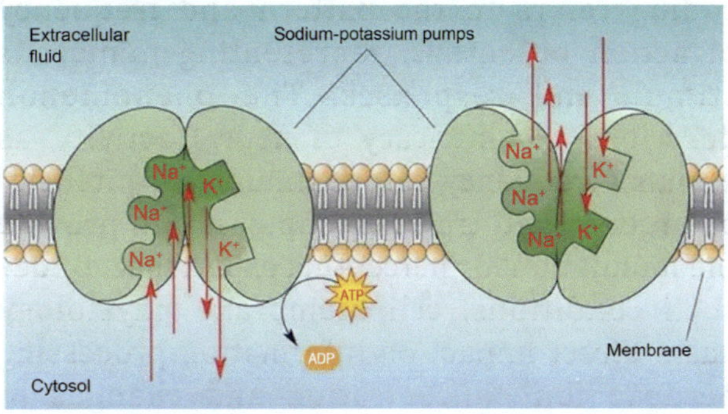

Figure 2.13. Difference between ion channels and ion pumps.

Source: https://qph.cf2.quoracdn.net/main-qimg-fe96d0faa1523ac2d870b72e73020db8.webp.

2.4.3. Importance in Nerve Impulse Transmission

The transmission of nerve impulses is a fundamental process that enables communication in the nervous system, as it enables the transmission of signals rapidly over relatively long distances. At the center of the transmission process is the cell membrane, and it functions as a selective barrier indispensable for the maintenance of electrochemical gradients behind action potentials. When the nerve impulse occurs, it is triggered by a stimulus that opens up the sodium channels of the neuron's membrane and hence leads to depolarization. The movement of sodium ions results in an action potential, which propagates along the axon through a series of membrane repolarization and depolarization. The role of the cell membrane in carrying out the transition is essential, as it offers an immediate and efficient pathway for the nerve impulses necessary for prompt physiological responses. Additionally, the transmission of nerve impulses is not a mere communication issue; it constitutes the root of all thought processes and physiological responses. The ability of neurons to encode and convey information comes about through the process of impulse transmission. Neural coding refers to the pattern and frequency of action potentials, representing numerous stimuli and responses. The phenomenon describes the intricacy of neural activity, as impulse frequency can communicate intensity or urgency and trains of impulses can provide the foundation for perceptual experience. Under such conditions, cell membrane physiology has a direct impact on information processing because ion concentration and changes in membrane potential regulate the rhythms of firing of neurons. This complicated mechanism highlights the necessity of understanding cell membrane dynamics in the context of overall neural function and cognition. Moreover, the impact of deranged nerve impulse transmission is widespread, with both motor and sensory functions being involved. Disruptions in the ion channels, and therefore the integrity and function of the cell membrane, can lead to a variety of neurological diseases. For instance, conditions , such as multiple sclerosis are characterized by demyelination of myelin sheaths, which insulate axons and facilitate the rapid transmission of impulses. This leads to an abrupt decline in velocity and efficiency of nerve impulses, which is manifested in terms of motor deficit and sensory perversion. Appreciation of nerve impulse transmission mechanisms not only sheds light on normal physiology but also emphasizes possible therapeutic avenues to treat numerous neurological diseases. The intersection of cell membrane physiology and nervous signal integrity reveals the delicate balance required for normal neural function and overall organismal wellness (Bullock & Perkel, 1968; Mohamed et al., 2011).

Test Your Knowledge

1. What is the membrane potential and how is it generated across the plasma membrane of a cell?
2. How do the sodium-potassium pump and ion channels allow the resting membrane potential?

2.5. Cell Membrane and Homeostasis

Learning Outcome

1. Explain the regulation of internal environment;
2. Define the role in the uptake of nutrients and the removal of waste;
3. Explain the effect on cellular metabolism.

The structure and function of the cell membrane are of most significance in maintaining homeostasis in cellular environments. Composed of a bilayer of phospholipids embedded with proteins, the membrane is a selective barrier that manages the movement of materials in and out of the cell to maintain internal stability. In addition to cellular integrity protection, selective permeability also allows for the efficient transport of required ions and molecules. Homeostasis relies on various processes, , such as passive transport, facilitated diffusion, and active transport, through which cells can regulate nutrient intake and waste elimination effectively. The intricate relationship between these transport mechanisms emphasizes the importance of the structure of cell membranes in ensuring life processes, hence a unifying theme for cellular physiology knowledge. Moreover, homeostasis also involves the process of ion transport across the cell membrane, an important aspect being the transport of calcium ions (Ca2+). Toxicity may arise due to excess Ca2+, and therefore, regulation is necessary for cell health. Na+/Ca2+ exchanger and plasma membrane Ca2+-ATPase are a few specialized proteins that play pivotal roles in maintaining intracellular Ca2+ levels, particularly in sensitive cells like lens epithelial cells. The Na+/Ca2+ exchanger actively expels Ca2+ in exchange for sodium ions, which maintains an inward-directed gradient that needs to be carefully regulated to prevent Ca2+ overloading. This delicate balance is necessary for optimal cellular function and reflects the important interdependence between membrane transport processes and cellular homeostasis, emphasizing the sophisticated level of cellular regulation. In addition, the consequences of disturbed ion homeostasis on cellular function can be spectacular. For instance, protein depletion like LETM1, which regulates mitochondrial K+/H+ exchange, upsets monovalent cation homeostasis and prevents regular Ca2+ flows and induces cellular malfunction (Mattarei et al., 2017). Regular calcium signaling is necessary for several cellular processes, including the contraction of muscle, the release of neurotransmitters, and cell survival pathways. Ca2+ interference can trigger pathological consequences , such as cell death or disease progression, as discovered in diseases , such as cataracts, where deregulation of Ca2+ is the cause of opacification of the lens (Rhodes et al., 2008). Therefore, the discovery of the role of the cell membrane in the transport and ion homeostasis is important not just for its biological relevance but also for possible therapeutic remedies against many diseases related to improper cellular regulation (Figure 2.14).

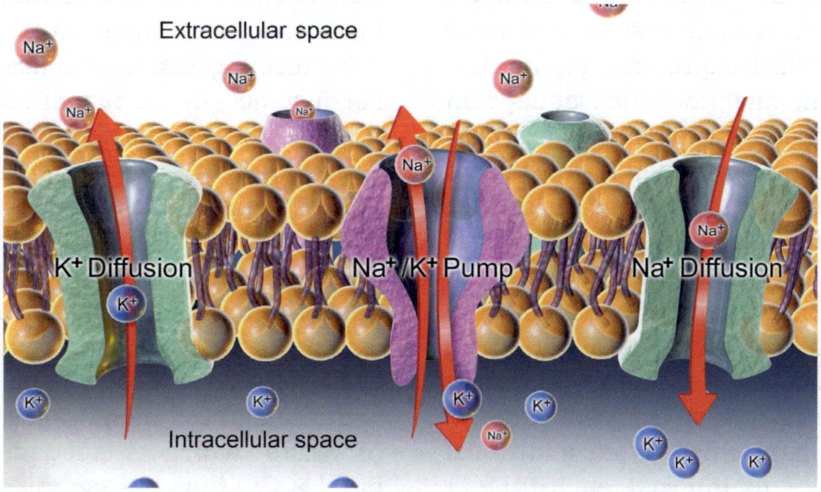

Figure 2.14. Cells maintain homeostasis.

Source: https://biologydictionary.net/wp-content/uploads/2018/04/Sodium-potassium-pump-and-diffusion.jpg.

2.5.1. Regulation of Internal Environment

Regulation of a cell's internal environment is core to maintaining homeostasis, a state vital to the existence and operation of the cell. At the core of this, the cell membrane has a selective permeability that facilitates controlled exchange of ions, nutrients, and waste products. This selective permeation is, to a large extent, facilitated by membrane proteins that can function as transporters or channels to route the movement of substances based on the individual needs of the cell. For instance, the concentration of required ions , such as potassium and sodium must be tightly regulated to maintain electrochemical gradients required for cellular metabolism and signaling. Thus, each failure in these control systems can have detrimental effects on cell functionality, underscoring the cell membrane's essential role in ensuring that the internal environment remains optimally balanced and functional for cellular functions. In plants, the activity of aquaporins, a particular family of membrane proteins, illustrates the complex regulatory mechanism that preserves internal environment equilibrium. Aquaporins facilitate the passive movement of water and small solutes across the cell membrane and thus have a direct impact on water homeostasis and nutrient acquisition. It has been demonstrated that aquaporin expression, e.g., HvPIP2;1, is controlled to counteract stressful environments like salinity, which causes down-regulation to prevent cellular dehydration and damage. Higher CO2 conductance and assimilation rates in transgenic HvPIP2;1-expressing plants also demonstrate the manner in which aquaporin regulation supports not just cellular homeostasis but also plant productivity under various stress conditions. It demonstrates the need for further studies on aquaporin functions to promote stress tolerance as well as productivity, reaffirming in turn the vital relationship between cell membrane physiology and environmental acclimation. In addition, the introduction of mimetic compounds for major nutrients, , such as phosphite in the case of phosphate, imposes an additional layer of complexity to internal environment regulation. Phosphite affects plant physiological responses by disturbing the typical homeostasis of phosphate, a central molecule that participates in energy transfer and cellular communication. Experiments have shown that the phosphite-treated plants failed to react to phosphate starvation as would be anticipated, illustrating a picture of intricate interaction between different regulatory mechanisms within the cell. Alteration of the pools of metabolites induced by phosphite treatment, particularly amino acids like glutamate and aspartate, illustrates how stress signals might alter internal conditions and potential resistance to pathogens. These facts point to the importance of understanding how different substances can influence internal regulation, thus lending power to the common understanding of cell membrane physiology and its use in maintaining the internal environment in various biological systems.

2.5.2. Role in Nutrient Uptake and Waste Removal

The role of the cell membrane in the uptake of nutrients and the excretion of waste plays a critical role in cellular function and well-being. It is a discriminatory barrier that controls the passage of ions, nutrients, and waste products in and out of the cell to maintain homeostasis. The primary process of nutrient influx is by processes , such as facilitated diffusion and active transport, in which individual proteins in the membrane offer channels for the movement of substances against their concentration gradients. For instance, in the fungal cells, the membrane proteins are pivotal to nutrient transport and assimilation, an important aspect for biomass increase and growth, as outlined in Boswell et al. (2017). The lack of the complex architecture would hinder cells from gaining essential nutrients for metabolism and energy production, leading to compromised cellular activities and eventually to cell death. Of no lesser importance is the role of cell membranes in the elimination of waste, which is needed to prevent toxic build-up within the cytoplasm. Cells utilize a variety of mechanisms for transport, including exocytosis, to eliminate waste material, thus regulating the optimum internal conditions. This role is especially relevant in organisms , such as Escherichia coli, where differential partitioning of organic acids during metabolic activity facilitates efficient removal of waste. For example, research has shown that electrodialysis enhances organic acid recovery, which not only aids the removal of waste but also recycles these products for future metabolic activities, e.g., biohydrogen production, as stated in Majewski et al. (2011). Such transport processes under control emphasize the role of the cell membrane in establishing the delicate balance between nutrient uptake and waste expulsion. The physiological functions of the cell membrane in the excretion of waste and uptake of nutrients are significant across all organisms. Multicellular organisms possess specialized cells to demonstrate the synergistic function of the membranes in the absorption of nutrients and the excretion of waste. Intestinal epithelial cells employ microvilli to enhance the surface area to ensure the effective uptake of nutrients to supply the organism with vitamins and minerals. Alternatively, in fungi, membrane dynamics are pivotal in vegetative growth, where nutrients are transported into cells and maintain anabolic processes and help with growth and reproduction, as illustrated in Boswell et al. (2017). This double role of cell membranes in nutrient uptake and waste removal testifies to the complexity of cellular physiology as well as to the potential significance for cell function in health and disease, and indicates the necessity for extended research in these important fields (Figure 2.15).

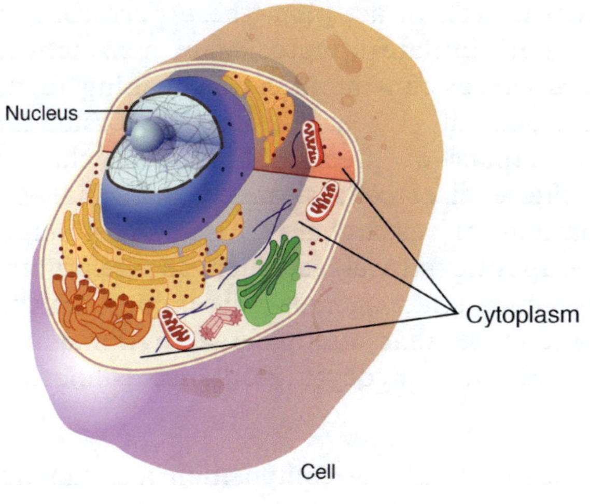

Figure 2.15. Cytoplasm.

Source: https://www.genome.gov/sites/default/files/tg/en/illustration/cytoplasm.jpg.

2.5.3. Impact on Cellular Metabolism

The role of cellular membrane physiology in influencing metabolism is well rooted in the ability of cells to react to environmental changes and to preserve homeostasis. Central to this interaction is the role of cholesterol in cellular membranes, which has evolved to regulate the diffusion of molecules, most importantly oxygen. The presence of cholesterol makes possible the formation of specialized membrane domains known as caveolae, which play a critical role as signaling centers. These adaptations play a significant role in controlling cellular responses to varying oxygen levels, especially during hypoxia. By controlling the diffusion of oxygen, caveolae enhance cellular respiration and, hence, optimize energy production and overall metabolic efficiency. The presence of these adaptations in membranes underscores the importance of cellular structures in ensuring metabolic processes. This intricate interaction bears witness to the significance of membrane composition in the evolution of oxidative management and energy metabolism (Zuniga-Hertz & Patel, 2019). The cell-metabolism interaction is even more intricate when the environment is heart failure, where the integrity of the membrane is modified to have a direct impact on metabolic function. Heart failure involves extensive remodeling, dysfunction, and stress caused by hundreds of external stimuli , such as drug therapies. Specifically, cardiotoxic agents like doxorubicin significantly compromise mitochondrial function and alter cellular energy metabolism. For instance, these agents elicit alterations in oxidative phosphorylation and glycolysis, which are essential pathways for ATP production. These alterations in the metabolic processes may lead to contractile dysfunction and increased cell apoptosis, ultimately exacerbating symptoms of heart failure. Understandings of the drug effects provide hints at possible therapeutic interventions, with particular emphasis on having regard for cellular membrane physiology in developing ways to oppose drug-induced metabolic perturbation (Ganeshan, 2019). In addition, current research indicates that the protective agents, , such as melatonin, reverse harmful metabolic consequences induced by cardiotoxic drugs by normalizing cellular signaling processes. Melatonin has been found to restore mitochondrial function and control primary metabolic genes that govern cell energy processes. Its administration in cardiomyocyte models shows promise in reversing doxorubicin-induced oxidative stress-related alterations and drug-caused apoptosis. Through restoration of homeostasis in metabolic signaling cascades, melatonin enhances cardiac cells' stress resistance, thereby illustrating the interaction between cellular membranes, metabolic health, and disease remission. This highlights an important area of research, with emphasis placed on the importance of the fact that interventions in pathways involving the membrane may prove highly therapeutic in the treatment of metabolic derangement of heart failure as well as other cardiopathies. This interaction places particular importance on the maintenance of membrane function and integrity in the facilitation of best cellular metabolism (Ganeshan, 2019).

Test Your Knowledge

1. How does the cell membrane regulate the cell's internal environment to attain homeostasis regardless of external changes?
2. What is the role of selective permeability of the cell membrane in regulating ion and nutrient balance?

2.6. Pathological Conditions Related to Cell Membrane

Learning Outcome

1. Describe the membrane disorder in disease;
2. Define the toxin action on membrane integrity;
3. Describe the role of the membrane in drug delivery systems.

Cell membrane integrity and function are vital to cellular homeostasis, and any impairment can be the cause of pathological conditions, particularly in cardiac physiology. Heart failure (HF) is a classic example of a complex interaction of malfunctioning cellular mechanisms initiated by an alteration of cell membrane dynamics. As cardiomyocytes undergo structural and electrical remodeling, they are made more susceptible to stress. Different research works have depicted that cardiotoxic substances like doxorubicin (DOX) induce colossal mitochondrial dysfunction by modifying energetic pathways important for maintenance of membrane potential and cell survival. In addition, these perturbations not only initiate apoptosis but also activate gene expression modification leading to the development of heart disease. Understanding the impact of these pathological changes at the level of cellular membranes makes it possible for researchers to examine potential therapeutic strategies, such as melatonin's protective effect against drug-induced cardiac malfunction that minimizes arrhythmias and fosters cardiomyocyte resilience (Ganeshan, 2019).

Cell membrane composition and function are also essential in other pathologies, such as vascular disease in hypertension and obesity. A key component of this process is the uncoupling protein 2 (UCP2), which is found in the inner mitochondrial membrane and is engaged in the regulation of oxidative stress and bioenergetics of mitochondria. Regulation of UCP2 has significant implications for the prevention of vascular damage; downregulation of UCP2 has been established to be a factor leading to development of atherosclerosis and complications of hypertension. Experiments indicate UCP2 deficiency involvement in atherosclerotic lesion development, reaffirming its protective nature in cellular and systemic contexts. This association highlights the cell membrane's function as an action site as well as that of a functional barrier, suggesting targeting UCP2 may offer new therapeutic options against cellular dysfunction in a variety of vascular pathologies (Pierelli et al., 2017). Moreover, it is of significance to identify cell membrane dysfunction and disease progression in designing successful treatments. Therapeutic agents and natural compounds that upregulate UCP2 are capable of averting the effects of hypertensive organ damage. By enhancing UCP2 expression, therapeutic agents are capable of improving endothelial function and fighting oxidative stress, hence acting as a protective mechanism for vascular complications. These findings illustrate the importance of cell membrane integrity and reveal potential therapeutic paths for diseases like hypertension and diabetes. As research continues to define the intricate relationships between cell membrane physiology, pathology, and therapeutic targets, we are in a better place to concoct treatments that not only alleviate symptoms but also address cellular dysfunctions underlying the diseases (Pierelli et al., 2017) (Figure 2.16).

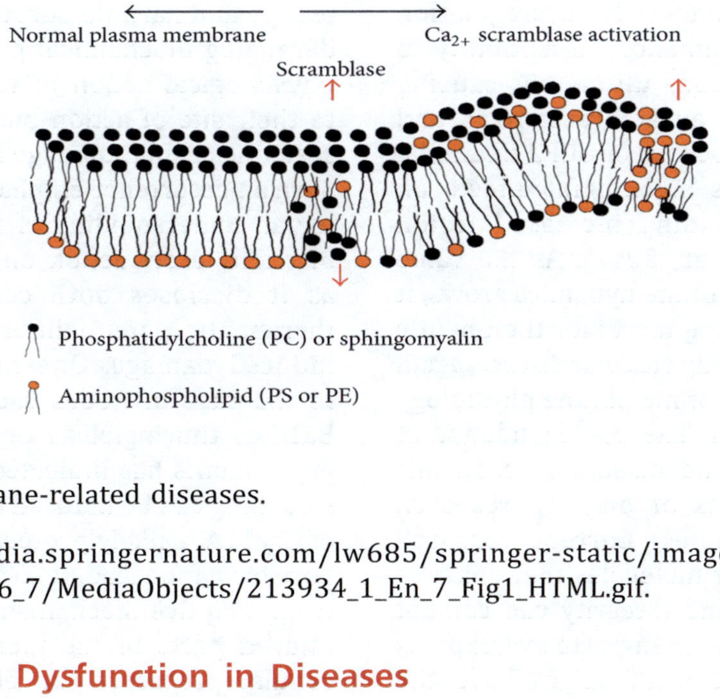

Figure 2.16. Membrane-related diseases.

Source: https://media.springernature.com/lw685/springer-static/image/chp%3A10.1007%2F978-3-642-16105-6_7/MediaObjects/213934_1_En_7_Fig1_HTML.gif.

2.6.1. Membrane Dysfunction in Diseases

Cellular membrane structure and functioning are responsible for maintaining homeostasis in cells. Dysfunction of the membranes typically presents itself as cause or consequence of a multitude of diseases, and most commonly in the cardiovascular and metabolic fields. Oxidative stress typically results in dysfunction of the membranes, degrading lipid moieties such that pathways of signal transmission and cell communication are compromised. For instance, in heart failure, the altered membrane dynamics disrupt the electrical and mechanical properties of cardiac cells, resulting in arrhythmias and contractile dysfunction. Coupling mitochondrial dysfunction, commonly induced by drugs , such as doxorubicin, enhances these complications by heightening oxidative stress and triggering apoptosis of cardiomyocytes, reflecting a complex interplay between drug interactions and membrane health (Ganeshan, 2019). Comprehension of these mechanisms is of great importance in designing therapeutic approaches with the aim of maintaining or restoring membrane integrity in disease situations. Furthermore, studies identify the contribution of membrane-associated proteins in disease conditions. A case in point is UCP2, which plays a critical role in mitochondrial function and regulation of membrane potential. UCP2 has protective effects against oxidative stress and is involved in several vascular disorders that are associated with obesity and diabetes. Its dysregulation has the potential to enhance susceptibility to endothelial dysfunction, ultimately causing complications , such as atherosclerosis and hypertension. The knockout of UCP2 in animal models demonstrates meaningful effects on vascular health, including increased lesion formation (Pierelli et al., 2017). As the value of UCP2's role in membrane dynamics grows, it emerges as a compelling target for therapeutic interventions for relieving vascular disease, again highlighting the value of membrane physiology to disease and health. The co-dependence of membrane function and disease mechanisms underlines the merits of ongoing research into potential therapies. Current research aims to elucidate how molecules that enhance membrane function and integrity can combat disease. As an example, attempts to overexpress defense proteins like UCP2 might have the double benefit of augmenting mitochondrial function while at the same time safeguarding membranes against oxidative destruction. This set of questions is extremely relevant in the context of drug-induced toxicity, where the drugs like doxorubicin cause cellular damage through compromised membrane integrity (Ganeshan, 2019). Ultimately, knowledge of the multifaceted roles of membrane dysfunction in the onset of disease can inform novel treatment paradigms, resulting in novel solutions with the aim of addressing membrane-associated deficits in various diseases.

2.6.2. Effects of Toxins on Membrane Integrity

Cell membrane integrity is essential in maintaining homeostasis of the cell. Toxins can eliminate this equilibrium by compromising membrane integrity, and thereby cellular function and survival. For instance, certain toxins can disrupt the lipid bilayer, making the membrane permeable and ultimately result in cell lysis. Once the membrane is compromised, essential ions and molecules escape and harmful substances penetrate, thus deranging biochemical processes. Notably, the physiological action of toxins is not confined to their site of action but, instead, can extend systemic cellular damage throughout the tissue. Such an occurrence emphasizes the requirement for an understanding of how different classes of toxins exert action on membrane integrity, as it discloses both cellular response and therapeutic potentialities for reversing toxin-induced damage. One important instance is in the case of Aedes cadherin and the toxin Bacillus thuringiensis Cry11A. Evidence from experiments has indicated that cell membrane sloughing can be induced by low concentrations of Cry11A, a likely protective response to toxin pore formation leading to cell damage. Sloughing is an adaptive mechanism by which cells shed injured parts of the membrane so that vital cellular processes can be continued. Besides that, the cry toxins can also bind to receptors within cells and hence possess specific cellular responses. For the Aedes mosquito, localized AaeCad in certain midgut areas allows localized action in the event of exposure to Cry toxins, showing the delicate interaction between toxin-receptor affinity and membrane stability without exerting extensive cytotoxicity (Aimanova et al., 2020). Studies of the biochemistry of toxin-disrupted biochemical pathways have enhanced our understanding of membrane dynamics under the influence of toxins. Disruption of mitochondrial membrane potential can trigger a cascade of cellular events toward cell death as in the case of agents causing damage to respiration. Such findings are essential to the understanding of the overall consequences of toxin exposure to cellular metabolism and lifespan. Also, in recent years, progress in mitophagy modulator chemistry has given new prospects for exploration of cellular response regulation mechanisms to toxin-induced membrane injury. Through the study of interaction between protective repair processes and irreversible damage, researchers are then able to extend their knowledge about cellular responses induced by toxic environments and thus develop the tools for potential therapeutic interventions aimed at preserving membrane integrity (Brunet et al., 2017) (Figure 2.17).

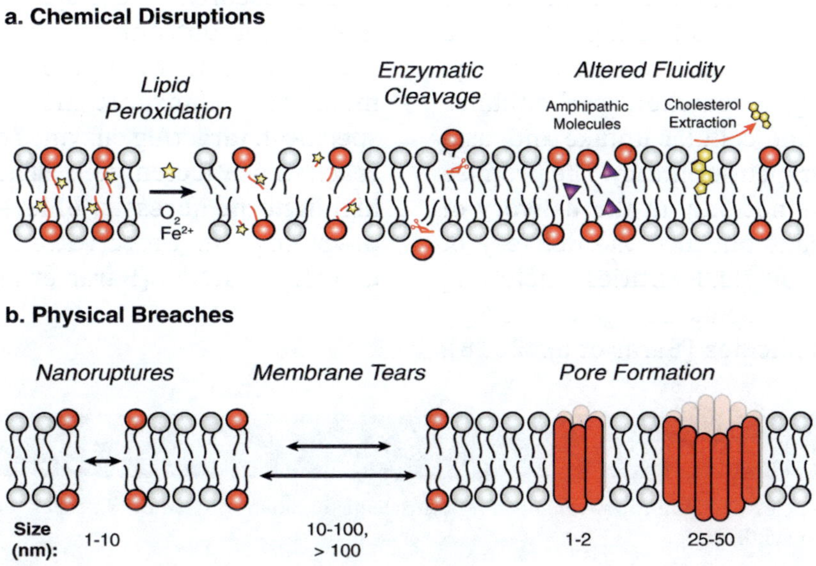

Figure 2.17. Plasma membrane integrity: implications for health and disease.

Source: https://media.springernature.com/lw1200/springer-static/image/art%3A10.1186%2Fs12915-021-00972-y/MediaObjects/12915_2021_972_Fig1_HTML.png.

2.6.3. Role of Membrane in Drug Delivery Systems

The cell membrane plays a critical role in drug delivery systems as it is a selective barrier that controls the access of therapeutic entities to cells. By doing this, it ensures effective targeting of drugs so that they reach the point of desired location and not have unwanted side effects systemically. For effective drug delivery, there has been exploitation of membrane dynamics, e.g., receptor-mediated endocytosis. For instance, transferrin, a serum glycoprotein, utilizes its receptor on the proliferating cell to facilitate the internalization of iron, which has been rediverted for application as a drug carrier. By conjugating drugs or other therapeutic compounds to transferrin or anti-transferrin receptor antibodies, scientists can enhance cell entry, making it an intriguing method in the creation of new drug delivery systems, as indicated in studies of membrane facilitation by such targeting mechanisms (Akiyama et al., 1994). Furthermore, enhancements to drug delivery systems often involve the creation of nanoparticles or vesicles that are designed to mimic natural cellular structures. Such drug carriers, such as liposomes or micelles, are designed to encapsulate drugs and protect them from degradation during transportation to the target location. The interaction between these drug carriers and the cell membrane also plays a very critical role; it controls the kinetics of release of loaded drugs. By adjusting the surface properties of these drug carriers, such as charge and hydrophobicity, researchers can enhance membrane fusion and cellular uptake and, as a result, improve therapeutic efficacy. The promise of these systems is not only in the delivery of small-molecule drugs but also the delivery of the more bulky biological entities, including proteins and nucleic acids, for gene therapy and customized medicines (Barar et al., 2018).

There remains the challenge of drug delivery system developments regarding biodistribution and cellular uptake of therapeutic materials, particularly where complex diseases like lysosomal storage disorders are involved. The limitations of conventional enzyme replacement therapy underscore the need for new delivery modalities. The majority of conventional therapies are hampered by difficulties , such as immunogenic responses and limited penetration into target tissues, e.g., the central nervous system. To overcome these difficulties, the development of targeted enzyme delivery systems (EDSs) has become paramount in recent research. These systems aim to enhance therapeutic outcomes with reduced unwanted side effects through the process of making membrane transport mechanisms extremely specific in targeting enzymes or drugs to directly reach the affected cells. These developments highlight the necessity of leveraging membrane physiology in the creation of effective drug delivery systems (Barar et al., 2018).

Test Your Knowledge

1. What can deficiencies of membrane transport proteins lead to cause to develop diseases , such as cystic fibrosis or Liddle syndrome?
2. What are the consequences of impaired membrane integrity by oxidative stress or lipid peroxidation in neurodegenerative disorders?

SUMMARY

Physiological processes of cell membranes are closely interwoven with varied cellular activities, varying from volume regulation to signal transduction. The delicate equilibrium of such membranes facilitates the required ion exchanges favorable to homeostasis. For instance, research in Amphiuma red blood cells has demonstrated that they have the ability to perform regulatory volume decrease (RVD) and regulatory volume increase (RVI), wherein the membranes dynamic responses to osmotic stress are manifested. These processes involve active transport of ions like K+ and Cl-, highlighting the electroneutral function of such channels in volume regulation, as evidenced by findings suggesting the significance of Na/H and K/H exchange mechanisms towards maintaining cellular integrity (Cala et al., 1983). Such understanding helps to propound the significance of ion channels and transporters in supporting cellular physiology through a complex interplay between cellular responses to environmental stimuli. Furthermore, the role of signaling molecules, such as vasopressin, cannot be underestimated in membrane physiology. Vasopressin enables osmotic water permeability to be controlled by regulating the trafficking of water channels in cell membranes. Studies have shown that vasopressin-stimulated endosomal vesicles have a very high water permeability compared to other biological membranes, which emphasizes their crucial role in cellular hydration dynamics (Shi et al., 1990). The activation of protein kinase cascades is another illustration of the capacity of signaling cascades to modulate membrane function in accord with the physiological needs of the organism. The knowledge of these interactions not only provides insight into cellular homeostasis but also presents us with a very important clue for potential targets of therapy for water balance disease and membrane dysfunction. Briefly, advances in cell membrane physiology underscore the sophistication and adaptability of such systems in maintaining cellular health and function. The study of ion transport mechanisms and signaling pathways underscores the orchestration required to respond to changing demands of the environment. The results of this research have implications that transcend the confines of basic cellular biology, informing therapeutic intervention in a variety of pathologies that occur as a result of membrane dysfunction. Therefore, detailed knowledge of cell membrane physiology remains essential not only to scientific investigation but also to the practice of medicine and biotechnology, paving the way for inventions based on our expanding comprehension of these vital cellular components.

A correct understanding of cell membrane physiology is key to appreciating how cells react to their surroundings and gain homeostasis. Major highlights note the critical roles played by cell membranes in regulating substance movement, signaling, and structural integrity. The phospholipid bilayer of the membranes functions as a selective barrier that facilitates the passage of some molecules while inhibiting others, thus contributing to cellular compartmentalization. Second, membrane-embedded proteins enable many functions , such as transport, signal transduction, and communication with other cells. This multi-dimensional property of the membrane is a critical part of cellular function, and any malfunction will lead to aberrant cell processes that influence overall physiological processes. In addition, astrocytes, the glial cells, also demonstrate the complexity of membrane physiology within the non-neuronal cell. The glial cells take up neurotransmitters and control extracellular potassium levels, which in turn affect neuronal excitability and communication. New computational models have shown that the new astrocyte structure contributes to their ability to regulate local concentration fluctuations of ions. Astrocytes, for instance, can generate Ca2+ signals used to control neural circuitry by mechanisms that are often experimentally out of reach. The results derived from such a study emphasize the importance of membrane dynamics within the frame of the general neural physiology, suggesting that astrocytic processes are more intricate than previously understood, as evidenced in studies like Araque et al. (2018).

Also, understanding the dynamics of the myometrial smooth muscle layer provides further indications of spatial heterogeneity importance in the realm of membrane physiology. Recent mathematical models have shown how fluctuations in coupling strengths between cells can increase global excitability, which is necessary for efficacious uterine contractions during parturition. The models show that localized stimulation may travel through a network of myometrial cells, depending on the physical connections formed through gap junctions. The balance of spatial organization seems to be crucial in achieving synchronous excitation in the muscular tissue, and this implies that cell-to-cell interactions at the membrane level can have profound influences on higher levels of physiological function. Therefore, studying these properties not only enhances knowledge of the cell membrane physiology but also emphasizes its role in a variety of biological processes, as observed in research findings like Shmygol et al. (2013).

KEY TERMS FROM THIS CHAPTER

- Active Transport
- Endocytosis
- Facilitated Diffusion
- Integral Proteins
- Lipid Rafts
- Membrane Proteins
- Passive Transport
- Phospholipid Bilayer
- Selective Permeability
- Diffusion
- Exocytosis
- Fluid Mosaic Model
- Ion Channels
- Membrane Potential
- Osmosis
- Peripheral Proteins
- Receptor-Mediated Endocytosis
- Signal Transduction

CRITICAL THINKING QUESTIONS

1. **What is the fundamental composition of the cell membrane?**
   a. DNA and RNA
   b. Phospholipid bilayer
   c. Protein chains
   d. Polysaccharide walls
2. **Which of the following is one of the functions of membrane proteins?**
   a. DNA replication
   b. Protein synthesis
   c. Transport of molecules
   d. Energy storage
3. **What is the role of cholesterol in the cell membrane?**
   a. Breaks down lipids
   b. Increases membrane fluidity and stability
   c. Synthesizes ATP
   d. Activates DNA transcription
4. **What type of transport employs ATP to move substances across the membrane?**
   a. Diffusion
   b. Facilitated diffusion
   c. Active transport
   d. Osmosis
5. **What is the normal resting membrane potential in most animal cells?**
   a. +70 mV
   b. –70 mV
   c. 0 mV
   d. –120 mV

Short Answer Questions

1. What is the main component of the cell membrane?
2. Define selective permeability.
3. What is the function of membrane proteins?
4. What is cholesterol's function in the cell membrane?
5. Distinguish between passive and active transport of the cell membrane.
6. Explain different types of passive transport (diffusion, osmosis, facilitated diffusion) with examples.
7. Explain the sodium-potassium pump and its role in creating membrane potential.
8. Explain receptor-mediated endocytosis with an example.
9. Describe the signal transduction process across the cell membrane.
10. Describe how ion channels influence membrane physiology and nerve signaling.

Answers to Critical Thinking Questions

1. (b); 2. (c); 3. (b); 4. (c); 5. (b)

REFERENCES

1. Aimanova, K. G., Chen, J., & Gill, S. S. (2020). *Aedes* cadherin receptor that mediates *Bacillus thuringiensis* Cry11A toxicity is essential for mosquito development. https://core.ac.uk/download/323067607.pdf (accessed on 16th June 2025).

2. Akiyama, A., Andreason, A., Ariatti, N., Armentano, D., Bailey, C., Bali, R., et al. (1994). Delivery of drugs, proteins and genes into cells using transferrin as a ligand for receptor-mediated endocytosis. https://core.ac.uk/download/12164936.pdf (accessed on 16th June 2025).

3. Alawak, M. (2019). *Immune Magnetic Thermosensitive Liposomes for Cancer Therapy*. https://core.ac.uk/download/288436500.pdf (accessed on 16th June 2025).

4. Antollini, S. S., & Fabiani, C. (2019). Alzheimer's disease as a membrane disorder: Spatial cross-talk among beta-amyloid peptides, nicotinic acetylcholine receptors and lipid rafts. https://core.ac.uk/download/287882156.pdf (accessed on 16th June 2025).

5. Araque, A., Chvatal, A., Grosche, A., Panatier, A., Verkhratsky, A., Volterra, A., Wallraff, A., et al. (2018). Disentangling astroglia physiology with a realistic cell model *in silico*. https://core.ac.uk/download/161233176.pdf (accessed on 16th June 2025).

6. Barar, J., Khiavi, M. A., Mousavi, R., & Rafi, M., et al. (2018). Enzyme replacement therapies: What is the best option? https://core.ac.uk/download/213441626.pdf (accessed on 16th June 2025).

7. Bartol, T., Bell, M., Rangamani, P., Sejnowski, T., et al. (2019). Dendritic spine geometry and spine apparatus organization govern the spatiotemporal dynamics of calcium. https://core.ac.uk/download/323064209.pdf (accessed on 16th June 2025).

8. Berkowitz, O., Fenske, R., Finnegan, P. M., Hardy, A., et al. (2013). Acclimation responses of *Arabidopsis thaliana* to sustained phosphite treatments. https://core.ac.uk/download/11245159.pdf (accessed on 16th June 2025).

9. Bernardoni, P., Di Sano, F., & Piacentini, M. (2012). The reticulons: Guardians of the structure and function of the endoplasmic reticulum. https://core.ac.uk/download/pdf/53849973.pdf (accessed on 16th June 2025).

10. Bich, L., Moreau, J. F., & Pradeu, T. (2019). Understanding multicellularity: The functional organization of the intercellular space. https://core.ac.uk/download/228134961.pdf (accessed on 16th June 2025).

11. Bosia, C., Campa, C. C., & Ferro, E. (2021). Rab11-mediated trafficking and human cancers: An updated review. https://core.ac.uk/download/524606886.pdf (accessed on 16th June 2025).

12. Boswell, M., Carlile, J., Daniel, J., Deacon, R., Deak, M., Falconer, A., Feldmann, H., et al. (2017). *Introduction to Fungal Physiology*. https://core.ac.uk/download/228177974.pdf (accessed on 16th June 2025).

13. Brunet, A., Cassidy-Stone, A., Hoshino, A., Hoshino, A., Jain, A., Kazlauskaite, A., Khaminets, A., et al. (2017). The pharmacological regulation of cellular mitophagy. https://core.ac.uk/download/76981017.pdf (accessed on 16th June 2025).

14. Budin, I., Lee, C., & Venkatraman, K. (2024). Setting the curve: The biophysical properties of lipids in mitochondrial form and function. https://core.ac.uk/download/622529448.pdf (accessed on 16th June 2025).

15. Bullock, T. H., & Perkel, D. H. (1968). Neutral coding–A report based on an NRP work session. Contractor Report (CR), Document ID

16. https://ntrs.nasa.gov/citations/19690022317 (accessed on 16th June 2025).

17. Bultynck, G., D'hondt, C., Himpens, B., Iyyathurai, J., et al. (2014). Cx43-hemichannel function and regulation in physiology and pathophysiology: Insights from the bovine corneal endothelial cell system and beyond. https://core.ac.uk/download/55846647.pdf (accessed on 16th June 2025).

18. Cafferty, P., Casagrand, J., Co, E., Flemming, R., et al. (2023). Creating the HAPS Physiology Learning Outcomes: Terminology, eponyms, inclusive language, core concepts, and skills. https://core.ac.uk/download/590971416.pdf (accessed on 16th June 2025).

19. Cala, P. M. (1983). Cell volume regulation by *Amphiuma* red blood cells. The role of Ca+2 as a modulator of alkali metal/H+ exchange. https://core.ac.uk/download/323071325.pdf (accessed on 16th June 2025).

20. Carlsson, A., Cooper, J. M., Glidle, A., Li, D., et al. (2013). Rheology at the micro-scale: New tools for bio-analysis. https://core.ac.uk/download/16459334.pdf (accessed on 16th June 2025).

21. Catalá, Á. (2019). Lipid peroxidation modifies the assembly of biological membranes: "The lipid whisker model." https://core.ac.uk/download/pdf/296425968.pdf (accessed on 16th June 2025).

22. Chowdhury, F., Maruthamuthu, V., & Muhamed, I. (2017). Biophysical tools to study cellular mechanotransduction. https://core.ac.uk/download/84112663.pdf (accessed on 16th June 2025).

23. Destexhe, A., Louveau, A., Gardner-Medwin, A. R., Smith, A. J., Thrane, A. S., Frankenhaeuser, B., Lu, B., et al. (2019). Astrocytic ion dynamics: Implications for potassium buffering and liquid flow. https://core.ac.uk/download/479749716.pdf (accessed on 16th June 2025).

24. Eisenberg, R. S., Liu, C., & Mori, Y. (2011). A model of electro diffusion and osmotic water flow and its energetic structure. https://core.ac.uk/download/pdf/81131622.pdf (accessed on 16th June 2025).

25. Farquhar, M. G., & Palade, G. E. (1998). The Golgi apparatus: 100 years of progress and controversy. https://core.ac.uk/download/323062257.pdf (accessed on 16th June 2025).

26. Fomovska, A., Topolska, A. E., Lige, B., Shen, B., Kafsack, B. F., Luft, B. J., Lord, C., et al. (2013). Protein trafficking through the endosomal system prepares intracellular parasites for a home invasion. https://core.ac.uk/download/19785875.pdf (accessed on 16th June 2025).

27. Pierelli, G., Stanzione, R., Forte, M., Migliarino, S., Perelli, M., Volpe, M., & Rubattu, S. (2017). Uncoupling Protein 2: A Key Player and a Potential Therapeutic Target in Vascular Diseases. *Oxidative medicine and cellular longevity, 2017*, 7348372. https://doi.org/10.1155/2017/7348372(accessed on 16th June 2025).

28. Fushimi, K., Shi, L. B., & Verkman, A. S. (1991). Solvent drags measurement of transcellular and basolateral membrane NaCl reflection coefficient in kidney proximal tubule. https://core.ac.uk/download/323075180.pdf (accessed on 16th June 2025).

29. Kasi Ganeshan, T. 2019. *Investigating the protective role of the natural hormone Melatonin, in reducing drug-induced cardiotoxicity in the therapy of chronic diseases.* PhD thesis University

of Westminster School of Life Sciences https://doi.org/10.34737/qy74w (accessed on 16th June 2025).

30. Kim, M., Krasnopeeva, E., Le, D., Pilizota, T., et al. (2021). Active efflux leads to heterogeneous dissipation of proton motive force by protonophores in bacteria. https://core.ac.uk/download/458057167.pdf (accessed on 16th June 2025).

31. Krishnamoorthy, G., Lu, S., Ntreh, A., Zgurskaya, H. I., et al. (2011). Mechanism and function of the outer membrane channel TolC in multidrug resistance and physiology of *Enterobacteria*. https://core.ac.uk/download/pdf/8617318.pdf (accessed on 16th June 2025).

32. Kurniawati, N. D., Machmudin, D., & Sanjaya, Y. (2010). Histological study of SlNPV infection on body weight and peritrophic membrane damage of *Spodoptera litura* larvae. https://core.ac.uk/download/12346573.pdf (accessed on 16th June 2025).

33. Maini, P. K., Dallon, J. C., & Sherratt, J. A. (2005). A multiscale model for collagen alignment in wound healing. https://core.ac.uk/download/pdf/96773.pdf (accessed on 16th June 2025).

34. Majewski, A. J., Bisaillon, M., Clark, S., Gest, T., Hallenbeck, J., Hewitt, J., KiBeom, K., et al. (2011). Electro-extractive fermentation for efficient biohydrogen production. https://core.ac.uk/download/pdf/1631309.pdf (accessed on 16th June 2025).

35. Mattarei, A., Pfeiffer, C., De Stefani, D., Seifert, J., Nowikovsky, K., Zoratti, M., Zoratti, M., et al. (2017). LETM1-mediated K+ and Na+ homeostasis regulates mitochondrial Ca2+ efflux. https://core.ac.uk/download/132266357.pdf (accessed on 16th June 2025).

36. Mori, Y. (2011). Mathematical properties of pump-leak models of cell volume control and electrolyte balance. http://arxiv.org/abs/1104.4097 (accessed on 16th June 2025).

37. Zuniga-Hertz, J. P., & Patel, H. H. (2019). The Evolution of Cholesterol-Rich Membrane in Oxygen Adaption: The Respiratory System as a Model. *Frontiers in physiology*, *10*, 1340. https://doi.org/10.3389/fphys.2019.01340 (accessed on 16th June 2025).

38. Quintana, A., Raffaello, A., Rasola, A., Tosatto, A., Varadi, A., Rowland, A. A., Tarasov, A. I., et al. (2017). The mitochondrial Ca(2+) uniporter: Structure, function, and pharmacology. https://core.ac.uk/download/129191720.pdf (accessed on 16th June 2025).

39. Rhodes, J. D., & Sanderson, J. (2008). The mechanisms of calcium homeostasis and signalling in the lens. https://core.ac.uk/download/2773039.pdf (accessed on 16th June 2025).

40. Shi, L. B., Wang, Y. X., & Verkman, A. S. (1990). Regulation of the formation and water permeability of endosomes from toad bladder granular cells. *The Journal of general physiology*, *96*(4), 789–808. https://doi.org/10.1085/jgp.96.4.789(accessed on 16th June 2025).

41. Shmygol, A., Blanks, A. M., Challis, J. R. G., McCloskey, C., Hodgkin, A. L., van den Berg, H. A., Kao, C. Y., et al. (2013). Spatial heterogeneity enhances and modulates excitability in a mathematical model of the myometrium. https://core.ac.uk/download/16663999.pdf (accessed on 16th June 2025).

42. Silvis, M. R. (2009). *RAB GTPase Regulation of Apical Cystic Fibrosis Transmembrane Conductance Regulator Recycling in Polarized Intestinal Epithelial Cells*. https://core.ac.uk/download/12209596.pdf (accessed on 16th June 2025).

43. Zhu, C., Clarkson, D. T., Luu, D. T., Zelazny, E., Chaumont, F., Cooper, G. J., Bienert, G. P., et al. (2008). Barley plasma membrane intrinsic proteins (PIP aquaporins) as water and CO_2 transporters. https://core.ac.uk/download/12528699.pdf (accessed on 16th June 2025).

MUSCLE PHYSIOLOGY

3

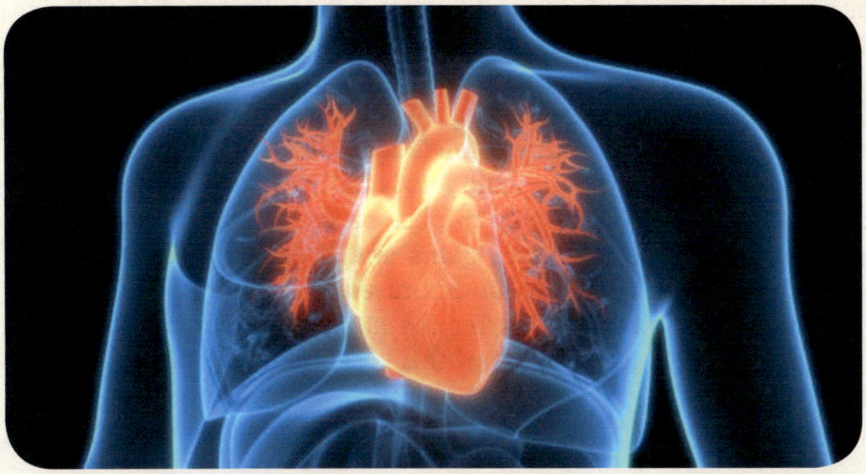

LEARNING OBJECTIVES

After studying this chapter, you will be able to:

1. Define muscle tissue types;
2. Describe the muscle structure;
3. Explain the mechanism of muscle contraction;
4. Highlight the muscle metabolism;
5. Discuss muscle growth and adaptation;
6. Evaluate the muscle disease and disorder.

Introduction

The muscle physiology consists of the intricate mechanisms behind muscle functioning and performance. Understanding how muscles contract, generate force, and react to various stimuli is essential for sports performance improvement and muscle disorder treatment. Muscle physiology integrates aspects of biochemistry, biomechanics, and neural control to give a comprehensive overview of the functioning of muscles within the human body. The relationship between muscular strength and power is specifically important for sport excellence given that, in most instances, athletes require both attributes to perform at their best. Whereas strength measures the maximum force a muscle can apply, power also measures the velocity at which force is applied, highlighting the importance of velocity in athletic competition. This distinction is important because research has demonstrated that varying velocities of contraction can alter muscular power adjustments and performance levels, thus requiring specialized training techniques (Brenneman et al., 2016). In addition to an understanding of the variables influencing muscular power, neuromuscular coordination is at the core of muscle physiology. The central nervous system coordinates a group of muscles with many different tasks, and effective postural control relies on the intricate neural exchange between them. A study of these exchanges reveals that muscle function is not merely a mechanical affair but involves a lot of neural control. With high-density multichannel electromyography (EMG) analysis, the researchers have demonstrated that muscle network and coordination changes come about due to various postural tasks. This highlights the importance of understanding the variation of muscle activity under different conditions, which can find application in training protocols to achieve peak performance and prevent injury. By knowing the neural bases of muscle interaction, researchers can better understand the logic for effective strength and power training, consolidating the need for a multi-dimensional approach to muscle physiology (Boonstra et al., 2019). As muscle physiology evolves, it only becomes more critical that new training approaches are needed to maximize muscular adaptation. The traditional training methods, e.g., isotonic and isometric training, have provided the fundamentals; new methods , such as inertial load training, however, need to be scrutinized more closely. They are promising to grow muscular power through novel methods of loading that control speed and force delivery in ways different from dominant paradigms. Given the knowledge base to be improved on according to the needs as determined by the research community, it is an urgent necessity to systematically review these novel modalities. Future research would focus on creating procedures for inertial loading that might yield greater muscle performance gains and broader application to various sporting activities. Ultimately, expanding our knowledge of muscle physiology will not only result in improved athletic performance but also in rehabilitation methods in individuals with muscular impairment, demonstrating the fundamental importance of this research (Brenneman et al., 2016; Boonstra et al., 2019) (Figure 3.1).

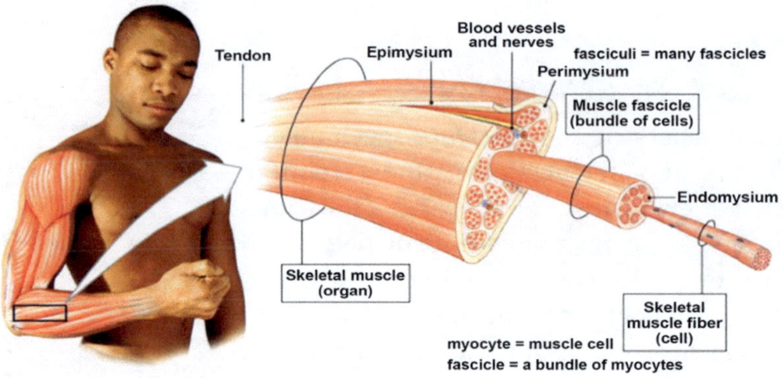

Figure 3.1. Muscle physiology diagram.

Source: https://o.quizlet.com/AnBdQ7EXJlFdamBaAmO-dA_b.png.

Definition of Muscle Physiology

Essentially, muscle physiology is the examination of muscle structure, function, and biochemical processes behind muscle activity. It is a discipline that crosses biology and medicine that explains how muscles contract, relax, and generate force needed to move. To learn about muscle physiology is to learn about the various types of muscle tissue, skeletal, smooth, and cardiac, and their corresponding functions within the human body. Every muscle type possesses unique features that define how they respond to stimuli and add to the processes of the body. The intricate interaction between muscle fibers, motor neurons, and biochemical mechanisms regulating energy metabolism only adds more depth to our study. As researchers study the molecular mechanisms of muscle contraction, they learn about the impact of exercise, hormonal changes, and injury on muscle function and integrity and generally the ability of the body and the quality of life. There is a deep understanding of muscle physiology, which depends on an appreciation of the neuromechanical dynamics governing muscle activity. Muscles are not independent structures; rather, they function as components of systems involving the nervous system and connective tissues. The motor unit, the motor neuron and the skeletal muscle fibers innervated by it, occupies a central position in this interaction. When the motor neuron is activated, it generates an electrical impulse that causes the contraction of muscle fibers, which is closely linked with the availability of energy substrates. Natural variation among people makes this system more difficult, with each individual's neuromechanical characteristics affecting their reaction to muscle. For instance, variations in muscle fiber types can significantly affect strength and endurance results, and reinforce the necessity for individualized approaches in rehabilitation and training (Alicea et al., 2009). Lastly, integration with other biological systems demonstrates the integrated nature of this discipline. The enteric nervous system (ENS) or the brain-in-the-gut is an ideal example of such integration because it controls the functioning of smooth muscles in the gut and influences overall health and well-being (Zizzo et al., 2011). With our greater understanding, researchers are increasingly fascinated with the interactions between response of skeletal muscle and systems like the cardiovascular, respiratory, and immune systems. These interactions emphasize how muscle activation affects metabolic functions beyond mere movement, affecting energy expenditure and recovery. By deconstructing these advanced relationships, muscle physiology offers valuable data for performance improvement, rehabilitation procedures, and prevention of musculoskeletal diseases, thus making it significant in health and exercise disciplines.

Importance of Studying Muscle Physiology

Studying muscle physiology is crucial to learn the intricate mechanisms of muscle function and adaptation. As they are the prime movers, muscles are not only responsible for voluntary and involuntary movements but play a vital role in maintaining overall well-being. Muscle physiology helps to account for how muscular systems respond to stimuli including exercise, environment, and disease. This knowledge is vital in the development of effective training and rehabilitation programs. In addition, research in muscle physiology drives sporting science progress so that athletes can optimize their performance but minimize the risk of injury. Muscle physiology research gives immediate information input into medicine and kinesiology practice with important information regarding the behavior of muscles in health and disease. Muscle physiology research also enhances our knowledge about the process of aging and its influence on muscle function. Sarcopenia, the age-associated loss of muscle strength and mass, represents challenging geriatric medicine problems, and therefore research in the area becomes even more critical. Knowledge of the biological mechanisms leading to muscle wasting can guide the development of interventions that will help ensure the preservation of muscle integrity in older people. In addition, exploring the neuromechanics of muscle contractions shows the complexity of motor control and the nervous system's function in facilitating movement (Santello et al., 2017). Such a nuanced understanding informs the development of therapeutic interventions for diseases that affect muscle performance, such as stroke, multiple sclerosis, and muscular dystrophies, and testifies to integrative research within muscle physiology. Lastly, the results of muscle physiology have broader implications than just the clinical setting to extend into more universal applications in robotics and biomechanics. For instance, understanding gained through the analysis of biological motion can be used to guide the creation of advanced robotic systems that mimic human muscular action, resulting in more effective and efficient machines. The crossing of biological and engineering concepts is enabled to produce new solutions to mechanical challenges, bridging the two areas. Such cross-disciplinary investigations not only enhance muscle physiology knowledge but also trigger technology advancements that can lead to increased quality of life in various sectors, e.g., rehabilitation and assistive technology. Thus, a firm grasp of muscle physiology serves not only scientific inquiry but also practical application that may lead to societal benefit (Figure 3.2).

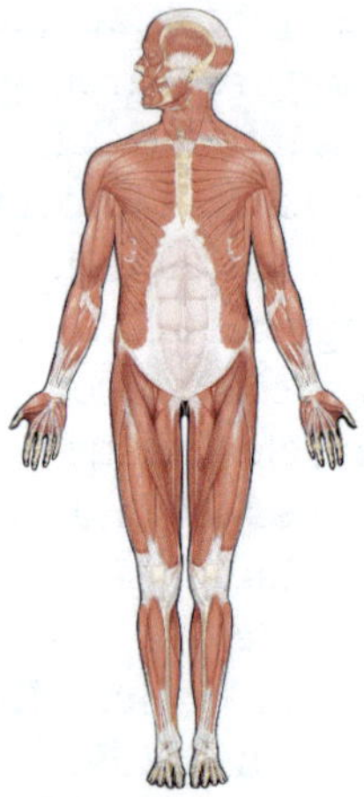

Figure 3.2. Human body muscular system.

Source: https://cdn.britannica.com/24/252524-049-AAD44065/interactive-human-body-muscular-system.jpg.

Overview of Muscle Types

Muscle tissue is essentially separated into three various categories: skeletal, cardiac, and smooth muscle, each with unique functions in the body. Striated-looking skeletal muscle is fixed to the bone and responsible for voluntary movement. It is under conscious control and can execute purposeful actions , such as walking, lifting, or posture maintenance. Skeletal muscle fibers possess a remarkable plasticity for adaptation to varying physical demands. This adaptability is evidenced by the metabolic transition that occurs in certain species, such as the Weddell seal, wherein a shift in gene expression facilitates the realignment of muscle function as animals grow and adapt to accommodate new habitats, demonstrating the relationship between the physiology of muscle and the demands of behavior (Ptitsyn & Kanatous, 2009). Unlike skeletal muscle, cardiac muscle is striated muscle and an involuntary muscle present only in the heart. Its primary function is to contract rhythmically to pump the blood around the circulatory system and maintain vital functions that are critical for life. Cardiac muscle cells, or cardiomyocytes, are specifically tailored to allow repeated contraction and are connected by intercalated discs, which allow coordinated electrical signaling. This property facilitates the natural rhythmicity and anti-fatigue of the heart, separating it from skeletal muscle. This description of the physiological properties of cardiac muscle gives us essential information about the health of the heart and how stressors , such as microgravity and disuse influence muscle performance and induce states of atrophy or hypertrophy (Blottner et al., 2017). Smooth muscle, the third one, is also involuntary and occurs predominantly in hollow organ walls , such as the intestines, blood vessels, and bladder. Smooth muscle lacks striations and is controlled directly by the autonomic nervous system. This muscle type is designed to facilitate involuntary action, including peristalsis of the digestive system as well as blood circulation regulation via vasoconstriction and vasodilation in the circulatory system. The functional variability of smooth muscle is demonstrated through its ability to adapt to various demands and external conditions. The appreciation of the complex relationship between these categories of muscles and their unique physiological function is essential to a full appreciation of muscle physiology, allowing for eventual advancements in medical and rehabilitative therapy for muscular disorders and injuries.

3.1. Types of Muscle Tissue

Learning Outcome

1. Define the skeletal muscle;
2. Describe the cardiac muscle;
3. Discuss the smooth muscle.

Muscle tissue is basically broken down into three distinct types: skeletal, cardiac, and smooth muscle, each having unique characteristics and functions. Skeletal muscle is voluntary, striated, and directly under the control of the somatic nervous system, causing movement by contraction and relaxation. Skeletal muscle is fixed to bones by tendons and is involved in locomotion and posture. The contractile fibers of skeletal muscle are found in bundles, which increase their force-generating capacity. Understanding the anatomy and physiology of skeletal muscle is relevant in certain specialties, including sports medicine and rehabilitation, as it is typically the reference point when considering muscle pathology or injury. Cardiac muscle, found solely in the heart, possesses both involuntary control and certain structural features, such as intercalated discs that facilitate coordinated contractions. Unlike skeletal muscle, cardiac muscle is striated but exists perpetually throughout the life of a person, nourished by intrinsic pacemaker cells that regulate heart rate. As it is involuntary, this allows the heart to rapidly respond to shifting physiological demands, like increased activity during exercise or at rest. The single mode of calcium regulation in cardiac muscle cells is the solution to a majority of cardiac pathologies and, therefore the focus of significant research effort in cardiovascular health. This form of muscle is studied to uncover complex physiological mechanisms, crucial to homeostasis and understanding disease processes. Smooth muscle tissue, found in hollow organ walls , such as the alimentary tract and blood vessels, is mostly involuntary and non-striated. It offers slow, sustained contractions critical in managing flow through these systems. Smooth muscle contraction is autonomic and locally regulated by hormonal and nervous stimuli, in contrast to skeletal and cardiac muscle, and influences functions, such as digestion, blood pressure, and respiratory rate.

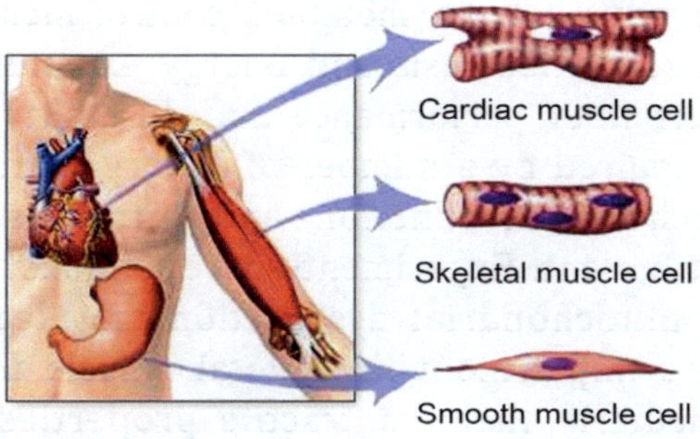

Figure 3.3. Types of muscle tissue.

Source: https://medlineplus.gov/ency/images/ency/fullsize/19917.jpg.

Physiological properties of smooth muscle differ significantly from the rest of the muscles, especially with regard to adaptation and maintaining tension for a prolonged period of time. Research on the function and regulation of smooth muscle, particularly with respect to diseases , such as hypertension, highlights its function in maintaining overall health alongside a better understanding of muscle physiology (Subramaniam et al., 2012; Carter et al., 2019) (Figure 3.3).

3.1.1. Skeletal Muscle

Skeletal muscle is essential to human physiology as it is used for movement, posture, and overall metabolic health. Comprised of multinucleated fibers of significant length with a history of powerful contraction, skeletal muscle is crucial for voluntary and reflexive movement. The fibers are divided into different types based on their speeds of contraction and metabolic capabilities, mainly Type I (slow-twitch) and Type II (fast-twitch). Type I fibers are also less susceptible to fatigue and are utilized primarily for endurance activities, while Type II fibers are utilized for short periods of strength and power. This difference emphasizes the importance of skeletal muscle in determining individuals' physical capacities, which can be influenced by training regimens, age, and nutrition. In addition, skeletal muscle is directly related to metabolic control, including glucose homeostasis and energy expenditure. Muscle fiber performance and durability may be impaired by a number of factors, including mitochondrial function and intramuscular environment. Experiments have demonstrated that mitochondrial dysfunction may lead to severe impairment in skeletal muscle fibers, particularly their contractile properties and overall performance. It is significant to explore how diseases like mitochondrial myopathy may impair muscle function since such dysfunction also occurs in aging and neuromuscular disease. Understanding such interactions is critical for the development of therapeutic interventions to treat the consequences of such disorders, as well as the promotion of muscle health in the aged (Bernardino Gomes et al., 2023). With age, there is sarcopenia, characterized by declining muscle strength and mass. This condition is also being recognized as a global health issue, as it has been associated with reduced physical function and elevated risk for disability and mortality in older individuals. Notably, sarcopenia is more than the loss of muscle mass, but in proportion, the quality of muscle also reduces, typically exacerbated by the re-distribution of body fat, notably in skeletal muscle itself. Excess adipose tissue in non-fat tissues can be detrimental to muscle contractility, and therefore, a context-specific understanding of muscle physiology is required. Research into the interaction between muscle function and adipose tissue can contribute to an understanding of mechanisms underlying sarcopenia and guide the development of appropriate interventions to preserve muscle integrity and promote healthier aging (Carter et al., 2019) (Figure 3.4).

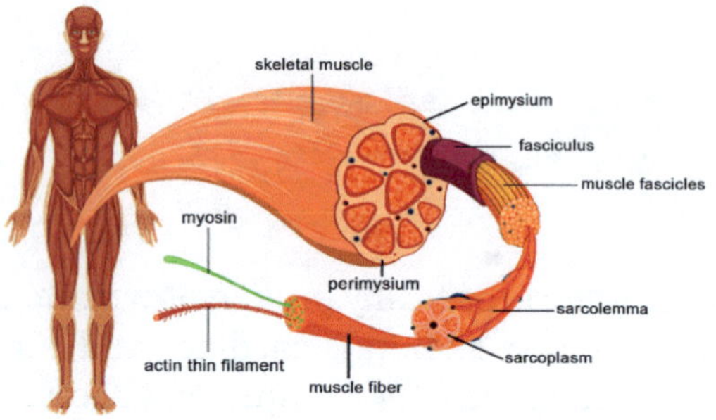

Figure 3.4. Skeletal-muscle.

Source: https://media.geeksforgeeks.org/wp-content/uploads/20240219161024/Skeletal-Muscle.png.

3.1.2. Cardiac Muscle

The cardiac muscle, or myocardium, is a special form of striated muscle found only in the heart. It is not voluntary muscle like skeletal muscle; cardiac muscle is involuntary and operates automatically without consciousness. The structure of the cardiac muscle is extremely organized, in which the myofibrils are spread out in the form of branches and connected by intercalated discs. These discs allow for speedy electrical conduction, enabling synchronized contractions required for effective pumping of the blood. Cardiomyocytes, or cardiac muscle cells, have a high density of mitochondria to maintain their energy demand in the process of long-term contraction. Key proteins like myosin play critical roles in cardiac muscle contraction, and it has been reported that chaperone action like that of UNC-45 is required for efficient myosin folding and accumulation, particularly during heart tissue maturation as well as in the context of most cardiomyopathies (Cammarato et al., 2011). Functionally, cardiac muscle is distinguished by its ability to maintain rhythmic contraction throughout one's life. This rhythmicity is regulated primarily by the pacemaker cells of the heart's sinoatrial node. Cardiac muscle contraction and relaxation are regulated by many physiological factors, including neural and hormonal inputs. In the event of dynamic exercise, the body requires enhanced cardiovascular output, and this evokes adaptations in heart rate and contractility through mediation by the autonomic nervous system. Particularly, sympathetic activation increases contractility and heart rate, while parasympathetic withdrawal tones down. These adjustments facilitate efficient delivery of oxygenated blood to respond to muscular requirements during exercise, considering the intricate interaction between cardiac muscle physiology and overall body function as a whole (Crisafulli et al., 2014). Cardiac muscle integrity is paramount to cardiovascular health since deficits are known to result in different types of cardiomyopathy, a condition related to abnormal heart muscle function. Indications exist of the role that certain chaperone proteins, including UNC-45, play in ensuring cardiac performance; disturbances in these mechanisms may cause decreased myofibrillar content and faulty contractility (Cammarato et al., 2011). Understanding the molecular and physiological processes of cardiac muscle activity is central to developing targeted therapeutic strategies against cardiovascular disease. Therefore, cardiac muscle research today extends beyond the mechanical to embrace molecular biology, genetics, and environmental influences on muscle physiology, requiring an interdisciplinary strategy for the study of muscle physiology. In order to do so, ongoing research in the molecular chaperones for myosin stability could also be an essential unlock to heart disorder prevention and treatment (Figure 3.5).

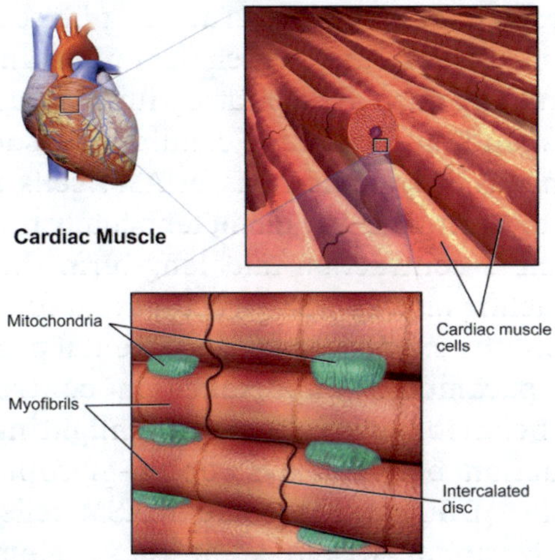

Figure 3.5. Cardiac muscle.

Source: https://cdn.storymd.com/optimized/RoeJ7Bcadv/original.jpg.

3.1.3. Smooth Muscle

Smooth muscle is a highly significant part of the muscular system, and it plays a considerable role in the physiological functions of most organ systems. Unlike skeletal muscle, which is voluntarily regulated, smooth muscle operates involuntarily to regulate vital processes , such as digestion, blood pressure, and respiration. Smooth muscle contractions are more prolonged in nature, permitting smooth muscle to maintain tension for extended periods, which is crucial for such activities as the regulation of the caliber of blood vessels and peristalsis within the gastrointestinal tract. The intricate structure of smooth muscle cells accommodates these multifunctional contractions, which include a lattice structure of actin and myosin filaments that allows efficient development and relaxation of tension. This built-in plasticity accommodates smooth muscle adaptation to different physiological requirements and is an interesting area of study in the field of muscle physiology. It has been found in research that smooth muscle cells possess high phenotypic plasticity, particularly true for airway smooth muscle (ASM). The cells can change between contractile and proliferative phenotypes at a very fast rate, which is important for maintaining normal respiratory function as well as responding to disease conditions , such as asthma. The dynamic roles of ASM cells allow them to control airway diameter acutely through reversible contraction and long-term through remodeling airway wall structure and function. Notably, the expression of fundamental proteins is of paramount importance in controlling ASM behavior, with studies highlighting the interaction between dystrophin-glycoprotein complex (DGC) and caveolae in ASM cells. The organizational structure of these elements within the cellular framework is of critical significance in regulating intracellular calcium mobilization and thereby influencing ASM tissue contractility properties as well as overall airway physiology (Sharma et al., 2012). Control of contraction and reactivity in vascular smooth muscle is also complex and has a significant impact on cardiovascular status. Hypertension is an example of how dysregulation of smooth muscle function may lead to severe health consequences. Vascular smooth muscle cells undergo phenotypic remodeling, moving from a quiescent to a proliferative phenotype, which can enhance vascular resistance and reduce arterial diameter. Remodeling is influenced by numerous interrelating systems, including the renin-angiotensin-aldosterone system and oxidative stress pathways. In addition, the changes in intracellular calcium not only cause contraction of the smooth muscle but also influence the gene expression and cellular function. For that reason, the mechanisms controlling the behavior of vascular smooth muscle must be understood to develop therapeutic methods for combating hypertension and related diseases (Alves-Lopes et al., 2018).

Test Your Knowledge

1. What are the three major kinds of muscle tissue, and how do they differ structurally, where are they found, and how do they move?
2. How does skeletal muscle fiber contract at the molecular level, and what is the role played by actin and myosin in it?

3.2. Muscle Structure

Learning Outcome

1. Explain the muscle fibers and the myofibrils;
2. Explain the sliding filament theory and sarcomeres;
3. Learn about the elements of connective tissue.

Muscle structure is a highly evolved organization of cellular elements, tissues, and fibers, all intricately designed to give movement and support posture in the body. Macroscopically, skeletal muscle is composed of clusters of muscle fibers, which are made up of myofibrils—thin filaments and thick filaments for contraction. Each muscle fiber is enclosed within a membrane called the sarcolemma and has more than one nucleus because of its origin in fetal life. Fibers may be organized in various manners; for instance, muscles involved in the production of explosive bursts of force tend to have a pennate arrangement. This structural organization influences the function and effectiveness of the muscle, pointing to the fundamental principle of form corresponding to function in muscle physiology. Understanding these structural elements is important in the exploration of muscle contraction mechanisms at a more advanced level and the muscle performance dynamics in health and disease. Intracellular muscle fiber organization also accounts for their physiological roles. In the sarcoplasm, the cytoplasm of the muscle fibers, the mitochondria are accountable for generating energy through aerobic metabolism. Plenty of mitochondria are also particularly vital to endurance-trained individuals since they enhance the muscles' capacity to utilize oxygen efficiently. Additionally, the alignment and order of myofibrils that contain sarcomeres, the units of contraction, are free from disorganization and express a well-organized structure to allow for successful force development and mechanical efficiency. Extreme mitochondrial dysfunction, as occurs in many neuromuscular diseases, has been demonstrated to disrupt this highly regulated system, leading to substandard muscle performance and structural integrity, highlighting the importance of maintaining the health of mitochondria in skeletal muscle physiology (Bernardino Gomes et al., 2023). Unraveling this interaction is essential for developing therapeutic interventions to correct muscle function in disease states. Last but not least, the interaction between muscle architecture and the nervous system plays a central role in the regulation of muscle activity. Muscle contractions are coordinated by the brain through neural impulses directed to motor units that consist of motor neurons and the muscle fibers these innervate.

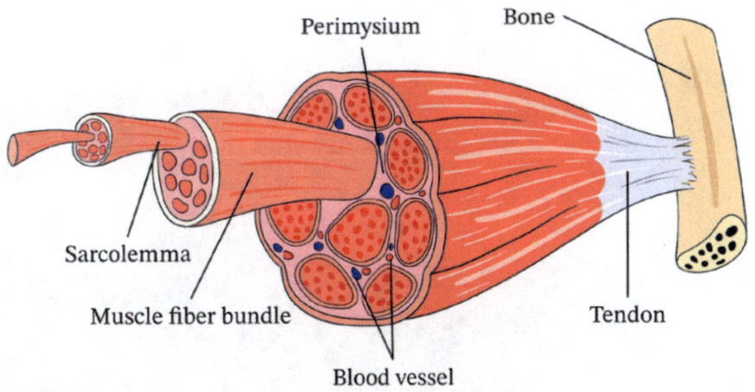

Figure 3.6. Structure of muscles.

Source: https://images.nagwa.com/figures/explainers/174167281012/2.svg.

Recent research has unfolded the diversity of brain rhythm coordination with muscle activation across various physiological states and the complexity of neuromuscular control (Ivanov et al., 2020). The neuro-muscular interactivity, besides giving precise movements, also controls muscle tone and responsivity based on body needs and tasks. For instance, the cortico-muscular network's strength and connectivity are significantly altered in resting conditions, showing an energy-saving and recovery-promoting adaptation mechanism. This reveals more about muscle structure and emphasizes the need to study neural effects on muscle physiology in greater detail, particularly in relation to movement and health (Figure 3.6).

3.2.1. Muscle Fibers and Myofibrils

Muscle fibers are the fundamental cellular components of muscle tissue, each functionally adapted to carry out specific physiological functions in movement and stability. Classified primarily into two types, slow-twitch (Type I) and fast-twitch (Type II), muscle fibers exhibit varied metabolic properties and functional profiles. Slow-twitch fibers have high mitochondrial content and myoglobin to conduct endurance activities by means of aerobic respiration. In contrast, fast-twitch fibers are adapted for rapid, powerful contractions and make greater use of anaerobic metabolism. This classification reflects the elasticity and adaptability of muscle fibers to perform various forms of physical activity and training protocols and rehabilitation interventions, as well as optimization for performance. Understanding the biochemical and physiological content of muscle fibers, energy systems, velocity of contraction, and fatigue resistance, provides insight into their response to acute and chronic exercise stimuli, further evidence of the complexity of muscle physiology. The important component of muscle fibers is the myofibril, a structured assembly of bundles of actin and myosin filaments, the contractile proteins of the muscle. Myofibrils are ordered very structurally, with the formation of sarcomeres, the units of contraction.

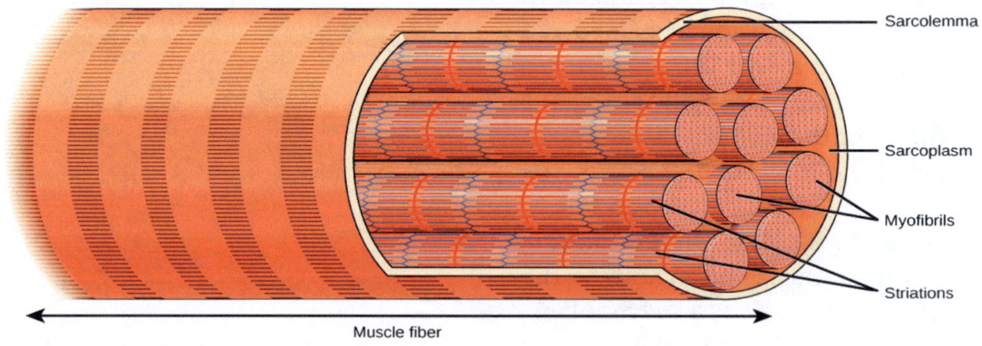

Figure 3.7. Types of muscle tissue and fibers.

Source: https://s3-us-west-2.amazonaws.com/courses-images/wp-content/uploads/sites/1223/2017/02/08002651/Figure_38_04_02-1024x401.jpg.

The alignments allow for the sliding filament mechanism that governs the process of contraction at a microscopic level. Myofibrils have been demonstrated to undergo dramatic structural alterations when there are changes in loading conditions, e.g., immobilization states. For instance, studies of hypokinesis-induced muscle atrophy have revealed that restricted motility leads to dystrophic myofibril changes like an increase in sarcoplasmic reticulum size and increased oedema in the surrounding interfibrillar space (Belak et al., 2025). These findings underscore the crucial role of myofibrils in conferring structural stability to muscles and their support for muscle fiber adaptive processes to activity and rest. Also, myofibrillar plasticity and muscle fiber plasticity are prone to numerous physiological statuses, e.g., exposure to microgravity. Studies on rats placed in zero gravity revealed that myofibrillar yields were profoundly lower in slow-twitch muscle fibers due to preferential slow-myosin isoform degradation (Baldwin et al., 2025). This reveals that muscle fibers with higher slow-twitch fiber content are particularly sensitive to protein degradation of myofibrils due to atrophy-inducing conditions. The simultaneous increase in myofibril ATPase activity in such muscles underscores the inherent biochemical adaptations occurring under conditions of stress. Understanding such processes is essential for designing purpose-specific interventions to maintain and recover muscle under clinical and athletic settings, reiterating again the fine interdependence between muscle physiology and muscle fiber function (Figure 3.7).

3.2.2. Sarcomeres and the Sliding Filament Theory

The basic building block of skeletal muscle, the sarcomere, is responsible for the muscle tissue's overall function. Sarcomeres are made up of varying proteins, primarily actin and myosin, that function throughout muscle contraction. The sliding filament theory is the most prevailing description of muscle contraction on a microscopic level. This theory proposes that myosin filaments travel along actin filaments, shortening the sarcomere and the entire muscle. The contraction process is powered by the release of calcium ions and ATP hydrolysis, which provides energy for the myosin heads to attach to actin and pull filaments inward. It is important to realize the intricate sarcomere anatomy in order to know how muscle movement is generated and regulated throughout a variety of diverse physical exercises. The sliding filament theory, while widely accepted, fails to illustrate all of muscle physiology. For instance, occurrences , such as eccentric contraction, where a muscle generates tension as it is lengthening, are counter to the sliding filament model's simplicity. Recent research suggests that other processes, such as force enhancement during stretching and the actions of other proteins like titin, also contribute to muscle function. All these complications make the length-force relation of muscles not a straightforward property but rather an emergent property of a vast number of interacting variables, such as activation level and recruitment of motor units.

The organization of muscle fibers and their arrangement and distribution introduce further complexity into the interaction of muscle force and length. Hence, more integrative consideration of muscle physiology is required, one that includes both its timing and environmental variables that affect muscle dynamics (Huijing et al., 1995). New models of muscle physiology, such as the "popping sarcomeres" and "winding filament" models, try to explain functionalities that the sliding filament model omits. Such models provide insights into how intricate combinations of protein structures in the sarcomere can carry out new patterns of contraction, especially during those movements involving quick or explosive movements. The role of titin, a giant protein responsible for passive elasticity and sarcomere stability, has also gained particular importance.

Through the integration of titin in the mechanics of eccentric contraction and emphasizing its interaction with actin-myosin dynamics, researchers are able to more accurately describe the physiological laws of muscle contractions. This general awareness is significant, especially in fields like sports medicine and rehabilitation, where precise muscle control and recovery processes are crucial (Massa et al., 2020) (Figure 3.8).

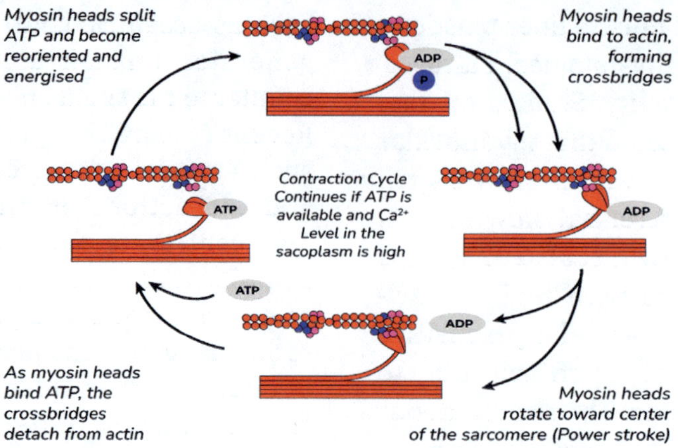

Figure 3.8. Sliding filament theory.

Source: https://media.geeksforgeeks.org/wp-content/uploads/20240402173408/Sliding-Filament-Theory.png.

3.2.3. Connective Tissue Components

The connective tissue components play a role in the general function and physiology of muscles. Composed predominantly of elastin and collagen fibers, such tissues obtain structural support through the transmission of forces generated by the muscle fibers. Extracellular matrix (ECM), a type of connective tissue, not only provides structural support but also influences cell function in the guise of biochemical communication. In the case of skeletal muscle, endomysium, a type of connective tissue sheath surrounding single myofibers, facilitates maximum diffusion of nutrients and serves as a scaffold for the architecture of muscle fibers. This organization is of essential importance to optimal muscle contraction and performance overall, in that it facilitates more even tension distribution with movement. To create methods for maintaining muscle function, it is essential to appreciate the function of connective tissue elements in muscle physiology, as conditions , such as aging or disuse negatively affect the efficiency of these supportive structures. When muscles age, changes in the properties and composition of connective tissue can have a significant impact on muscle function. Research indicates that the volume ratio of connective tissues increases with age, potentially making the muscle stiffer and less force-producing. Specifically, the stiffening of connective tissues like the endomysium will add to greater resistance under concentric contraction, thus limiting the muscle's ability for force production with shortening. In contrast, eccentric contractions are less adversely affected, which suggests that age-related modifications in connective tissue do impair certain types of muscle activity. It is vital to be aware of such microstructural changes occurring with age because it highlights the intricate interaction of the ECM and the functioning of the muscle, thus informing us on how we can prevent muscle performance decline as one grows older (Zhang et al., 2020). Adding to the intricacy of connective tissue behavior in muscle physiology is the influence of extrinsic conditions like weightlessness brought about in long-term space flight. The musculoskeletal system is highly adaptive and plastic to mechanical loads. However, prolonged loss of gravity can generate significant impairments in the structure and function of muscle and connective tissue. This state emphasizes the necessity of investigating how adaptations of connective tissues would develop under both conditions of disuse and overload. In-depth research into the compensatory mechanisms of connective tissues could steer the development of effective countermeasures to maintain muscle function during space missions and determine rehabilitation protocols on Earth. Finding a balance between researching the biological foundations of connective tissue and optimizing measures to maintain musculoskeletal integrity is essential for astronauts and the elderly (Zhang et al., 2020).

Test Your Knowledge

1. Describe the organization and function of a sarcomere. How is it divided, and how does this connect to the muscle contraction process?
2. How do layers of connective tissue (perimysium, epimysium, endomysium) organize and stabilize skeletal muscle tissue?

3.3. Muscle Contraction Mechanism

Learning Outcome

1. Describe the function of calcium ions;
2. Define actin and myosin interaction;
3. Describe the energy utilized for muscle contraction.

The multifaceted process of muscle contraction is ultimately reliant on the excitation-contraction coupling process, an event that relates neural impulses to body muscle movement. It comes about as a motor neuron-created action potential is transmitted into muscle fibers, initiating the discharge of calcium ions from the sarcoplasmic reticulum. Calcium is sequestered by troponin, inducing a conformation shift opening up binding sites on actin filaments. This exposure enables myosin heads, which are equipped with adenosine triphosphate (ATP), to bind to actin to create cross-bridges. The resulting power stroke pulls in the actin filaments, eventually shortening the muscle fiber and creating contraction. It is important to understand this process for muscle physiology to explain how muscles develop force and respond to different types of physical activity, which is why studying muscle physiology is so important in both health and disease. Muscle contraction is not strictly structural, though. It is also intimately linked to numerous regulatory variables that may influence performance. Among these regulators, the most vital one is the autonomic nervous system, particularly during dynamic exercise. Neural reflexes , such as the arterial baroreflex and exercise pressure reflex, regulate cardiovascular variables to provide the contracting muscles with the necessary oxygen while simultaneously removing metabolic by-products. Under exercise, such regulatory feedback enables blood to be routed to contracting muscles, limiting potential harm from ischemic conditions. Consequently, interference with these neural control mechanisms can have the very serious consequence of not only impacting muscular effectiveness but also cardiovascular wellness in general, demonstrating the significant interconnection between muscle contraction mechanics and systemic physiological reactions under exercise (Crisafulli et al., 2014). Furthermore, the inclusion of muscle fatigue serves to provide another level of sophistication to the mechanism of contraction by highlighting the failing performance of skeletal muscle under prolonged or high-level effort. Research has demonstrated that muscle fatigue correlates with loss of amplitude of the myoplasmic calcium transient by reduced flux of calcium through the ryanodine receptor. This reduction accumulates to diminished force production, impacting athletic function and overall physical fitness. Certain causes of this attenuated release of Ca2+ include inactivation of dihydropyridine receptors, and alterations of communication between these receptors and ryanodine receptors that cause release of calcium from the sarcoplasmic reticulum. It is essential to comprehend such cellular impairments in order to organize plans to combat fatigue and enhance muscular performance, thereby dictating better performance outcomes in sports as well as rehabilitative settings (Fitts et al., 2011) (Figure 3.9).

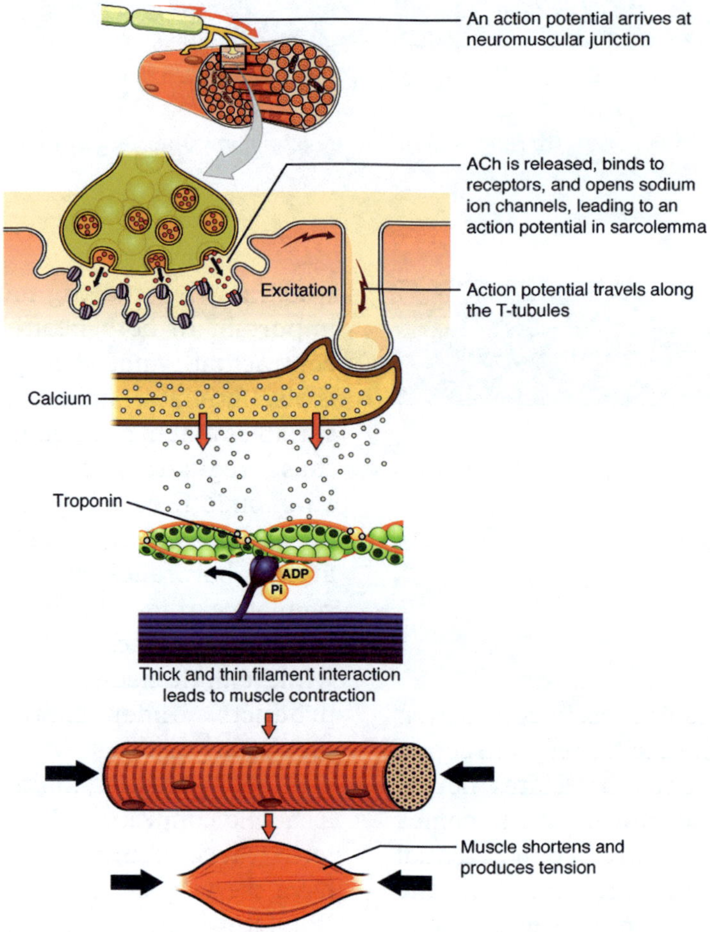

Figure 3.9. Muscle fiber contraction and relaxation.

Source: https://pressbooks-dev.oer.hawaii.edu/anatomyandphysiology/wp-content/uploads/sites/29/2017/09/1010a_Contraction_new.jpg.

3.3.1. Role of Calcium Ions

Calcium ions (Ca^{2+}) play the role of initiating the contraction of the muscles, basically spanning the electrical stimuli of muscle fibers to mechanical force generation. On muscle fiber stimulation by an action potential, it causes the release of Ca^{2+} from the sarcoplasmic reticulum, a specialized organelle for calcium storage. The release of the calcium ions gets bound to troponin, a regulatory protein present on the actin filaments. Binding causes conformational change in the troponin, which further leads to tropomyosin, another regulatory protein, shifting position and exposing binding sites on the actin filaments. This opens up active sites that allow myosin heads to bind, leading to the formation of cross-bridges and ultimately muscle contraction. The sophisticated interaction among these proteins opens up the precise regulation of calcium ion levels, as essential to normal muscle function, forming the foundation of related physiologic mechanisms in muscle physiology. Besides their role in inducing contraction, intracellular calcium ion concentration also has a crucial role in the ability of skeletal muscle to generate force and perform. As the quantity of Ca^{2+} varies, the level of activation of the muscle fiber becomes a function of various interrelated factors like structure and length of the muscle. Research has shown that muscle activation's short-term history may influence the efficacy of calcium ions to cause contraction, especially through avenues , such as potentiation and fatigue. This highlights that muscle force is not a fixed characteristic but a dynamic response that is influenced by the complex interplay of calcium with other physiological variables. The degree of activation modulates the excitability of muscles to calcium, highlighting its significance in adjusting muscle strength and endurance capacity within a given context of muscular activity (Huijing et al., 1995). Calcium ions also contribute to the mechanism of fatigue in muscles, which can significantly decrease a muscle's functional capacity by prolonged use. Accumulation of metabolic by-products like phosphate (Pi) and protons (H^{+}) has been shown to be linked with reduced calcium sensitivity levels, and therefore with reduced force production. Elevated concentrations of such ions have the potential to directly diminish myosin and actin interaction, discourage the efficacy of cross-bridge cycling, and lower the muscle's overall power production capacity. Consequently, when calcium ion availability and sensitivity are affected, the ensuing muscle contraction becomes less effective, indicating a relationship between calcium ions and muscle function during fatigue (Debold et al., 2016). Such a relationship therefore demonstrates the need for maximum levels of calcium to facilitate continued muscle function, especially in demanding circumstances.

3.3.2. Interaction of Actin and Myosin

The coordination between actin and myosin forms the basis for muscle physiology, facilitating the process of muscle contraction. Actin filaments are protein strands that are thin in nature and form part of a structural framework within muscle cells, while myosin filaments are thicker with motor functions that drive contraction. The sliding filament mechanism is the process by which the myosin heads attach to specific points on the actin filaments on stimulation by an increase in intracellular calcium level and contract by a series of force-producing power strokes. The process not only requires the hydrolysis of ATP to provide the force for the movement but is also tightly regulated by troponin and tropomyosin, the activity of which makes the myosin heads available to or unavailable from actin. Lastly, this intricate interaction enables muscles to generate force and facilitates a wide range of movement required for physiological function. Regulation of actin-myosin interaction is highly influenced by a range of intracellular signaling pathways that modulate muscle contraction. For example, calcium ion signaling pathways are responsible for initiating contraction; elevated calcium concentration augments actin-myosin cross-bridge formation, leading to contraction. Moreover, the advancement of studies reveals the role of various kinases, such as RhoA-

Rho kinase (ROCK) and protein kinase C (PKC), in the regulation of smooth muscle contraction independently of calcium levels. The intricate dynamics of such a regulatory process highlight the mechanisms by which the tone of vascular smooth muscle is modified, consequently influencing total vascular resistance and hence blood pressure.

This data draws out the pathophysiological changes that are associated with hypertension, and the abnormal control of such pathways has the potential to lead to increased vascular contraction and supports the central role of actin and myosin interactions in maintaining cardiovascular health (Alves-Lopes et al., 2018). In disuse and muscle atrophy, the role of actin and myosin interactions is also highlighted. One general model under which to examine such adaptations is hindlimb unloading (HU), which simulates disuse of skeletal muscle. Under such conditions, a decline in the properties of myosin heavy chain (MHC) fibers is extremely marked, with large diminutions in rate of contraction and force production. This emphasizes the dependence of muscle performance upon maintenance of optimal actin-myosin interactions. Interestingly, interventions that promote myosin light chain (MLC3f) elevation have shown promise to counteract the detrimental effect of disuse on the velocity of muscle contraction, indicating that therapeutic interventions can augment muscle performance during inactivity. Thus, understanding molecular mechanisms that regulate the actin-myosin interaction is imperative in formulating interventions to preserve muscle integrity and function during states of disuse (Asakura et al., 2019) (Figure 3.10).

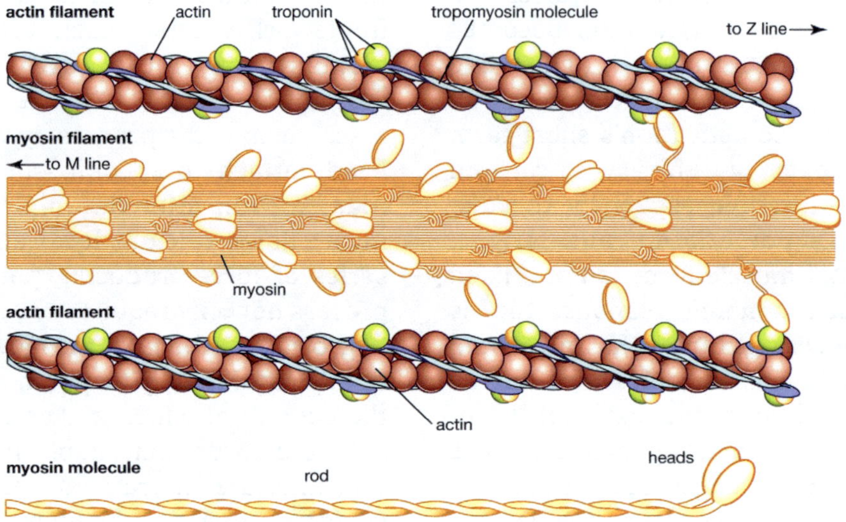

Figure 3.10. Structure-actin-myosin-filaments.

Source: https://cdn.britannica.com/65/54165-050-C4C8B933/structure-actin-myosin-filaments.jpg.

3.3.3. Energy Sources for Muscle Contraction

Muscle contraction fundamentally relies on multiple sources of energy that provide the body's physiological requirements for movement. At the cellular level, ATP plays a central role in muscle contraction. ATP serves as the energy currency directly engaged in the actin and myosin filament interaction during the contractile cycle. But the depletion of ATP reservoirs during prolonged activity forces the activation of alternative routes of energy supply. The regeneration of ATP involves anaerobic glycolysis when oxygen is absent, which provides a rapid but limited source of energy from glucose or glycogen. As muscle contraction continues, aerobic respiration becomes increasingly important, using oxygen to generate ATP from carbohydrate and fat stores with maximum efficiency, thus allowing constant muscle activity and long-term endurance. In addition to ATP, phosphocreatine is a core reservoir of energy that helps regenerate ATP in the initial stages of high-force muscle contraction.

This energy-rich molecule donates a phosphate group to adenosine diphosphate (ADP), rapidly converting it into ATP, thereby providing the energy for sudden bursts of activity. Phosphocreatine plays its vital role in the fast-twitch muscle fibers, which rely crucially on rapid energy production for short, explosive movements. Moreover, the transition from phosphocreatine usage to glycolysis and aerobic metabolism also highlights the flexibility of muscle energetics, with energy demand governing metabolic routes. All in all, such information regarding metabolic sources provides insight into how muscle fibers adjust and react towards varying physical demands and demarcates performance and recovery. Research has highlighted that variables , such as muscle fiber type, exercise intensity, and duration determine patterns of energy usage during muscle contraction. For instance, fast-twitch fibers are highly reliant on anaerobic energy systems in generating power at a rapid moment, while slow-twitch fibers are more dependent on aerobic metabolism, which is in accordance with their capacity to sustain longer. Moreover, environmental factors, such as microgravity, can alter normal muscle physiology, leading to muscle atrophy and diminished functional capacity. Studies of muscle atrophy in prolonged weightlessness, including the investigation of physiological and biochemical changes, have focused on the need for countermeasures to attenuate muscle strength and endurance loss (Herbison et al.). In general, a complete picture of muscle energy sources for contraction not only explains fundamental muscle biology but also reveals how to construct training to optimize sports performance and to avoid muscle wasting in disease, including that described in the investigation of gastrointestinal motility and its connection to muscle (Atabai et al., 2016).

Test Your Knowledge

1. What is the sliding filament theory, and how do actin and myosin filaments interact to produce muscle contraction?
2. How is ATP used in the contraction and relaxation of muscle fibers.

3.4. Muscle Metabolism

Learning Outcome

1. Identify the anaerobic vs. aerobic metabolism;
2. Define the ATP production and usage;
3. Describe the lactic acid and muscle fatigue.

Muscle metabolism is accountable for playing a central role in the world's physiology of skeletal muscle, with energy production being an inherent component of muscular function and activity. The mechanisms of muscle metabolism can be divided into two primary pathways: anaerobic and aerobic metabolism. Anaerobic metabolism provides instant energy for short, high-intensity activity via glycolysis, the process of glucose to lactate conversion. Aerobic metabolism utilizes oxygen to produce ATP from fatty acids and glucose over longer periods, supplying a long-term energy solution for prolonged effort. This double role allows the muscle to acclimate to altered demands, supporting performance over a spectrum of physical effort, ranging from sprinting to endurance activities. These metabolic pathways should be understood because they influence training programs, rehabilitative processes, and the management of muscle-related conditions, revealing how muscle function and the energy systems interact. Aging and muscle metabolism is a critical field of research, particularly on sarcopenia's causation, muscle loss and strength loss that occurs with advancing age. Existing evidence affirms that impaired myogenesis, muscle development, and mitochondrial damage are key contributors to sarcopenia (Belli et al., 2019). Muscle quality loss can lead to reduced physical activity capacity, further exacerbating the problem of aging. Mechanisms to reverse muscle metabolism with pharmacological interventions, including the use of metabolic modulators like trimetazidine, have been demonstrated to stimulate myogenic gene expression and enhance oxidative metabolism in senescent skeletal muscle. These measures, in that they improve mitochondrial protein synthesis, could reverse the effect of aging on muscle function and the quality of life of elderly adults. In addition, the adaptability of the musculoskeletal system reveals the importance of knowledge on muscle metabolism in various circumstances, particularly in disuse, such as long-duration space travel. It is evident from research that weightlessness results in extensive musculoskeletal unloading, which has adverse effects on muscle function and structure (N/A). The changes that occur under such conditions are of utmost relevance to examine, as they offer insights into the processes of muscle metabolism and its recovery. Effective countermeasures need to be designed to protect muscle function from sustained inactivity. For this reason, acquiring knowledge from disuse effects on metabolism increases the complexity of our understanding of muscle physiology, as it offers avenues for training improvement, rehabilitation, and overall musculoskeletal health (Figure 3.11).

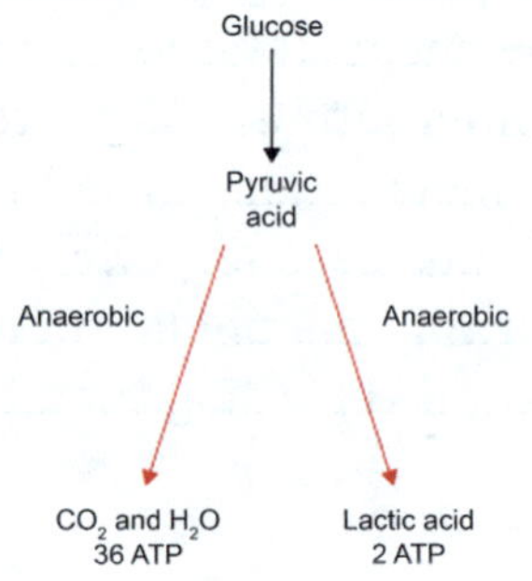

Figure 3.11. Muscle metabolism.

Source: https://ars.els-cdn.com/content/image/3-s2.0-B9780128042540000053-f05-20-9780128042540.jpg.

3.4.1. Aerobic Versus Anaerobic Metabolism

The distinction between aerobic and anaerobic metabolism lies at the heart of an understanding of muscle physiology, particularly as it relates to energy production during exercise. Aerobic metabolism uses oxygen to convert substrates, mainly carbohydrates and lipids, into ATP, which supplies energy for long-term, lower-intensity exercise. This process occurs in the mitochondria and is highly efficient, generating a great deal of ATP from every molecule of glucose. Anaerobic metabolism, conversely, takes place without oxygen and is primarily employed during high-energy activities that exceed the aerobic system's limit. This pathway allows for rapid generation of ATP through glycolysis but is accompanied by the creation of lactate, which will lead to muscle fatigue and dulled performance. Understanding of these two pathways helps to shed light on the ways different kinds of training and exercise shape overall muscle function and endurance. The shift from anaerobic to aerobic metabolism also helps in determining an athlete's performance in different activities. During brief intervals of high-intensity exercise, like sprint or weightlifting exercises, the body's anaerobic mechanisms are used to meet short-term energy demands, confirmed by the rapid decline in muscle glycogen stores. It has been shown through research that some training modalities like Sprint Interval Training (SIT) have the ability to bring about adaptations in aerobic and anaerobic capacity, perhaps supporting overall performance while minimizing time investment (Hurst et al., 2014). For instance, SIT athletes possess greater maximal oxygen uptake (VO2max), which leads to improved endurance function. Consequently, a balanced training regimen consisting of anaerobic and aerobic exercise can optimize physiological adaptation and performance at various intensities. Furthermore, metabolic processes regulating muscle fatigue offer important information regarding sustainability during long-duration exercise. Research has shown anaerobic endeavors provide transient bursts of strength and power but are unsustainable due to the accumulation of metabolic by-products , such as lactate, which can have a detrimental effect on performance (Bundle et al., 2017). The relationship between muscular force and endurance illustrates how fatigue changes based on the energy systems being utilized, with aerobic metabolism allowing for greater exercise durations and recuperation through its efficiency at resynthesizing ATP. This provides understanding of the importance of training procedures that develop both metabolic pathways, so athletes may engage in both high-intensity sprinting and longer endurance activities. Lastly, it is within the interaction between aerobic and anaerobic metabolism that training programs need to be tailored to optimally enhance sport performance while optimally improving capacities for recovery.

3.4.2. Adenosine Triphosphate (ATP) Production and Usage

ATP is the predominant energy currency of muscle physiology, supplying energy for muscle contraction, biochemical events and cellular function. The production of ATP occurs in three large routes: substrate-level phosphorylation, oxidative phosphorylation, and the creatine phosphate system. In striated muscle, especially in terms of increased energy demand, the production of ATP is primarily based on oxidative phosphorylation by the mitochondria. Not only does this yield enormous amounts of ATP, but also contributes to determining the muscle's endurance and exercise adaptability as it aligns substrate supply with oxygen supply. Understanding the intricate processes of ATP synthesis and regulation is key to understanding how muscular energy demands are met during varying exercises, ranging from aerobic exercise to anaerobic short bursts of explosive strength. Efficiency of ATP utilization is also key in muscle physiology and has direct implications on muscle function as well as recovery. ATP is used quickly in contraction; during muscle fiber contraction, hydrolysis of ATP provides energy for the cross-bridge cycling process for actin and myosin filaments to interact appropriately. Magnesium, the second highest intracellular cation, complexes with ATP, thereby influencing its bioavailability and utilization in enzymatic processes. Within muscle tissue, the role of magnesium is not only the stabilization of ATP but also affects enzyme activity for energy production and regulates ion transport across cell membranes, ultimately controlling muscle contractility and metabolic activities. The intracellular ratio of magnesium may significantly affect not only the efficacy of ATP but also the function of muscle per se, exhibiting the prominence of the mineral in energy metabolism (Nassiri et al., 2024). Recent work has shown that growth factors, such as insulin-like growth factor 1 (IGF1), have the ability to further enhance ATP production in skeletal muscle, especially in training adaptations. By inducing differentiation of myoblasts to mature myotubes, IGF1 induces physiological transformation which not only adds to contractile protein quantity but also triggers mitochondrial biogenesis. This results in higher ATP production and higher oxidative capacity, enabling the skeletal muscle to sustain activity for longer durations without exhaustion. Additionally, IGF1 has been found to be responsible for enabling the muscles to respond to insulin, thus enabling glucose uptake necessary in the generation of ATP. These findings demonstrate a relationship between parameters of ATP production and muscle metabolism, which may be addressed for therapeutic purposes in pathologies like type 2 diabetes and muscle disease, demonstrating the broader potential of ATP dynamics in health and disease (Dreher et al., 2023) (Figure 3.12).

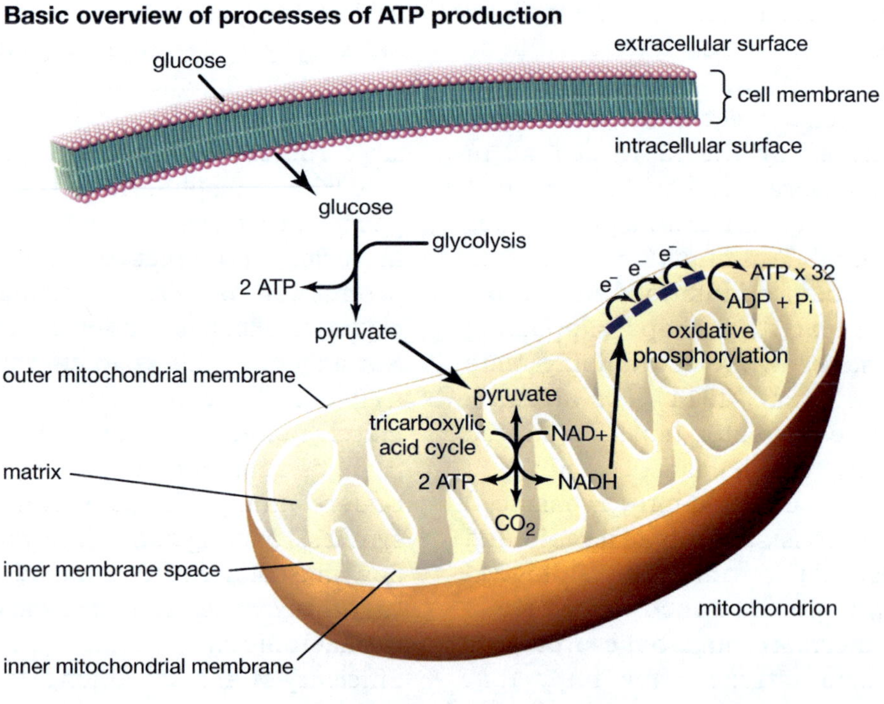

Figure 3.12. Processes-production- Adenosine triphosphate (ATP)-glycolysis-tricarboxylic-acid-cycle.

Source: https://cdn.britannica.com/78/117278-050-576B132B/processes-production-ATP-glycolysis-tricarboxylic-acid-cycle.jpg.

3.4.3. Lactic Acid and Muscle Fatigue

The muscle and lactic acid physiology has been an area of interest in muscle physiology research. During high-intensity effort by muscles, the anaerobic metabolism comes with a high reliance on the body during the activity and yields lactic acid by quick formation. It is a chemical that results from the incomplete oxidation of glucose when there is insufficient oxygen and rises in the blood during strenuous work. As lactic acid accumulates, it may impair muscle function by interfering with metabolic processes and altering pH levels, producing the sensation of fatigue. Interestingly, the accumulation of lactic acid is not solely to be blamed for muscle fatigue; other processes , such as the depletion of energy and ionic imbalance, also have important roles. Consequently, while lactic acid has been associated with the decline in muscle performance, it is important to view it in the broader context of a number of mechanisms contributing to the decline. There has been a notable advance in what is known about the role of lactic acid in fatigue of muscles, with specific reference to recovery. Active recovery, whereby exercise of low intensity is done, has been seen to facilitate faster elimination of lactic acid than passive rest. It is during active recovery that the level of blood lactate decreases more rapidly, a factor significant in enabling efficient recovery after maximal exercise. A study indicates that engaging in activities that cause a heightened heart rate enables enhanced metabolic lactate clearance and hence minimizes symptoms of fatigue and enhances future performance. Lactic acid's physiological response is also further complicated by the level of exercise; higher levels of lactate equate to increased muscular effort, which in turn acts to accentuate the need for personalized recovery programs based on one's physical exertion levels and metabolic demands. As such, an appreciation of the relationship is paramount to maximizing athletic performance and recovery protocols. Furthermore, studies on the effects of various recovery modalities on lactic acid levels have yielded important results. For instance, low-level laser therapy has been evaluated in terms of its effectiveness in diminishing muscle fatigue based on modulation of biochemical indices like blood lactate and levels of cortisol. However, evidence suggests that laser therapy is not highly effective in clearing lactic acid, and this result demonstrates the need for future research in the field. The interactions between exercise, lactic acid accumulation, and muscle fatigue are complex, influenced by numerous variables , such as age, sex, nutrition, and exercise type. Elucidation of the dynamics requires an integrated approach to training and recovery in both sport and clinical populations, with the ultimate impact of furthering muscle physiology research and its translation to exercise science. As the mechanisms are researched further, there remains a need to devise effective strategies for regulating lactic acid production and minimizing muscle fatigue.

Test Your Knowledge

1. What are the principal energy systems utilized by muscle cells in short, moderate, and long exercise?
2. How do muscle cells control lactic acid accumulation during exhausting exercise?

3.5. Muscle Adaptation and Growth

Learning Outcome

1. Describe the hypertrophy vs. atrophy;
2. Define the function of resistance training;
3. Explain the influence of diet on muscle growth.

Muscle adaptation and growth are mostly the byproducts of the mechanotransduction process, which refers to the mechanism by which muscle cells respond to mechanical stress through physiological adaptation. Muscles, once subjected to resistance training or stress, undergo microtearing, resulting in a cascade of biological events aimed at repairing and hypertrophying. This adaptive response is characterized by increased synthesis of muscle proteins and satellite cell recruitment, effectively enlarging and strengthening muscle fibers. These are reflections of the muscles' inherent plasticity, an important feature that allows it to survive with varying conditions of mechanical loading or unloading. Understanding these processes is essential to developing successful training interventions with ensuing superior muscle remodeling and performance improvement. In states of prolonged weightlessness, such as during space travel, the musculoskeletal system is faced with the extreme unloading condition, leading to decreased muscle activity with subsequent atrophy.

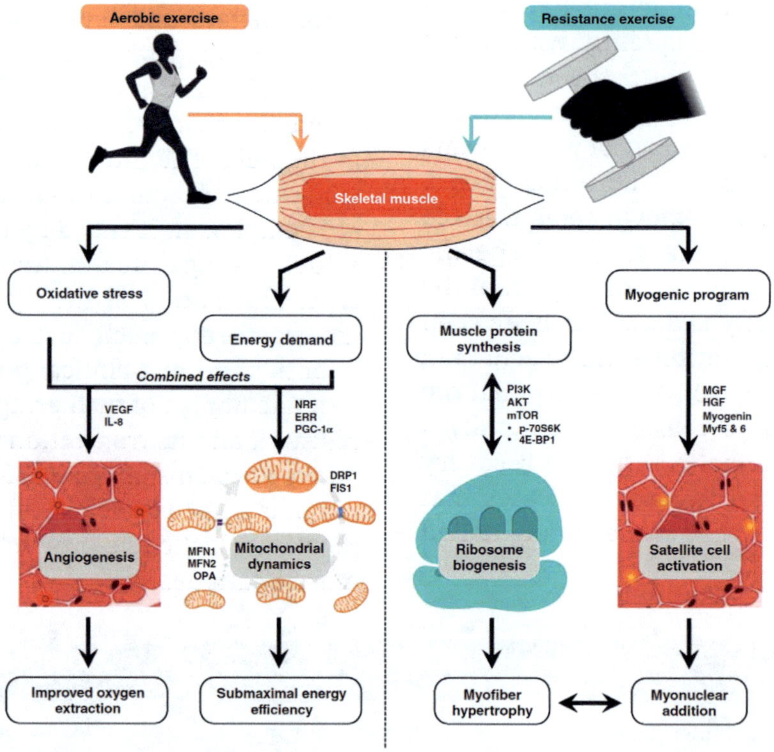

Figure 3.13. Key skeletal muscle adaptations to aerobic and resistance exercise, highlighting the role of molecular transducers of these effects.

Source: https://www.researchgate.net/profile/Liliana-Baptista-2/publication/359123021/figure/fig2/AS:1133151460036616@1647175769946/This-figure-illustrates-key-skeletal-muscle-adaptations-to-aerobic-and-resistance.png.

The adaptive muscle response under such conditions is an indication of the system's ability to alter its functional and structural characteristics under decreased stimuli. In fact, the prevailing NASA studies emphasize the need for countermeasures to defend against the harmful effects of muscle disuse in long-duration missions. The findings highlight that in the absence of physical activity, skeletal muscle can rapidly transition to a state of disuse, creating functional impairments. The above information is not only significant when considering space travel but also serves to highlight the importance of ensuring that muscle integrity is retained through appropriate physical interventions in any occupation where muscle unloading presents a problem (Zhang et al., 2020). The development of sarcopenia, or the wasting of muscle that occurs through the aging process, further indicates that muscle adaptation is multifaceted. As age increases, the acquisition of adiposity is usually coupled with muscle loss, and this twinning is clinically significant. The coexistence of muscle loss with fat gain has been shown to independently correlate with compromised physical function and enhanced risk of illness in the elderly. Remarkably, studies over the past few years have shown that muscle quality, as measured by the muscle's contractile efficiency and muscle fiber composition, can be more significant than muscle amount. The regional effects of increased adiposity around skeletal muscle can disturb the environment of the muscle, increasing the processes of muscle degeneration and putting emphasis on interventions aimed not just at muscle preservation but also at overcoming the stressors of adiposity to effectively treat sarcopenia (Carter et al., 2019) (Figure 3.13).

3.5.1. Hypertrophy Versus Atrophy

It is crucial in the context of muscle physiology to understand the contrast between hypertrophy and atrophy as both are significant to the adaptation and maintenance of muscle mass. Hypertrophy refers to the increase in muscle fiber diameter due to an assortment of stimuli, most commonly resistance training, while atrophy is a reduction in muscle mass that is often induced by disuse or other harmful forces , such as disease or aging. The relative equilibrium between these mutual processes is largely governed by factors like diet, hormonal content, and the applied mechanical loads on the muscle, which demonstrates the plasticity of the skeletal muscle. Hypertrophic capacity demonstrates the adaptive nature of muscle tissue, as it adjusts to increased loads by developing more myofibrillar proteins and cellular components, which thereby improves muscle fibers' strength and overall strength. Alternatively, muscle atrophy is a significant issue, especially for populations who experience long times of inactivity, such as the elderly or space travelers with zero-gravity exposure. Reports indicate that aging can accelerate disuse-induced loss of strength and muscle mass by reducing the recovery of muscles after disuse periods. One study revealed that older rats recovered muscle mass from a hindlimb unloading phase more slowly than their young counterparts, further indicating the role played by neuromuscular transmission and proteostasis in recovery in muscle (Baar et al., 2016). The generation of markers of stress and disruption of protein degradation pathways also impede the process of recovery, indicating how extended disuse leads to structural and functional impairment of muscle tissue. Furthermore, muscle atrophy is significantly exacerbated by conditions that involve severe unloading, such as in extended-duration space flights. The musculoskeletal system is highly resilient, with an ability to react to stimuli; however, prolonged weightlessness induces detrimental structural changes (Zhang et al., 2020). The physiological implication of this process is dire, with astronauts being able to lose muscle mass and strength, necessitating effective countermeasures against these effects.

Understanding the subtle distinctions between hypertrophy and atrophy not only informs the prescription of training and rehabilitation programs but also indicates increased focus on building muscular health through targeted interventions within ground and space environments (Figure 3.14).

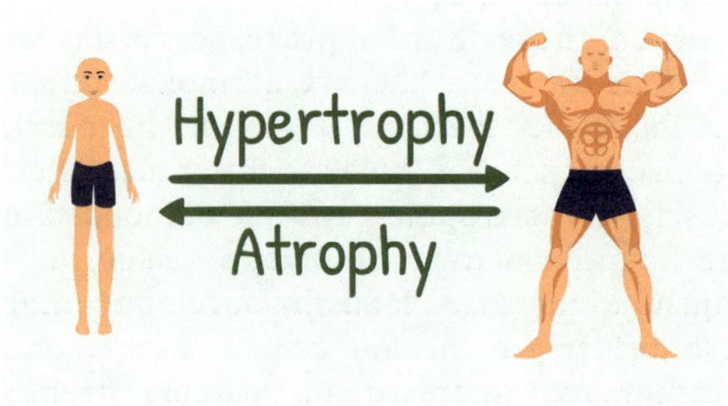

Figure 3.14. Hypertrophy and atrophy essential within the framework of muscle physiology.

Source: https://i.ytimg.com/vi/9Mo-7HCs1Rs/maxresdefault.jpg.

3.5.2. Role of Resistance Training

Resistance training has a particularly prominent influence on muscle physiology through its capacity to induce muscle hypertrophy and enhance muscular strength. By regular resistance training, the muscle fibers experience microtrauma that induces a cascade of biological processes that culminate in muscle repair and growth. Muscle protein synthesis is induced by mechanical tension and metabolic stress, which stimulate various signaling pathways like the mTOR pathway that is required for muscle protein synthesis. The adaptation to increased resistance not only increases growth but also increases the effectiveness and efficiency of muscle contractions and, in turn, increases the overall functional ability of individuals. As has been seen in ongoing research, force-velocity peak power can lead to improved sporting performance, and thus varied training methods based on specific muscular adaptations are essential (Brenneman et al., 2016). Furthermore, resistance training is an important intervention for the prevention and attenuation of the effects of physical inactivity, which is associated with various health issues, including obesity and cardiovascular disease. Resistance exercise participation, systematic in nature, enhances skeletal muscle function, thereby positively influencing metabolic rates and energy expenditure. The aspect is of special significance in light of rising issues associated with sedentary behavior. Resistance training not only enhances muscular strength but also enhances endurance and metabolic well-being, providing a multifaceted approach to fitness and overall health.

Additionally, the efforts to generate exercise mimetics have also gained recognition as a potential alternative for people who are unable to execute traditional forms of exercise, and it emphasizes the role of resistance training in creating optimum muscle physiology and overall health (Handschin et al., 2014). In addition, the function of resistance training goes beyond physical adjustments, having an impact on mental and emotional health. Strength training in a regular capacity has been shown to be associated with enhanced mood as well as fewer symptoms of depression and anxiety. This psychophysical relationship is critical, as the advantages of resistance training are transcendent, carrying over into many areas of an individual's life, such as enhancing self-efficacy and body image. The discipline of abiding by a consistent resistance training program builds up resilience and a sense of accomplishment that can be translated to other aspects of life. As muscle physiology is still a focal point of scientific inquiry, the combination of resistance training concepts not only enhances physical health but also brings about a whole-person approach to health, proving the extensive impact of this exercise mode on human physiology and psychology (Figure 3.15).

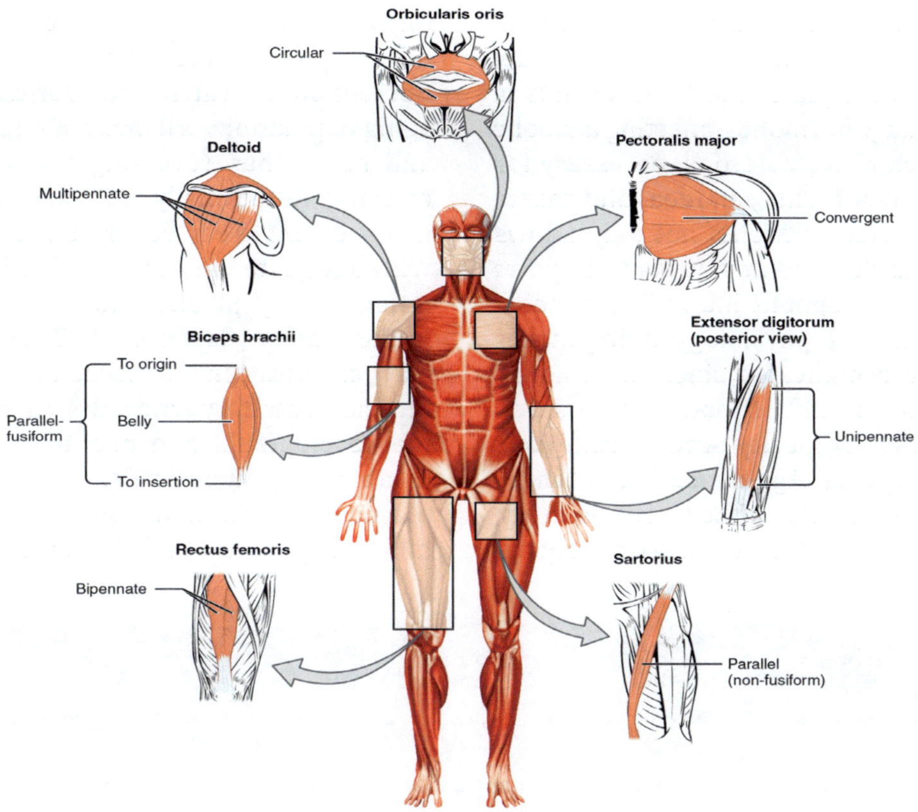

Figure 3.15. Role in shaping muscle physiology.

Source: https://nurseslabs.com/wp-content/uploads/2017/07/Thyroid-and-Parathyroid-Glands-Muscular-System.jpg.

3.5.3. Impact of Nutrition on Muscle Growth

Nutrition plays a key role in muscle development since it serves as the primary stimulus for muscle hypertrophy and overall health. As the body undergoes resistance training, physiological adjustment entails micro-tears in muscle fibers that need optimal nutritional support for their repair and construction. Proteins are a central part, as they provide the amino acids that are used for muscle protein synthesis. Appropriate macronutrient consumption, and indeed of protein and carbohydrates in particular, is necessary following exercise, as these assist with the replenishment of muscle glycogen and optimization of muscle recovery. Some food constituents have also been shown to modulate anabolic signaling pathways, which amplify the muscle-building response. For instance, the timing of nutrient intake relative to exercise can profoundly affect muscle adaptation, and this points towards the important aspect of nutrient timing for optimizing sporting performance and the development of the muscle. The function of micronutrients in muscle physiology cannot be overemphasized, given that they have supporting roles in enzymic reactions that are relevant to energy metabolism and muscle recovery. Vitamins and minerals support metabolic functions for the contraction, repair, and growth of muscles. For instance, vitamin D and calcium are important to muscle function, while antioxidant vitamins C and E can curtail oxidative stress from intense exercises and therefore help maintain muscle tissue. Additionally, good equilibrium between fats is required to manage hormones, affecting anabolic hormones , such as testosterone, necessary for muscle development. Thus, an ideal diet that is rich in many varied nutrients not only allows for optimal muscle growth but also supports muscle quality throughout life and is hence a component of muscle physiology. Aging makes nutrition more complicated since, with aging, muscle loss and a shift in body composition towards increased adiposity occur, putting one at risk of sarcopenia. Age-dependent changes in the quality of muscle, rather than quantity, have been hypothesized to be due to inadequate nutrition and can themselves lead to reduced physical performance and enhanced risk of disability as observed in research on sarcopenia. Correction of nutritional deficiencies among aging populations will maintain muscle function and mass, thus reversing the adverse effects of aging. Additionally, personalized nutritional management to correct protein intake in tandem with adequate caloric intake will enhance the inflammatory profile and metabolic response in the elderly (Carter et al., 2019). In the same way, clarification of mechanisms that govern muscle growth, particularly in terms of early life development and nutritional optimization in animals , such as fish, highlights the role played by nutrition in muscle physiology during different phases of life (Valente et al., 2013).

Test Your Knowledge

1. What cellular and molecular adjustments occur in muscle tissue due to resistance training-induced hypertrophy?
2. How do endurance and strength training affect various muscle fiber types and metabolic pathways differently?

3.6. Muscle Disorders and Diseases

Learning Outcome

1. Describe the most common muscle disorders;
2. Define the effect of aging on muscle function;
3. Specify the rehabilitation and treatment of muscle injury.

Muscle disorders and diseases encompass a wide range of conditions that significantly impact muscle function and overall well-being. Muscle disorders are often caused by genetic mutation, autoimmune processes, or neurodegenerative processes that alter muscle physiology. For instance, myopathies, or muscle tissue diseases, can be brought about by hereditary diseases , such as muscular dystrophy or acquired diseases , such as polymyositis. The manifestations of such diseases are often characterized by muscle cramps, atrophy, and weakness and severely compromise an individual's mobility and quality of life. It is necessary to know the mechanisms behind these conditions to create effective therapeutic interventions and treatment plans that are capable of restoring muscular function and alleviating symptoms, pointing to the intricate interrelationship between muscle wellness and greater body systems. Further, understanding of muscle disorders also necessitates consideration of the interaction between the muscular system and hormonal control of the body. Hormonal shifts, and most notably those concerning sex hormones , such as estrogen and progesterone, have been identified to alter the physiology of muscles, with potential for influence over the symptomatology of various muscular ailments. For example, recent research indicates that hormonal imbalances may exacerbate symptoms of muscle disorders by some effect on muscle metabolism and regeneration. Investigation of the role of such hormones in muscle disease has the potential to reveal novel targets for therapy, symptom alleviation as well as the correction of hormone imbalance underlying muscle pathology. The hormonal profile thus provides an essential background against which to evaluate the subtleties of muscle disease and how it affects overall well-being (Linson et al., 2013). Also, modern research stresses the interdependence of psychological and motor systems in muscle disorders as postulating a triadic relationship between mind, brain, and body. As per this psychomotor theory, movement disturbances may express concealed psychological states and, inversely, psychological states may be reflected in consequent movement disturbances, determining the need for an integrated treatment strategy.

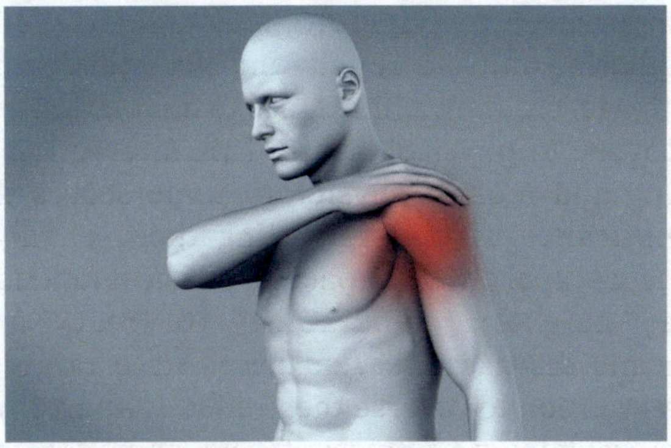

Figure 3.16. Muscle diseases.

Source: https://lonestarneurology.net/wp-content/uploads/2024/05/1-Top-10-Muscle-Diseases-List-Symptoms-Treatments.jpg.

For instance, neurologic diseases that impinge on motor function are invariably linked with psychological disturbance, and this implies that interventions for stimulating muscle strength are also likely to increase mental health. Via this psychomotor relationship, practitioners can develop more integrated treatment regimens that address the motor and psychological aspects of muscle disorders and eventually develop a more integrated approach to patient management in muscle physiology (Tan et al., 2007) (Figure 3.16).

3.6.1. Common Muscle Disorders (Muscular Dystrophy)

Muscle disorders , such as muscular dystrophy have a significant impact on muscle function and lead to progressive weakening and degeneration of skeletal muscle fibers. Of all the types, Duchenne muscular dystrophy (DMD) is very severe, occurring mostly in boys and characterized by early presentation of symptoms. This condition is caused by mutations in the dystrophin gene, which is essential for preserving muscle fiber structural integrity. Lack of dystrophin makes fibers more susceptible to fibrillational stress, leading to damage and necrosis of muscles. In advanced stages, chronic inflammation is a key factor in pathophysiological changes. Infiltration by inflammatory cells, with subsequent release of cytokines and chemokines, contributes to the enhancement of muscle fiber damage and complicates regeneration processes. Understanding the dynamics of such inflammatory processes is of greatest relevance for the creation of specific therapeutic strategies to prevent disease progression in DMD patients (De Paepe & De Bleecker, 2013). Besides DMD, all other muscular dystrophies come under the category of dystroglycanopathies, where alpha-dystroglycan glycosylation is typically impaired. The conditions indicate the significant role that glycosylation plays in muscle function and stability. LARGE is one of the most important enzymes that facilitate proper glycosylation of alpha-dystroglycan, and its dysfunction is associated with several muscular dystrophies. Experiments have indicated that overexpression of LARGE has been capable of causing hyperglycosylation of alpha-dystroglycan, potentially restoring it to function within the diseased tissues. Model organism research indicates that intramuscular delivery of the LARGE enzyme not only improves glycosylation but also is a promising therapeutic avenue for individuals suffering from such specific muscular conditions. The importance of the implications of such results illustrates the valuable line of future investigation and treatment of muscular dystrophies (Brockington et al., 2010).

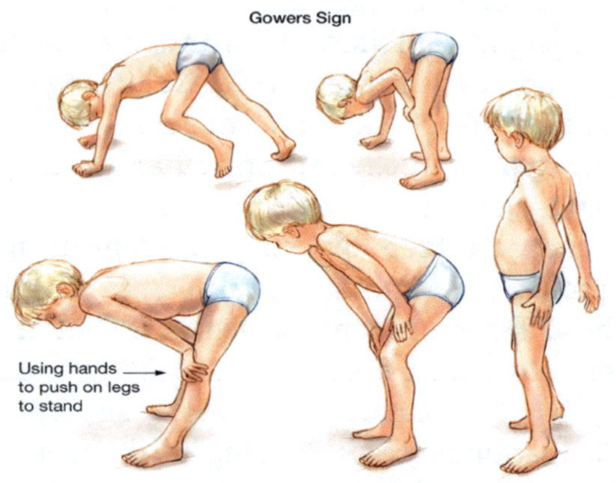

Figure 3.17. Duchenne muscular dystrophy (DMD).

Source: https://ordindia.in/wp-content/uploads/2021/12/DMD.png.

It is essential to overcome the issues posed by common muscle disorders through a multifaceted strategy in both research and treatment models. Considering that inflammation, structural integrity, and enzymatic function are all integral to creating a comprehensive understanding of the intricacies of muscular dystrophies. Future therapies can be facilitated by intervention in the resulting biochemical pathways of these disorders. As an example, pharmacologic therapies that are aimed at raising LARGE expression have the potential to correct glycosylation processes and possibly reconstitute muscle function. Furthermore, knowledge on the relationship between inflammation and muscle degeneration could offer opportunities for immunomodulatory therapies. Later on, with research still unfolding, the focus will be directed on how to translate these scientific discoveries into effective treatments, transforming the landscape of patient care for those afflicted with muscular diseases (Figure 3.17).

3.6.2. Impact of Aging on Muscle Function

As age overtakes an individual, there is a remarkable decline in muscle function, largely characterized by a diminishment of muscle mass and strength, terms applied together referred to as sarcopenia. This age-dependent effect is also exacerbated by alterations in muscle fiber makeup, a change from fast-twitch fibers that facilitate rapid movement to slow-twitch fibers, which are endurance-oriented. These alterations lower the overall functioning of muscles for contractile force required during daily activities, thus affecting quality of life negatively. Furthermore, physiological mechanisms regulating muscle repair and growth decline with age, creating a hindrance to adaptation and recovery to physical stress. This interaction of aging and muscle physiology underscores the significance of understanding these changes because, apart from impacting physical function, they heighten vulnerability to injury and chronic disease and also necessitate targeted intervention to reverse these effects. Apart from the breakdown of muscle tissue, aging directly correlates with mitochondrial dysfunction in skeletal muscle fibers. Mitochondria play a crucial role in energy production, and when they are impaired, muscle function suffers profoundly as energy demands during physical performance increase. The overall impact of mitochondrial inefficiency can lead to dysfunctional muscle metabolism, which in turn is related to a high risk for metabolic disease. Mitochondrial disease in skeletal muscle is not only troubling in the context of aging but also coincides with a number of neuromuscular illnesses, revealing an intricate interaction between muscle fibers and energy-producing apparatuses. Such interactions suggest that therapeutic manipulations that maximize mitochondrial functioning can produce beneficial effects not only within clinical samples but also in the aging population trying to maintain muscle function and quality of life (Bernardino Gomes et al., 2023). Evidence from recent research indicates that exercise interventions, particularly strength training, are able to reverse the deteriorating impact of aging on the function of muscles. Anticipatory maneuvers can stimulate muscle hypertrophy, enhance strength, and improve general physical function.

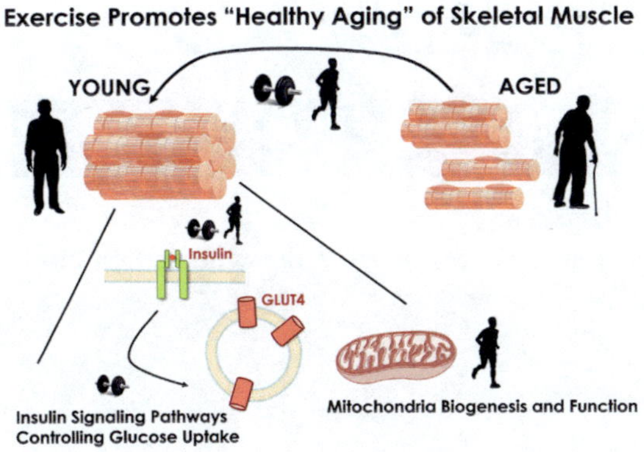

Figure 3.18. Exercise promotes healthy aging of skeletal muscle.

Source: https://www.cell.com/cms/10.1016/j.cmet.2016.05.007/asset/2e252275-7e37-4276-a013-3a62536f5f21/main.assets/gr1_lrg.jpg.

Creatine supplementation has been an adjunctive option, with potential to augment lean muscle mass and maximize strength even in older adults who have a tendency to lose muscle. With this in mind, regular resistance training accompanied by dietary interventions emerges as a holistic approach to treat sarcopenia. By doing this, not only can one retain muscle function into older age, but also improve tolerance to treatment-related adverse effects, especially in patients with underlying illness. Thus, meeting the challenges of aging and muscle physiology with multi-component interventions is essential for fostering active and independent aging (Fairman et al., 2018) (Figure 3.18).

3.6.3. Rehabilitation and Treatment Options

Rehabilitation and treatment options for muscle injury are gaining more attention in clinical and academic circles because they play a crucial part in recovery and functionality. A complete rehabilitation program most commonly includes physical therapy, with an emphasis on gradual recovery of strength, flexibility, and proprioception. The evidence shows that impairment of balance is particularly significant, as instability can be a time-waster and can contribute to a higher risk of subsequent injury. Patients with chronic symptoms following injury, e.g., post-concussion syndrome (PCS), are more likely to experience issues with balance control, which may also impede the rehabilitation process. Thus, specifically targeted interventions to enhance postural muscle activation are essential to maximize results in this population. Rehabilitative protocols using consideration of muscle physiology are able to offer tailored strategies, which may greatly improve functional recovery and guarantee longevity of musculoskeletal system health (Cinelli et al., 2017). In addition to standard physical therapy, new treatment modalities are becoming increasingly significant as integral components of rehabilitation protocols. One potential choice is the use of platelet-rich plasma (PRP) injections, which have received attention for their capacity to enhance healing in the majority of muscular and tendon injuries. This biological treatment capitalizes on the capacity of a patient's own blood for healing, done by concentrating growth factors and other constituents that facilitate tissue regeneration. Its application in the therapy of conditions like rotator cuff tears reveals its significance in rehabilitation because it can result in improved outcomes and potentially shorten the number of surgical interventions. PRP therapy is not only a form of conservative management but also reflects the growing convergence of muscle physiology and regenerative medicine (Loccisano et al., 2016). The integration of these innovative methodologies into the conventional rehabilitative techniques emphasizes the active process of muscle recovery procedures. Moreover, rehabilitative program success is highly dependent on a multidimensional rehabilitation approach suited to the individual patient and the corresponding conditions of injury. A clear understanding of the mechanical and physiological processes involved in muscle function and recovery is critical for clinicians in developing effective rehabilitation protocols. Variables like age, activity level, and severity of injury should be taken into account to ensure the highest possible effectiveness of treatment protocols. For example, older people who are experiencing rotator cuff injuries can react differently to conservative versus operative treatments because the risks of surgery become greater with advancing age. Thus, meticulous consideration of each patient's unique case in combination with evidence-based interventions can lead to more pleasing outcomes. Lastly, rehabilitation for restored muscle function needs to be as diverse and adaptable as the injury it poses difficulties, reinforcing that in muscle physiology individualized care is paramount (Loccisano et al., 2016).

Test Your Knowledge

1. What are the primary causes and manifestations of muscular dystrophy?
2. How does myasthenia gravis interfere with neuromuscular transmission, and what is the contribution of autoantibodies to the disease?

SUMMARY

A thorough understanding of muscle physiology is a prerequisite for many purposes, ranging from the optimization of sporting performance to the prevention and rehabilitation of injury. Advances over the last decade or so have proved the sophistication of muscle function, where the type of muscle fiber, recruitment of motor units, and energy metabolism are central concerns. The findings point to the significance of personalized training programs for athletes, according to their specific needs in their sport as well as to individual physiological responses. This tacit knowledge assists in the development of an adequate conditioning plan that optimizes performance while protecting against risks of injury, as evidenced by the deep contrasts between running requirements of field hockey players and the associated developments in training regimes for their individual playing roles, according to Van der Merwe & Haggie (2018). Moreover, the growing popularity of using various forms of stimuli, such as menthol, in sports performance training is indicative of a shift towards cross-disciplinary models of muscle physiology research. Research has discovered that menthol application can enhance performance outcomes by triggering a perceptual cooling response with a positive impact on physical and psychological exercise parameters. This suggests that sensory interventions will be effectively incorporated into training and competition settings to maximize athlete performance. As demonstrated in Barwood et al. (2019), the ability to customize these methods in line with particular response profiles emphasizes the importance of continued investigation into the way in which different physiological processes react to sensory stimulation in generating positive outcomes on muscle function and overall sporting performance. Finally, interaction between various physiological and psychological factors needs to be resolved through subsequent muscle physiology research by demonstrating how and why these factors are susceptible to manipulation for further optimizing athletic performance. Investigation into the exact mechanisms by which different interventions, for instance, menthol or other cooling interventions, influence muscle function can yield significant data for optimization of both training and competitive strategies. As the field continues to evolve, it will be important to integrate a coordinated view, such as emerging technologies and approaches, to better understand muscle function in various situations. The combined approach will ultimately result in more effective and research-based practice in sports science, enabling enhanced outcomes in athletes and the capacity to preserve their long-term health and performance durability.

The understanding of the fundamental components of muscle physiology becomes crucial in unraveling the complexity of muscle function and pathologies. Of significance is the appreciation of the application of certain animal models , such as the dystrophic mdx mice on the DBA/2J (D2) background for research in DMD. These models carry a polymorphic genetic background that encapsulates enhanced dystropathology compared to the conventional mdx mice, and they therefore constitute a platform for therapeutic intervention assessment. Such models are more than observationally relevant; they contain disease modifiers present in man, providing a good foundation for drug efficacy research and drug development. This collective study seeks to synthesize pathological features of such novel mice and assess their potential applications in preclinical studies, as is evident from findings suggestive of their applicability in comparative studies and identification of knowledge gaps (Aartsma-Rus et al., 2018). In addition, studies on glucocorticoid receptors offer critical insights into non-genomic pathways influencing muscle physiology. The localization of these receptors in various aspects of skeletal muscle cells highlights their multifaceted functions, from myoblasts to myotubes, and even to the extracellular matrix that surrounds adult muscle fibers. Evidence points out that these receptors not only exist at certain sites within cells but also play a key role in mediating fast intramuscular signaling events, including the activation of the mitogen-activated protein kinase (MAPK) pathway. These interactions have the potential to have profound physiological effects, particularly when delivered together with synthetic glucocorticoids like beclomethasone dipropionate. Collectively, these findings significantly aid in the understanding of signaling processes involved in muscle physiology that are not dependent on genomic alterations, further confirming the dynamic nature of muscle responses to hormonal regulation (Steverding et al., 2015).

The global insights achieved through these studies constitute a holistic body of knowledge in muscle physiology. It brings together data from animal models and hormone receptor signaling, pointing out the complexity of the muscular reaction to environmental and genetic conditions. As researchers proceed in exploring the multi-faceted interactions in muscle cells, it is evident that the interaction of genetic components, receptor location, and hormonal regulation remains at the center. Such comparative investigations not only discover the mechanisms involved in muscle function but also inform potential therapeutic interventions towards diseases like DMD and other related diseases. Ultimately, advancing our knowledge in such areas promises us a brighter future of increased treatment modalities regarding muscle wellness and disease prevention, thereby laying the grounds for future advancements in research on muscle physiology.

KEY TERMS FROM THIS CHAPTER

- Acetylcholine (ACh)
- ATP (Adenosine Triphosphate)
- Cross-Bridge Cycle
- Muscle Contraction
- Muscle Twitch
- Neuromuscular Junction
- Sarcomere
- Sliding Filament Theory
- Tetanus
- Troponin
- Actin
- Calcium Ions (Ca^{2+})
- Motor Unit
- Muscle Fatigue
- Myosin
- Sarcolemma
- Sarcoplasmic Reticulum
- Summation
- Tropomyosin
- T-Tubules

CRITICAL THINKING QUESTIONS

1. **What is the functional unit of a skeletal muscle fiber?**
   a. Sarcolemma
   b. Sarcomere
   c. Myofibril
   d. Actin
2. **Which ion is essential for initiating muscle contraction?**
   a. Sodium (Na^+)
   b. Potassium (K^+)
   c. Calcium (Ca^{2+})
   d. Chloride (Cl^-)
3. **Which protein does calcium bind to in initiating muscle contraction?**
   a. Actin
   b. Myosin
   c. Troponin
   d. Tropomyosin
4. **What neurotransmitter is released at the neuromuscular junction?**
   a. Dopamine
   b. Acetylcholine
   c. Serotonin
   d. Norepinephrine
5. **What type of muscle contraction occurs when muscle tension increases but the muscle is not shortened?**
   a. Isotonic contraction
   b. Eccentric contraction
   c. Isometric contraction
   d. Concentric contraction

Short Answer Questions

1. Provide the three categories of muscle tissue.
2. What is the functional unit of a muscle fiber?
3. What protein binds with calcium to facilitate muscle contraction?
4. Describe the similarities and differences among skeletal, cardiac, and smooth muscle in structure, function, and control.
5. Describe the physiological changes that occur in muscles during prolonged exercise.
6. Describe the different types of muscle contractions: isotonic and isometric.
7. Describe the causes and effects of muscle fatigue.
8. Describe the excitation-contraction coupling process in skeletal muscles.

Answers to Critical Thinking Questions

1. (b); 2. (c); 3. (c); 4. (b); 5. (c)

REFERENCES

1. Aartsma-Rus, A., Bogdanik, L., Davies, K., De Luca, A., et al. (2018). "Of mice and measures": A project to improve how we advance Duchenne muscular dystrophy therapies to the clinic. https://core.ac.uk/download/161772638.pdf (accessed on 16th June 2025).
2. https://core.ac.uk/download/61514843.pdf Valente, L.M.P., Moutou, K.A., Conceição, L.E.C., Engrola, S., Fernandes, J.M.O. and Johnston, I.A. (2013), What determines growth potential and juvenile quality of farmed fish species?. Rev Aquacult, 5: S168-S193. https://doi.org/10.1111/raq.12020 (accessed on 16th June 2025).
3. Alicea, B. (2009). Natural variation and neuromechanical systems. https://core.ac.uk/download/pdf/87287.pdf (accessed on 16th June 2025).
4. Alves-Lopes, R., Anagnostopoulou, A., Arner, A., Camargo, D. L., et al. (2018). Vascular smooth muscle contraction in hypertension. https://core.ac.uk/download/150600176.pdf (accessed on 16th June 2025).
5. Asakura, A., Graber, T. G., Kim, J. H., Liu, L., et al. (2019). Increasing myosin light chain 3f (MLC3f) protects against a decline in contractile velocity. https://core.ac.uk/download/304658533.pdf (accessed on 16th June 2025).
6. Atabai, K., Azary, S., Ha, A., Hart, J., et al. (2016). α8β1 integrin regulates nutrient absorption through an Mfge8-PTEN dependent mechanism. https://core.ac.uk/download/323073398.pdf (accessed on 16th June 2025).
7. Baar, K., Baehr, L. M., Bodine, S. C., De Sousa, T. A., et al. (2016). Age-related deficits in skeletal muscle recovery following disuse are associated with neuromuscular junction instability and ER stress, not impaired protein synthesis. https://core.ac.uk/download/323070264.pdf (accessed on 16th June 2025).
8. Baldwin, K., Herrick, R., & Oganov, V. (2025). Experiment K-6-10. Effects of zero gravity on myofibril protein content and isomyosin distribution in rodent skeletal muscle. https://core.ac.uk/download/pdf/42822704.pdf (accessed on 16th June 2025).
9. Barwood, M., Best, R., Gillis, J., Jeffries, D., et al. (2019). Oral application of L-menthol in the heat: From pleasure to performance. https://core.ac.uk/download/287723714.pdf (accessed on 16th June 2025).
10. Zhang, Y., Chen, J. S., He, Q., He, X., Basava, R. R., Hodgson, J., Sinha, U., & Sinha, S. (2020). Microstructural analysis of skeletal muscle force generation during aging. *International journal for numerical methods in biomedical engineering*, *36*(1), e3295. https://doi.org/10.1002/cnm.3295(accessed on 16th June 2025).
11. Belak, M., Boda, K., Kocisova, J., Marcanik, J., et al. (2025). Electron microscopical and histochemical studies on the transverse striated muscles of birds after prolonged hypokinesis. https://core.ac.uk/download/pdf/42858615.pdf (accessed on 16th June 2025).
12. Belli, R., Bonato, A., Caruso, M., Costelli, P., et al. (2019). Metabolic reprogramming promotes myogenesis during aging. https://core.ac.uk/download/231747052.pdf (accessed on 16th June 2025).
13. Bernardino Gomes, T. M., Di Leo, V., & Vincent, A. E. (2023). Interactions of mitochondrial and skeletal muscle biology in mitochondrial myopathy. https://core.ac.uk/download/595485533.pdf (accessed on 16th June 2025).

14. Blottner, D., Ciciliot, S., Furlan, S., Gambara, G., et al. (2017). Gene expression profiling in slow-type calf soleus muscle of 30 days space-flown mice. https://core.ac.uk/download/84921730.pdf (accessed on 16th June 2025).

15. Boonstra, T. W., Faes, L., Kerkman, J. N., Marinazzo, D., et al. (2019). Information decomposition of multichannel EMG to map functional interactions in the distributed motor system. https://core.ac.uk/download/225020486.pdf (accessed on 16th June 2025).

16. Brenneman, M. T. (2016). *Training for Muscular Power Adaptations: The Role of Contraction Type and Velocity*. https://core.ac.uk/download/211333301.pdf (accessed on 16th June 2025).

17. Brockington, M., Brown, S. C., Cirak, S., Liu, L., et al. (2010). Transgenic overexpression of LARGE induces alpha-dystroglycan hyper glycosylation in skeletal and cardiac muscle. https://core.ac.uk/download/1730280.pdf (accessed on 16th June 2025).

18. Bundle, M. W., Hunter, S. K., & Sundberg, C. W. (2017). Rates of performance loss and neuromuscular activity in men and women during cycling: Evidence for a common metabolic basis of muscle fatigue. https://core.ac.uk/download/213083105.pdf (accessed on 16th June 2025).

19. Cammarato, A., Oldfors, A., Knowlton, A. A., Brand, A. H., Monier, B., Zeitouni, B., Stanley, B. A., et al. (2011). The UNC-45 chaperone is critical for establishing myosin-based myofibrillar organization and cardiac contractility in the *Drosophila* heart model. https://core.ac.uk/download/pdf/8598858.pdf (accessed on 16th June 2025).

20. Carter, C. S., Justice, J. N., & Thompson, L. (2019). Lipotoxicity, aging, and muscle contractility: Does fiber type matter? https://open.bu.edu/bitstream/2144/40625/7/carter_justice_thompson_Lipotoxicity_paper_04302019.pdf (accessed on 16th June 2025).

21. Cinelli, M. E., Kalmar, J. M., Kaster, A., et al. (2017). Task-dependent modulation of cortical excitability and balance control in individuals with post-concussion syndrome. https://core.ac.uk/download/143689897.pdf (accessed on 16th June 2025).

22. Crisafulli, A., Marongiu, E., Nobrega, A. C. L., O'Leary, D. S., et al. (2014). Neural regulation of cardiovascular response to exercise: Role of central command and peripheral afferents. https://core.ac.uk/download/pdf/54599119.pdf (accessed on 16th June 2025).

23. De Paepe, B., & De Bleecker, J. L. (2013). Cytokines and chemokines as regulators of skeletal muscle inflammation: presenting the case of Duchenne muscular dystrophy. *Mediators of inflammation, 2013*, 540370. https://doi.org/10.1155/2013/540370h(accessed on 16th June 2025).

24. Debold, E. P., Fitts, R. H., Nosek, T. M., Sundberg, C. W., et al. (2016). Muscle fatigue from the perspective of a single crossbridge. https://core.ac.uk/download/213062126.pdf (accessed on 16th June 2025).

25. Dreher, S., Grubba, P., von Toerne, C., Moruzzi, A., Maurer, J., Goj, T., Birkenfeld, A., et al. (2023). Engineering of human myotubes toward a mature metabolic and contractile phenotype. *bioRxiv*. https://www.semanticscholar.org/paper/80c92b50a72955dfda7a4cd2fdd7e3492646397d (accessed on 16th June 2025).

26. Fairman, C. M., Galvão, D. A., Hart, N. H., Kendall, D., et al. (2018). The potential therapeutic effects of creatine supplementation on body composition and muscle function in cancer. https://core.ac.uk/download/213607833.pdf (accessed on 16th June 2025).

27. Fitts, R. H. (2011). New insights on sarcoplasmic reticulum calcium regulation in muscle fatigue. https://core.ac.uk/download/213085414.pdf (accessed on 16th June 2025).

28. Freeman, C. (2019). *The Effects of Pre and Post Exercise Low-Level Laser Therapy on Biochemical Markers of Skeletal Muscle Fatigue in Equines*. https://core.ac.uk/download/215464245.pdf (accessed on 16th June 2025).

29. Garzia Zizzo, M., Mastropaolo, M., & Serio, R. (2011). The enteric nervous system: New developments and emerging concepts. https://core.ac.uk/download/46602300.pdf (accessed on 16th June 2025).

30. Handschin, C., & Svensson, K. (2014). Modulation of PGC-1α activity as a treatment for metabolic and muscle-related diseases. https://core.ac.uk/download/33298388.pdf (accessed on 16th June 2025).

31. Herbison, G. J., & Talbot, J. M. (2025). Research opportunities in muscle atrophy. https://core.ac.uk/download/pdf/42848744.pdf (accessed on 16th June 2025).

32. Huijing, P. A. (1995). Parameter interdependence and success of skeletal muscle modelling. https://core.ac.uk/download/pdf/11461276.pdf (accessed on 16th June 2025).

33. Hurst, R. A. (2014). *The Effects and Differences of Sprint Interval Training, Endurance Training and The Training Types Combined on Physiological Parameters and Exercise Performance*. https://core.ac.uk/download/29841767.pdf (accessed on 16th June 2025).

34. Ivanov, P. C., Lombardi, F., Rizzo, R., Wang, J. W. J. L., & Zhang, X. (2020). Network physiology of cortico–muscular interactions. https://core.ac.uk/download/576922455.pdf (accessed on 16th June 2025).

35. Kemi, O. J., McIntyre, L., Menzies, C., Menzies, J., et al. (2010). Blood lactate clearance during active recovery after an intense running bout depends on the intensity of the active recovery. https://core.ac.uk/download/80930.pdf (accessed on 16th June 2025).

36. Linson, E. A. (2013). *The Interplay Between Hormones and Irritable Bowel Disease*. https://open.bu.edu/bitstream/2144/12149/6/Linson_Elyse_2013_nosig_nocv.pdf (accessed on 16th June 2025).

37. Loccisano, A. (2016). *Platelet-Rich Plasma for The Treatment of Partial Rotator Cuff Tears*. https://open.bu.edu/bitstream/2144/14355/9/Loccisano_bu_0017N_10415.pdf (accessed on 16th June 2025).

38. Massa, B., Mazzeo, F., Montesano, P., Palermi, S., et al. (2020). From "sliding" to "winding" filaments theory: A narrative review of mechanisms behind skeletal muscle contraction. https://core.ac.uk/download/333885124.pdf (accessed on 16th June 2025).

39. Nassiri, O., Belmahi, S., Amrani, A., Sebbar, E. H., & Choukri, M. (2024). Verification of the analytical performance of the serum magnesium assay on Abbott Architect ci8200. *World Journal of Biology Pharmacy and Health Sciences*. https://www.semanticscholar.org/paper/bdbba1305e53172e85939e446b989ad7a55b4fed (accessed on 16th June 2025).

40. Ptitsyn, A., & Kanatous, S. (2009). Transformation of metabolism with age and lifestyle in Antarctic seals: A case study of systems biology approach to cross-species microarray experiment. https://core.ac.uk/download/pdf/1569887.pdf (accessed on 16th June 2025).

41. Santello, M., & Valero-Cuevas, F. J. (2017). On neuromechanical approaches for the study of biological grasp and manipulation. http://arxiv.org/abs/1710.08557 (accessed on 16th June 2025).

42. Sharma, P. (2012). Role of caveolae and the dystrophin glycoprotein complex in airway smooth muscle phenotype and lung function. https://core.ac.uk/download/644028896.pdf (accessed on 16th June 2025).

43. Steverding, D., Akujuru, E., Protasi, F., Mutungi, G., Goldberg, A. L., Arthurton, L., Boncompagni, S., et al. (2015). Membrane glucocorticoid receptors are localized in the extracellular matrix and signal through the MAPK pathway in mammalian skeletal muscle fibers. https://core.ac.uk/download/41988926.pdf (accessed on 16th June 2025).

44. Subramaniam, S., Wang, Y., & Winters, J. (2012). Functional classification of skeletal muscle networks. I. Normal physiology. https://core.ac.uk/download/213080019.pdf (accessed on 16th June 2025).

45. Tan, Ü. (2007). The psychomotor theory of human mind. https://core.ac.uk/download/pdf/86857.pdf (accessed on 16th June 2025).

46. Van der Merwe, Frans & Haggie, Marrin (2018). *GPS Analysis of a Team Competing at A National Under 18 Field Hockey Tournaments.* https://www.strengthandconditioning.org/jasc-27-5/2377-original-scientific-research-study-gps-analysis-of-a-team-competing-in-a-national-under-18-field-hockey-tournament https://core.ac.uk/download/187724717.pdf (accessed on 16th June 2025).

NERVE PHYSIOLOGY

4

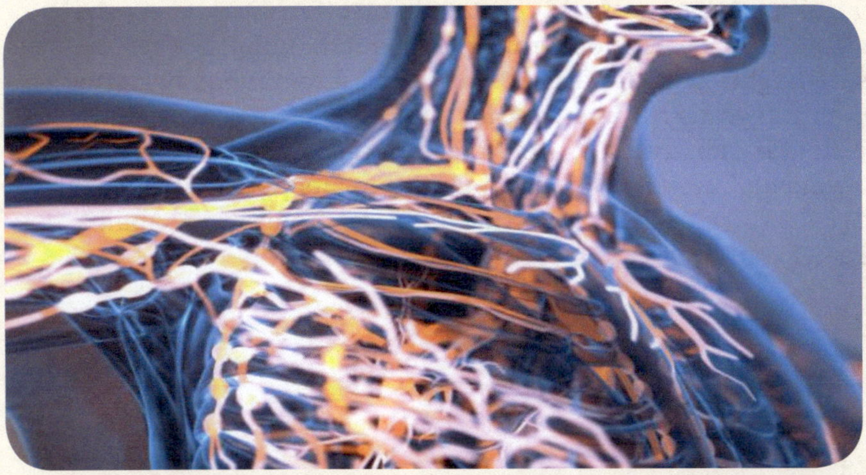

LEARNING OBJECTIVES

After studying this chapter, you will be able to:

1. Explain the structure of neurons;
2. Explain the action potentials in nerve physiology;
3. Explain the synaptic transmission;
4. Identify neurotransmitter systems;
5. Study the propagation of nerve impulses;
6. Evaluate the disorders of nerve physiology.

Introduction

The understanding of nerve physiology is crucial for describing how neural systems operate and respond to stimuli. Nerve cells, or neurons, are the building blocks of the nervous system, with the task of transmitting electrical impulses all over the body. These are specialized cells with their own structure, such as the cell body, dendrites, and axons. The process of signal transmission begins with the generation of action potentials—short electrical alterations in membrane potential by which neurons communicate and talk with other types of cells. This elaborate system of communication allows for the coordination of physiological functions and responses, further establishing the significance of nerve physiology in sustaining homeostasis and ensuring interactions with the outside world, hence forming the basis of broader arguments in neuroscience and similar fields. A significant branch of nerve physiology is synaptic transmission processes, which form the basis of nerve propagation of signals. Once the action potential has arrived at the axon terminals, action potentials cause neurotransmitters to be released into the synapse's cleft. The chemical messengers bind to receptors on the postsynaptic neuron and have a variety of excitatory or inhibitory effects that decide whether further action potentials are generated. This process is far from a straightforward relaying of information, but rather a tightly controlled, dynamic interaction influenced by a number of different factors, including what kind of neurotransmitter. For example, it has been discovered that some neurotransmitters can modulate responses in a differential way, and understanding these nuances is important for understanding neurological disease and health, especially when neurotransmission is compromised. In exploring the physiological foundations of nerve function, research in similar disciplines has begun to uncover the complexities of neural contribution to indices of health. For instance, more recent research has focused on fetal heart rate variability (fHRV) as an index for measuring neural function and health in developing organisms. These experiments have identified specific measures of vagal modulation of fHRV with promise for discovering the neural processes underlying important periods of development. The understanding of the role of the vagus nerves in such measures highlights feedforward and feedback interactions in nerve physiology, underscoring the utility of an integrative framework for the study of neural systems. Such continued investigation into the neural substrates of physiological response, therefore, is crucial not only for furthering our knowledge of nerve physiology but also for its potential clinical applications, as outlined in the trajectories of bioelectronic medicine and fetal monitoring (Abbink et al., 2025; Burns et al., 2019) (Figure 4.1).

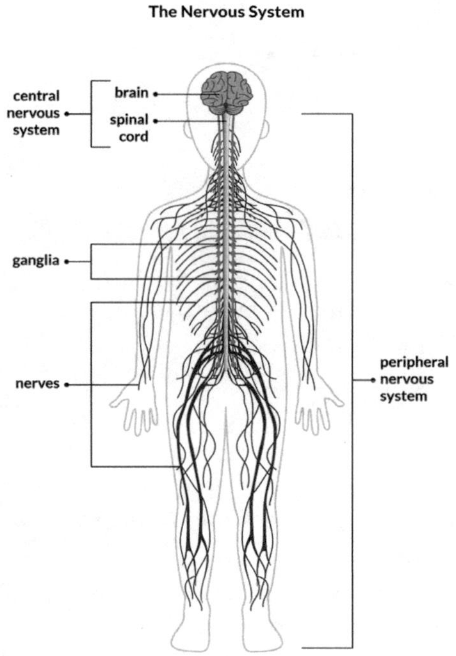

Figure 4.1. Physiology of the nervous system.

Source: https://cdn.cancer.ca/-/media/cams/neuroblastoma/39c12c90-5312-11eb-8c37-0242902869b1-en.png?h=619&iar=0&mw=543&w=543&rev=e9d2dababc544e3cbe71865f43540f0c&hash=20C958E9DE38B602807E9BA2508B0BBA.

Definition of Nerve Physiology

The field of nerve physiology encompasses the intricate science of the process and function of nerves within the nervous system. Nerve physiology examines the fundamental operations of the neurons, specialized cells that transmit electrical impulses to other areas of the body. It entails understanding how action potentials are generated and propagated down axons to facilitate rapid communication between different areas of the body. Furthermore, nerve physiology delves into synaptic transmission, where it places significance on the significant interaction between neurons that facilitates neurotransmitter release and transmission of signals. This connectivity puts a focus on the complexity of neural transmission and acts as a fundamental foundation for studies of various neurological processes and conditions. Among the important aspects of nerve physiology is the investigation of ion channels, which play a significant role in generating the electrical signals that characterize neuronal function. These ion channels are selectively permeable to ions like sodium, potassium, calcium, and chloride, which respond to changes in membrane potential. Repolarization and depolarization reactions, powered by ion movement across the membrane, are pivotal for action potential conduction on nerve fibers. The exact dynamics and kinetics of these ion channels are studied intensively to gain insight into their function in nerve excitability and neurotransmission. Along with that, disruption of these processes can cause a variety of neurological diseases, and the importance of sound knowledge in nerve physiology toward the formulation of a therapeutic approach and intervention. Nerve physiology study also encompasses proper methodologies for the quantification of neuronal behavior and characteristics. The advances in technology, such as electrophysiological recording techniques and imaging methods, have significantly widened the ability to experiment with the function of nerves in the living organism. For instance, the creation of computerized equipment that measures aspects of neuronal morphology makes it possible to subject the influence of structural variation on functional parameters to more stringent testing. Such equipment, which can detect bifurcation geometry subtleties, provides a refinement over usual hand-operated methods, and this suits predictions in modern neuroscience literature very well. Through the combination of experimental data with computational approaches, scientists can better describe the complexity of nerve physiology and its relationship to clinical illness (Kling et al., 1939; Al-Diri et al., 2010).

Importance of Studying Nerve Physiology

The significance of research in nerve physiology extends beyond academic curiosity. It is a foundation for understanding a lot of physiological processes that specify human health and behavior. By studying the way neurons talk to and signal one another in intricate networks, researchers can uncover the causes of neurological disease. This information is useful in designing treatments for diseases , such as Alzheimer's disease, multiple sclerosis, and epilepsy, to name a few. Further, an understanding of nerve physiology can reveal the impact of stress on the body and how chronic stressors influence everything from hormone secretion to immune function. Such multidisciplinary insight underscores the need for an integrated health care approach that combines understanding of brain function with body physiology, as noted by the report of the existence of a gap between brain-based and body-based practitioners in health care (Estrine & DeLisle, 2006). Besides, research in nerve physiology provides critical information regarding the role played by environmental factors in modulating neural function. Various stressors, whether physical, emotional, or environmental in origin, will have a strong impact on the nervous system, producing alterations in behavior and health. By understanding the mechanics of nerve impulses and synaptic transmission, researchers can have a better appreciation of the mechanisms by which extrinsic variables affect stress response. Understanding this is growing more critical in a time of heightened anxiety and stress disorders and requires measures that promote neural integrity. As the brain integrates the body's response to thousands of experiences, understanding nerve physiology becomes critical in controlling the effects of chronic stress on health and integrated practice in medicine (Estrine & DeLisle, 2006).

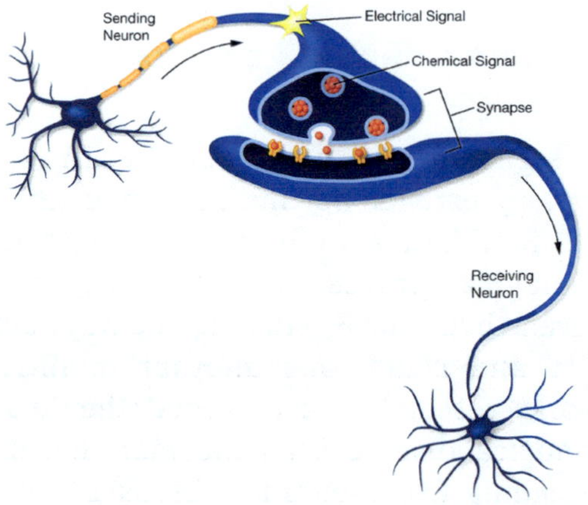

Figure 4.2. Neurons transmit messages in the brain.

Source: https://learn-genetics.b-cdn.net/neuroscience/neurons/neurons-2.jpg.

Lastly, the implications of a study into nerve physiology extend towards the development of new therapeutic approaches to ensure maximum nerve repair and regeneration. Advances in neuroscience have been promising for regenerative medicine, with knowledge of the cellular mechanisms of nerve injury being central. Insights derived from nerve physiology inform the design of targeted therapies, e.g., biomaterials or neuroprotective agents, that can potentially restore function to injured nerves. In light of the increasing frequency of neurological injury and degenerative illnesses, the significance of such studies cannot be overemphasized. Interdisciplinary research in this area promotes a paradigm shift towards more holistic treatments, addressing the preeminent interaction among various body systems and the nervous system as a whole, in keeping with the perception that nerve physiology needs to be comprehensively understood at all levels of scale if human health is to be advanced (Figure 4.2).

Overview of the Nervous System

The nervous system is the body's main headquarters and communication center, and it is vital to maintaining homeostasis and brokering interactions with the environment. The brain, spinal cord, and peripheral nerves constitute the intricate network that enables organisms to detect stimuli, interpret information, and respond through motor systems. Functionally, the nervous system is subdivided into two large units: the central nervous system (CNS) and the peripheral nervous system (PNS). CNS, comprising the brain and spinal cord, consolidates sensory input and organizes voluntary and involuntary movement, while PNS connects CNS to limbs and organs and allows body communication. It is crucial to be aware of the structural and functional hierarchy of the nervous system in an effort to comprehend its function in disease as well as health, illuminating research and clinical avenues.

Within this complex web, nerve cells or neurons are elementary building blocks that provide for the transmission of electrical impulses and facilitate communication across extensive distances within the body in an instant. Neurons are dedicated cells with the ability to generate action potentials, or short electrical discharges. They possess specialized structures, like dendrites, to receive messages, and axons, to transmit impulses to other neurons or effects , such as muscles and glands. The neurons communicate with each other at synapses—these are special links that allow neurotransmitters to bridge between neurons, indicating the function of chemical communication within the nervous system. The balance between neurotransmitters and proper neurological operation is very critical; disturbances could lead to disorders that demonstrate the delicate balance present within this biological system. This intricacy becomes particularly important when used in explanations of nerve physiology because it shows how complex processes are involved in perception and response. Advances in neurobiology have now detailed the role of glial cells as well as neurons in supporting and regulating nervous system activity. Glial cells used to be thought of as supporting structures, but they are now found to actually regulate neuronal functions, homeostasis, and respond to damage. For instance, astrocytes, a family of glial cells, contribute to the blood-brain barrier integrity, regulate the recycling of neurotransmitters, and regulate synaptic plasticity, which is necessary for learning and memory. The increasing realization of the dynamic interaction between the neuron and glial cells emphasizes the importance of studying the nervous system as an integrated and dynamic system, rather than as a static aggregation of various cell types. This perspective explains the pathological processes of various neurological illnesses and emphasizes the necessity of correlated research and therapeutic approaches in nervous system disease. In addition, recent findings on glial cell functions fall into harmony with contemporary glycomics advances, demonstrating that glycosylation processes are able to influence neurological well-being as well as disease progression (Alavi & Axford, 2008).

4.1. Structure of Neurons

Learning Outcome

1. Define the types of neurons: sensory, motor, and interneurons;
2. Highlight anatomy of a neuron: dendrites, axon, and synapse;
3. Understand myelination and why it is crucial.

The structure of neurons is very specialized to enable their simplest function of carrying electrical impulses in the nervous system. One neuron has three distinct parts: the cell body (soma), dendrites, and the axon. The cell body contains the nucleus and organelles needed for cellular metabolism and the synthesis of neurotransmitters. Dendrites extend from the cell body and are laden with specialized receptors that receive information coming in from other neurons. This branching enables the neurons to integrate synaptic inputs. The axon is a long, slender process that carries electrical impulses away from the cell body, ending at the axon terminals, which release neurotransmitters in order to convey information to nearby neurons. All these components constitute a system that is well adapted to information processing and transmission, and thus neurons are central to nerve physiology. Myelination is another vital aspect of neuronal structure that has a significant impact on the velocity of conduction of signals. Axons are usually wrapped in myelin sheaths—lipid-based coverings released by glial cells, such as oligodendrocytes in the central nervous system and Schwann cells in the peripheral nervous system. These sheaths are insulating and prevent any loss of the electrical signal as it passes down the axon. The myelinated regions alternate with naked regions, or internodes, with nodes of Ranvier in between them. Dense clusters of ion channels at these nodes facilitate the rapid re-establishment of action potentials through a phenomenon known as saltatory conduction. This mode of conduction is not only efficient but also energy-conserving, emphasizing the evolutionary advantage gained with myelination for accelerating communication within the nervous system. Organization of axonal and myelin structure is a part of their normal function, consistent with the overall dynamics of nerve physiology. Furthermore, the presence of specialized ion channels within the neuronal membrane is essential for neurotransmission. For instance, channels , such as potassium channels TRAAK have been identified as the significant subunits that regulate resting membrane potentials and action potentials in neurons. In the nodes of Ranvier, TRAAK channels contribute to the leak K+ current, which plays a critical role in hyperpolarizing the membrane and increasing the availability of sodium channels for depolarization during the conduction of an action potential. This nuanced interrelation of excitability and membrane stability reflects the complexity of neuronal architecture in its facilitation of physiological function. The remarkable ability of neurons to rapidly convey information through synapses is an immediate effect of both the structural properties of the neurons and the particular ion channels controlling their electrical properties, and this very significantly increases our understanding of nerve physiology and neuronal communication (Ghaninia et al., 2007; Brohawn et al., 2019) (Figure 4.3).

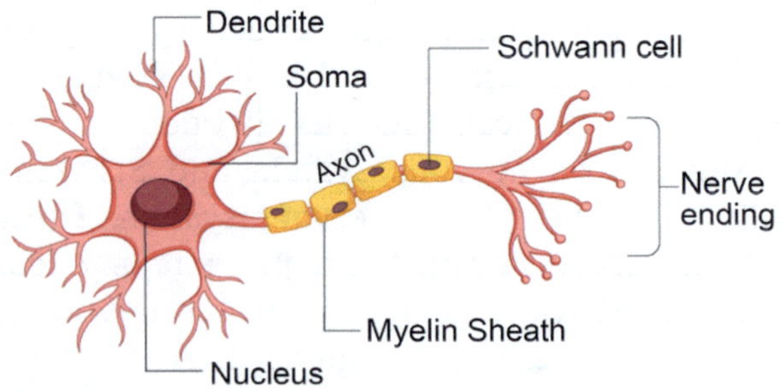

Figure 4.3. Structure of a neuron.

Source: https://cdn1.byjus.com/wp-content/uploads/2020/02/STRUCTURE-OF-NEURON.png.

4.1.1. Types of Neurons: Sensory, Motor, and Interneurons

The nervous system is essentially made up of three principal forms of neurons: sensory, motor, and interneurons, all with varying but connected functions. Sensory neurons are the very first contact with the external environment. They transmit various types of sensory information, such as touch, pain, temperature, and spatial sense, from peripheral receptors to the CNS. They form an integral part of the information necessary for the CNS to process the stimuli and generate appropriate responses. Significantly, sensory neurons convert environmental stimuli into electrical impulses such that the organism is in a position to respond and adapt to variations in the environment and thus play an important role in perception and response to stimuli. Motor neurons, on the other hand, play the key role of conveying impulses from the central nervous system to muscles and glands throughout the body. These neurons serve primarily to induce voluntary and involuntary movement, bearing commands capable of enabling muscle contraction and the secretion of glands. There are two broad categories of motor neurons: upper motor neurons, found within the brain and influencing voluntary movement, and lower motor neurons, which actually innervate skeletal muscles. The communication between such neurons is critical to orderly movement, as documented in disease studies , such as amyotrophic lateral sclerosis (ALS), when motor neuron loss upsets this fragile equilibrium and leads to severe functional deficits (Swash, 2022). Interneurons act as the central facilitators between sensory and motor neurons, combining sensory data and creating the appropriate motor response. They occur mostly in the central nervous system and form the nucleus of reflexes, communication between neurons, and modulation of complex networks in the spinal cord and brain. The variety of types of interneurons renders them capable of exercising different functions like inhibition and excitation of motor pathways, which is essential to ensure coordinated and controlled movements. Stein's work on intersegmental coordination accounts for the critical roles of interneurons to coordinate body segment signals, indicating their role in movement pattern control (Macmillan et al., 1983). The collaborative action of sensory, motor, and interneurons illustrates the intricacy and finesse of the nervous system (Figure 4.4).

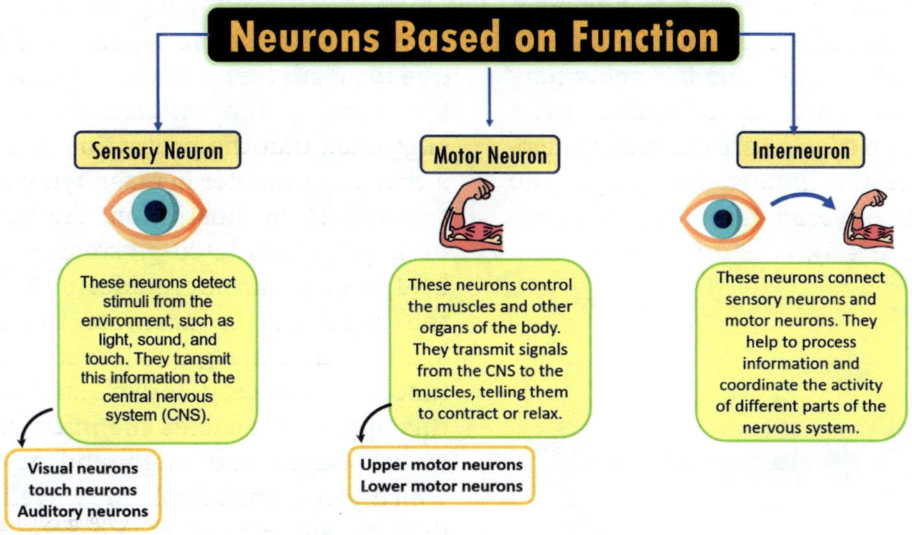

Figure 4.4. Neurons based on function.

Source: https://i.ytimg.com/vi/zqfs38DOBfY/maxresdefault.jpg.

4.1.2. Anatomy of a Neuron: Dendrites, Axon, and Synapse

The anatomy of a neuron has several integral components functioning together to contribute to the neuron's function in the nervous system's complex system. Branching structures that project from the soma of the neurons, dendrites are instrumental to the reception of synaptic input from other neurons. The structures have a large surface area, allowing them to integrate information from many sources. The dendritic spines' morphological complexity enhances synaptic plasticity, which is essential to memory and learning. Furthermore, the spine density and location may significantly influence the efficiency and neuronal communication, as it highlights their functional and structural importance in propagating the nerve impulse. Attached directly to the soma is the axon, a thin extension that is long and transmits electrical impulses away from the cell body. The axon typically ends in specialized structures known as axon terminals, where the neurotransmitters are released into the synaptic cleft to act on adjacent neurons. Myelination, where oligodendrocytes or Schwann cells encircle axons, plays a vital role in accelerating electrical conduction through saltatory conduction. This enables neuronal signals to travel quickly and efficiently throughout the nervous system and maintains the fidelity of neuronal communication. Since (N/A) explains the complexities of synaptic transmission and membrane structure, the structure of the axon is the most relevant in facilitating efficient signalling between neurons. The synapse is the most important spot where communication occurs between neurons. It is a complicated arrangement where the presynaptic neuron releases neurotransmitters and these are received by receptors on the postsynaptic neuron. Synaptic plasticity, or the weakening or strengthening of synapses over time, is a requirement for many physiological processes, including reflexes and motor coordination. Synaptic development is not haphazard; it's governed by developmental rules, as indicated by models intended to investigate neuronal networks in animals like the Xenopus tadpole (al Azad et al., 2014). These models show how elongation of axon and synapse formation can mimic the operation of an entire nervous system, and thus indicate the importance of synaptic architecture in the overall game plan of nerve physiology (Figure 4.5).

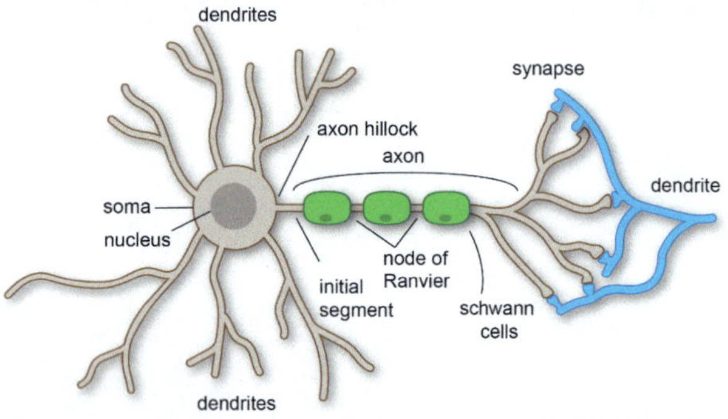

Figure 4.5. Anatomy of a neuron.

Source: https://upload.wikimedia.org/wikipedia/commons/9/9e/Anatomy_of_neuron.png.

4.1.3. Myelination and Its Significance

Myelination is an essential nervous system physiological process that allows impulse conduction to be rapid over axons. This fat insulation, consisting primarily of lipids, separates nerve fibers and significantly enhances the speed and efficiency of electrical impulse conduction. The myelin not only increases the conduction velocity of action potentials but also has an integral role in overall axon stability. Disruption or deterioration of myelination, as with many neurological diseases, can result in disabling functional impairment, demonstrating the importance of this physiological process. Myelination is therefore an active characteristic that is necessary for normal nerve conduction, indicating its key role in overall nerve health and function. In spinal cord injury (SCI), the importance of myelination is further emphasized. Following an SCI, the nervous system's regenerative capacity will be depressed due to an adverse microenvironment illustrated by scarring and inflammation. It has been suggested that the promotion of myelination is a critical parameter in magnifying recovery after trauma. As an illustration, the transplantation of a poly(lactide-co-glycolide) multichannel bridge in a chronic model of SCI has shown the capability to promote the extension of axons and remyelination, leading to improved functional recovery. As explained in recent work, this approach enables the interaction between macrophages and oligodendrocytes, both of which play a crucial role in remyelination. Thus, myelination-enhancing interventions can likely reverse the long-term implications of SCI and make myelination a crucial point for therapeutic intervention in neurotrauma. Furthermore, interactions involving myelination and functional recuperation from neurological injury highlight the importance of oligodendrocytes and axonal health maintenance functions. Oligodendrocytes not only provide the myelin sheath but also engage in support of neuronal metabolism, influencing axonal viability and function. Recent studies have brought into focus how blocking proinflammatory signaling and enhancing components supportive of myelination can lead to significant increases in tissue regeneration. For example, coordinated delivery systems, such as polycistronic vectors to deliver neuroprotective factors, have shown enhanced axonal density and myelination in SCI model systems. These findings suggest that modulation of myelination using appropriate strategies may present effective avenues for augmenting recovery and reestablishing nerve function, further emphasizing the role of myelination in nerve physiology.

Test Your Knowledge

1. What are the chief structural components of a neuron?
2. In what ways does the structure of the axon allow for transmission of nerve impulses over long distances?

4.2. Action Potentials

Learning Outcome

1. Explain the characteristics of action potentials
2. Explain the mechanism of action potential generation
3. Understand the role of ion channels in action potentials

Action potentials are a significant event in nerve physiology because they permit the conduction of electrical signals along neurons. These rapid, short changes in membrane potential permit communication in the nervous system, which is required for such functions as reflexes and voluntary movement. When a neuron attains a threshold potential, a chain of ion channel openings takes place, mainly involving sodium ions.

The entry of sodium depolarizes the neuron, and an action potential is generated. This phenomenon does not simply translate to a mere electrical change; its complexities include intricate interactions among different concentrations of ions and dynamics of channels, which illustrate a sophisticated system that supports neural communication. Understanding action potentials is central to studying how we perceive and respond to stimuli, and thus, they are central to cognitive function and behavioral responses. The transmission of action potentials along the axon of a neuron is facilitated by the myelination of axons. Myelin sheath, formed by oligodendrocytes in the central nervous system and Schwann cells in the peripheral nervous system, is an insulating layer that allows saltatory conduction, raising the transmission speed of electrical signals significantly. Nodes of Ranvier, the gaps in the myelin sheath, give the action potential the convenience of hopping from node to node. This mechanism not only accelerates signal transmission but also renders it energy efficient, reducing the metabolic cost of maintaining ionic gradients through the neuron's membrane.

Thus, both the structure of neurons and myelination are closely associated with the efficacy of action potentials, suggesting the evolutionary significance of such mechanisms in the nervous system. Action potentials are more than mere electrical activity; they are also components of conscious experience and the control of behavior. The coincidence between action potentials and higher-order functions, such as cognition and emotional processing, demonstrates the interdependence of physiological processes and outcome behavior. According to cognitive science, although brain structures do exhibit specific responses to stimuli, the hypothesis that the brain is simply in existence to process information lacks immediate evidence. In addition, consciousness emerges from the dynamic interplay of cellular membrane potentials within the entire body, and not just in the brain (Burock et al., 2010). This further insight adds to the role of action potentials in sensation and emotional experience, toward an integrated conception of consciousness grounded in physiological mechanisms (Jerath et al., 2015) (Figure 4.6).

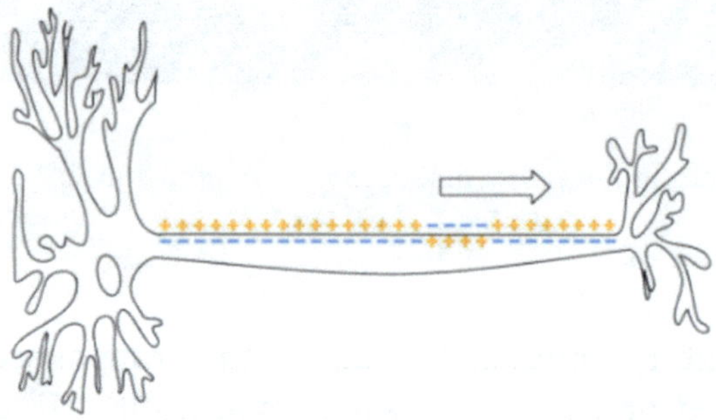

Figure 4.6. An action potential travels down an axon.

Source: https://upload.wikimedia.org/wikipedia/commons/9/95/Action_Potential.gif.

4.2.1. Definition and Characteristics of Action Potentials

The definition of action potentials is crucial for the understanding of nerve physiology since these events are the fundamental mechanism by which the neuron transmits information. An action potential is a transient, short-lived change in the membrane potential of a neuron that consists of depolarization followed by repolarization. This electrical impulse occurs when a neuron reaches a certain threshold potential, typically brought about by the entry of sodium ions through voltage-gated ion channels. The positively charged ions thus bring about the change in the membrane potential, leading to an all-or-nothing response should the threshold be met. Hence, action potentials not only conduct signals along neurons but also permit calcium-dependent neurotransmitter release to enable inter-synaptic communication and neural circuit operation. The nature of action potentials highlights their dynamic nature for effective nerve transmission. Action potentials possess a typical waveform with well-defined phases: the depolarization phase, the repolarization phase, and the hyperpolarization phase. During depolarization, the great influx of sodium leads to a positive voltage deflection; repolarization is brought about by potassium ion efflux, restoring a negative membrane potential. Interestingly, action potential duration and amplitude can be altered by a number of physiological and pharmacological interventions, as illustrated in experiments on cardiac myocyte action potential modulation through engineered ion channels (Muhammed Sönmez et al., 2025).

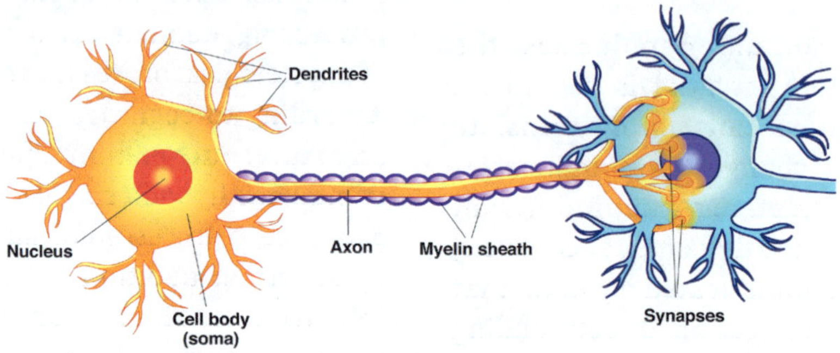

Figure 4.7. Neurons communicate.

Source: https://ugc.futurelearn.com/uploads/assets/9d/cd/9dcdd082-dcf7-461c-ada0-ee63578778bc.jpeg.

These characteristics highlight the intricacies of membrane excitability, underscoring the role of action potentials in neuronal as well as muscle tissues in maintaining homeostasis and responding to inner as well as outer stimuli. In addition, firing patterns of action potentials are pertinent in understanding the physiological consequences of various substances on the nervous system. Existing research has shown how exogenous factors, such as acute cannabis consumption, are able to alter sympathetic nervous function through interference in the firing patterns of action potentials. One such example is that one study found that following smoking of cannabis, both the amplitude and frequency of sympathetic action potentials were reduced in a manner that suggests that exogenous factors possess the potential to disrupt normal neuronal firing processes and lead to alteration of neural communication (D'Souza et al., 2025). This is to emphasize the need for both cellular and physiological consideration of action potential properties. The importance of being able to assess the influence of various stimuli on action potential properties is a significant discovery in terms of interaction between external and internal neural processes, highlighting the significance of knowing action potentials as part of nerve physiology (Figure 4.7).

4.2.2. Mechanism of Action Potential Generation

The mechanism of action potential generation is the focal point of studying nerve physiology because it encapsulates the mechanisms underlying the fact that neural communication is possible. An action potential starts when a neuron undergoes massive depolarization, a change in membrane potential that occurs following the passage of a stimulus across a threshold. This depolarization is caused primarily by the influx of sodium ions (Na^+) through voltage-gated sodium channels, which open during the initial stimulus. After the voltage reaches approximately -55 mV, there's a rapid spike where there's a temporary reversal of membrane potential that reaches a peak at around +30 mV typically. This kind of depolarization is significant as it initiates further physiological responses, enabling neuronal communication and signaling. Without such a specific process, the neuronal ability to deal with and conduct information would be substantially reduced. Following the initial phase of rapid depolarization, there is a secondary phase of repolarization, whereby the membrane potential returns to resting. This phase is significantly controlled by the efflux of potassium ions (K^+) through voltage-gated potassium channels, opened as a result of the initial depolarization. The efflux of K+ contributes to the reduction of membrane potential by a large magnitude, thus allowing the neuron to regain its negative resting potential. Repolarization is required for the neuron's electrical state to be restored, hence making it ready for the succeeding stimulus. After-hyperpolarization phase also occurs, in which the membrane potential becomes slightly more negative than at rest, which is mostly brought about by sustained permeability of the membrane to the potassium ion.

This process is essential to blocking the neuron from becoming excitable for a brief period of time, thereby maintaining signaling in homeostasis in neural circuits. The intricate properties of sympathetic preganglionic neurons (SPNs) illustrate the nuances of action potential generation and their physiological relevance. Recent studies on SPNs have indicated that different classes possess different intrinsic firing properties that correlate with their respective functional roles within the autonomic nervous system. Muscle vasoconstrictor-like SPNs, for instance, exhibit higher baseline firing rates and distinct temporal patterns of action potential than cutaneous vasoconstrictor-like SPNs. They highlight the significance of the generation of action potential not as a simple yes or no occurrence, but as a complex process that enables neurons to adjust their output following physiological requirements. Such information informs us on the role of SPNs in crucial processes, like cardiorespiratory reflex integration, thereby emphasizing the general effect of action potential mechanisms on overall neural functioning (Mohamed et al., 2011; Stalbovskiy et al., 2014) (Figure 4.8).

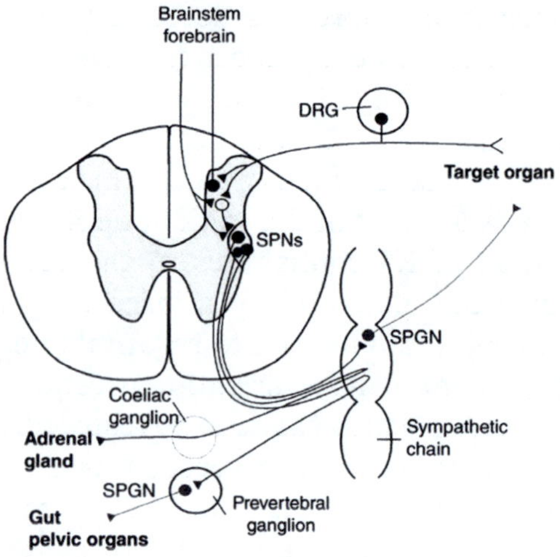

Figure 4.8. Sympathetic preganglionic neurons.

Source: https://onlinelibrary.wiley.com/cms/asset/c827f435-51e3-49a5-951c-6e6c855694e9/nc14002001.jpg.

4.2.3. Role of Ion Channels in Action Potentials

Reliance on the pharmacology of ion channels is essential to the pharmacologically triggered action potentials, i.e., peak voltage-gated Na+ and K+ channels. Once the threshold potential of the neuron, approximately -55 mV, is attained, the voltage-gated Na+ channels rapidly open and Na+ ions enter the cell. This causes a drastic depolarization of the neuron's membrane potential, which quite commonly reaches +30 mV. The speedy transition of resting potential to depolarization is essential to the development of the action potential due to the rapid flip in membrane potential that enables the signal to travel along the neuron.

Following this initial period of depolarization, the Na+ channels close, while the K+ channels open to repolarize the membrane and restore the resting potential. This complicated process emphasizes how vital ion channels are to the development and passing on of neural signals. In addition to voltage-gated channels, leak K+ channels play an important role in maintaining the neuron's resting membrane potential, which is necessary for action potential initiation. Recently, a study has identified the central role of the TRAAK potassium channel in nodes of Ranvier, where it contributes to part of the leak K+ current in myelinated nerve fibers. Specifically, TRAAK hyperpolarizes the resting membrane potential, thus making more Na+ channels available for subsequent action potentials, allowing rapid conduction of signals in myelinated axons (Brohawn et al., 2019).

Such a mechanism is particularly important in the context of mechanical nociception, where action potential generation is regulated and ultimately determines pain signaling pathways. Thus, the presence and operation of various ion channels directly influence the extent and efficiency by which action potentials are propagated in the nervous system. The spatial distribution of ion channels also impacts the functional properties of neuronal signaling. The density of various ion channels, including both sodium and potassium channels, varies not only for various types of neurons but also at varying locations within a given neuron. For instance, while voltage-gated Na+ channels are in high density at the axon hillock, where action potentials are usually generated—K^+ channels like TRAAK are also located at sites , such as the nodes of Ranvier with the aim of optimizing signal transmission efficiency. In this manner, action potentials can propagate efficiently and rapidly along extended axons, a critical condition for successful transmission between neurons (Mohamed et al., 2011). The differential distribution and kinetic characteristics of ion channels represent their critical functions in modulating the physiological behaviors of neurons, expressing their critical roles in both normal and pathological states of nerve physiology.

Test Your Knowledge

1. How do voltage-gated sodium and potassium channels contribute to the generation and conduction of an action potential?
2. What is the role of the refractory period, and how does it guarantee one-way transmission of nerve impulses?

4.3. Synaptic Transmission

Learning Outcome

1. Identify the mechanism of neurotransmitter release;
2. Describe the nature of the types of neurotransmitters and their roles;
3. Explain the mechanisms of synaptic plasticity.

Synaptic transmission is the mechanism by which neurons communicate with one another, an integral part of nerve physiology upon which all neural function relies. It begins at the presynaptic terminal, with the action potential triggering release of neurotransmitters into the synaptic cleft. These messenger chemicals diffuse across the thin gap between neurons and bind to specific receptors on the postsynaptic membrane. This binding initiates a chain of intracellular events that can produce either excitatory or inhibitory postsynaptic potentials. The balance of these two contrary tendencies is crucial to the integration of signals in the nervous system, ultimately determining behavior, mood, and body function. Normal functioning of synapses is thus critical since any defect would lead to a range of neurological abnormalities, which points to the importance of understanding synaptic dynamics in the context of overall nerve physiology. The dynamic richness of synaptic transmission is more than just neurotransmitter release and receptor binding. It is an intricate interaction of various ion channels, second messenger systems, and the local cell environment of the neuron. New findings show that the extracellular environment is a strong determinant of synaptic efficacy and patterns of neurotransmitter release. Specifically, the biochemical composition of the immediate surroundings affects not only the magnitude of the postsynaptic response but also the plasticity modifications that are responsible for learning and memory. The interdependence of cells and the surrounding environment means that an expanded physiological context needs to play a larger role in the investigation of synaptic transmission. In this context, the traditional conception of neural coding as a categorical notion is dismissed, as the effects of extrinsic factors mirror a more comprehensive model of information processing by the nervous system, particularly in terms of concepts of mass action in the nervous system (Werner, 2012). Moreover, synaptic transmission is controlled by various mechanisms of modulation that affect the efficacy and plasticity of synaptic interfaces. Synaptic facilitation, depression, and long-term potentiation (LTP) or long-term depression (LTD) significantly alter the manner synapses respond to repetitive stimulation. The modulations are involved in processes , such as learning and memory by altering the strength and connectivity of synapses with time. The dynamics of synaptic plasticity illustrate the flexibility of the system, a level of complexity that needs to be investigated through various theoretical frameworks. In general, encoding by impulse and by train can account better for how various channels convey information to process it and how this communication can be regulated by the chemical environment (Bullock & Perkel, 1968). Understanding these principles of synaptic transmission is not merely essential to explaining neurophysiological mechanisms but also to designing therapeutic strategies to treat synaptic dysfunction observed in neurological disease (Figure 4.9).

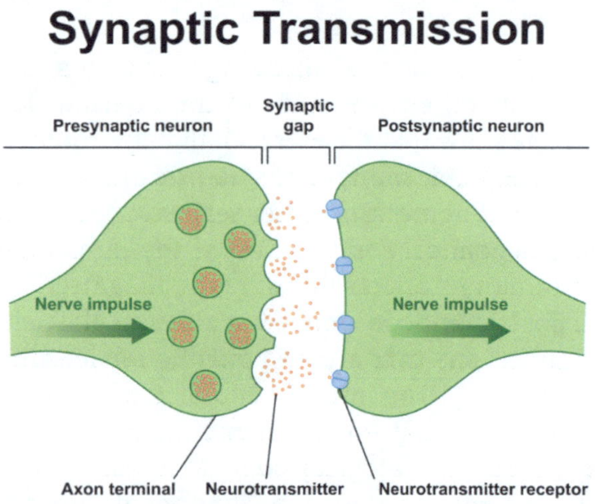

Figure 4.9. Synaptic transmission.

Source: https://www.simplypsychology.org/wp-content/uploads/Chemical-synapse.png.

4.3.1. Process of Neurotransmitter Release

Neurotransmitter release process is vital in developing communication between the neurons in the nervous system. This intricate process begins at the terminal of the axon, where the action potential depolarizes the voltage-gated calcium channels and allows calcium ions to enter. This rapid increase in intracellular concentration of calcium is a critical signal that initiates the fusion of the synaptic vesicles with the presynaptic membrane. The fusion of such vesicles, which contain neurotransmitters, allows the contents to be released into the synaptic cleft. Not only does this procedure ensure that neurotransmitters reach their target receptors on the postsynaptic neuron, but it also establishes synaptic strength and efficacy of transmission. Therefore, research on neurotransmitter release is crucial in understanding broader concepts of nerve physiology like synaptic plasticity and overall neural function. Following the initial release of neurotransmitters, synaptic efficacy and recovery are controlled by a complex interaction of control mechanisms. Vesicles that have released their neurotransmitters are either recycled through endocytosis or refilled with neurotransmitters synthesized within the presynaptic neuron. Furthermore, the release of neurotransmitters is modulated by many factors like presynaptic receptors and local signal molecules, thus indicating the dynamic regulation of synaptic milieus. Evidence suggests that there are different release mechanisms for different neurotransmitters, highlighted by individual neurotransmitter receptors, as seen in experiments on neuronal synapses. For instance, augmented release of neurotransmitters upon calcium influx can create a more robust postsynaptic response to enhance synaptic strength. The process is analogous to depolarization-activated potentiation observed in synapses, where persistent activation results in the strengthening of efficacy in neurotransmitter release and, by association, benefits neural circuit operation (Lin et al., 1993). Neurotransmitter release is not only applicable in physiological settings but can be conceptualized in pathophysiological settings as well, highlighting its applicability in both health and disease. For instance, dysregulation of the processes of neurotransmitter release can cause neurological disorders , such as depression, schizophrenia, and neurodegenerative diseases. Moreover, the role of calcium dynamics in the release of neurotransmitters is critical, as alteration of calcium mobilization is likely to result in altered synaptic functions. Experiments have shown hypoxia and local inflammation to be capable of negatively affecting the synaptic release process, implying an interesting overlap between neurotransmitter dynamics and general cellular health. Furthermore, the cross-talk among sympathetic innervation, which may affect the neurotransmitter release at the level of pericytes in the renal circulation, points to the multifaceted roles that neurotransmitters play in local regulatory pathways (Crawford et al., 2013). Understanding these processes gives potential routes for therapeutic interventions aimed at restoring normal nerve function (Figure 4.10).

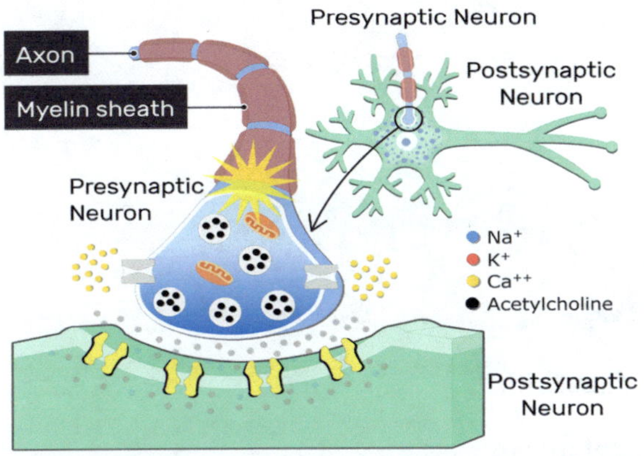

Figure 4.10. Neurotransmitter release at cholinergic synapses.

Source: https://www.getbodysmart.com/wp-content/uploads/2017/10/Action-potential-impulses-imageActionPotential0010-Neurotransmitter-Release-At-Cholinergic-Synapses.-1024x796.png.

4.3.2. Types of Neurotransmitters and Their Functions

One of the key roles of neurotransmitters is to enable communication in the nervous system and influence different physiological and psychological processes. Of the major neurotransmitter types, amino acids like glutamate and gamma-aminobutyric acid (GABA) are interesting for their opposite functions. Glutamate is the primary excitatory neurotransmitter of the brain and is accountable for synaptic plasticity as well as cognitive functions like learning and memory. GABA, on the other hand, is the primary inhibitory neurotransmitter and acts to regulate neuronal excitability throughout the nervous system. Proper nervous function and homeostasis rely on the balance of excitatory and inhibitory messages, thereby influencing behavior, mood, and cognitive health. Dysregulation of these neurotransmitter systems can lead to neurological diseases, so it is vital to become aware of their specialized roles in nerve physiology. Another very important class of neurotransmitters are monoamines, such as dopamine, norepinephrine, and serotonin, all of which are implicated in mood regulation and emotional responses. Dopamine, often referred to as the feel-good neurotransmitter, has a significant role in reward circuits, modulating motivation, pleasure, and motor control. Norepinephrine, which is linked to the body's response to stress, assists in the regulation of arousal and alertness. Serotonin, which affects mood, sleep, and appetite, is commonly researched in the depression and anxiety disorders, implying that serotonin imbalance might be the cause of these disorders. The interaction between these monoamines is crucial to emotional stability, and their mechanisms of action can provide a clue to possible targets for therapeutic intervention for mood disorders and thereby enhance the role of neurotransmitter mechanisms in clinical practice. Furthermore, neuropeptides, a heterogeneous group of neurotransmitters, have been of interest due to their roles in modulating various physiological functions, like pain, stress, and metabolic functions. Neuropeptides , such as substance P and endorphins are major factors in pain perception and moods. Substance P is employed in the transmission of pain signals, while endorphins are involved in the diminishment of pain and inducing euphoria. The complexity of these neuropeptides is illustrated in their interaction with other neurotransmitter systems, showing a multidimensional strategy for understanding nerve physiology. Their effect can be seen in many conditions, as emphasized in recent research that points to the neurotransmitters' involvement in both physical and emotional aspects of health and disease, supporting the position that psychosocial factors might affect not only psychological resilience, but also physiological conditions, as discussed in cases , such as digestive neoplasms, for example, in Jerath et al. (2015); Caragea et al. (2016) (Figure 4.11).

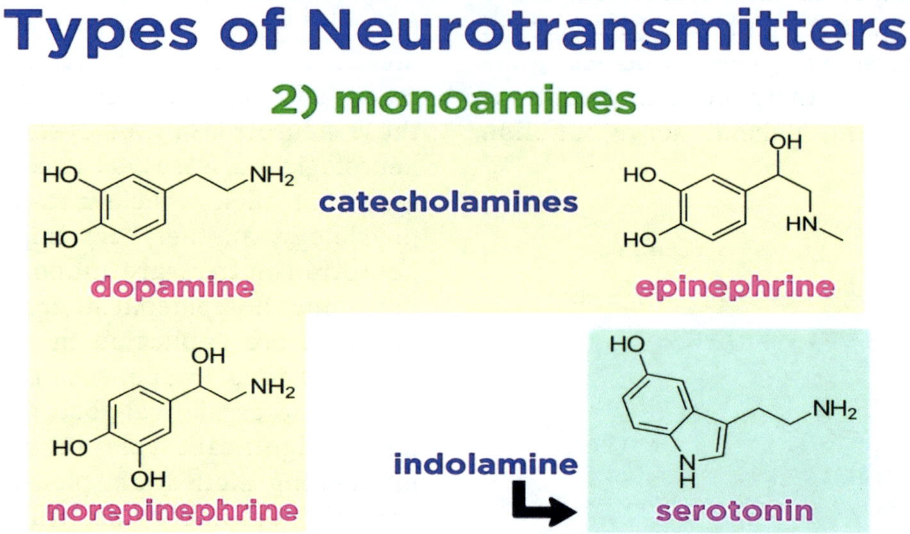

Figure 4.11. Neurotransmitters: Type, structure, and function.

Source: https://i.ytimg.com/vi/LOHKVp8hn7o/maxresdefault.jpg.

4.3.3. Mechanisms of Synaptic Plasticity

Synaptic plasticity is a fundamental mechanism of learning and memory, consisting of modifications of synaptic efficacy as synaptic activity varies. A form well known is depolarization-activated potentiation (DAP), documented in the blue crab T fiber synapse. In this model, brief presynaptic depolarization leads to large excitatory postsynaptic potential (EPSP) amplitudes, indicating direct proportionality between calcium levels and synaptic increase. Specifically, the amplitude of DAP is controlled by the amplitude of conditioning pulse, while its decay is linearly exponential in time. This calcium-based mechanism demonstrates how transient increases in the strength of synaptic transmission can remain so, hence enabling communication between neurons for short periods, which is crucial for dynamic processing within the neuron (Lin et al., 1993). Another crucial element of synaptic plasticity is presynaptic homeostatic plasticity (PHP), which maintains equilibrium in synaptic transmission across a broad range of species. This type of process ensures that the neuron can maintain stable signaling regardless of fluctuating levels of activity. Recent studies have revealed the molecular mechanisms of PHP, in particular with the identification of Multiple C2 Domain Proteins with Two Transmembrane Regions (MCTP). The protein is ER-localized in various neuronal compartments and plays a pivotal role in calcium entry mediation. MCTPs are a calcium sensor that is important for stabilizing neurotransmission and controlling short-term release dynamics, hence supporting the homeostatic accommodations required in the regulation of synaptic efficacy (Davis et al., 2017). The integration of varied mechanisms of synaptic plasticity ensures the plasticity of neuronal circuits against activity and experience. DAP and PHP are both examples of how adjustments of the presynaptic environment may exert a vastly beneficial impact on synaptic output. While DAP brings to the fore the rapid and transient shifts that reinforce synaptic efficacy under some conditions, PHP requires the preservation of long-term stability in neural activity. Together, these processes reflect the complexity of synaptic adaptivity, demonstrating that the ability to modify synaptic transmission is not only important for rapid adaptation but also essential to preserving long-term stability in neurological processes. Understanding these processes will continue to shed light on the intricacies of nerve physiology and its importance to learning, memory, and neurological disease.

Test Your Knowledge

1. How do neurotransmitters like acetylcholine, dopamine, or GABA influence the membrane potential of the postsynaptic cell?
2. What is the role of calcium ions in neurotransmitter release from the presynaptic terminal?

4.4. Neurotransmitter Systems

Learning Outcome

1. Name the major neurotransmitter systems: dopaminergic, serotonergic, and cholinergic;
2. Define the impact of neurotransmitters on mood and behavior;
3. Describe the effects of neurotransmitter imbalance.

Neurotransmitter systems play a crucial role in carrying out neuron-to-neuron signaling and consist of a vital component of nerve physiology. They contain various neurotransmitters that have certain functions to perform and mechanisms that affect numerous physiological processes. For instance, excitatory neurotransmitters glutamate and dopamine allow nerve impulses to be transmitted, while inhibitory neurotransmitters GABA regulate neural impulses, creating homeostasis in the nervous system. It is the carefully adjusted balance of these inhibitory and excitatory signals that is necessary to ensure cognitive processes, mood regulation, and coordination of motor activity. As a result, any interference with these neurotransmitter systems can cause significant neurological diseases and highlights the importance of finding their intricate dynamics in the broad framework of nerve physiology. Adenosine, a neuromodulator, acts upon neurotransmitter systems especially by altering neuronal responses. It acts by interacting with adenosine receptors on the surfaces of neurons, and subsequently altering the levels of second messengers in cells. This modulation is either excitatory or inhibitory, depending on cellular background and activated receptors.

The appearance of adenosine leads to increased inhibition of neuronal firing, thereby modifying various neurological functions and signaling pathways. The action of adenosine is tightly regulated by nucleoside transporters to deliver the appropriate influx and efflux of adenosine within the cellular microenvironment. These dysfunctions may be brought about by substances like alcohol, which interfere with adenosines normal function, bringing about alterations in motor coordination and sedation, thereby underscoring the significance of these systems in both health and illness (Diamond et al., 1997). Moreover, the reciprocal interaction of emotional state and neurotransmitter systems points to the intimate connection of physiological state and psychological well-being. The feedback processes of the autonomic nervous systems, especially when under stress, significantly influence the release of neurotransmitters and, subsequently, emotional reactions. With negative emotional states, decreases in cardiorespiratory coherence can shift the dynamic to sympathetic dominance, thus enhancing feelings of distress and anxiety. Positive emotional states are associated with increased coherence and parasympathetic shift, provoking a feeling of relaxation and calmness. These interactions all point to the limbic system and its connection to neurotransmitter systems as being key to understanding how emotions are processed and controlled within the brain. Such information not only facilitates our understanding of auditory and motor responses but also suggests avenues for therapeutic intervention in mood disorders, making the study of neurotransmitter systems clinically relevant (Crawford et al., 2015) (Figure 4.12).

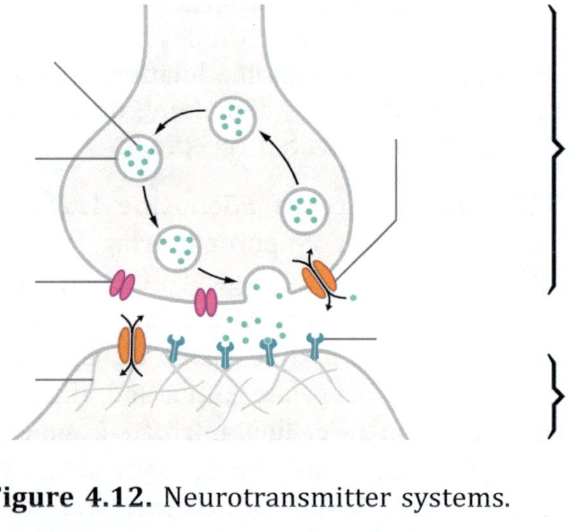

Figure 4.12. Neurotransmitter systems.

Source: https://upload.wikimedia.org/wikipedia/commons/d/d7/SynapseSchematic_lines.svg.

4.4.1. Major Neurotransmitter Systems: Dopaminergic, Serotonergic, and Cholinergic

The dopaminergic system is tasked with regulating several of the most significant physiological processes, including mood, reward, and control of motor function. Dopamine, the principal neurotransmitter, is synthesized in numerous brain regions, particularly the substantia nigra and ventral tegmental area. Its projections target key locations , such as the striatum and prefrontal cortex. Dysregulation of dopaminergic signaling has a direct relationship with neurodegenerative disease like Parkinsons disease (PD), where extensive loss of dopaminergic neurons leads to characteristic motor symptoms like tremor and rigidity. Also of interest has been the interaction of dopamine with other neurotransmitter systems in explaining the intricacy of mood regulation, since alterations in its function can be detected in clinical disorders like depression and anxiety and suggest the fine balance necessary for efficient neurotransmission in the central nervous system. The serotonergic system, which is primarily mediated through serotonin (5-HT), is highly involved in mood, cognition, as well as modulation of emotional response. Synthesis occurs in raphe nuclei neurons that are serotonergic, and serotonin is widely distributed throughout the brain, influencing diverse psychological activities. From clinical studies, the role of serotonin in mood disorders has been observed, particularly with the administration of selective serotonin reuptake inhibitors (SSRIs). The amount of serotonin not only influences emotional stability but is also implicated in appetite and circadian rhythms. Abnormalities in serotonergic transmission have been linked to a wide range of psychiatric diseases, indicating the neurotransmitter's function in producing not just stability in mood but overall neurophysiological health and hence its importance in neurobiological research and treatment. The cholinergic system, characterized by the action of acetylcholine (ACh), is utilized for vital functions in peripheral as well as central nervous systems. It participates in neuromuscular junction muscle contraction and also has a vital function in attention, memory and learning mechanisms within the brain. The basal forebrain and brainstem contain significant cholinergic populations of neurons with projection to cortical and subcortical destinations. Dysregulation of cholinergic signaling has been noted in neurodegenerative diseases, most notably Alzheimer's disease, wherein cholinergic neuronal depletion accompanies cognitive decline. As well, the interaction among the cholinergic system and other systems of neurotransmitters, such as those using dopamine and serotonin, delineates the neurochemical complexity involved in controlling behavioral and physiological response. Knowledge of these interactions is necessary in order to continue with the development of therapeutic strategies for neurological illness that disrupt cholinergic function (Figure 4.13).

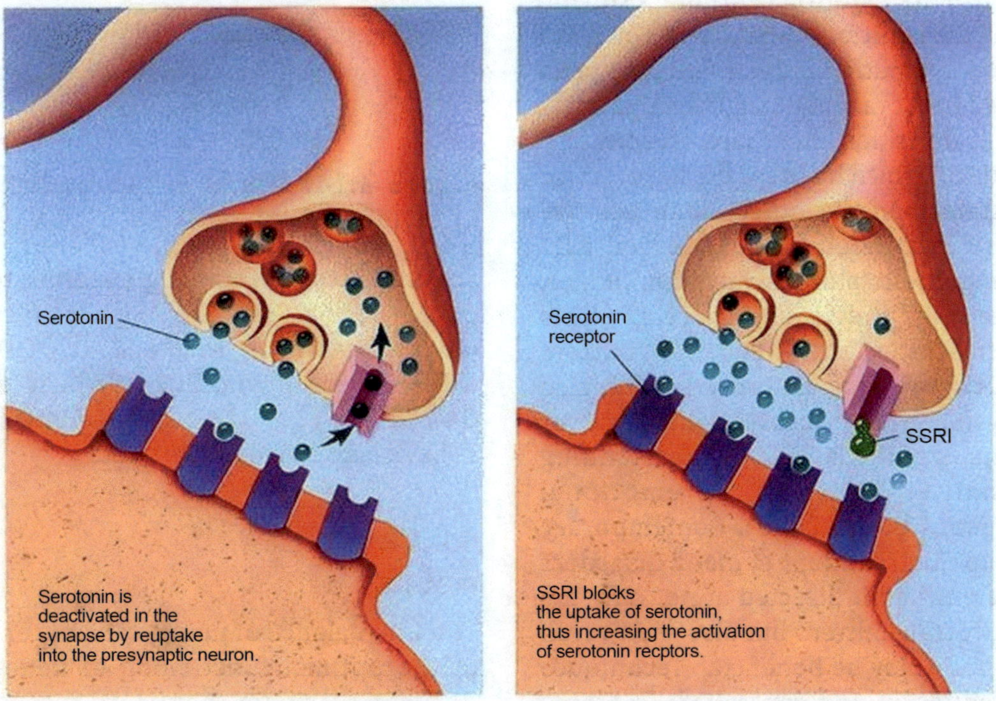

Figure 4.13. Selective serotonin reuptake inhibitors (SSRIs) work.

Source: https://www.ocduk.org/wp-content/uploads/2018/05/howSSRIwork2.jpg.

4.4.2. Effects of Neurotransmitters on Behavior and Mood

The intricate relationship between neurotransmitters and behavior is a central theme of nerve physiology. Neurotransmitters serotonin, dopamine, and norepinephrine have essential regulatory functions in maintaining mood and emotional states. For instance, serotonin, or the happy neurotransmitter, has been linked to feelings of happiness and contentment. Low serotonin levels have also been associated with mood disorders like depression and anxiety, a testament to its crucial function in emotion regulation. Dopamine, on the other hand, is central to the brain's reward system, having an influence not only in the elevation of mood but also in motivation and pleasure response. Observing how such neurotransmitters interact with various neural circuits is essential for understanding the biological foundation of mood and behavior, demonstrating the strength of biochemical activities in shaping psychological states. Beyond their roles in mood, neurotransmitters are deeply integrated with the body's physiologic response to stress and emotion. The autonomic nervous system (ANS), which includes the sympathetic and parasympathetic branches, is controlled by neurotransmitter activity, thereby regulating body response to emotional stimuli. During stress, neurotransmitter imbalances can lead to heightened sympathetic dominance, as seen by heightened heart rate and heightened arousal response. This transition alters cardiorespiratory coherence (CRC), which happens during aversive emotional states. On the other hand, positive emotions are associated with increased CRC and parasympathetic shift toward dominance, which causes an individual to relax. This dynamics illustrates how neurotransmitters not only affect psychological processes but also mediate physiological processes, which further supports the significance of understanding neurotransmitter function in emotional health (Crawford et al., 2015). Contemporary approaches to the treatment of mood disorders suggest that treatment directed at not only the levels of neurotransmitters but also the overall state of the body may be beneficial. Techniques , such as meditation and controlled breathing have emerged as potential ways of reversing the deleterious effect of stress and anxiety by restoring homeostatic equilibrium. By focusing on the interplay between emotion and breathing, individuals can employ these practices to enhance autonomic control and emotional well-being. Research reveals that these practices are capable of increasing CRC and allowing for transition to parasympathetic dominance, and this contributes to enhanced emotional regulation (Jerath et al., 2015). Such studies provide the potentiality of non-pharmacological treatments for mood disorders, which state that a holistic treatment through neurotransmitter modulation and behavior techniques would be a more successful treatment for emotional issues (Figure 4.14).

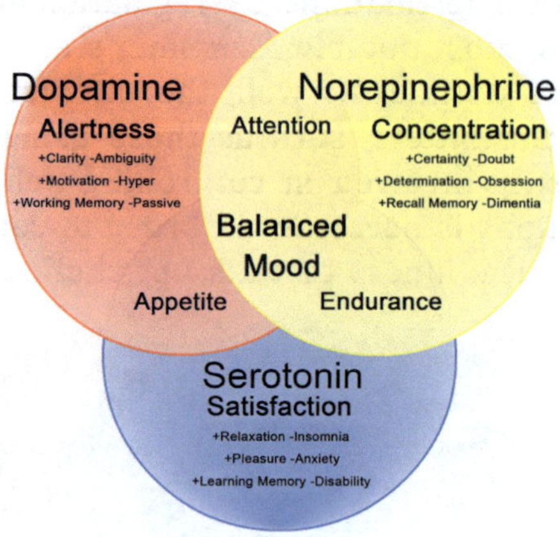

Figure 4.14. Effects of neurotransmitters on behavior and mood.

Source: https://lh6.googleusercontent. com/proxy/qk5DJ3KsfU3 gprrY03eha4n0w HRYtwpq4Nf4Lo_Aiz74ZZmc QDkUmtdyv KUUN0T0SgnipjwnolEG2 b9B14ACIy7SyXoiCqj G4YZUezoyq UBDov LZeaQswo8e4cs EsLavkaaa8Twr9IydqRpKuLt5.

4.4.3. Implications of Neurotransmitter Imbalances

The fine balance of neurotransmitters is crucial to the optimal functioning of neural circuits. A disequilibrium between these chemical messengers has been seen to bring about extreme disturbances in the process of communication between neurons, ultimately materializing as varied neurological and psychological disorders. For instance, deficiencies in serotonin have been traced to affective disorders , such as depression and anxiety, highlighting the need for balanced levels of neurotransmitters in regulating emotions. Additionally, imbalances may affect cognition and memory, where glutamate and GABA are replete with roles in learning and memory functions. Consequently, understanding the consequence of neurotransmitter imbalances is significant in that it points to their inherent role in the preservation of not only mood stability but cognitive health as well, and it paints a broad spectrum of physiological and psychological impact that deserves more studies. Research has tended to explore the effects of neurotransmitter imbalance beyond the conventional neurological pathway to the gut-brain axis. More recent evidence suggests that gut microbiota is implicated in the regulation of levels of neurotransmitters, hence modulation of mood and cognitive functions. Certain bacteria, for instance, can synthesize neurotransmitters exogenously or regulate the hosts synthesis of these molecules, suggesting a complex interaction between diet, gut integrity, and brain physiology. The findings indicate a paradigm shift in understanding how the physical health may influence mental health. As the balance of the microbiomes is shifted by an array of factors, such as diet and environment, the maintenance of a healthy microbiome might reverse effects concerning neurotransmitter imbalance. This points towards an integrative approach to treating related disorders. This interrelatedness offers new therapeutic avenues that would greatly improve mental health interventions, as the literature (Bhattacharyya et al., 2023) has noted. As life expectancy rises, the consequences of neurotransmitter imbalance become increasingly urgent, particularly in relation to age-related neurodegenerative disorders , such as Alzheimer's. Literature shows that age-related alterations in ion channel activity can contribute to neurotransmitter dysregulation, leading to the pathogenesis and progression of these diseases. Notably, amyloid-beta (Aβ) plaques have been discovered to cause disruptions in ionic balances within neurons, which directly affect neurotransmitter signal pathways (Sadegh-Zadeh et al., 2019). These interruptions emphasize the necessity of early detection and treatment of these diseases because even minor imbalances have the potential to enhance neurodegeneration. As such, continued investigation into the identification of precursors to neurotransmitter disturbances offers a promising path for the development of more advanced therapeutic strategies and improved quality of life among older populations. The significance of such an understanding emphasizes the urgent interface of neurobiology and public health and necessitates further investigation in both scientific and clinical contexts.

Test Your Knowledge

1. What is the main role of neurotransmitters in the nervous system?
2. Identify two excitatory and two inhibitory neurotransmitters and their net effects.

4.5. Nerve Impulse Propagation

Learning Outcome

1. Describe the saltatory conduction in myelinated fibers;
2. State the determinants of nerve impulse velocity;
3. Discuss comparison of conduction in myelinated and unmyelinated fibers.

The intricate process of nerve impulse transmission is ultimately reliant on the dynamic characteristics of neuronal membranes, which are barriers and channels for the electrical messages traveling through the nervous system.

The mechanism of producing an action potential begins when a neuron is activated past its threshold, which leads to rapid depolarization caused by the entry of sodium ions (Na^+). The process of repolarization follows, as potassium ions (K^+) exit the neuron. Coordination of the rapid rise and fall in the membrane potential is done through the sequential opening and closing of ion channels.

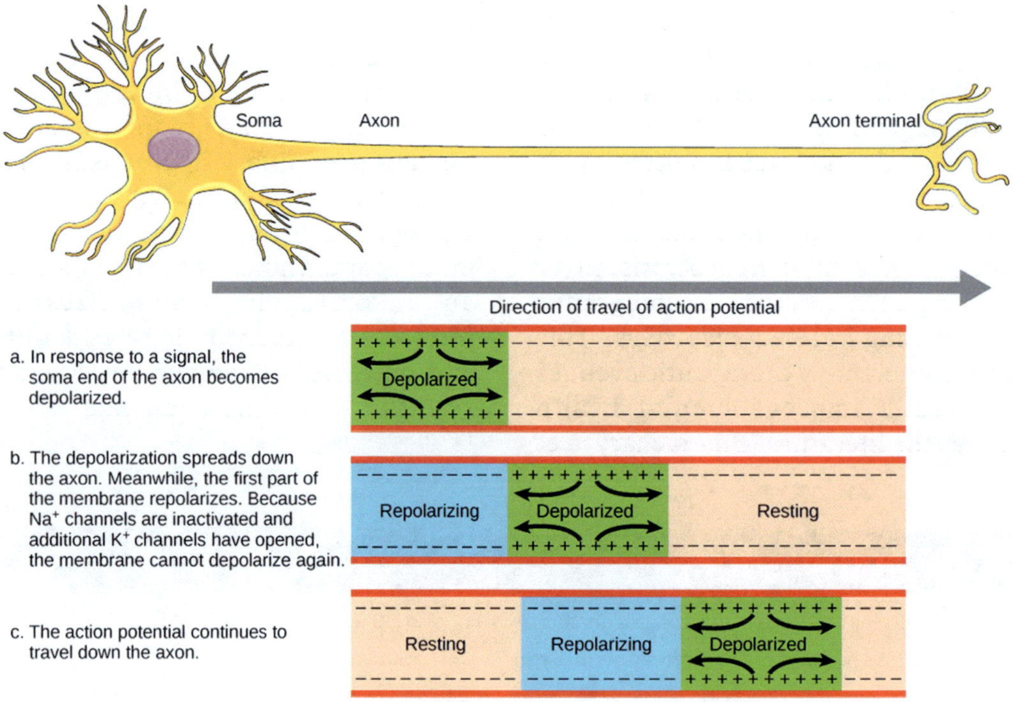

Figure 4.15. Nerve impulse propagation.

Source: https://files.mtstatic.com/site_4463/1893/0?Expires=1748426133&Signature=eOpdzho6Vei-~bHutNIs7tBfPV0E6VgLRK8NbMq6n7Q5j6Jfakc3dTwMjLFfDbclgFgYbC~fADJGyl1OYmlt10ruMsm7YUtSmiJ0Cex25GzO6PASOY1bIi3C~dm~aNupxLc8gqEbPpCNaEqhXTK5dFV1OEoCr3zQ56Eo8ImjMqw_&Key-Pair-Id=APKAJ5Y6AV4GI7A555NA.

The coordination between such electrical changes and the structural makeup of the neuron is crucial to efficacious transmission as the physical structure of lipid bilayers and specialized proteins governs ion transport through the membrane and therefore preserves neural function and communication. Transmission is also reliant on the myelination process, which has a significant effect of enhancing speed of conduction. Myelinated axons, characterized by covering sheaths produced by oligodendrocytes in the central nervous system or Schwann cells in the peripheral nervous system, support an action referred to as saltatory conduction. The mechanism offers for impulses to jump between the nodes of Ranvier, where ion channels are highly concentrated, rather than moving continually along the axon.

The result is a tremendous speeding up and efficiency of signal conduction, emphasizing the importance of cellular structures in nerve physiology. Without these adjustments, coordination and rapid transmission of neural messages would be greatly impaired, and the interdependence of anatomy and function in the nervous system is ensured. Recent studies have improved our knowledge of the biophysical mechanisms behind nerve impulse propagation and shown that these events are not restricted to electrical and biochemical processes alone. The Hodgkin-Huxley model forms a basic framework for understanding neuronal excitability, yet it fails to cover a number of mechanical factors that affect action potentials and propagating nerve impulses.

Experiments indicate that forces , such as reversible heat exchange and axonal expansion are primary mechanisms for impacting neuronal behavior, pointing to the necessity of integrating such divergent forces into contemporary neurophysiological paradigms. Emphasis on the mechanical basis of neuronal signaling necessitates a shift in paradigm that promotes a more integrated concept of nerve function, including thermodynamic and materials science principles to better manage and control nervous system activity (Figure 4.15).

4.5.1. Saltatory Conduction in Myelinated Fibers

The complex process of saltatory conduction in myelinated fibers is crucial to the effective workings of the nervous system. Myelin sheaths, made up of layers of lipids that surround the axons of neurons, form isolated segments surrounded by nodes of Ranvier. Action potentials, the electrical impulses that make communication between neurons possible, leap from node to node, not along the entire axon length. This organized "skipping" greatly increases the speed of transmission, making it possible for almost instantaneous response to stimuli. Myelin sheathing not only decreases ion exchange across the membrane but also conserves energy to be expended in the restoration of ionic balance following action potential, giving it a central role in nerve function maintenance and effective neurotransmission. Further, the mechanism of ephaptic coupling, which involves the capacity of neighboring neurons to phase-lock their action potential, is intriguingly similar to the physiology of saltatory conduction. The coordination would be particularly reasonable in the case of densely packed neurons, where the electrical activity of one could affect the excitability of adjacent fibers, thereby making nerve conduction more efficient and rapid. This is a reference to the complex interactions of neural tissue, where both single and population behaviors contribute to performance. By understanding these mechanisms, researchers can better appreciate myelinated fiber dynamic structural-functional interaction and implications that reach beyond neural communication to world neurophysiological well-being, as suggested by recent models proposing an approximate scale of correlation between neuron bundles (Pekker et al., 2015). Despite well-proven rules that guide action potential transmission, recent research has raised the issue of relationships between biological channels and membrane characteristics in myelinated axons. Current models demonstrate that alterations in electric potential across lipid bilayers are not the sole contributing forces to the conduction of signals; instead, there is a more nuanced appreciation for the role of intra-membrane electric field propagation. This approach can explain the phenomenon of saltatory conduction, both for the leaping of action potentials from node to node and for the consistent delay incurred regardless of distance between nodes of Ranvier as suggested by newly emerging research. This emphasis on the electrochemical dynamics within myelinated fibers has wide-ranging implications for both clinical application and general neuroscience, and it emphasizes the value of further research into these basic transmission mechanisms, as outlined in Boadas et al. (2018).

4.5.2. Factors Affecting Nerve Impulse Speed

Speed of conduction of the nerve impulse is governed by two principal determinants: myelination and diameter of the axon. Myelination greatly enhances conductivity due to the insulating sheaths on the axon, the myelin sheath. Not just does the sheath avoid the dissipation of electrical charge, but it facilitates the process of saltatory conduction, in which impulses leap from one node of Ranvier to another. It results in a very greatly enhanced transmission velocity relative to unmyelinated fibers. Moreover, larger axon diameters provide greater speed by decreasing the internal resistance to ion flow and allowing for a faster transmission of action potentials. All of these structural characteristics are an evolutionary trade-off that maximizes neural efficiency in an array of physiological contexts, which sheds light on the richness of nerve impulse dynamics and the pivotal role they play in sensory and motor abilities. Temperature is another important determinant of the velocity of nerve impulses. Biochemistry supporting transmission of nerve impulses is dependent upon temperature, in that higher thermal energy increases ion movement and enzymatic activity used to generate action potentials. More importantly, higher temperatures can increase the depolarization and repolarization phases of the action potential, consequently accelerating the process down the nerve fibers. Conversely, lower temperatures may slow down these processes at the cost of nerve signal conduction and even have functional impairments. This interaction underlines the need to have efficient body temperatures to secure efficient nervous system functioning, for instance, in response to extreme environmental temperatures during physiological responses.

For this reason, health practitioners and biologists have to be aware of the impact of temperature on nerve conduction for appreciation of the susceptibility of neural processes to the environment. Finally, ionic concentration within intracellular and extracellular spaces plays a significant role in nerve impulse velocity regulation. Movement of ions, particularly sodium (Na^+) and potassium (K^+), plays a crucial role in creating as well as propagating action potentials. Ion concentration fluctuations can significantly affect the excitability of the neural membrane and consequently signal transmission speed. For example, alterations in the concentration of extracellular sodium have the capacity to alter threshold for action potential, both influencing frequency and amplitude of impulses transmitted down the axon. Calcium ions also contribute significantly to the release of neurotransmitters from synapses and influence global efficacy of neuronal transmission. These ionic interactions further indicate the importance of homeostatic conditions within the nervous system, and as such, it is important to realize how such factors contribute towards neural functionality, especially in pathological states when imbalances of ions may occur, as in neurological disease (Bullock & Perkel, 1968; Bewick et al., 2018).

4.5.3. Comparison of Conduction in Myelinated Versus Unmyelinated Fibers

The mechanism of conduction of nerve impulses varies widely between unmyelinated and myelinated fibers primarily due to the differences in structure inherent in the two. Myelinated fibers have a cover made of fatty material known as myelin, which protects the axon and enables fast transmission of the impulse through the process of saltatory conduction. This procedure allows the action potentials to "hop" from one Node of Ranvier, where the myelin sheath does not exist, to another, with a conduction velocity of as much as 120 meters per second. In unmyelinated fibers, it does not exist, and impulses move more slowly, typically between 0.5 and 2 meters per second. The presence of myelin not only enhances speed but also conserves energy, as fewer ions must be exchanged in the transmission of the action potential, and myelinated fibers are particularly efficient at transmitting signals over large distances. Moreover, the difference between conduction of myelinated and unmyelinated fibers has significant physiological ramifications, particularly on sensory operations. For instance, the rapid conduction speed of myelinated Aδ fibers is crucial to rapidly identify sharp pain, while unmyelinated C fibers transmit slow, dull pain sensation. This functional segregation can be observed in studies demonstrating how stimulation of Aδ fibers induces an immediate, acute pain sensation, and activation of C fibers induces a late, throbbing pain sensation. This interaction may be observed in experimental paradigms in which laser stimulation is applied to the skin. With sophisticated techniques, researchers can selectively activate the different fiber types to elucidate their unique roles in pain perception and advance our understanding of sensory processing streams and their resultant behavior (Carmon et al., 2012). In general, the difference between conduction in unmyelinated and myelinated fibers not only indicates a difference in speed but also a general subtlety of how the nervous system receives information. The varying threshold for activation in the fibers, for instance, suggests a nuanced function of interaction with the environment, reacting to the types of stimuli the body receives. It has been evident that myelinated fibers are made for rapid response, more likely to endure crucial situations, and unmyelinated fibers have a function in estimating continuous sensory inputs. Such knowledge attained by exploring differences facilitates the potential of clinical application, particularly in the release of pain and treatment for neurophysiological disorders, highlighting the need for intervention according to certain nerve fiber types (Binder et al., 1977) (Figure 4.16).

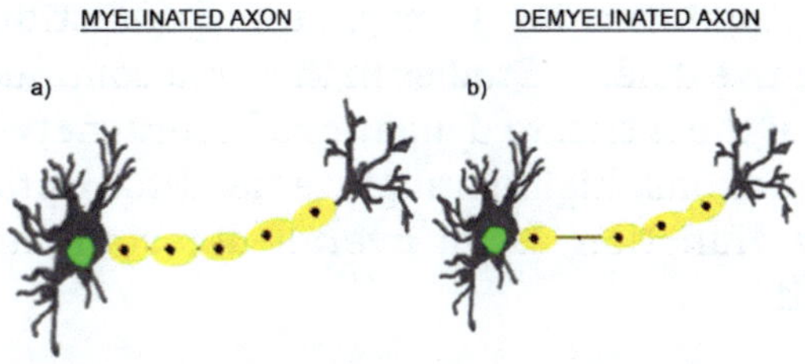

Figure 4.16. Myelinated and unmyelinated axons.

Source: https://cdn-ccnli.nitrocdn.com/hPbgvskpJmIfLTeYLYGdGpfRfGKbrYYq/assets/images/optimized/rev-9bf19a8/alevelbiology.co.uk/wp-content/uploads/2020/12/Myelinated_and_demyelinated_axons.png

Test Your Knowledge

1. What is saltatory conduction, and why is it faster than continuous conduction?
2. How do myelination and axon diameter affect the speed of transmission of the nerve impulse?

4.6. Disorders of Nerve Physiology

Learning Outcome

1. Describe the commonest neurological disorders: Parkinson's disease, multiple sclerosis, and epilepsy;
2. Define how the impact of nerve disorders on physiology and function;
3. Describe the current research and treatment modes.

Understanding of nerve physiology disorders must entail careful consideration of the intricate mechanisms controlling neuronal function. Nerve physiology encompasses normal and diseased conditions, variations giving rise to several neurological disorders. For instance, disruptions in ionic currents through nerve membranes can lead to disorders , such as multiple sclerosis or amyotrophic lateral sclerosis. Coordination of neurotransmitter discharge with ion channel function is essential to neuronal homeostasis. Dysregulation of these processes can lead to symptoms ranging from motor dysfunction to cognitive defects. Studies in this area continue to reveal the intricate dynamics of neural network interactions, highlighting the need for optimal nerve function as an overall determinant of health.

The respiratory system provides a special insight into how nerve physiology affects body function. Breathing disorders illustrate how disruptions in nerve signaling can have extensive effects. In particular, control of heart rhythms and blood pressure according to breath patterns serves the function of maintaining homeostasis. Understanding the physiological changes that occur with the process of inspiration and expiration, such as total small hyperpolarization in inspiration and depolarization during expiration, gives insight into how nerve impulses are closely related to breath mechanisms. As highlighted by current research, the relation between respiration and the autonomic nervous system further points towards the significance of nerve physiology in the management of several medical conditions, including stress disorders and respiratory disorders (Jerath et al., 2015). Moreover, emotional states play a far-reaching role in nerve physiology as expressed in various levels of CRC during various emotional states. Negative effects are associated with decreased CRC, reflecting a movement toward sympathetic dominance that can exacerbate existing nerve disorders or introduce new physiological issues. Conversely, positive affect enhances parasympathetic function, favoring a more balanced autonomic response. This dynamic process illustrates how the brain, through the modulation of its governing mechanisms, integrates sensory feedback to regulate emotional experience, highlighting the importance of knowing the neurological stakes for mental health. Therapeutic practices , such as pranayama and meditation can perhaps capitalize on these physiological findings to cure mood disorders, symbolizing the interdependence between emotional and nerve physiology (Crawford et al., 2015) (Figure 4.17).

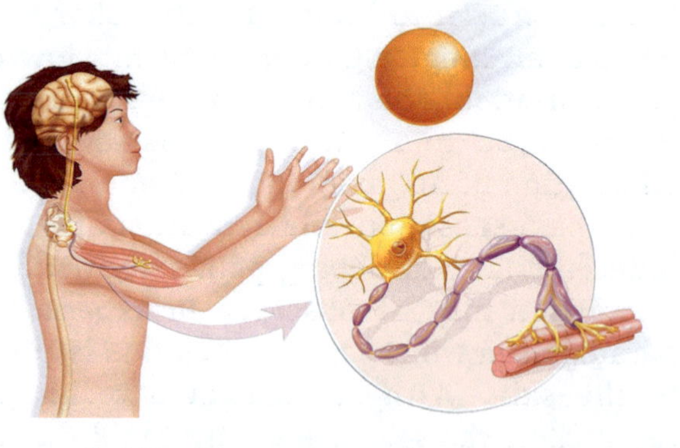

Figure 4.17. Neuromuscular system and diseases.

Source: https://media.healthdirect.org.au/images/inline/original/neuromuscular-system-illustration-a57386.jpg.

4.6.1. Common Neurological Disorders: Multiple Sclerosis (MS), Parkinson's Disease (PD), and Epilepsy

The physiology of nerves is such that it is imperative to know general neurological disorders , such as MS, PD, and epilepsy, because they graphically illustrate the impact of neural dysfunction on human health. Multiple sclerosis is an autoimmune condition in which the myelin sheaths surrounding nerve fibers become degenerated, so that neurons are unable to communicate with each other properly. The resulting symptoms can be very varied, ranging from fatigue and motor dysfunction to cognitive impairment. The pathophysiology of MS makes it important to value neural signaling processes and immune response mechanisms because both play crucial roles in its disease process and its regulation. In contrast to multiple sclerosis, Parkinson's disease primarily affects the basal ganglia, where the degeneration of dopaminergic neurons results in typical symptoms of tremor, rigidity, and bradykinesia. The neurodegenerative feature of PD provides insightful knowledge on neurotransmitter loss processes, in this example, dopamine, that is crucial for regulating motor function. The illness not only disables motor circuits but can also trigger cognitive and emotional disturbances. Advancement in neuroimaging is directed at revealing the basic structural changes in the brain that accompany PD, shedding light on the potential of specific therapeutic intervention to mitigate symptoms and enhance the quality of life (Jayaraman et al., 2023). Epilepsy, another prevalent neurological disorder, results from the abnormal electrical activity of the brain, leading to various types of seizures and degrees of severity. Epilepsy research poses a challenge to an investigation of the excitatory and inhibitory mechanisms of neurons, highlighting the delicate balance required for normal brain function. Biophysics of neuron research shows how abnormalities in synaptic transmission result in seizure activity, and it encourages more effective anticonvulsant treatments. Additionally, new research into natural products, e.g., those of *Achillea millefolium* L. (Yarrow), has been effective in epilepsy control through its antioxidant and anti-inflammatory properties, pointing towards the significance of neuroprotective strategies in the treatment of neurological conditions (Shamsizadeh et al., 2017). These relationships point towards the potential that a deep understanding of nerve physiology might lead to new ways of addressing conditions , such as MS, PD, and epilepsy.

4.6.2. Impact of Nerve Disorders on Physiology and Function

The intricate system of nerve physiology and function is severely compromised by nerve disorders, which have a profound impact on the overall functioning of the body. Nerve disorders like neuropathy, multiple sclerosis, and Parkinson's disease illustrate how impairment in nerve signal conduction can be manifested through alterations in physiological response. For instance, neuropathy patients lose sensation, feel weakness, and aches, reflecting the need to keep the function of nerves intact to convey effectively within the nervous system. Additionally, nerve diseases can trigger cascade phenomena affecting numerous body systems, from muscular coordination to visceral regulation. As natural feedback mechanisms are disrupted, the individual may experience not only physical but also psychological symptoms that further complicate their health. The relationship of nerve disorders to physiological function extends to the field of respiratory regulation. Mechanics of breathing are inevitably linked to autonomic nervous control, where disruptions can initiate serious health disorders. Since nerve function is compromised, as with certain respiratory illnesses and breathing disorders of a nervous origin, coordination between the inhalation and exhalation processes is compromised. This is best seen with illnesses involving the peripheral or central nervous system, leading to reduced respiratory drive and compromised gas exchange. Second, there should be an appreciation of such physiological modulation because disease states like breath-holding or impaired hyperventilation can compound underlying disease states. The physiological nuances of these interactions underscore the importance of nervous health in managing and addressing respiratory complications more effectively (Jerath et al., 2015). The impact of nerve disorders on mental and emotional conditions should also not be downplayed. A healthy nervous system is tasked with emotional balance through its management of responses to stress and anxiety, while disorders may result in overreactions that disrupt everyday functioning. Emerging evidence suggests that breathing training and meditation can be effective interventions that help restore homeostasis upset by emotional disturbances. By enhancing better neural regulation of the breathing pattern, such interventions can potentially forestall the physical as well as mental manifestations of diseases , such as depression and anxiety.

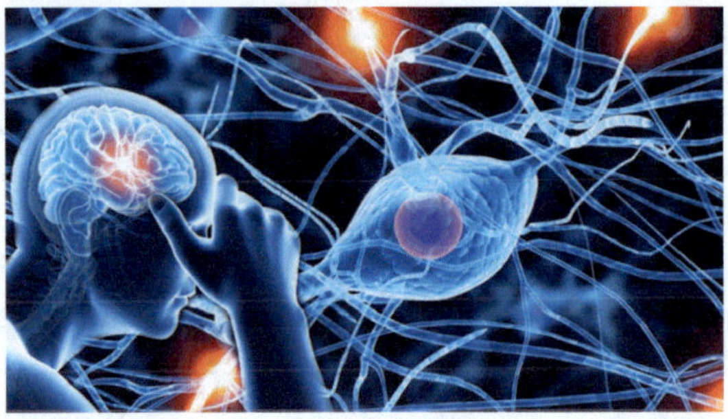

Figure 4.18. Nerve disorders.

Source: https://www.chaudharyhospital.in/wp-content/uploads/2020/05/Neurologicaldisorders-1-1.png.

Therefore, the understanding of the interplay between nerve physiology and emotional well-being not only draws from the awareness of such complex interactions but also opens up the possibility of integrative treatment modalities. The identification of the multi-faceted nature of nerve disorders makes it possible to adopt a more integrative mode of healthcare that addresses both the physiological and the emotional dimensions (Barnes et al., 2015) (Figure 4.18).

4.6.3. Current Research and Treatment Options

Recent studies on the physiology of nerves have yielded fundamental findings on how neural paths are modulated and influence various health conditions. Research has indicated that the dynamics of respiration play a vital role in shaping cardiovascular and **nervous** system function, and this is a coming together of respiratory methods and nervous system well-being. Specifically, the phenomenon of minor hyperpolarization with inspiration and minor depolarization with expiration shows potential therapeutic avenues towards the treatment of respiratory and stress diseases. Such information regarding the effect of respiration on cellular membrane potential is a new paradigm for the design of non-invasive therapy for diseases with nerve function , such as anxiety and hypertension. These developments indicate the necessity for holistic approaches to nerve physiology by valuing the interdependence between neural and respiratory processes (Jerath et al., 2015). In a study of modern erectile dysfunction (ED) therapies, it is apparent that the condition is often facilitated by neuropathological mechanisms. The intricate relationship between sexual function and the physiology of nerves has seen a lot of work directed towards pharmacological and non-pharmacological interventions. Recent research emphasizes how the prevalence of ED, which impacts as many as 150 million men worldwide, can be informative with respect to its neurological mechanisms. With increased knowledge regarding nerve-mediated mechanisms for erection, newer approaches like phosphodiesterase type 5 inhibitors and novel nerve stimulation methods are being tested to advance efficacy. Greater insight into the neurophysiological basis of ED also allows clinicians to adopt a holistic approach to management that involves nerve health alongside traditional approaches (Kalsi et al., 2013). Current research further emphasizes the therapeutic potential of neuroregenerative approaches to the management of nerve pathologies. Understanding of nerve plasticity, complemented by advances in molecular biology, has precipitated exciting advancements in regenerative medicine. The continued investigation into neurotrophic factors aims at inducing the regeneration of nerves as well as improving the functionality of damaged neuronal circuits. Stem cell therapy and targeted electrical stimulation are also on the radar to determine whether they have any role to play in facilitating nerve regeneration and functional recovery. By bringing together the most recent research on cellular and molecular processes coupled with therapeutic intervention, the physiology of nerves can potentially transform the management of neurologic and other similar disorders to provide improved quality of life to the affected group. Hence, further research and advancement remain at the top of nerve health and therapeutic management.

Test Your Knowledge

1. How does multiple sclerosis distort the myelin sheath, and what impact does this have on the transmission of the nerve impulse?
2. What is the physiological basis of neuropathic pain, and how is it different from normal pain signaling?

SUMMARY

An excursion into nerve physiology, it is necessary to synthesize the convoluted connection between nerve function and the general principles of neural signaling. The appreciation of how neurons convey information by means of complicated electrochemical phenomena is not only informative about physiological mechanisms but also suggestive of the possibility for technological innovations in medicine and neuroscience. As can be noted in many research questions, the multidimensional perspective to nerve physiology, ranging from molecular interactions at synapses to broader implications of neurotransmitter dynamics, unravels a rich fabric of biological function. Such research is characterized by the creativity and endurance necessary for deciphering the enigmas of neural communication, supporting the notion that a quantitative program of intense rigor can give fundamental insight into this field of inquiry (Traill, 2007).

Additionally, the advance of knowledge in nerve physiology recalls combining theoretical models with empirical data. The interdependence of idealistic and empirical viewpoints, highlighted in Helmholtz's accounts, contributes towards a more complete explanation of the underlying processes of perception and thought. Through studies today, the incorporation of varied theoretical views allows us to appreciate the complexity of nervous systems and their adaptive functions. It underscores the importance of multidisciplinary collaboration in accelerating our understanding of neural behavior and mechanisms, an activity that sparks innovation in cognitive models as well as therapeutic approaches (Bell et al., 2014). This convergence will be invaluable in cracking the puzzles introduced by neurological disorders and advancing groundbreaking research in neuroscience. Briefly, the physiology of nerves not only illuminates simple biological phenomena, but it also engenders a wider debate on the significance of such findings for science as a whole and for society generally. By emphasizing the worth of nuanced appreciation in the domain of neuroscience, we establish the foundation for the prospect of forthcoming research endeavors encompassing the specifics of neural processes and the broader questions of consciousness and perception. An interest in interdisciplinarity coupled with theory-heavy analysis becomes a common thread for future research. Ultimately, the search for knowledge in the field of nerve physiology is not merely an intellectual exercise but an endeavor that can have the potential to revolutionize our comprehension of the human experience and enhance our capacity to treat neurological illness on multiple fronts.

Nerve physiology captures the complexities of signal conduction and processing within the nervous system, specifically the roles of neurons and support cells. The electrochemical gradient that prevails at the nerve center is sustained by ion channels, sodium and potassium channels in particular, that are necessary for the formation of action potentials. An action potential is a short, transient change in membrane potential that propagates along axons, allowing communication between neurons. The mechanism of saltatory conduction, occurring at myelinated nodes of Ranvier, has the extraordinary effect of enhancing signal velocity, demonstrating the advanced structural adaptations of nerve fibers. Familiarity with these fundamental properties is essential to learn how nerve impulses generate reflexes and motor functions and how such disorders can lead to neurological diseases, pointing out the relevance of maintaining neuronal structure and function in disease and health. The function of the sympathetic nervous system in modulating peripheral vasculature, particularly in stress responses, has been explained in recent studies. Quantitative estimates of sympathetic nerve activity (SNA) between different regions of the body, i.e., core and periphery, have been offered in research studies using photoplethysmography during cold exposure tests. For example, significant reductions in Pulse Transit Time (PTT) were identified, indicating elevated sympathetic activity with cold immersion. The core-periphery differential sympathetic response circulating underscores the adaptive body processes of homeostasis. Results , such as these not only enhance our understanding of physiological responses to environmental stimuli but also inform us of autonomic dysregulation-related conditions, illustrating the critical interaction between nerve physiology and systemic physiological adaptability in varying contexts, as highlighted through SNA research (Ainslie et al., 2019). Also, the neural input to such physiological parameters as fetal heart rate variability (fHRV) offers an intriguing window on nerve physiology in the clinical setting. Recent research illuminates the vagus nerve in modulating fHRV, offering insight into the autonomic control of the developing fetus. Using complex analytical techniques, indices have been found to be specific for vagal regulation of fHRV, and they inform us as to how nerve activity can be quantified in terms of heart rate dynamical changes. This knowledge is vital for monitoring in utero, especially during clinical interventions, as it takes into account the underlying physiology of disease and health during fetal development. Applying this knowledge to practice enhances our ability to assess fetal health, illustrating the broad impact of nerve physiology in medicine and healthcare, including research into neural contribution to fHRV (Burns et al., 2019).

KEY TERMS FROM THIS CHAPTER

- Acetylcholine
- Axon
- Depolarization
- Myelin Sheath
- Neurotransmitter
- Refractory Period
- Resting Membrane Potential
- Schwann Cells
- Sodium-Potassium Pump
- Synaptic Cleft
- Action Potential
- Dendrites
- Hyperpolarization
- Neuron
- Nodes of Ranvier
- Repolarization
- Saltatory Conduction
- Signal Transmission
- Synapse
- Voltage-Gated Channels

CRITICAL THINKING QUESTIONS

1. **What is the resting membrane potential of a typical neuron?**
   a. +30 mV
   b. 0 mV
   c. –70 mV
   d. –30 mV
2. **Which ion primarily enters the neuron during the phase of depolarization of an action potential?**
   a. Potassium (K^+)
   b. Sodium (Na^+)
   c. Calcium (Ca^{2+})
   d. Chloride (Cl^-)
3. **What is the function of the myelin sheath in nerve fibers?**
   a. Slow down nerve impulse conduction
   b. Create action potentials
   c. Increase the speed of nerve impulse conduction
   d. Release neurotransmitters
4. **Which part of the neuron accepts incoming messages?**
   a. Dendrites
   b. Axon
   c. Axon terminals
   d. Myelin
5. **What occurs at the synapse in nerve transmission?**
   a. Electrical impulses are stored
   b. Nerve cells divide
   c. Myelin is created
   d. Neurotransmitters are released to the next neuron

Short Answer Questions

1. What is the resting membrane potential of a neuron?
2. Name the two chief types of nerve cells.
3. What is an action potential?
4. What ion primarily enters the neuron in depolarization?
5. Compare and contrast myelinated and unmyelinated nerve fibers.
6. Outline the steps in the conduction of the nerve impulse down a myelinated axon.
7. Describe the process of refractory periods in nerve conduction.
8. Describe the function of calcium ions in neurotransmitter release at the synapse.

Answers to Critical Thinking Questions

1. (c); 2. (b); 3. (c); 4. (b); 5. (c)

REFERENCES

1. Abbink, W., Geurds, F., Roques, J., Vis, H., et al. (2025). Differential responses of Nile tilapia (*Oreochromis niloticus*) to fin clip wounding and related stress: Perspectives. https://core.ac.uk/download/pdf/29249634.pdf (accessed on 16th June 2025).
2. Ainslie, D., Anderson, M., Appelhans, B., Billman, G., Budidha, K., et al. (2019). Photoplethysmography for quantitative assessment of sympathetic nerve activity (SNA) during cold stress. https://core.ac.uk/download/169434493.pdf (accessed on 16th June 2025).
3. al Azad, A. K., Borisyuk, R., Buhl, E., Conte, D., et al. (2014). Can simple rules control development of a pioneer vertebrate neuronal network generating behavior? https://core.ac.uk/download/153536060.pdf (accessed on 16th June 2025).
4. Alavi, A., & Axford, J. S. (2008). Glyco-biomarkers: potential determinants of cellular physiology and pathology. *Disease markers*, *25*(4-5), 193–205. https://doi.org/10.1155/2008/863032(accessed on 16th June 2025).
5. Al-Diri, B., Habib, M., Hunter, A., Steel, D., et al. (2010). Manual measurement of retinal bifurcation features. https://core.ac.uk/download/53983.pdf (accessed on 16th June 2025).
6. Alvarez-Curto, E., Caltabiano, G., Liste, M. J. V., Marsango, S., et al. (2015). Defining the organizational structure of dopamine and muscarinic acetylcholine receptors. https://core.ac.uk/download/46558276.pdf (accessed on 16th June 2025).
7. Anderson, A. J., Ciciriello, A. J., Cummings, B. J., Dumont, R. J., et al. (2019). PLG bridge implantation in chronic SCI promotes axonal elongation and myelination. https://core.ac.uk/download/286361703.pdf (accessed on 16th June 2025).
8. Anderson, A. J., Ciciriello, A. J., Cummings, B. J., Dumont, R. J., et al. (2020). Polycistronic delivery of IL-10 and NT-3 promotes oligodendrocyte myelination and functional recovery in a mouse spinal cord injury model. https://core.ac.uk/download/305124291.pdf (accessed on 16th June 2025).
9. Jerath, R., Crawford, M. W., Barnes, V. A., & Harden, K. (2015). Widespread depolarization during expiration: a source of respiratory drive?. *Medical hypotheses*, *84*(1), 31–37. https://doi.org/10.1016/j.mehy.2014.11.010(accessed on 16th June 2025).
10. Bell, M., Bernfeld, B., Boring, B., Bradley, D., Cahan, S., Crary, M., Daston, L., et al. (2014). Hermann von Helmholtz's empiric-transcendentalism reconsidered: Construction and constitution in Helmholtz's psychology of the object. https://core.ac.uk/download/55764436.pdf (accessed on 16th June 2025).
11. Bewick, G., Smith, L., Lomo, T., Martinov, V. N., Nja, A., et al. (2018). Activity-dependent plasticity of transmitter release from nerve terminals in rat fast and slow muscles. https://core.ac.uk/download/177222.pdf (accessed on 16th June 2025).
12. Bhattacharyya, D., Ghosh, J., & Mukhopadhyay, S. (2023). From gut to gray matter: The surprising links between the microbiome and brain. https://core.ac.uk/download/603896988.pdf (accessed on 16th June 2025).
13. Binder, M. J., Brill, M. H., Gruberg, E. R., Joyner, R. W., et al. (1977). *Neurophysiology*. https://core.ac.uk/download/4421009.pdf (accessed on 16th June 2025).
14. Bologna, M., & Dirkx, M. F. (2022). The pathophysiology of Parkinson's disease tremor. https://core.ac.uk/download/599500557.pdf (accessed on 16th June 2025).

15. Brohawn, S., Campbell, E., Handler, A., MacKinnon, R., et al. (2019). The mechanosensitive ion channel TRAAK is localized to the mammalian node of Ranvier. https://core.ac.uk/download/323081529.pdf (accessed on 16th June 2025).

16. Bullock, T. H., & Perkel, D. H. (1968). Neutral coding–A report based on an NRP work session. Contractor Report (CR), Document ID

17. https://ntrs.nasa.gov/citations/19690022317 (accessed on 16th June 2025).

18. Burns, P., Cao, M., Desrochers, A., Durosier, F., et al. (2019). Vagal contributions to fetal heart rate variability: An omics approach. http://arxiv.org/abs/1901.06431 (accessed on 16th June 2025).

19. Burock, M. (2010). Evidence for information processing in the brain. https://core.ac.uk/download/11923040.pdf (accessed on 16th June 2025).

20. Caragea, D., Florescu, C., Pirici, D., Târtea, G. C., et al. (2016). The substrate of the biopsychosocial influences in the carcinogenesis of the digestive tract. https://core.ac.uk/download/144552990.pdf (accessed on 16th June 2025).

21. Carmon, A., Mouraux, A., Zaitsev, A. V., Bromm, B., et al. (2012). Thermal detection thresholds of Aδ- and C-fiber afferents activated by brief CO_2 laser pulses applied onto the human hairy skin. https://core.ac.uk/download/pdf/8718659.pdf (accessed on 16th June 2025).

22. Crawford, C., Kelly, M. C., Kennedy-Lydon, T. M., Peppiatt-Wildman, C. M., et al. (2013). Sympathetic nerve-derived ATP regulates renal medullary vasa recta diameter via pericyte cells: A role for regulating medullary blood flow? https://core.ac.uk/download/30712001.pdf (accessed on 16th June 2025).

23. Crawford, M. W., & Jerath, R. (2015). How does the body affect the mind? Role of cardiorespiratory coherence in the spectrum of emotions. https://core.ac.uk/download/131207333.pdf (accessed on 16th June 2025).

24. Davis, G. W., Dickman, D. K., Fetter, R. D., Genç, B., et al. (2017). MCTP is an ER-resident calcium sensor that stabilizes synaptic transmission and homeostatic plasticity. https://core.ac.uk/download/323063498.pdf (accessed on 16th June 2025).

25. Diamond, I., Dohrman, D., & Gordon, A. (1997). The role of the neuromodulator adenosine in alcohol's actions. https://core.ac.uk/download/323079180.pdf (accessed on 16th June 2025).

26. D'Souza, A. W., Thiessen, J. S., Cheung, C. P., Nardone, M., Lee, J. B., Baker, R. E., Shoemaker, J. K., et al. (2025). Inhibition of muscle sympathetic action potential firing and recruitment patterns following cannabis inhalation in humans. *Journal of Applied Physiology*. https://www.semanticscholar.org/paper/b2e75d2de4fb474c9bea969877e92dd59c9b8ebf (accessed on 16th June 2025).

27. Estrine, J., & DeLisle, L. (2006). Stress: Putting the brain back into medicine. https://core.ac.uk/download/71356692.pdf (accessed on 16th June 2025).

28. Ghaninia, M. (2007). *Olfaction in Mosquitoes*. https://core.ac.uk/download/11695204.pdf (accessed on 16th June 2025).

29. Jayaraman, C., & Joseph, A. (2023). Preprocessing techniques for neuroimaging modalities: An in-depth analysis. https://core.ac.uk/download/553310232.pdf (accessed on 16th June 2025).

30. Kalsi, J., & Muneer, A. (2013). Erectile dysfunction–An update of current practice and future strategies. https://core.ac.uk/download/29416259.pdf (accessed on 16th June 2025).

31. Kling, I. H. (1939). *The Hormones of Invertebrates*. https://open.bu.edu/bitstream/2144/4470/1/Kling_1939_web.pdf (accessed on 16th June 2025).
32. Lin, J. W., & Llinás, R. (1993). Depolarization-activated potentiation of the T fiber synapse in the blue crab. https://open.bu.edu/bitstream/2144/27851/1/Depolarization-activated%20potentiation%20of%20the%20T%20fiber%20synapse%20in%20the%20blue%20crab.pdf (accessed on 16th June 2025).
33. Macmillan, D., Altman, J., & Kien, J. (1983). Intersegmental coordination in the crayfish swimmeret system reconsidered. *Journal of Experimental Zoology, 228*, 157–162. https://www.semanticscholar.org/paper/05bb251481627c06fb153e1829f1dd9ded5bb9aa (accessed on 16th June 2025).
34. Madrenas Boadas, J., Martí Cabarrocas, A., & Pérez González, J. J. (2018). Action potential propagation: Ion current or intramembrane electric field? https://core.ac.uk/download/210528928.pdf (accessed on 16th June 2025).
35. Mohamed, A., & Abdalwahab, M. (2011). A comparative study fourth order Runge–Kutta-TVD scheme and Fluent software case of inlet flow problems. https://core.ac.uk/download/12007634.pdf (accessed on 16th June 2025).
36. Mueller, J., & Tyler, W. J. (2013). A quantitative overview of biophysical forces governing neural function. http://arxiv.org/abs/1309.6277 (accessed on 16th June 2025).
37. Pekker, M., & Shneider, M. N. (2015). Correlation of action potentials in adjacent neurons. http://arxiv.org/abs/1505.03385 (accessed on 16th June 2025).
38. Sadegh-Zadeh, S. A. (2019). Computational methods toward early detection of neuronal deterioration. https://core.ac.uk/download/556180728.pdf (accessed on 16th June 2025).
39. Shamsizadeh, A., Vakilian, A., Moghadam-Ahmadi, A., Ayoobi, F., Hassanshahi, G., Fatemi, I., & Allahtavakoli, M. (2017). Bio-effectiveness of the main flavonoids of *Achillea millefolium* in the pathophysiology of neurodegenerative disorders–A review. https://core.ac.uk/download/88230086.pdf (accessed on 16th June 2025).
40. Sönmez, M., Stüdemann, T., Manthey, C., Covic, A., Shehata, N., Im, J., Schwarzová, B., et al. (2025). Modulation of cardiomyocyte contractility and action potentials with chemo genetic chloride currents. *The Journal of Physiology, 603*, 1399–1415. https://www.semanticscholar.org/paper/9be8921f0adc1e97217e20ba2d87abe4e5934a97 (accessed on 16th June 2025).
41. Stalbovskiy, A. O., Pickering, A. E., Paton, J. F. R., Leslie, J., Briant, L. J. B., Robertson, D., & Schramm, L. P. (2014). Mapping the cellular electrophysiology of rat sympathetic preganglionic neurons to their roles in cardiorespiratory reflex integration: A whole cell recording study *in situ*. https://core.ac.uk/download/29027049.pdf (accessed on 16th June 2025).
42. Swash, M. (2022). Modulation of spinal inhibition in amyotrophic lateral sclerosis. *Acta Physiological, 234*. https://www.semanticscholar.org/paper/bfdf8bf8770e23958a8637f0b47abb6b0d15048d (accessed on 16th June 2025).
43. Traill, R. R. (2007). The gulf between behavioral psychology and fundamental physiology: A systematic attempt to bridge the gap. Monograph 15: Brunel University, Institute of Cybernetics, UK. https://core.ac.uk/download/333454.pdf (accessed on 16th June 2025).
44. Werner, G. (2012). *Excitable Media Seminar*. https://core.ac.uk/download/pdf/13598664.pdf (accessed on 16th June 2025).

AUTONOMIC NERVOUS SYSTEM

5

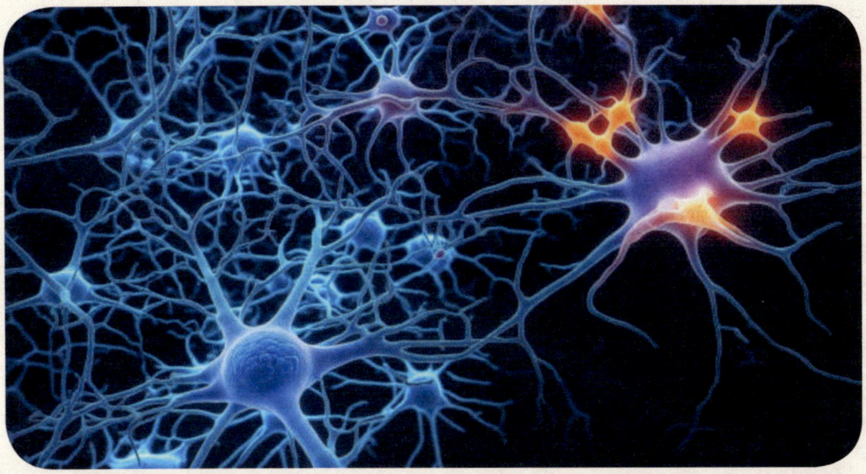

LEARNING OBJECTIVES

After studying this chapter, you will be able to:

1. Discuss the structure of the autonomic nervous system;
2. Describe the functions of the autonomic nervous system;
3. Discuss the neurotransmitters of the autonomic nervous system;
4. Highlight the autonomic nervous system and health;
5. Study diagnostic tools for autonomic nervous system testing;
6. Assess the treatment and management of autonomic disorders.

Introduction

The autonomic nervous system (ANS) maintains homeostasis in the body, its functioning largely beneath the level of our awareness. It regulates involuntary functions like heart rate, blood pressure, breathing, digestion, and sexual arousal. The ANS is broadly divided into three divisions: the sympathetic, parasympathetic, and enteric nervous systems. All of these branches work together to control physiological function, from the fight-or-flight response initiated by the sympathetic system right through to the rest-and-digest processes provided by the parasympathetic system. An understanding of the complexity of the ANS is not only critical in grasping fundamental human physiology, but in examining the interaction between mental and physical health, as this system is closely associated with stress and emotional regulation. Recent research indicates a promising connection between such practices as yoga and the enhancement of its adaptability, highlighting its potential use in mental health and stress management. For instance, regular practice of yoga has been shown to promote neural adaptability and adaptive processes regarding the ANS, offering potentially novel therapeutic strategies in mental illness. Studies have indicated that yoga can significantly influence the nervous system's adaptive capacity, leading to enhanced physical and mental well-being. As detailed in the literature, yogic practices, particularly respiratory maneuvers, have been linked to reductions in cortisol levels, a stress hormone, thereby enhancing autonomic function and emotional regulation (Biesok et al., 2024). This suggests that lifestyle interventions in the ANS can lead to substantial health gains. In addition, the significance of autonomic dysfunction implications in various chronic illnesses should not be overlooked. For example, fibromyalgia, which affects an estimated 2% of the population, illustrates the intricate autonomic nervous system relationship with mechanisms of chronic pain. The disease is characterized by a wide range of symptoms, including fatigue, migraines, and sleep disturbances, whose treatment regimens may be tricky (Dorsher, 2008). A neuroendocrinologic model of fibromyalgia places emphasis on the need to recognize the pathophysiology of interdependency among mental and physical well-being in managing this condition. A grasp of the potentials of the ANS in such cases further enables clinicians to develop holistic interventions not just for treatment of symptoms but also to target the core autonomic mechanisms, resulting finally in improved patient care and resistance to chronic health issues (Figure 5.1).

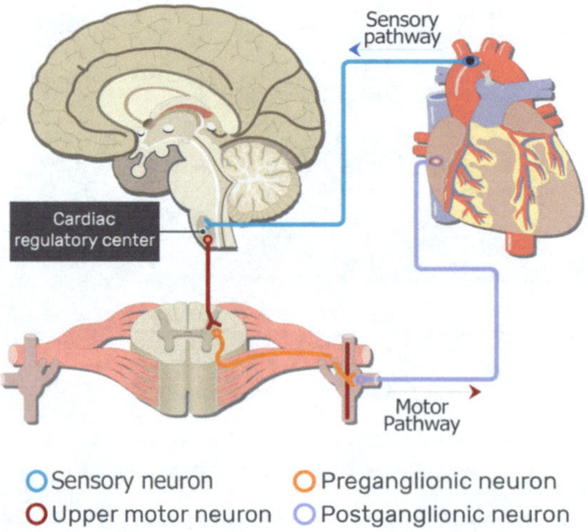

Figure 5.1. Sample-autonomic-nervous-system (ANS)-pathways.

Source: https://www.getbodysmart.com/wp-content/uploads/2017/10/Sample-Autonomic-Nervous-System-Pathways-Labeled-1024x1024.png.

Definition of the Autonomic Nervous System (ANS)

The ANS is the body's central homeostatic regulatory mechanism that oversees a vast range of involuntary physiological activities. Working below consciousness, it is responsible for critical processes , such as heart rate, breathing rate, digestion, and blood pressure. The intricate system is essentially made up of three primary parts: the sympathetic, parasympathetic, and enteric nervous systems. Each component contributes in an individual way to body regulation; for instance, the sympathetic system invokes the fight or flight response during stress, and the parasympathetic system becomes active during relaxation, allowing recovery and energy conservation. The ANS not only, therefore, creates a constant internal environment but also enables adaptive responses of the body to both endogenous and exogenous stimuli, thereby indicating its pivotal role in human physiology. The autonomic nervous system definition expands far beyond mere regulation of visceral functions; it is a complex interplay between neural and hormonal responses that adjust to address various needs of the body. The complexity of the ANS is typical of the principles of distributed cognition in which multiple sensors and neural elements work together to produce homeostasis without an executive mechanism controlling every movement. This distributed system of organization requires a revision of volition and choice in physiological terms. Christensen (2006) reported that the lack of a single all-encompassing integrated control center means that controlling internal states is a process that arises from the dynamic interactions among the simpler cognitive systems rather than being derived from a centralized volitional force. The implications of this perspective extend into the concept of disease and disorder wherein such neural communications are interrupted to the point of impairing autonomic function. Further, the convergence of the ANS with higher-order cognitive processes places this nervous system at center stage for psychological and neurological discourse, particularly for the mind-body issue. (Motofei et al., 2017) contends that the difference between physical brain activity and nonphysical mental operations leaves room to explore how autonomic processes collaborate with cognitive experience , such as reasoning and judgment. Because various autonomic responses may influence emotional states and processes of decision-making, the understanding of the ANS must encompass both its physiological and psychological dimensions. This dual consideration not only adds depth to the definition of the autonomic nervous system but also propels subsequent studies to seek to understand how these complex interactions affect our minds and overall well-being. The ANS is thus given a call for a multidisciplinary approach that will recognize its invaluable contribution to both physical and mental wellness.

Importance in Human Physiology

The ANS is pivotal to the homeostatic process in the human body, and this is crucial for survival. ANS regulates the involuntary functions of the body, including heart rate, digestion, and respiratory rate. Through its two divisions, the sympathetic and parasympathetic nervous systems, the ANS generates a dynamic balance that is crucial in stressful as well as tranquil states. The sympathetic branch prepares the body for "fight or flight" responses, activating mechanisms , such as heightened heart rate and heightened alertness. The parasympathetic branch allows for "rest and digest" mechanisms, allowing for recuperation and energy storage. By controlling a delicate balance between these opposing functions, the autonomic nervous system directly regulates physiological processes that promote health, illustrating the intricate interaction between the body's systems necessary to human physiology. Further, the significance of the autonomic nervous system can be observed in the complexity of heart rate regulation and cardiovascular health. In modern studies, the pathways through which inhibitory heterotrimeric G proteins may modulate heart rate by altering the activity of ion channels highlight the biochemical mechanisms of cardiac regulation. Modulating the frequency by which the heart will beat, the ANS directly affects blood pressure, oxygenation, and metabolic processes in the body. This interaction is particularly important with respect to exercise, stress, and relaxation, in which the heart's response must be rapid and suitable to the body's shifting needs. Understanding how the ANS regulates heart rate and cardiovascular health provides valuable insight into arrhythmia and hypertension and further supports the system's importance in the context of human physiology (Ang et al., 2012).

In addition, ANS is an integral component of the complex relationship between neurophysiology and higher body functions. The link between visceral systems and neurophysiology comes to highlight the importance of such autonomic control to mental and physical health. For instance, the regulation of visceral organs is not merely a physical function but also influences psychological states to highlight the interconnection among psychosomatic entities. Autonomic nervous system disorders may manifest themselves in broad-ranging symptoms, some of which are anxiety, gastrointestinal disturbance, and changes in blood pressure. The study of these relationships further illuminates physiological science and can lead to new therapies. By exploring areas , such as physiological cybernetics and artificial intelligence application in health monitoring, scientists can acquire a greater understanding of the regulatory control of the ANS in health and disease and how its crucial importance is expressed in human physiology (Lange et al., 2025) (Figure 5.2).

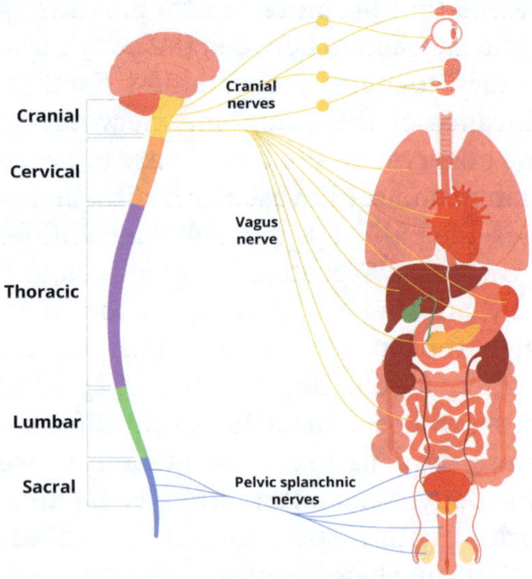

Figure 5.2. Structure-of-the-parasympathetic-system.

Source: https://teachmeanatomy.info/wp-content/uploads/Structure-of-the-Parasympathetic-System-949x1024.png.

5.1. Components of the Autonomic Nervous System (ANS)

Learning Outcome

1. Describe the sympathetic nervous system;
2. Emphasize parasympathetic nervous system;
3. Learn about enteric nervous system.

The autonomic nervous system (ANS) is a complex and integral component of human physiology that regulates involuntary behavior maintaining homeostasis. The ANS is typically divided into three functional systems: the sympathetic, parasympathetic, and enteric nervous systems. The sympathetic nervous system prepares the body for stress-fight or flight responses through increased heart rate, dilatation of the pupils, and discharge of adrenaline. In contrast, the parasympathetic nervous system controls rest and digest functions, promoting relaxation and recuperation through decreased heart rate and increased digestive activities. The enteric nervous system, or so-called second brain, independently governs gastrointestinal function but also talks to the remaining two systems, exemplifying the intricate harmony needed for maintaining health and responding dynamically to changing conditions of the environment. Observing the function of heart rate variability (HRV) is an informative prism through which to view the operation of the autonomic nervous system. HRV indicates the balance of autonomic input from sympathetic and parasympathetic components and holds prognostic value for an individual's cardiovascular status. HRV alterations have also been correlated with several conditions, such as chronic cerebral ischemia and angina pectoris, emphasizing the way autonomic regulatory disturbances can be of clinical importance. For instance, parasympathetic diminishment, typically found in patients with underlying disease conditions like chronic cerebral ischemia, can be accompanied by an increase in low-frequency spectral components of heart rate variability. These results emphasize the importance of measuring autonomic function through HRV analysis to define potential risks and tailor treatment interventions in cardiovascular patients (Inhula, 2018). Further research into the variability of physiological responses caused by the autonomic nervous system across body positions proves its essential role in maintaining cardiovascular homeostasis. Research using methods , such as wavelet transformations has revealed that different body orientations invoke disparate responses in heart rate and blood pressure variability and refer to how the ANS changes to provide equilibrium. Specifically, comparisons in trials involving subjects in supine versus head-down tilt positions have illustrated large discrepancies in low-frequency and very low-frequency components of heart rate and blood pressure and suggest a dynamic response to changing external stimuli and internal needs. The ability of the ANS to adjust cardiovascular parameters adaptively in relation to posture change underlines its pivotal role in preserving the body's capability to respond effectively to changes in the environment to ensure optimal functioning under various states of the body (Federici et al., 2005) (Figure 5.3).

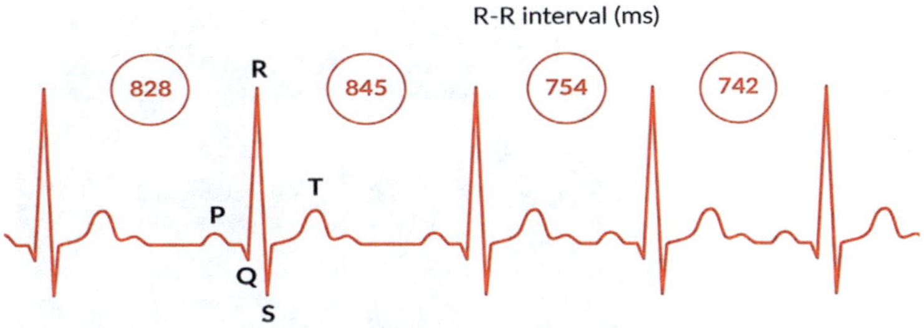

Figure 5.3. Heart rate variability (HRV).

Source: https://www.firstbeat.com/wp-content/uploads/2018/04/heart-rate-variability-firstbeat.jpg.

5.1.1. Sympathetic Nervous System (SNS)

The SNS, a key component of the autonomic nervous system, is primarily responsible for the body's fight or flight response, enabling rapid physiological accommodations when in danger or under stress. This highly intricate system functions within a network of pathways that radiate from the thoracic and lumbar regions of the spinal cord. When triggered, the SNS releases catecholamines, namely adrenaline and norepinephrine, which result in an increased heart rate, elevated blood pressure, and heightened mobilization of energy. These responses place the body in a state of instant response for survival in risky situations. The SNS not only operates during acute stress but also has a central role to play in regulating body processes under basal conditions, such as digestion and temperature regulation, to demonstrate its dual role in emergency as well as homeostatic processes. Psychologically and physiologically, the sympathetic nervous system may have both favorable and unfavorable effects. Persistent activation of the SNS, typically because of chronic anxiety or stress, may lead to a variety of health issues, from cardiovascular diseases, metabolic disorders to psychiatric disorders. For instance, over-activation of the SNS can result in persistent raised blood pressure and heart rate, which are highly risky. Besides, this hyperactivity can affect the autonomic balance, disrupting the harmony with the parasympathetic nervous system (PNS), which is in charge of rest and digestion. Understanding the influence of sympathetic activation on health is important to develop good interventions in stress management and integrative treatment planning that address both psychological and somatic expression of stress disorders (Li et al., 2025).

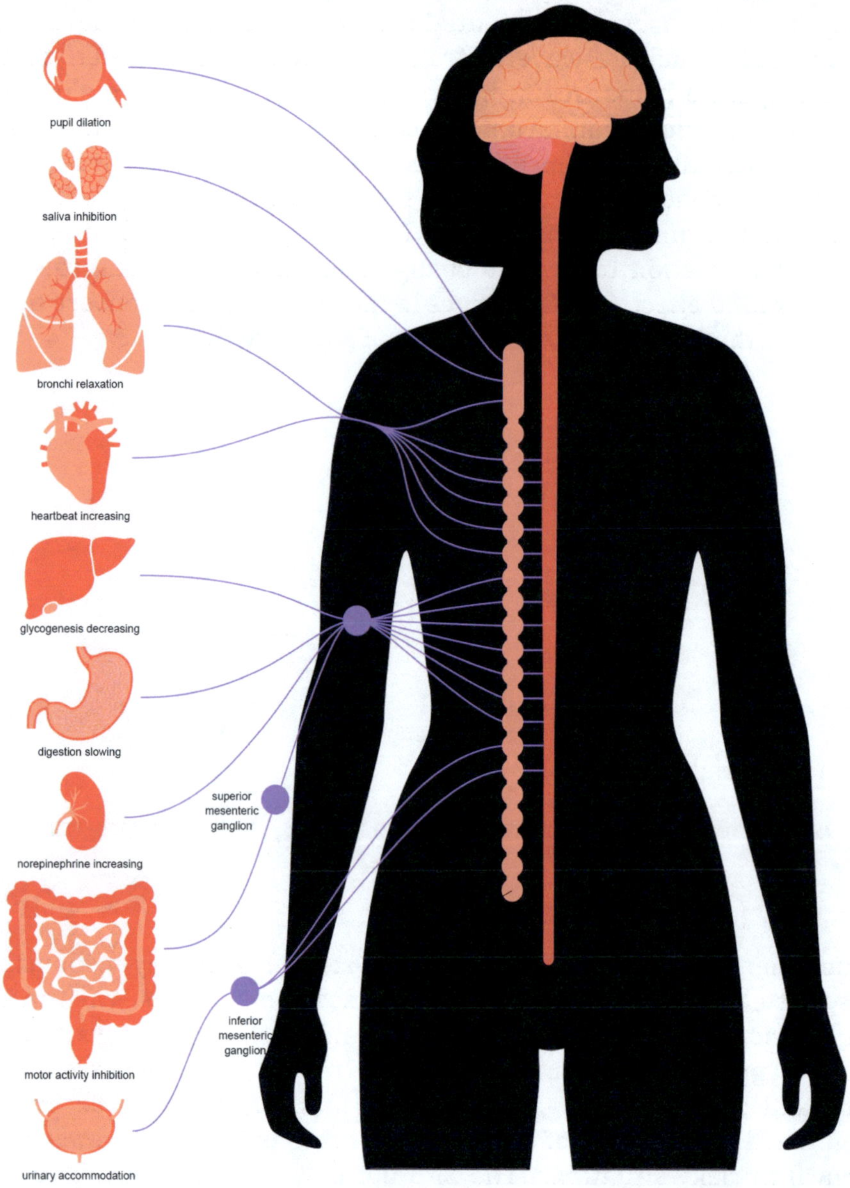

Figure 5.4. Sympathetic-nervous-system (SNS).

Source: https://www.simplypsychology.org/wp-content/uploads/Sympathetic-Nervous-System.jpeg.

Furthermore, the interaction between the sympathetic nervous system and other therapeutic treatments, including the use of psychedelics, has been the focus of recent studies. Past studies have postulated that psychedelics can modulate autonomic regulation by changing SNS activity, giving interesting insight into cardiovascular health and stress response (A D L and Raju, 2023). This connection underscores the significance of a deeper understanding of the SNS not only about traditional physiological principles but also for the development of new psychiatric treatments. By shedding light on the mechanisms by which chemicals might interact with the SNS, scientists can design targeted treatments that capitalize on the natural interrelationships between physiological states and mental well-being. Such developments may finally lead to new ways of health care, based on the integrated character of the autonomic nervous system and its function in an all-around approach to human health (Figure 5.4).

5.1.2. Parasympathetic Nervous System (PNS)

The PNS is a key feature within the larger scheme of the ANS, whose main function is to provide a state of rest and digest. This component of the ANS conserves energy by relaxing and sustaining digestive processes after the body has been subjected to stress. The PNS achieves this through neurochemical communication, with acetylcholine as its primary neurotransmitter, which acts on a variety of target organs. By reducing heart rate, exciting intestinal and glandular activity, and the unfastening of sphincter muscles, the PNS reverses the condition of heightened arousal due to its opposing counterpart, the SNS. This highly fine adjustment between the parasympathetic and sympathetic branches to the body is what is accountable for homeostasis, and therefore it emphasizes the importance of the PNS to health and well-being. Experiments have established that impaired function of the PNS can lead to severe health issues, particularly in obese and metabolic disease populations. A study with 100 volunteers revealed that obese individuals showed very low parasympathetic activity, as reflected by a highly impaired standing-to-laying ratio, which is one of the significant indicators of autonomic dysfunction (Grewal et al., 2011). This reduction in parasympathetic control can make an individual susceptible to diverse cardiovascular complications because the body cannot maintain its resting state and respond suitably to stimuli from the environment. It is thus very important to understand the PNS dynamics not just to treat current health issues but also to design preventive mechanisms aimed at safeguarding cardiovascular function. Furthermore, the impact of chronic stress on the PNS prevents mental health and physical well-being from communicating. Stress activates the SNS, typically forming sympathetic-dominant responses that can suppress parasympathetic function in the long term.

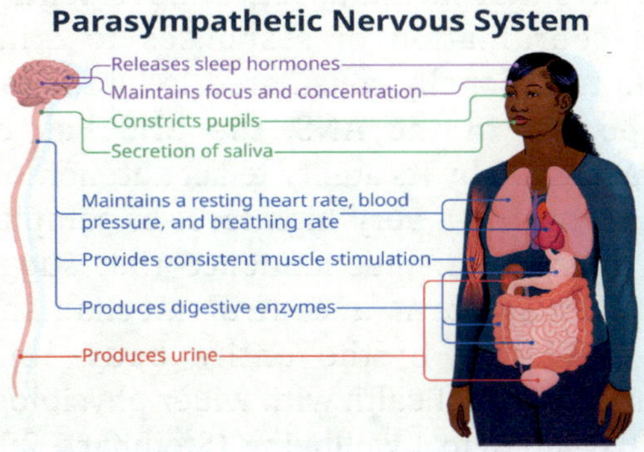

Figure 5.5. Parasympathetic nervous system.

Source: https://www.verywellhealth.com/thmb/H7h3nagrjjGQqcMjxcd4NkqJ__g=/1500x0/filters:no_upscale():max_bytes(150000):strip_icc()/ParasympatheticNervousSystemPSNS-v1-8992348880a4400aa46680b8113b4433.png.

The imbalance could be involved in the pathogenesis of most stress-related disorders, thus interventions that will enhance the performance of the PNS must be a high priority in clinical practice. Interventions , such as mindfulness, relaxation therapies, and controlled breathing have been found to stimulate PNS activity and thus lower the ill effects of chronic stress. This understanding is in line with the understanding that interventions for health must target both the psychological and physiological sides, bridging the gap between different health care practices targeting the body-mind interaction (Estrine & DeLisle, 2006) (Figure 5.5).

5.1.3. Enteric Nervous System (ENS)

The ENS or "second brain" plays a role in the ANS in that it regulates gastrointestinal function autonomously of the central nervous system (CNS). The complex network of neurons, incorporated into the walls of the gastrointestinal tract, regulates such functions as peristalsis, blood flow, and secretory functions. The ENS is composed of approximately 100 million neurons that transmit signals through intricate pathways that facilitate reflex movements and local coordination of responses to stimuli. While traditionally considered to be the lesser component of the ANS, the ENS has been characterized by its ability to act autonomously, demonstrating a very high level of complexity and operational independence that suggests that it may form a central mechanism in the regulation of the entire body, linking gastrointestinal health with wider physiological and psychological wellbeing (Steinhart, 2001). As more research is done on the ENS, its function in disease and health is still under investigation. The bidirectional dialogue between the ENS and CNS is highlighted by their interaction, which paves the way to understanding more about the functions of the gut-brain axis. A great deal of understanding has been achieved about the function of enteric neurotransmitters like serotonin and ATP that play specific functions in gut motility and sensory. Of special interest is the suggestion of purinergic signaling, where ATP is a cotransmitter in the peripheral and central nervous systems. This affects not just gastrointestinal disease, but also depression and anxiety, as the neurochemical milieu of the ENSs can directly impact mood and cognitive states (Burnstock, 2009). Thus, the disentanglement of the complex interactions between ENS function and mental well-being is a significant subject of continued research. Identification of the its possible roles in a multitude of disease states is confounded by its involvement in the autonomic regulating system. Dysregulation in enteric circuits can lead to functional gastrointestinal disorders, including irritable bowel syndrome and inflammatory bowel disease, demonstrating the very existence of the causal relationship between the ENS and overall well-being. Investigation has shifted more and more in the direction of the neuron-glial interactions of the ENS and their implications for neuropathologies, propounding that alterations in this neural circuit can be associated with alterations in gut bacteria or inflammation. The degree to which the ENS can adapt to stressors or damage opens up optimistic therapeutic strategies, emphasizing its integrative role within the ANS. The ENS not only contributes to gut health but also forms a vital component of the interdependent system of organs responsible for homeostasis in the entire organism (Steinhart, 2001).

Test Your Knowledge

1. What are the two main subdivisions of the autonomic nervous system?
2. Which division of the ANS is responsible for the 'fight or flight' response?

5.2. Functions of the Autonomic Nervous System (ANS)

Learning Outcome

1. Explain control of involuntary body functions;
2. Explain its function in stress response;
3. Gain insight into the effect on homeostasis.

The ANS has a significant role that is regulating involuntary physiological activities so that basic functions are carried out without being directly aware. It consists primarily of two divisions: the sympathetic and parasympathetic nervous systems, each regulating unique reactions to internal or external stimuli. The sympathetic nervous system is commonly referred to as the fight or flight system, which causes body functions to start during stressful periods. For instance, this system increases heart rate, opens airways, and pumps blood into essential organs, thereby ensuring that the body can respond immediately. The parasympathetic system, referred to at other times as the rest and digest system, prefers resting and restoration.

Functions of ANS

Sympathetic	Parasympathetic
► Heart	► Heart
► ↑ heart rate	► ↓ heart rate
► ↑ force of contraction	► ↓force of contraction
► Blood vessels	► Blood vessels
► *Constriction*	► No effect
► Lungs	► Lungs
► Bronchodilation	► Bronchoconstriction
► GIT	► GIT
► ↓ motility	► ↑ motility
► Sphincter contraction	► Sphincter relaxation
► Decreased secretions	► Increased secretions

Figure 5.6. Functions of autonomic nervous system (ANS).

Source: https://howmed.net/wp-content/uploads/2010/09/functions-of-autonomic-nervous-system.bmp.

It controls digestive processes, slows heart rate, and conserves energy, signifying a balanced interaction required for homeostasis. Awareness of its role highlights the ANS's active role in promoting balance within the organism. Apart from homeostasis, the ANS is equally complex in its role in modulating emotional and stress response through its physiological processes. The activation of the sympathetic nervous system by stress has the potential to create physiological alterations that can affect health, such as repeated stimulation of the sympathetic nervous system leading to elevated blood pressure and heightened cortisol secretion, with consequent health implications in the long term. The parasympathetic system, however, has the potential to counteract stress effects by inducing relaxation and recovery and thereby increasing overall health and well-being. Recent research has also looked at how people's variation in response to stress, depending on attachment style, affects physiological outcomes as well. For instance, individuals with secure attachment styles may experience more adaptive physiological responses to stress, while individuals with insecure attachment styles may exhibit heightened reactivity.

The nature of such interactions demonstrates the importance of the ANS not only in physical health but also in psychological and emotional resilience (Robles & Kane, 2014). In addition, ANS interacts with many other bodily systems, a testament to its character and the overlap of body function. That is, inhibitory heterotrimeric G proteins play an important role in cardiac function by controlling heart rate through the action of G protein-coupled receptors. These proteins can reduce heart rate in response to any number of stimuli, a testament to itscapacity to adaptively regulate cardiovascular health. Research indicates that disruptions in this signaling pathway may produce undesirable cardiovascular effects, further emphasizing the value of learning how the network of regulators governs heart function (Ang et al., 2012). All humans, broadly speaking, the activities of the ANS involve more than plain old regulation of involuntary reactions; they involve interplay with cognitive and emotional processes, further emphasizing the value of the system's crucial role in general well-being and adaptability in the face of the numerous challenges of life (Figure 5.6).

5.2.1. Regulation of Involuntary Bodily Functions

The ANS controls involuntary body functions in a very complicated way. The system, however, is operating primarily beneath conscious awareness. The system has two larger branches: the sympathetic and parasympathetic nervous systems. Sympathetic division is primarily responsible for the body's fight or flight response, enabling rapid physiological adaptation to stress through an increase in the heart rate, dilation of airways, and diversion of blood flow to vital organs. Parasympathetic division is responsible for rest and digest function, stimulating body functions , such as digestion and conservation of energy. The balance between these two divisions is central to the preservation of homeostasis in a way that the body can react to variation in physical and environmental stress but equally maintain necessary involuntary processes like respiration and cardiac regulation. Awareness of the biomechanical process of involuntary functions reveals the complexity of physiological regulation, particularly in relation to respiration. Not only does respiration sustain life by making gas exchange possible, but also has a significant impact on cardiac rhythms and blood pressure. For instance, changes in heart rate with inspiration and expiration can lead to changes in autonomic tone and cardiovascular health. Experiments demonstrate that respiration is a cellular membrane potential modulator such that inspiration is correlated with ubiquitous mild hyperpolarization and expiration with depolarization. This delicate interplay highlights respiratory drives potential as a therapeutic avenue for disease states , such as anxiety and hypertension, with robust emphasis given to studying these involuntary processes in an effort to uncover both physiological mechanisms and broader clinical applications (Jerath et al., 2015). Regulation of involuntary physiological processes exceeds mere automatic behavior, emphasizing the entwined nature of neural, hormonal, and environmental pressures. Dysregulation of the ANS can manifest in diverse clinical presentations, particularly among persons on the autism spectrum, where abnormal autonomic functioning can be suggestive of more widespread physiological challenge. The literature suggests that individuals with autism might face difficulties with central and peripheral nervous system functioning, which can explain the heterogeneity of their behaviors and coping mechanisms. Understanding these multilayered influences is central to developing effective assessment and intervention, as explanation of micro-movement's function and their association with autonomic responding may be explanatory for cognition development and regulation methods (Brincker et al., 2017). The study of involuntary functions thus engenders a rich interplay between basic biological mechanisms and their multifaceted implications for behavior and health (Figure 5.7).

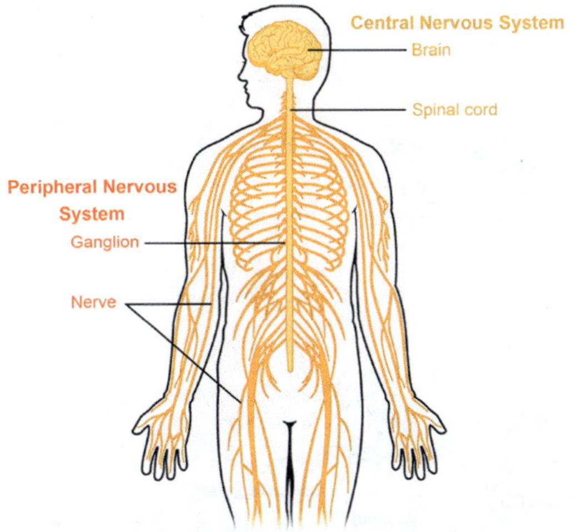

Figure 5.7. Peripheral nervous system (PNS) functions.

Source: https://qbi.uq.edu.au/files/38434/Nervous_System.jpg.

5.2.2. Role in Stress Response

The ANS plays a central part in the body's physiological response to stress, effectively managing several bodily functions. With two broad branches—the parasympathetic and sympathetic systems—the ANS regulates the body's involuntary responses to external and internal stimuli of stress. Sympathetic branch is primarily activated during stress, producing physiological responses , such as increased heart rate, elevated blood pressure, and sensitivity, all of which prepare the body for a fight or flight response. The parasympathetic branch, in contrast, regulates relaxation and recuperation, with the goal of returning to homeostasis. The delicate balance between the two branches is important not just for stress responses in the short term but also for long-term effects on health. Prolonged activation of the sympathetic nervous system may lead to the development of chronic stress states that clearly demonstrate the ANSs facilitation of overall well-being. Research points out the interrelation between stress responses and brain functions regulated by the ANS. In times of stress, the brain activates various neural pathways that subsequently trigger hormonal responses that are inherently linked to the ANS. This is best observed in the modulation of the hypothalamic-pituitary-adrenal (HPA) axis, which oversees mental release of cortisol, a major stress hormone. Hypercortisolism can affect numerous body systems, usually leading to mood disorders, cardiovascular disease, and impaired immunity. Furthermore, modulation of cardiac and respiratory functions, particularly during meditative conditions, demonstrates the ANSs regulation of stress responses (Jerath et al., 2015). Recognition of these dynamics offers the potential for future research into specifically targeted interventions that take advantage of the restorative powers of the ANS to reduce the negative consequences of stress. In the consideration of the clinical import of the ANS for stress management, it becomes imperative to recognize both the dual tracks of intervention to health: those that are centered upon neurological function and those that are centered upon the body's physical health. Conventional paradigms of history prefer the head-up model with treatments based on the brain, disregarding the intricate communication between the brain and body (Estrine & DeLisle, 2006). Nevertheless, an integrated approach taking into account bidirectional communication of the central nervous system and the ANS can optimize treatment models of stress disorders. Techniques , such as biofeedback, relaxation training, and meditation are good examples of techniques through which it is feasible to stimulate the parasympathetic system in order to minimize the impact of stress. Medical professionals can manage overall patients' needs concerning stress problems by understanding the general role of the ANS in stress reaction (Figure 5.8).

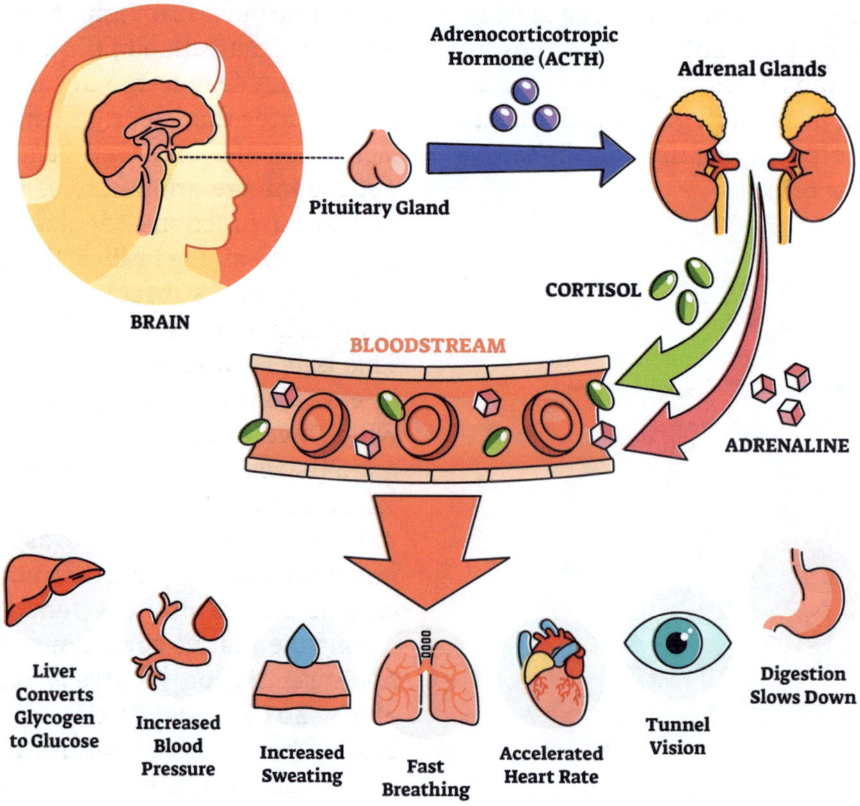

Figure 5.8. Stress response.

Source: https://www.simplypsychology.org/wp-content/uploads/hpa-stress-response.jpeg.

5.2.3. Impact on Homeostasis

Homeostasis, the ability of the body to maintain stable internal environments, is significantly influenced by the ANS. The ANS regulates involuntary bodily functions, including heart rate, digestion, and respiratory rate, which are crucial for the maintenance of homeostasis under changing external environments. Stressors activate the sympathetic division of the ANS to start the fight or flight response, whereby physiological reactions , such as heart rate and blood pressure rise. Although these adaptations ready the body for immediate response, they cause disruptions in homeostasis if the stress is sustained. Over time, recurrent stimulation of the sympathetic nervous system can lead to diseases like hypertension and metabolic disease, and thereby emphasize the need for adaptive mechanisms that restore balance within the body (Jerath et al., 2015). Conversely, the parasympathetic branch of the ANS is essential for aiding in recovery and re-establishment of homeostasis following stress. Relaxation activities , such as meditation stimulate parasympathetic activity, which has been shown to synchronize cardiorespiratory rhythms. This synchronization tends to modulate neuronal activity along autonomic pathways and can lead to beneficial physiological changes, e.g., reduced amygdala activity, associated with stress reactions. The induction of calm through parasympathetic stimulation not only facilitates emotional regulation but also maintains homeostasis by presenting a counterbalance to the effects of sympathetic stimulation. Parasympathetic dominance's ability to be reached is crucial in maintaining general functioning and health, encapsulating the fine balance the ANS has to navigate (Jerath et al., 2015). Also, new therapeutic approaches, such as INH, illustrate the plasticity of the ANSs in maintaining homeostasis within various clinical settings. Evidence shows that INH effectively enhances autonomic function, particularly in patients with illnesses , such as cerebral palsy and epilepsy, by restoring sympathetic-parasympathetic balance. The balance optimizes cardiovascular function and respiratory capacity, thereby allowing restoration of homeostasis. The potency of INH underscores the benefit of developing the ANS for its best functioning, particularly in communities that have been subjected to external stressors, such as those living in environments with high environmental pollution. Through stimulation of the higher vegetative centers, INH presents a valuable intervention in supporting homeostasis and returning biological equilibrium, underscoring the resourcefulness of the ANS in addressing diverse challenges.

Test Your Knowledge

1. How does the autonomic nervous system regulate heart rate and blood pressure?
2. What is the role of the parasympathetic division in digestion?

5.3. Neurotransmitters in the Autonomic Nervous System (ANS)

Learning Outcome

1. Explain the acetylcholine and norepinephrine;
2. Explain the neuropeptides and hormones.

The ANS regulates involuntary physiological processes like heart rate, digestion, and the rate of breathing, via the activity of many neurotransmitters. The primary neurotransmitters are acetylcholine, norepinephrine, and epinephrine which serve to mediate the communication of peripheral organs and the central nervous system. Acetylcholine, primarily functioning in the parasympathetic division, provokes the state of rest and relaxation, while norepinephrine and epinephrine, associated with the sympathetic division, prepare the body for emergency and stress reactions. They influence not only visceral functions but emotional and cognitive activities as well. Knowledge of the particular functions of these chemical messengers is critical for designing specific interventions for psychological disorders since neurotransmitter dysregulation in the ANS has been implicated in anxiety disorders and mood liability. In investigating the complex interaction between emotion and the autonomic nervous system, it becomes clear that neurotransmitters play a role not only in mediating physiological alterations but also in modulating affective experience. At stress episodes, increased levels of norepinephrine will result in an increase of sympathetic activity, creating a state of hyperarousal. In contrast, positive affect is typically associated with higher levels of acetylcholine, which activates the parasympathetic nervous system to promote relaxation and calmness. Research stresses the significance of cardiorespiratory coherence (CRC) in characterizing emotional states, whereby negative emotions reduce CRC as a symptom of sympathetic dominance and positive emotions enhance it as an indicator of parasympathetic dominance. This dynamic interaction suggests that regulating neurotransmitter activity by cognitive and behavioral approaches might be beneficial to the therapeutic management of mood and anxiety disorders, as are many forms of therapy. There has been recent research suggesting that holistic modalities , such as meditation and regulative breathing exercises, may be helpful adjuncts or alternatives to pharmacological interventions in managing emotional dysregulation under the conditions of neurotransmitter imbalance. By modulating the activity of the autonomic nervous system, these modalities can facilitate homeostasis and reverse stress-induced sympathetic dominance. Specifically, practitioners report that respiratory exercises and meditation enhance CRC, perhaps through limbic system and brainstem mechanisms involving feedback from somatic and emotional states.

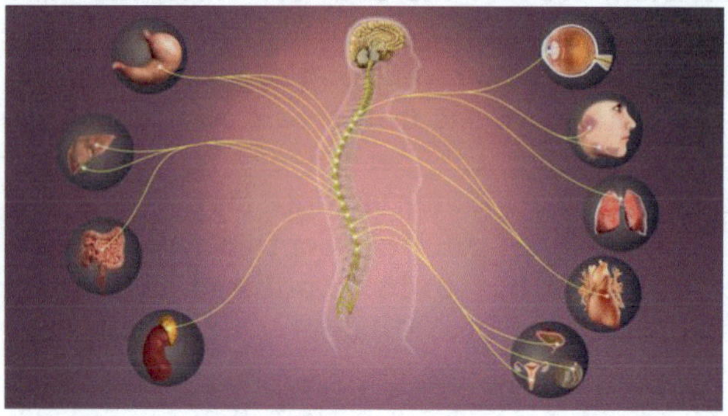

Figure 5.9. Sympathetic nervous system (SNS).

Source: https://www.physio-pedia.com/images/thumb/5/5c/Sympathetic_Nervous_System.jpg/550px-Sympathetic_Nervous_System.jpg.

The therapeutic effects of these interventions form the foundation for new treatments that are centered on the regulation of neurotransmitters in the ANS, in contrast to sole dependency on drugs. Consequently, further understanding of how neurotransmitters affect physiological as well as emotional states is essential in advancing therapeutic practice in the prevention and treatment of stress, anxiety, and related disorders, as highlighted in recent literature (Barnes et al., 2015; Crawford et al., 2015) (Figure 5.9).

5.3.1. Acetylcholine (Ach)

ACh is a fundamental neurotransmitter of the ANS, with a diverse range of physiological activities at its command. As one of the key components of both the parasympathetic and sympathetic divisions, ACh influences various processes, including heart rate, digestion, and glandular secretions. ACh is released in the synapse between the effectors and the neurons, where it attaches to cholinergic receptors, enabling transmission in the nervous system. Of note, its role is not merely transmittance; ACh is involved in the modulation of synaptic activity and consequently in the net efficacy of neural communication. This dual role hints at its role in homeostasis within the body and its discovery in reaction to environmental and intrabody equilibrium. Moreover, the specifics of its mechanism reinforce its many roles in the ANS. The neurotransmitter operates essentially through two receptor classes, which are nicotinic and muscarinic receptors. Ionotropic nicotinic receptors mediate fast synaptic transmission, particularly at neuromuscular junctions and autonomic ganglia. Muscarinic receptors, however, are metabotropic and primarily mediate slower, long-term signaling, simulating a variety of physiological responses in organs , such as the heart, lungs, and gastrointestinal tract. This receptor variability allows for complex control of body function, responses scaled to suit the exact demands of the situation. It also renders ACh a key mediator in functions , such as bronchoconstriction, slowing the heart, and gastrointestinal motility, again testifying to its central role in ANS function. Acetylcholine is crucial for normal autonomic function, but dysregulation can lead to extremely serious health issues. For instance, imbalances of ACh levels are implicated in neurodegenerative diseases , such as Alzheimer's disease, involving degeneration of the cholinergic neurons. Excessive activity of ACh can also lead to cholinergic toxicity effects, with implications on cognitive, respiratory, and muscle functions. Moreover, interaction between neurotransmitters, such as adenosine triphosphate (ATP), co-transmitter function in autonomic nerve transmission, demonstrates the complexity of ANS neurotransmission (Cunha et al., 2000). Understanding the pathways and actions of acetylcholine is paramount to grasping normal autonomic function, as well as the creation of therapeutic strategies for disorders including autonomic dysregulation (Brust et al., 2014) (Figure 5.10).

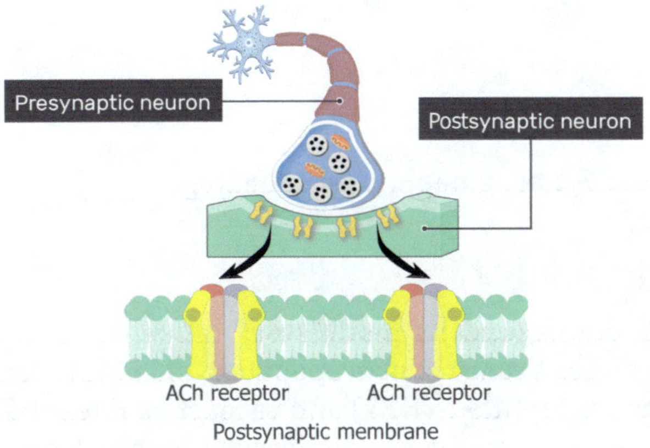

Figure 5.10. Acetylcholine (Ach) receptors.

Source: https://www.getbodysmart.com/wp-content/uploads/2017/09/Acetylcholine-Receptors-Labeled-1024x767.png.

5.3.2. Norepinephrine

Norepinephrine, a primary neurotransmitter of the autonomic nervous system, is essential in mediating the body's response to stress and maintaining homeostasis. As a key component of the sympathetic nervous system, norepinephrine is responsible for triggering the "fight or flight" response, characterized by increased heart rate, blood pressure, and energy metabolism. The response is essential for an organism survival because it enables people to respond quickly to danger. In the context of several disorders, such as postural orthostatic tachycardia syndrome (POTS), elevated levels of norepinephrine emphasize the complex interplay between neurotransmission and autonomic regulation. Specifically, POTS patients exhibit significant elevations in plasma norepinephrine with standing posture, reflecting augmented sympathetic drive that is implicated in symptomatology of these patients, such as tachycardia and fatigue (Raj et al., 2006). Understanding norepinephrine's multifaceted roles in the autonomic nervous system is important for deciphering its involvement in disease and health. Beyond its role in acute stress reactions, norepinephrine also plays a significant role in the modulation of metabolic functions, particularly in the context of overfeeding and obesity. Autonomic function, with alterations in sympathetic and parasympathetic outflow, has been found to be influenced by excessive caloric consumption in research. Increases in baseline plasma norepinephrine levels have been observed in hyperphagia-exposed animal models, suggesting a compensatory response with the intent of maintaining energy substrate homeostasis (Prins et al., 1996). The resultant increase in sympathetic tone is required for increased lipolysis and energy mobilization during times of excessive caloric loading. However, this compensatory response can be dampened, leading to reduced release of norepinephrine on exertion when overfed. Thus, the fine line of norepinephrine levels is critical in maintaining metabolic health and preventing the unpleasant side effects that often ensue with weight gain. In addition, dysregulation of norepinephrine signaling through the autonomic nervous system has significant consequences for cardiovascular health. The sympathetic nervous system, through the release of norepinephrine, not only modulates heart rate but also manages vascular tone and blood pressure. Chronic elevation of norepinephrine, as frequently encountered in hypertensive patients, can lead to sustained vasoconstriction and increased cardiac workload. This was highlighted by the importance of norepinephrine as a drug target in the management of autonomic dysfunction and cardiovascular disease. Furthermore, therapy aimed at restoring a normal balance of norepinephrine may stem the functional disabilities of many autonomic disorders, such as POTS. Overall, understanding norepinephrine's multifaceted impact on the autonomic nervous system lies at the heart of grasping the delicate balance between neurotransmission, metabolism, and cardiovascular health (Figure 5.11).

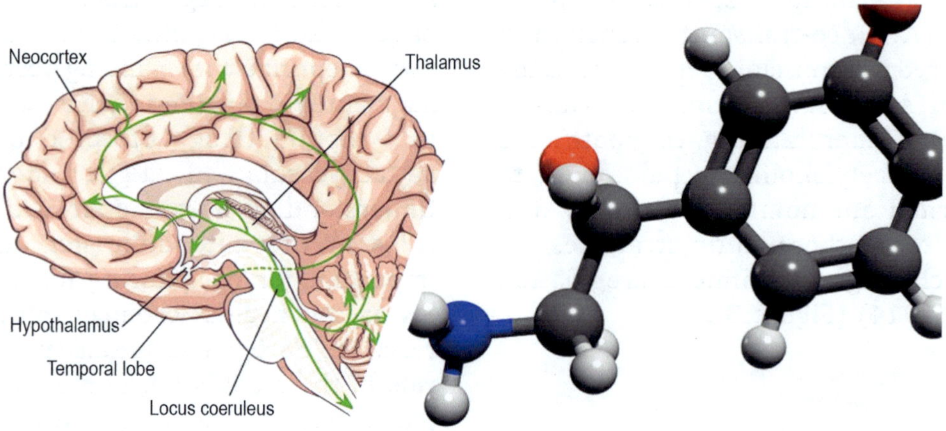

Figure 5.11. Norepinephrine function.

Source: https://draxe.com/wp-content/uploads/2019/07/norepinephrine-header.jpg.

5.3.3. Other Neuropeptides and Hormones

The ANS is key to regulating varied physiological functions, and its modulatory influence is not restricted to conventional neurotransmitters but also includes a range of neuropeptides and hormones. Particularly noteworthy are these molecules, such as neuropeptide Y (NPY) and vasoactive intestinal peptide (VIP), which figure prominently in functions , such as stress responses, circulatory regulation, and gastrointestinal functions. NPY, largely produced in sympathetic nervous system neurons, is a potent regulator of stress and anxiety by promoting energy conservation in stress responses. Similarly, VIP has also been found to modulate vascular tone as well as gastrointestinal motility, thus emphasizing its central role in coordination between the nervous and the gastrointestinal system. Collectively, these neuropeptides emphasize the intricate networks whereby the ANS influences not just autonomic but also emotional and cognitive processes, indicating the system's far-reaching implications. The research into other hormones , such as oxytocin and cortisol also reveals the complex interaction of the ANS. Oxytocin, or the bonding hormone, captures the neuroendocrine interconnections of the ANS and influences social behaviors and emotional responses. Cortisol, a key stress hormone, however, reveals the influence of the ANS on metabolic processes and cardiovascular state. Higher levels of cortisol, typically the consequence of prolonged sympathetic activation, cause an allostatic load state that can lead to many disease states, including hypertension and metabolic syndrome. This complicating interaction highlights the need for further investigation into the regulatory mechanisms of these hormones and their role in the regulation of autonomic function since their formation and discharge are typically responsive to environmental stimulation, influencing the ANS. The interaction between neuropeptides, hormones, and the ANS is essential for understanding the complicated responses of the human body. Existing research suggests an active role in the dissemination and efficacy of these neurochemical communications, which may indicate their possible impact on neuronal plasticity from chronic stress and environmental alterations. For instance, the neuroendocrine system is interlinked by means of positive and negative feedback loops, and they can lead to disease states if there are imbalances involved. Understanding this balance is crucial because this might be the key to new therapeutic mechanisms for conditions like anxiety disorders and metabolic diseases, which are rooted in dysregulation of these systems. Furthermore, researchers have proposed the theory of neurovisceral integration, theorizing that the autonomic pathways are not only conveying signals but are actually changing neurochemical states, thereby influencing gene expression and overall health outcomes (Martins et al., 2016; Domínguez Vías et al., 2021).

Test Your Knowledge

1. Which neurotransmitter do preganglionic neurons secrete in sympathetic and parasympathetic divisions?
2. What is the primary neurotransmitter secreted by postganglionic sympathetic neurons?

5.4. Autonomic Nervous System (ANS) and Health

Learning Outcome

1. Enumerate the disorders of autonomic dysfunction;
2. Describe the effect of stress on the autonomic system;
3. Describe the contribution to chronic illness.

The ANS plays a crucial role in the maintenance of homeostasis, which is required for overall health. The ANS is divided into sympathetic and parasympathetic divisions, both of which influence physiological processes in opposite ways. The sympathetic branch initiates the "fight or flight" response to stress, preparing the body for immediate movement by increasing heart rate and directing blood flow to essential muscles. The parasympathetic branch produces a "rest and digest" state, facilitating ease and rest." When the balance between the two systems collapses, particularly through prolonged stress, pathological effects may follow. This dysregulation can lead to such conditions as hypertension, anxiety, and metabolic syndrome, hence depicting the role of the ANS in health maintenance and disease susceptibility. One of the notable factors influencing the activity of the ANS is chronic stress. Altered autonomic regulation can manifest in a variety of physical and mental well-being disorders, from emotional disorders to cardiovascular disease. Some studies indicate, there is a profound connection between the emotional health of individuals and the functional potential of their ANS. Specifically, if stress becomes a chronic aspect of life, then the sympathetic system can get overstimulated, as a result of which both physical and mental health can get worn out. This renders the following appreciation of how the brain controls stress reactions and what resulting impacts they have on body functions relevant. The difference between health approaches based on psychological or physiological considerations alone serves to accentuate the requirement for an overall knowledge of well-being and health, and the role of the ANS as a unifying factor in such complex interaction (Estrine & DeLisle, 2006). New ways of closing the gap between emotional well-being and the ANS have been established, emphasizing approaches , such as those presented by the Institute of HeartMath. Their research provides perspective into the physiological benefits of positive states and how they might influence autonomic functioning. A key aspect of what they identify is the concept of physiological coherence as a unique mode of functioning that occurs during prolonged positive emotions, which elicits positive health consequences. Techniques , such as Freeze-Frame® and Heart Lock-In® were found to be effective in reducing stress by creating a state of coherence, which impacts the mental, emotional, and physiological status of the state of a person's health. By changing the stress reactions and enhancing positive emotional experience, these processes reflect the importance of addressing emotional wellbeing as part of interventions aimed at enhancing the health of the autonomic nervous system (Childre & McCraty, 2002) (Figure 5.12).

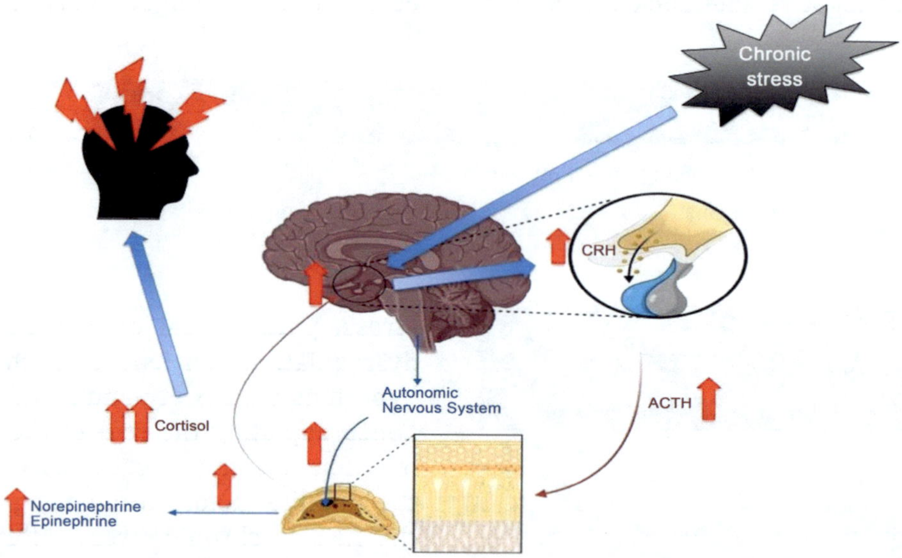

Figure 5.12. The role of the hypothalamic-pituitary-adrenal (HPA) axis and autonomic nervous system (ANS).

Source: Sic A, Bogicevic M, Brezic N, Nemr C, Knezevic NN. Chronic Stress and Headaches: The Role of the HPA Axis and Autonomic Nervous System. Biomedicines. 2025; 13(2):463. https://doi.org/10.3390/biomedicines13020463

5.4.1. Disorders Related to Autonomic Dysfunction

Disorders related to autonomic dysfunction are a group of clinical presentations that significantly impact quality of life. The ANS regulates involuntary physiological processes, such as heart rate, gastrointestinal peristalsis, and blood pressure. Dysregulation of this system will emerge as a variety of illnesses, including POTS and orthostatic hypotension. POTS, an inappropriately rapid increase in heart rate with standing, often leads to dizziness, fatigue, and palpitations. Orthostatic hypotension is a sudden drop in blood pressure that can lead to fainting and falls. The incidence of these disorders is highlighted by evidence that indicates as many as 25% of children and almost 70% of adults present with symptoms of autonomic dysfunction, which reflects a highly significant public health issue of note that deserves attention and ongoing research into mechanisms and management (Simonenko, 2017). The cross-talk between central disorders and autonomic failure, including those with symptoms of hypersomnolence, further illustrates the complexities of the ANS. Research in narcolepsy type 1 and other sleep disorders has demonstrated that most exhibit autonomic symptoms, such as alterations in cardiovascular function and disturbances in thermoregulation. Not only do these disrupt daily functioning, but they could also cause long-term health complications. The pathophysiological substrates for these autonomic dysfunctions remain unknown, but the literature has indicated that orexin/hypocretin neuronal deficits might be associated with such dysfunctions in narcolepsy.

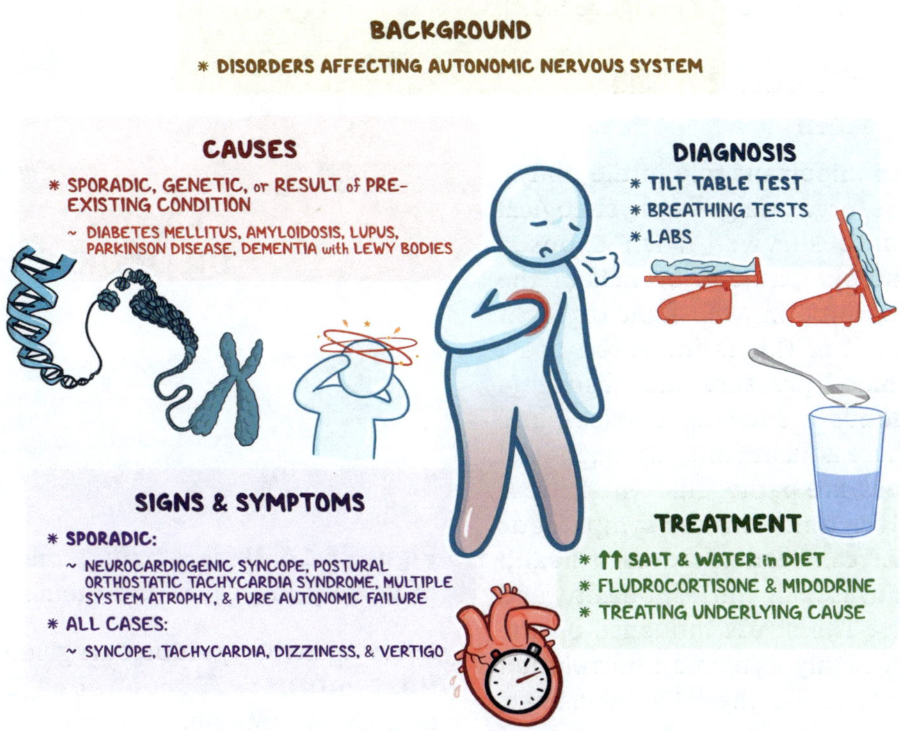

Figure 5.13. Disorders related to autonomic dysfunction.

Source: https://d16qt3wv6xm098.cloudfront.net/-r9bBRFoQ8qvuzJe-oa-sI-NRFe2vjU7/_.png.

Current treatments are largely symptom-oriented, employing wake-promoting agents, and this also raises questions about their impact on autonomic function and potential cardiovascular risks (Silvani et al., 2023). Clarifying such relationships is thus important to deliver comprehensive care to patients. Psychological factors also make significant contributions to the manifestation of autonomic dysfunctions. Group studies, such as with medical students, reveal correlations between psychological traits and autonomic reactivity. Studies have also shown that highly extraverted individuals are predisposed to present non-stability of higher nervous function, a condition that is marked by high autonomic responses like sympathicotonia. This would imply that distress may worsen autonomic disorders and initiate a vicious cycle of somatic complaints and psychological distress. The intersection between psychological health and autonomic dysfunction points to the importance of including psychological assessments in the diagnostic procedure. Thus, medical professionals can be made more aware of the multifaceted nature of autonomic disorders and modify interventions that address physiological as well as psychological aspects of patient health (Simonenko, 2017) (Figure 5.13).

5.4.2. Impact of Stress on the Autonomic System

The ANS plays an important role in the body's response to stress, organizing the physiological changes needed to survive. When exposed to a stressor, the sympathetic branch of the ANS is triggered, initiating the fight or flight reaction. The result of this is increased heart rate, increased blood pressure, and discharge of stress hormones , such as cortisol and adrenaline. All these adjustments, although vital during acute stress, are pathogenic when stress turns chronic. Over time, chronic sympathetic system activation can lead to adverse health effects like cardiovascular illness, obesity, and anxiety disorders. The stress influence on the ANS illustrates a highly dynamic interrelation between mental states and physiological change, which necessitates an integrated perspective of health encompassing both mental and physical sensations (Estrine & DeLisle, 2006). Chronic stress radically alters the balance between sympathetic and parasympathetic divisions of the ANS, and autonomic dysfunction results. Under normal conditions, the parasympathetic system, referred to as the rest and digest system, functions to counterbalance the effects of sympathetic arousal. Parasympathetic function is progressively exhausted by prolonged exposure to stress, resulting in inefficient recovery from stress and further inducing chronic physiological stress. This dysregulation also results in several other health issues, including gastrointestinal conditions and the suppression of the immune system. The relationship between stress and autonomic imbalance further highlights the importance of emotional well-being in ensuring physiological health. With prolonged chronic stress, the physical ability to achieve physiological coherence is lost, which is necessary for peak performance and the control of emotions (Childre & McCraty, 2002).

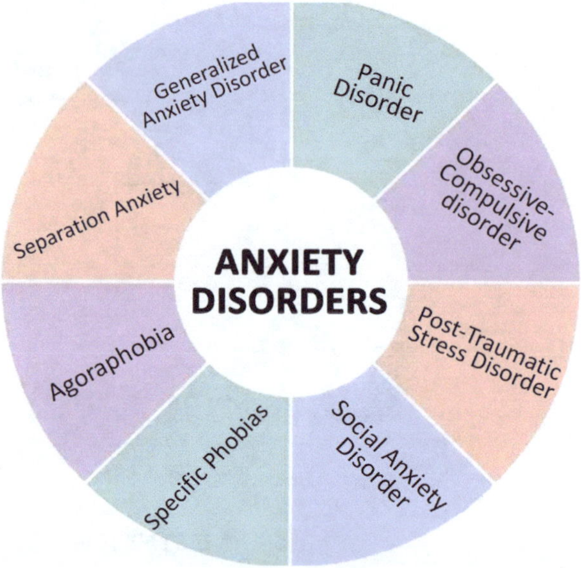

Figure 5.14. Understanding the different types of anxiety disorders and their symptoms.

Source: https://video.curegrid.co/dj/media/post_banners/Screenshot_2024-11-19_at_10.34.40AM.png.

Awareness of the impact of stress on the autonomic system also guides new interventions to minimize its negative impacts. Stress reduction and emotional regulation skills , such as the HeartMath techniques gained increasing popularity during the last two decades. They are reported to enhance physiological coherence, i.e., coordination among various systems in the body, which leads to improved emotional and physiological functioning. By inducing positive affective states, human beings are capable of activating the parasympathetic branch of the ANS to promote recovery and well-being. Lastly, this information identifies the critical role of the autonomic nervous system not only in responding to stressors but also in facilitating recovery and resilience in the face of life's challenges. As the link between stress and the ANS comes to light more and more, healthcare systems must embrace an integrated approach encompassing both emotional and physical health (Estrine & DeLisle, 2006) (Figure 5.14).

5.4.3. Role in Chronic Illnesses

Understanding the role of the ANS in chronic illnesses involves a careful consideration of its regulatory functions, particularly in sympathetic and parasympathetic dominance. The ANS has a critical function in maintaining homeostasis, while its pathological processes lead to a wide range of health conditions. Chronic diseases , such as hypertension, rheumatoid arthritis, and fibromyalgia are usually associated with augmented activity of the sympathetic nervous system, resulting in prolonged stress responses that exacerbate these disorders. Research has established that ANS modulatory interventions , such as hypnosis, reduce sympathetic activity significantly, thus offering new strategies for chronic health care. Specifically, hypnosis has been employed to lower skin conductance levels, supporting the notion that hypnosis can suppress symptoms reported in conditions dominated to a large extent by the sympathetic nervous system, changing the treatment strategies used in chronic illness (Kekecs et al., 2015). The incorporation of stress coping skills into treatment programs for chronic disease points towards the definitive role of emotional control in terms of physiological health. Chronic stress not only elevates sympathetic nervous system activity but could also disrupt parasympathetic functions essential to recovery and restoration. Programs that intervene in reducing emotional self-management, e.g., those made available to police officers, exhibit significant reductions in pathological physiological responses that are a product of chronic stress. Techniques fostering emotional equilibrium and empathy can carry over into improvements in areas of life that have considerable bearing on stress, such as interpersonal relationships and occupational functioning (Tomasino et al., 1999). This suggests the necessity of incorporating such techniques into chronic illness management to enhance overall well-being and perhaps disrupt the infinite loops of stress and illness. The prospect of bringing ANS-targeted interventions to the treatment of chronic disease is also underscored by the nervous system's plasticity to therapeutic intervention. As patients with chronic illness are often stuck in cycles of stress-induced worsening, interventions that target the ANS stand to not only alleviate symptoms but also improve quality of life. The reduction in sympathetic activity that accompanies treatments like hypnosis highlights the pivotal role of the ANS in chronic disease management, and the implication is that optimal modulation of its response can have long-term benefits. Furthermore, the use of holistic means by which understanding is gained of the interrelatedness of physical, psychological, and environmental factors is critical in the construction of overall treatment strategies for chronic diseases. Interacting with the nuances of the ANS allows both practitioners and patients to cultivate resilience and healing in chronic illness, maximizing therapy and patient outcomes.

Test Your Knowledge

1. How can dysregulation of the autonomic nervous system contribute to hypertension or heart failure?
2. What are common symptoms and physiological effects of autonomic neuropathy, and which diseases most commonly cause it?

5.5. Diagnostic Tools for Autonomic Nervous System Assessment

Learning Outcome

1. Describe the heart rate variability analysis;
2. Describe the tests for blood pressure response;
3. Discuss the autonomic reflex testing.

The assessment of ANS is extremely significant not just to understand physiological processes but also to diagnose numerous conditions related to autonomic dysfunction. There has evolved a broad range of diagnostic tests each of which provides unique information regarding the functioning of both parasympathetic and sympathetic subdivisions of the ANS. Earlier methods, including HRV analysis, are interested in the interaction between respiratory patterns and heart rate, which can be illuminating in terms of autonomic regulation during states of health and illness. Recent development has further made these methods more precise, such as the utilization of biofeedback technology to maximize awareness and volitional control of autonomic function, suggesting potential therapeutic avenues for diseases like anxiety and stress disorders. The delivery of accurate diagnostics is essential to recognize the underlying variables causing autonomic dysregulation, allowing for timely interventions.

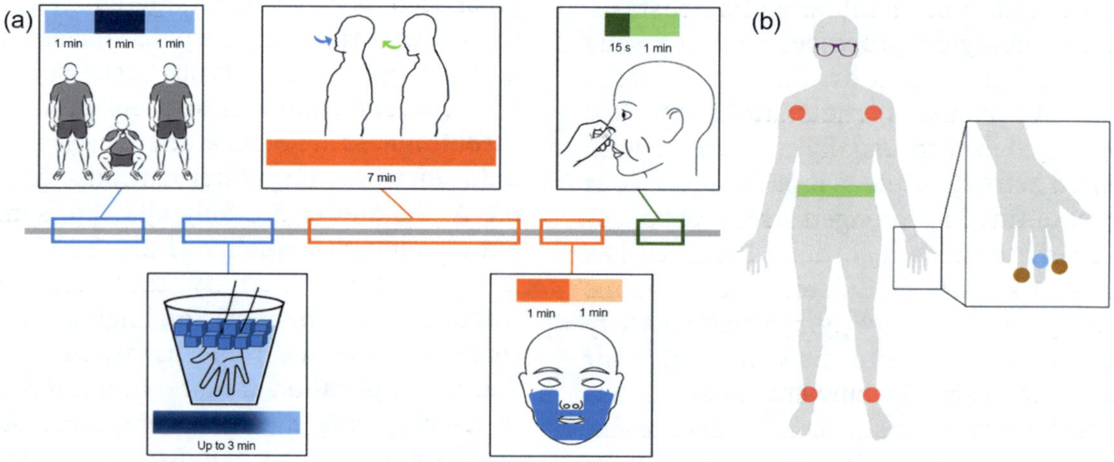

Figure 5.15. A method to quantify autonomic nervous system (ANS) function in healthy.

Source: https://media.springernature.com/lw1200/springer-static/image/art%3A10.1186%2Fs42234-021-00075-7/MediaObjects/42234_2021_75_Fig1_HTML.png.

Micro-movement analysis has been a useful tool to measure the ANS, particularly in disorders that have heightened physiological responsiveness, such as Autism Spectrum Disorder (ASD). Micro-movements have been discovered as markers of autonomic activity that reflect an objective measure of systemic responses that even standard methods of measurement may fail to detect. Notably, newer techniques combine continuous biometric monitoring with observation testing, as exemplified through studies using data from archives like the Autism Brain Imaging Data Exchange (ABIDE I-II). The identification of subgroups within autistic individuals based on the analysis of involuntary head movements and associated physiological rhythms has been achieved, revealing variability in severity and enhancing knowledge about movement behavior interactions and autonomic regulation. These findings indicate a call for new analytical modalities in an effort to understand the multifaceted nature of autonomic function across different populations. The use of advanced diagnostic modalities allows for a multidimensional understanding of the ANS, resulting in enhanced clinical outcomes through individualized interventions. Computerized cluster analysis of behavior data, for instance, can further refine the diagnostic process by differentiating among several phenotypes within disorders like autism, thereby disclosing subtle differences in symptom pattern. This interlinkage between observed behavior and underlying autonomic rhythm emphasizes the usefulness of integrated tests combining subjective and objective measures. As exemplified in studies using statistical models to compare data by sex in ASD, the utility of autonomic assessment extends beyond isolated diagnosis; it informs broad debates on developmental trajectory and the neurophysiological underpinnings of neurodiversity. Ultimately, the emergence of such tools underscores the pressing need for ongoing research and development aimed at elucidating the role of the autonomic nervous system in human health and behavior (Figure 5.15).

5.5.1. Heart Rate Variability (HRV) Analysis

The analysis of HRV is a critical method in quantifying the function of the ANS, i.e., its balance between sympathetic and parasympathetic activities. HRV reflects the body's adaptability to stressors, such as changes in heart rate over time, and can provide insight into physiological and psychological health. Through the examination of HRV with both time-domain and frequency-domain measures, researchers can determine information about autonomic regulation and forecast a variety of health outcomes. To illustrate, time-domain measurements , such as SDNN and RMSSD give insight into global autonomic tone. Frequency-domain measurements, by contrast, mirror the power distribution of oscillations in heart rate that give insight into sympathetic and parasympathetic division interaction, thereby revealing the dynamic nature of central nervous system modulation of heart rate. Further research highlights the correlation of HRV with cognitive performance, particularly in older individuals. A study on older patients found a significant positive relationship between higher scores in cognitive tests, for instance, Mini-Mental State Examination (MMSE), and increased sympathetic activity expressed by various indices of HRV, including SDNN and low frequency (LF) components. Interestingly, it was discovered in this study that increased sympathetic activation, rather than decreased vagal activity, was associated with better cognitive function in the elderly. These findings show that HRV is not just a cardiovascular well-being biomarker but an essential measure to gauge cognitive dynamics, and thus a more integrated view of how autonomic function impacts general mental acuity as a person grows older, favoring the salience of sympathetic effect on cognitive aging (Dalise et al., 2020). In addition to cognitive applications, HRV analysis has a key role in detecting autonomic maturation in risk populations , such as premature infants. The evidence suggests that HRV can be precisely measured in the immediate postnatal period and may represent ANS maturation in these newborns. A longitudinal study identified significant changes in HRV values throughout hospitalization, suggesting greater parasympathetic and sympathetic function. These findings suggest that HRV monitoring can be a sign of a non-invasive way to study autonomic maturation and predict long-term neurological outcomes of preterm infants because the variations of HRV values align with their clinical development. This is in accordance with the overall idea of ANS adaptation, which holds that heart rate dynamics have a central contribution to making judgments on development and maturation processes in a range of patient groups and, consequently, evolving predictive health strategies across a range of age groups (de Filho et al., 2019).

5.5.2. Blood Pressure Response Tests

Blood pressure response tests are a significant testing method in making a judgment on the operation of the ANS. These tests measure the body's ability to regulate blood pressure in response to a range of stimuli, a reflection of the interplay between parasympathetic and sympathetic factors. With methods , such as stress testing for position change or exercise, researchers can assess the effectiveness with which the ANS coordinates cardiovascular activity. As an example, the application of calibrated pressures in massage in rodent models had significant effects, in which graded pressure levels caused measurable systolic blood pressure changes. That is, 20 mm Hg and 40 mm Hg pressures made significant percentage decreases in blood pressure, pointing to its role in mediating cardiovascular control in response to exogenous stressors, which is in agreement with results on autonomic control in human studies. In addition to the capacity for understanding baseline and reflex blood pressure responses, testing is useful for the diagnosis of POTS. POTS is characterized by an inappropriately marked heart rate response to standing and is commonly associated with orthostatic intolerance along with other disabling symptoms. Blood pressure response tests prove to be effective in determining the autonomic dysfunction of POTS patients, often found to include high plasma norepinephrine levels coupled with a decreased blood volume. Coupling blood pressure response tests with clinical symptoms can provide a comprehensive picture of a patient's autonomic health, guiding therapeutic interventions toward achieving balance and alleviation of symptoms. Thus, these tests can be beneficial in clinical settings for the evaluation of autonomic dysregulation in various patient populations. Further, quantification of the response to blood pressure tests can uncover hidden information regarding the mechanism of autonomic control and how it impacts health. For example, the ratio of low-frequency to high-frequency, a critical indicator of autonomic tone, was seen to rise markedly with a specific pressure of massage. This enhancement suggests heightened sympathetic activity to higher mechanical stimuli, illustrating the capacity of the body to modify autonomic output to address cardiovascular demands. Such an observation not only provides enhanced pathophysiological understanding of blood pressure regulation but also makes it possible to initiate novel therapeutic approaches. Understanding the blood pressure response tests in the context of the ANS finally contributes to a clearer understanding of cardiovascular disease and health, with particular focus on autonomic balance in the maintenance of homeostasis (Figure 5.16).

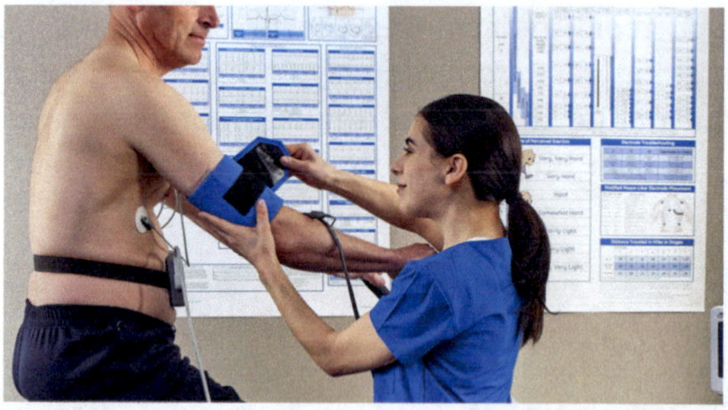

Figure 5.16. Blood pressure response during exercise stress testing.

Source: https://clinicalview.gehealthcare.com/sites/default/files/styles/hero_fallback/public/Man%20in%20a%20treadmill%20800x600.png?h=6416edf4&itok=YBdRzgNg.

5.5.3. Autonomic Reflex Testing

The subtleties of autonomic reflex testing are at the heart of understanding the operations of the ANS. This testing entails a series of tests designed to assess sympathetic and parasympathetic reflexes in response to various stimuli. Quantifying cardiovascular responses , such as heart rate and blood pressure in controlled settings allows clinicians to make inference regarding autonomic regulation. Tests like the Valsalva maneuver and deep breathing tests are standard components of autonomic testing and play an important role in patient diagnostics. Notably, there is no one test that can offer the full picture; thus, several tests are recommended to achieve diagnostic precision and validity. As such, autonomic reflex testing emerges as a vital test tool that clarifies patients' neurophysiological status, particularly when tailored based on conditions and responses (Siepmann & Ziemssen, 2019). Of the various measures obtained from autonomic reflex testing, sudomotor function is one important area of study. Sudomotor reflex testing assesses sympathetic nervous system function in the production of sweat, which is compromised in numerous diseases , such as autonomic neuropathies and neurodegenerative diseases. Studies like the quantitative sudomotor axon reflex test not only provide data regarding sweat gland function but also are sensitive markers of more generalized autonomic impairment. This feature of testing is especially enlightening because impaired sweating can have a tremendous impact on a patient's quality of life. Therefore, sudomotor testing is a valuable addition to cardiovascular assessment, providing a greater insight into autonomic well-being and the diverse impact of autonomic dysfunction (Siepmann & Ziemssen, 2019). Refinements in autonomic reflex testing techniques highlight ongoing refinement of diagnostic approaches in assessing autonomic nervous system function. Examining technologies like the Quantitative Direct and Indirect Axon Reflex Testing and Sudoscan, scientists try to minimize technical constraints that have long hampered these tests. Besides having the potential for more accurate diagnosis, these technologies also seek to minimize interindividual variance, further refining patient evaluation. Early studies of conditions , such as primary Sjögrens syndrome have revealed quantifiable correlations between autonomic symptoms and cardiovasculer reflex outcomes, and the prognostic value of such tests in many clinical situations. Increasing activity on this subject will likely further the use of advanced autonomic reflex testing in both the understanding and treatment of varied pathologies, ultimately to the advantage of patient care and outcome.

Test Your Knowledge

1. What is a tilt table test for, and how does it help diagnose autonomic dysfunction?
2. How are heart rate variability (HRV) tests used to assess autonomic nervous system balance?

5.6. Treatment and Management of Autonomic Disorders

Learning Outcome

1. Describe the pharmacological management;
2. Describe the lifestyle modifications of the autonomic nervous system (ANS);
3. Describe the Alternative therapies of the autonomic nervous system (ANS).

Treatment and management of autonomic disorders are quite intricate and require a very good understanding of the complex functions of the autonomic nervous system. Various therapeutic approaches have evolved to manage these disorders, addressing a specific dysfunction in the autonomic pathway. Neuromodulation procedures, such as vagus nerve stimulation (VNS) and sphenopalatine ganglion (SPG) stimulation, have also been very promising for the therapy of illnesses , such as migraines, which typically entail autonomic dysfunction. They are performed by modulating the neural circuits, thereby potentially decreasing symptoms related to autonomic dysregulation. New evidence indicates that these therapies are not only effective treatment options but also, in the majority of situations, well tolerated by patients, providing a strategic shift in autonomic disorder treatment in clinical practice (Puledda & Goadsby, 2016). In addition to neuromodulation, pharmacological treatments also play a significant role in the treatment of autonomic disorders. These drugs can be employed to decrease symptoms and improve the quality of life of patients by acting on specific neurotransmitter pathways. Beta-blockers, for instance, are used in managing tachycardia due to dysautonomia, while anticholinergic drugs are used to counteract over-salivation or gastrointestinal hypermotility. These treatments, nonetheless, rely much on a clear identification of the patient's autonomic pattern and processes that cause the disease. This individualized approach is essential since it helps in the administration of treatment plans using pharmacological and non-pharmacological methods effectively. Finally, no consideration can be given to the correlation between autonomic illnesses and psychological problems when it comes to intervention in treatment. Evidence indicates how conditions , such as anxiety can act as precipitating factors for autonomic dysfunction, particularly in atrial fibrillation, where anxiety has a significant influence on quality of life (Ceccacci et al., 2019). Therefore, it is essential to address mental health with psychotherapy and coping for anxiety as an integral part of overall treatment for autonomic disorders. By acknowledging the dynamic interaction between the ANS and mental health, clinicians are more capable of creating comprehensive treatment regimens that ensure symptom control and improved general health outcomes. This holistic approach promotes a wider understanding of autonomic disorders and emphasizes the benefit of interdisciplinary treatment in achieving optimal patient outcomes.

5.6.1. Pharmacological Interventions

Pharmacological therapy of the ANS plays a critical role in the treatment of hypertension and cardiovascular disease complications associated with it. Antihypertensive drug therapy, i.e., adrenergic beta-receptor blockers, has emerged as an effective treatment choice because of their efficacy in inhibiting sympathetic nervous system activity. By the influence of catecholamine effects , such as norepinephrine, these agents can reduce heart and blood pressure, hence reducing the work burden to the cardiovascular system. From literature, pharmacological modulation of the ANS appropriately not only cures hypertension but also minimizes the risk of atrial fibrillation and heart failure and leads to an overall improvement in cardiovascular well-being (Gottlieb et al., 2024). Consequently, the strategy emphasizes the potential to target the ANS as a logical means of preventing end-organ injury in hypertensive patients. Aside from beta-blockers, other pharmacologic interventions have gained attention for their potential to shift autonomic balance. For instance, drugs that promote vagal activation, such as low-level stimulation of the vagus nerve, are under investigation for their therapeutic potential in disorders involving heightened sympathetic dominance. These therapies are meant to enhance parasympathetic activity, and subsequently, there is enhanced autonomic outflow in balance and better cardiovascular parameters. Results from other studies show that such pharmacologic treatments can contribute towards better results in the management of dysregulation of ANS, which is commonly faced by hypertensive patients (Gottlieb et al., 2024). With constant research, the relationship between pharmacological interventions and the ANS uncovers significant findings, ushering in new modes of treatment that can successfully treat complicated health conditions. Moreover, the integration of pharmacological interventions and non-pharmacological strategies serves to reflect the multidisciplinary approach in treating ANS disorders.

Recent studies have shown the benefit of interventions , such as sacroiliac joint manipulation for augmenting autonomic balance, particularly in patients with diseases , such as primary dysmenorrhea. Adding complementary therapies , such as these, to traditional pharmacologic management is a way clinicians can augment outcomes that are most related to autonomic dysfunction. The information reveals that with such combined therapy, there are significant improvements in pain relief and well-being, further validating the necessity of holistic treatment in resolving ANS -affected disorders. As information regarding the autonomic nervous system emerges, increasingly more becomes evident that new treatment methods, integrating pharmacological and non-pharmacological practices, have immense potential to improve patient care (Figure 5.17).

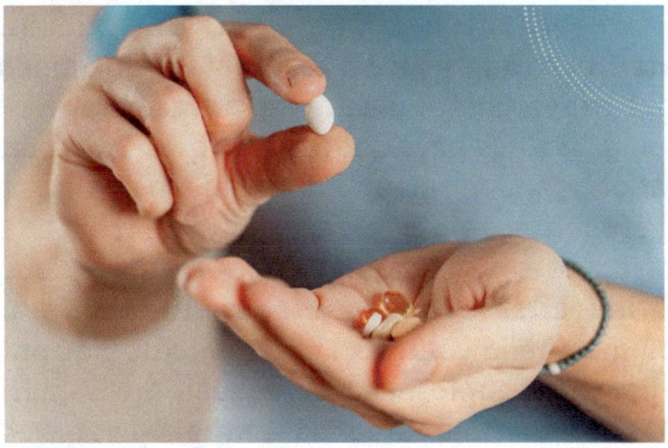

Figure 5.17. Treatment for autonomic dysfunction.

Source: https://lonestarneurology.net/wp-content/uploads/2023/06/1-Methods-of-Treatment-for-Autonomic-Dysfunction.webp.

5.6.2. Lifestyle Modifications

Lifestyle modifications play a significant role in the regulation of autonomic nervous functions and overall health. Physical exercise on regular basis is one of the most critical lifestyle adjustments that have been proven to influence autonomic regulation in a beneficial way. Exercise has been found to cause a paradigm shift in autonomic function by changing HRV to a positive value, which is a dominant indicator of autonomous regulation. In fact, studies have shown that during and after exercise, sympathetic activity may rise and parasympathetic activity may fall, which suggests dynamic interaction of these two systems in response to bodily stressors (Chiang et al., 2024). Through engagement in frequent aerobic and resistance training, individuals can achieve a lifestyle conducive to stress resilience, providing a gateway to improved cardiovascular and cognitive performance, which are central to maintaining an optimal ANS. In conjunction with exercise, dietary modification is also a critical element of lifestyle changes beneficial to the ANS. Eating a balanced, nutrient-rich diet can counteract the negative impact of stress on autonomic regulation. For instance, dietary intake of omega-3 fatty acids, antioxidants, and fiber can ensure a favorable environment for ANS regulation and cardiovascular well-being. Studies have shown that type 2 diabetic patients, and normally susceptible to autonomic dysfunction, were remarkably improved in terms of treatment satisfaction and quality of life after adopting dietary interventions for metabolic control. These benefits not only empower people but also reduce the somatic stress reactions due to inappropriateness of diet, which depicts the capacity of diet to effectively modulate autonomic balance (Hecquet et al., 2024). An overall plan including dietary modifications can then complement the general management of ANS disorders. Psychological considerations, such as stress-reducing interventions and mindfulness, are also crucial in developing a healthy autonomic nervous system. The contribution of chronic stress to the impact on autonomic balance is well established, with chronic stress having the potential to cause dysregulation of sympathetic and parasympathetic functions. Merging behavioral treatments , such as meditation, yoga, and biofeedback can decrease stress and produce relaxation, thereby promoting parasympathetic activity. These treatments not only promote a relaxing state but also improve attention, emotional control, and body recovery, therefore fortifying a lifestyle that promotes ANS well-being. Furthermore, interventions specifically to reduce stresses on the autonomic system show significant benefits for individuals with diseases like type 2 diabetes, where empowerment and quality of life improvement were observed in those actively engaged in such activities (Hecquet et al., 2024). Overall lifestyle modifications, therefore, spanning from exercise and dietary patterns to psychological well-being, are a multidisciplinary approach towards maximizing autonomic nervous system functioning (Figure 5.18).

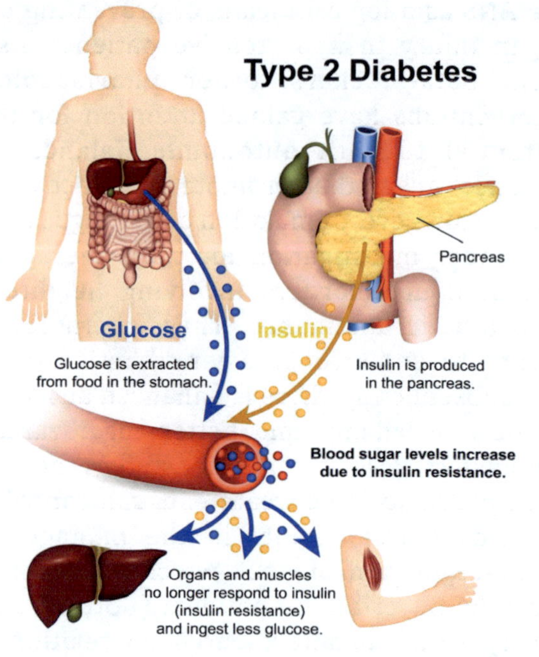

Figure 5.18. Type-2-diabetes.

Source: https://www.endocrineharmony.sg/wp-content/uploads/2024/10/Understanding-Type-2-Diabetes-854x1024.jpg.

5.6.3. Alternative Therapies

Alternative therapy has drawn increasing interest for its potential to control the ANS, particularly in managing stress and enhancing well-being. Reflexology is one method in which pressure is exerted on specific points on the body, primarily on the feet and hands, which are thought to correspond to organs and systems in the body. This practice refers to the idea that energy flows through certain paths, and blockages can lead to malfunctioning. By activating these reflex areas, reflexology might potentially normalize body functioning and lower stress levels, thereby affecting the sympathetic and parasympathetic branches of the ANS. Thus, relief in chronic pain and anxiety can be felt by an individual, making reflexology's role as a complementary approach to standard medical care for the management of autonomic dysregulation-related conditions evident. The potential of the practice in therapy has been discussed in extensive literature in various health scenarios, underscoring its role in the modern understanding of holistic health interventions (Quindlen, 2019). Breathing exercises and meditation have also risen to prominence in alternative therapy, especially with reference to their influence on the ANS. Current studies have brought to the limelight that these activities are capable of reversing homeostatic changes brought about by anxiety and stress. Through a focus on controlled breathing and awareness, these practices allow for a transition from sympathetic dominance to parasympathetic activation, enabling relaxation and emotional balance. This approach contrasts with conventional treatment approaches that typically seek to assault neurotransmitter imbalance using pharmacologic strategies. The hypothesis suggests that application of the body's own mechanism for self-regulation via breathing control could be of more benefit in treating emotional disease , such as anxiety and depression. The interaction between mood states and breathing also underlies the therapeutic benefit of including such techniques in treatment protocols for patients seeking to enhance overall mental well-being and stress resistance (Barnes et al., 2015). With complementary therapies increasingly finding their way into mainstream practice, understanding the mechanisms involved is ever more crucial to both professional and client. Reflexology's, meditation's, and the ANS's interactions reveal precious information about the body's response to psychological stresses. While their physiological mechanisms are yet to be completely demystified, current evidence supports their efficacy in the facilitation of well-being and prevention of stress diseases. The incorporation of alternative medicine in an integral practice can empower patients by providing them with a channel through which they actively assume responsibility for their well-being. With increasing popularity in these non-invasive methods, there is yet more research to be conducted to reveal the exact mechanisms through which they influence the ANS. While this study reaffirms the potential for alternative therapies to be employed alongside conventional interventions, it also builds up knowledge of the complex connection between body and mind in maintaining health (Barnes et al., 2015; Quindlen, 2019).

Test Your Knowledge

1. What are the difficulties in managing autonomic disorders with an effect on cardiovascular regulation, such as neurogenic hypertension?
2. How does multidisciplinary care and education of the patient aid in the effective management of chronic autonomic disorders?

SUMMARY

In regard to the intricate activities of the ANS, it is understandable that its implications far go beyond rudimentary physiological control. The findings derived from the research highlight the significance of understanding the ANS with respect to different health issues including psychiatric ailments and cancer. For instance, the dysfunction of the ANS, particularly in the case of schizophrenia, highlights the need for the implementation of individualized therapeutic interventions on an urgent basis. As intimated, the contrast between oral aripiprazole and its long-acting injectable variant suggests that formulation could bear significant influence on autonomic function, thus on treatment outcome and patient wellness. This becomes vital while seeking integrative management methods that not only address the mental health disorder symptoms but also underlying physiological derangements (Hattori et al., 2023). Moreover, the information regarding the ANSs function in cancer pathology and treatment response introduces a fascinating dimension to this analysis. The increased expression of the β-2-adrenergic receptors in lung cancer and the therapeutic benefit elicited by β-blocker therapy are reflective of the interplay between autonomic signaling and cancer biology. These issues bear not just on understanding lung cancer pathology but also on therapeutic approaches. The intersection of the ANS with pharmacology is a novel and burgeoning area of research with the potential to enhance patient care by potentially making integrative treatment regimens feasible that utilizes the inherent regulatory function of the ANS to improve prognostic results (Garramona et al., 2023). In short, the autonomic nervous system is at the center of the comprehension of numerous health conditions, particularly in its intricate balance with mental and physical illnesses. Since research continues to de-mythologize ANS functions, practitioners and researchers are given the opportunity to refine therapeutic processes more consistent with autonomic functioning. The ANS activity correlations with therapeutic outcomes in the disease conditions of schizophrenia and lung cancer emphasize the need for an interdisciplinary interaction between neurology, psychiatry, and oncology. Future research will be required to fill in the knowledge gaps and develop high-caliber, prospective clinical trials that can guide clinical interventions. Lastly, an enhanced understanding of the ANS not only has the potential to enhance the effectiveness of treatment but also break open new advances in the treatment of complex health conditions (Garramona et al., 2023; Hattori et al., 2023).

In consideration of the ANS, there is a need to establish some key points that attest to its complexity as well as significance to body function. The ANS is also divided further into the sympathetic and parasympathetic branches, which play distinct roles in homeostasis as well as the regulation of a myriad of physiological processes. Activation of the sympathetic nervous system, for example, elicits the fight or flight response that prepares the body to respond to harmful conditions by increasing heart rate and directing blood toward the muscles. The opposite is true with the parasympathetic nervous system, which promotes rest and digestion processes, lowering the heart rate and promoting recovery functions. The intricate balance maintained by ANS is significant in responding to environmental demands in order to enable the body to respond effectively to acute as well as chronic stressors. Additionally, the research has established the complex interaction between ANS and cardiac function with consequences for overall health. Autonomic control imbalance is involved in many cardiovascular diseases, such as heart failure and arrhythmias. Clarification of the mechanisms by which cardiac function is affected under the influence of autonomic stimulation is a major challenge due to the complexity of the neural interactions in various regions of the heart.

Emerging advances in neurocardiac modeling made it possible for scientists to predict the effects of sympathetic and parasympathetic stimulation on the heart, which could open up new therapeutic options. Development of this multiscale model incorporates various biological levels, from cellular signal transduction to tissue response, to better understand how autonomic imbalance may result in health complications and how interventions might reverse or prevent them (Clancy et al., 2023).

Practical applications of autonomic regulation techniques have also provided promising outcomes in improving quality of life and reducing stress-related impairments. For instance, interventions that target the enhancement of emotional self-regulation have been pilot tested in some populations, i.e., the police, and they reduced physiological stress responses and improved communication and inter-personal relationships. Such research indicates the importance of stress management strategies that target the ANS as a way of enhancing emotional and physiological balance in high-stress professions. By bridging the gap between theoretical research and practical implementation, these techniques can give rise to increased mental clarity, performance, and well-being, illustrating the importance of the autonomic nervous system in daily life (Tomasino et al., 1999).

KEY TERMS FROM THIS CHAPTER

- Acetylcholine (ACh)
- Autonomic Ganglia
- Blood Pressure Control
- Fight or Flight
- Homeostasis
- Muscarinic Receptors
- Norepinephrine (NE)
- Postganglionic Neuron
- Adrenergic Receptors
- Autonomic Nervous System
- Cholinergic Receptors
- Heart Rate Regulation
- Involuntary Control
- Nicotinic Receptors
- Parasympathetic Division
- Preganglionic Neuron

CRITICAL THINKING QUESTIONS

1. **Which division of the autonomic nervous system is involved in the "rest and digest" response?**
   a. Sympathetic nervous system
   b. Parasympathetic nervous system
   c. Somatic nervous system
   d. Central nervous system
2. **What is the primary neurotransmitter released by postganglionic sympathetic neurons?**
   a. Acetylcholine
   b. Norepinephrine
   c. Dopamine
   d. Serotonin
3. **Which cranial nerve is most associated with the parasympathetic nervous system?**
   a. Optic nerve (CN II)
   b. Vagus nerve (CN X)
   c. Trigeminal nerve (CN V)
   d. Facial nerve (CN VII)
4. **The "fight or flight" response is primarily mediated by which autonomic division?**
   a. Parasympathetic nervous system
   b. Enteric nervous system
   c. Sympathetic nervous system
   d. Somatic nervous system
5. **What kind of receptor does acetylcholine act upon in the target organs of the parasympathetic nervous system?**
   a. Adrenergic receptors
   b. Nicotinic receptors
   c. Muscarinic receptors
   d. Dopaminergic receptors

Short Answer Questions

1. What are the two primary subdivisions of the autonomic nervous system?
2. Which ANS subdivision is responsible for "fight or flight" responses?
3. Name the neurotransmitter released by the parasympathetic nervous system in the target organ.
4. What is the overall function of the sympathetic nervous system?
5. Describe the physiological effects on organs as a result of sympathetic stimulation.
6. Discuss the operation of the parasympathetic nervous system to regulate digestive processes.
7. Describe the pathway of autonomic nerve fibers from the CNS to target organs.
8. Compare the neurotransmitters and the receptors in the sympathetic and parasympathetic nervous systems.

Answers to Critical Thinking Questions

1. (b); 2. (b); 3. (b); 4. (c); 5. (c)

REFERENCES

1. Robles, T. F., & Kane, H. S. (2014). The attachment system and physiology in adulthood: normative processes, individual differences, and implications for health. *Journal of personality*, *82*(6), 515–527. https://doi.org/10.1111/jopy.12052https://core.ac.uk/download/294625964.pdf (accessed on 16th June 2025).
2. Alaerts, K., Brincker, M., Caballero, C., Whyatt, C. P., Chai, X. J., Cheng, C., et al. (2017). Stochastic signatures of involuntary head micro-movements can be used to classify females of ABIDE into different subtypes of neurodevelopmental disorders. https://core.ac.uk/download/287581413.pdf (accessed on 16th June 2025).
3. Alingh Prins, A., Scheurink, A., Steffens, A. B., et al. (1996). Overfeeding, autonomic regulation and metabolic consequences. https://core.ac.uk/download/pdf/12942087.pdf (accessed on 16th June 2025).
4. Ang, R., Opel, A., & Tinker, A. (2012). The role of inhibitory G proteins and regulators of G protein signaling in the *in vivo* control of heart rate and predisposition to cardiac arrhythmias. https://core.ac.uk/download/30697484.pdf (accessed on 16th June 2025).
5. Ashwini, D. L., & Raju, T. R. (2023). Autonomic nervous system and control of visual function. *Annals of Neurosciences, 30*(3), 151–153. https://doi.org/10.1177/09727531231176119 (accessed on 16th June 2025).
6. Jerath, R., Crawford, M. W., Barnes, V. A., & Harden, K. (2015). Widespread depolarization during expiration: a source of respiratory drive?. *Medical hypotheses*, *84*(1), 31–37. https://doi.org/10.1016/j.mehy.2014.11.010Biesok, M., Lewoniuk, N., Macherski, M., Szafraniec, R., et al. (2024). Analysis of the effects of regular yoga on the adaptive capacity of the nervous system. https://core.ac.uk/download/620863318.pdf (accessed on 16th June 2025).
7. Boundy, K., Cai, F. Z. J., Keen, H., Lester, S., et al. (2008). Mild autonomic dysfunction in primary Sjögren's syndrome: A controlled study. https://core.ac.uk/download/pdf/8114066.pdf (accessed on 16th June 2025).
8. Brincker, M., & Torres, E. (2017). Why study movement variability in autism? https://core.ac.uk/download/131210732.pdf (accessed on 16th June 2025).
9. Brust, P., Creeley, C., Feldman, R., Grandjean, P., Herken, H., Panzica, G., Parent, M., et al. (2014). Neurotoxicity. https://core.ac.uk/download/286729125.pdf (accessed on 16th June 2025).
10. Burnstock, G. (2009). Purinergic signaling: Past, present and future. https://core.ac.uk/download/1670991.pdf (accessed on 16th June 2025).
11. Ceccacci, A., Fedele, F., Lavalle, C., Maestrini, V., et al. (2019). Triggers for atrial fibrillation: The role of anxiety. https://core.ac.uk/download/188833222.pdf (accessed on 16th June 2025).
12. Chiang, J., Lin, Y. C., Hung, T. Y., Kao, H. H., & Kao, Y. H. (2024). The impact on autonomic nervous system activity during and following exercise in adults: A meta-regression study and trial sequential analysis. *Medicina, 60*. https://www.semanticscholar.org/paper/86e77d00199ec190289f8a8655267bab22b8ee89 (accessed on 16th June 2025).
13. Doc Childre, Rollin McCraty, 'The Grateful Heart: The Psychophysiology of Appreciation', in Robert A. Emmons, and Michael E. McCullough (eds), The Psychology of Gratitude, Series in Affective Science (New York, 2004; online edn, Oxford Academic, 22 Mar. 2012), https://doi.org/10.1093/acprof:oso/9780195150100.003.0012, accessed 26 July 2025.(accessed on 16th June 2025).

14. Christensen, W. (2006). The evolutionary origins of volition. https://core.ac.uk/download/pdf/87234.pdf (accessed on 16th June 2025).
15. Clancy, C. E., Dawson, J. R. D., DeMarco, K. R., Han, Y., et al. (2023). A multiscale predictive digital twin for neurocardiac modulation. https://core.ac.uk/download/617744749.pdf (accessed on 16th June 2025).
16. Crawford, M. W., & Jerath, R. (2015). How does the body affect the mind? Role of cardiorespiratory coherence in the spectrum of emotions. https://core.ac.uk/download/131207333.pdf (accessed on 16th June 2025).
17. Cunha, R. A., & Ribeiro, J. A. (2000). ATP as a presynaptic modulator. https://core.ac.uk/download/12427071.pdf (accessed on 16th June 2025).
18. Curras-Collazo, M. C., Dobyns, A., Gutierrez, R., Jha, S., et al. (2017). A calibrated method of massage therapy decreases systolic blood pressure concomitant with changes in heart rate variability in male rats. https://core.ac.uk/download/286361424.pdf (accessed on 16th June 2025).
19. Dalise, A. M., Prestano, R., Fasano, R., Gambardella, A., Barbieri, M., & Rizzo, M. (2020). Autonomic nervous system and cognitive impairment in older patients: Evidence from long-term heart rate variability in real-life setting. *Frontiers in Aging Neuroscience, 12*. https://www.semanticscholar.org/paper/da600a28a975a351e556c42c74bda495378b6a68 (accessed on 16th June 2025).
20. Domínguez Vías, G., & Ramírez Sánchez, M. (2021). Brain asymmetry: Towards an asymmetrical neurovisceral integration. https://core.ac.uk/download/493007120.pdf (accessed on 16th June 2025).
21. Dorsher, P. (2008). Fibromyalgia: A unifying neuroendocrinology model for understanding its pathophysiology. https://core.ac.uk/download/pdf/288173.pdf (accessed on 16th June 2025).
22. Judith Estrine, Lisa DeLisle. "Stress: Putting the Brain Back Into Medicine" International Longevity Center-USA, 2006, doi: https://core.ac.uk/download/71356692.pdf(accessed on 16th June 2025).
23. Federici, A., Zenzola, A., Xu, A., Akay, M., Aldroubi, A., Simone, F., Gonnella, G., et al. (2005). Response of autonomic nervous system to body positions: Fourier and wavelet analysis. http://arxiv.org/abs/physics/0310125 (accessed on 16th June 2025).
24. Garramona, F. T., Cunha, T. F., Vieira, J. S., Borges, G., Santos, G., de Castro, G., Ugrinowitsch, C., et al. (2023). Increased sympathetic nervous system impairs prognosis in lung cancer patients: A scoping review of clinical studies. *Lung Cancer Management, 12*. https://www.semanticscholar.org/paper/6fd58821e13984eed945c1686baa5401f57a2d14 (accessed on 16th June 2025).
25. Gottlieb, L. A., Mahfoud, F., Stavrakis, S., Jespersen, T., & Linz, D. K. (2024). Autonomic nervous system: A therapeutic target for cardiac end-organ damage in hypertension. *Hypertension (Dallas, Tex.: 1979), 81*, 2027–2037. https://www.semanticscholar.org/paper/e3432544b8a63aba6727392752bda65506eecf39 (accessed on 16th June 2025).
26. Grewal, S., & Gupta, V. (2011). Effect of obesity on autonomic nervous system. *International Journal of Current Biomedical and Medical Sciences*. https://core.ac.uk/download/pdf/14686.pdf (accessed on 16th June 2025).

27. Hattori, S., Suda, A., Kishida, I., Miyauchi, M., Shiraishi, Y., Noguchi, N., Furuno, T., et al. (2023). Differences in autonomic nervous system activity between long-acting injectable aripiprazole and oral aripiprazole in schizophrenia. *BMC Psychiatry, 23.* https://www.semanticscholar.org/paper/924ad99ec1e2d138a5a801d40f423c38e5378c79 (accessed on 16th June 2025).

28. Hecquet, S., Ballegaard, S., Eldrup, E., Hansen, C. S., Hansen, T., Harboe, G., Rossing, P., et al. (2024). New diabetic treatment by alleviation of autonomic nervous system dysfunction measured as periosteal pressure sensitivity at sternum improves empowerment, treatment satisfaction, and self-reported health of people with type 2 diabetes: A randomized trial. *Diabetes, Metabolic Syndrome and Obesity, 17*, 2519–2531. https://www.semanticscholar.org/paper/ace6b0308edd6218e01876ba84958becbd63222b (accessed on 16th June 2025).

29. Inhula, N. (2018). Variability of the heart rhythm as an additional marker for determining vegetative functions in patients with chronic cerebral ischemia. https://core.ac.uk/download/322516329.pdf (accessed on 16th June 2025).

30. Kekecs, Z., Szekely, A., & Varga, K. (2015). Alterations in electrodermal activity and cardiac parasympathetic tone during hypnosis. https://core.ac.uk/download/77011630.pdf (accessed on 16th June 2025).

31. Lange, K. A. (2025). *Physiology of Man and Animals in the Tenth Five-Year Plan: Proceedings of the Thirteenth Congress of the I. P. Pavlov All-Union Physiological Society*. https://core.ac.uk/download/pdf/42860886.pdf (accessed on 16th June 2025).

32. Li, H., Wang, H., & Wang, X. (2025). Psychedelics and the autonomic nervous system: A perspective on their interplay and therapeutic potential. *ACS Pharmacology & Translational Science, 8*(3), 899–902. https://www.semanticscholar.org/paper/5ddc94440df6424b0cf05f8e4c706089c6d0d931 (accessed on 16th June 2025).

33. Lisukha, L. (2017). The use of intermittent norm baric hypoxia in children's neurology (Review). https://core.ac.uk/download/301580754.pdf (accessed on 16th June 2025).

34. Martins, I. J. (2016). Anti-aging genes improve appetite regulation and reverse cell senescence and apoptosis in global populations. https://core.ac.uk/download/84887634.pdf (accessed on 16th June 2025).

35. Motofei, I. G., & Rowland, D. L. (2017). Psycho-physiologic emergentist; four minds in a body. https://core.ac.uk/download/144553869.pdf (accessed on 16th June 2025).

36. Park, S., Kim, H., Jung, J., & Lee, S. (2024). Effects of sacroiliac joint manipulation on autonomic nervous system and lower abdominal pain in women with primary dysmenorrhea: A randomized controlled trial. *Medicina, 60.* https://www.semanticscholar.org/paper/eda21b5e5c39f9468e3bcd03ca68320dcf8a975b (accessed on 16th June 2025).

37. Puledda, F., & Goadsby, P. J. (2016). Current Approaches to Neuromodulation in Primary Headaches: Focus on Vagal Nerve and Sphenopalatine Ganglion Stimulation. *Current pain and headache reports, 20*(7), 47. https://doi.org/10.1007/s11916-016-0577-5(accessed on 16th June 2025).

38. Quindlen, K. A. (2019). *Reflexology*. https://cupola.gettysburg.edu/cgi/viewcontent.cgi?article=1840&context=student_scholarship (accessed on 16th June 2025).

39. Raj, S. R. (2006). The postural tachycardia syndrome (POTS): Pathophysiology, diagnosis & management. https://core.ac.uk/download/pdf/86508.pdf (accessed on 16th June 2025).

40. Siepmann, T., & Ziemssen, T. (2019). The investigation of the cardiovascular and sudomotor autonomic nervous system—A review. https://core.ac.uk/download/201288195.pdf (accessed on 16th June 2025).

41. Silvani, A., Heidbreder, A., Lambert, I., Barateau, L., & Dauvilliers, Y. (2023). Autonomic dysfunction in hypersomnia. https://core.ac.uk/download/611892825.pdf (accessed on 16th June 2025).

42. Simonenko, G. (2017). Detection of autonomic dysfunctions in complex neuropsychological examination of NMU students. https://core.ac.uk/download/301580770.pdf (accessed on 16th June 2025).

43. Souza Filho, L. F. M., de Oliveira, J. C. D., Ribeiro, M. K. A., Moura, M. C., Fernandes, N. D., de Sousa, R. D., Pedrino, G., et al. (2019). Evaluation of the autonomic nervous system by analysis of heart rate variability in the preterm infants. *BMC Cardiovascular Disorders, 19*. https://www.semanticscholar.org/paper/daa59fffe74007a94702375e951c801542055101 (accessed on 16th June 2025).

44. Steinhart, E. (2001). Persons versus brains: Biological intelligence in human organisms. https://core.ac.uk/download/287611886.pdf (accessed on 16th June 2025).

45. Tomasino, D., Sundram, J., Atkinson, M., & McCraty, R. (1999). Impact of the Heart Math self-management skills program on physiological and psychological stress in police officers. https://core.ac.uk/download/71342457.pdf (accessed on 16th June 2025).

CENTRAL NERVOUS SYSTEM

6

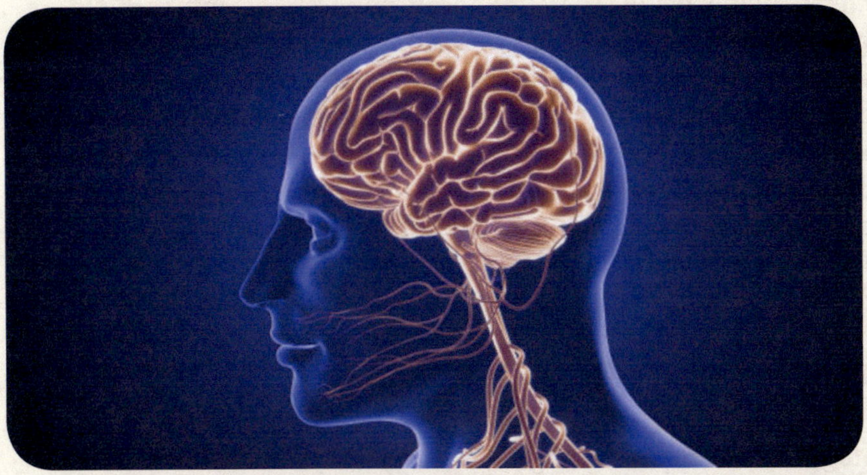

Introduction

The central nervous system (CNS), which consists of the brain and spinal cord, is vital in the processing and transmitting of neural information to the rest of the body. It is the master control center, not only regulating voluntary movements but also controlling involuntary processes that achieve homeostasis. Understanding the CNSs intricate structure and function is imperative for neuroscience, psychology, and medicine. The complexity of the CNS is further highlighted by its malleability or neuroplasticity, whereby it can reshape itself in response to injury or learning. By considering the primary functions of the different parts of the CNS, from the cerebral cortex through to the brainstem, an appreciation can be developed of integrated systems subserving cognitive as well as physiological processes, and this provides the background to more detailed examination of individual pathologies and what they imply with respect to health and disease management. Studies of CNS pathologies are supplemented by current research into how different pathologies affect brain structure and function.

LEARNING OBJECTIVES

After studying this chapter, you will be able to:

1. Explain the anatomy of the central nervous system;
2. Explain the functions of the central nervous system;
3. Explain the neurons and neurotransmission;
4. Highlight central nervous system disorders;
5. Study the diagnostic approach to the central nervous system;
6. Evaluate the treatment and management of the central nervous system.

For instance, CRPS patients illustrate the CNS involvement in pain perception and its potential alteration in chronic conditions. Recent studies using diffusion tensor imaging revealed structural connectivity abnormalities of CRPS patients, implying changes in white matter that could underlie their chronic pain experiences. Specifically, increased mean diffusivity and other parameters reflect disruptions of the neural transmission tracts essential for optimal brain function. These findings enlighten us regarding the intricate role of the CNS not only in the immediate response to pain but also in the long-term consequences of chronic pain syndromes and hence highlight the necessity to investigate neural pathways in designing effective therapy protocols (Acosta-Cabronero et al., 2017).

The emergence of the antiretroviral therapy (ART) in treating HIV/AIDS has pointed to the importance of understanding the CNSs development following pharma exposure, particularly in utero. With more HIV-1-infected mothers giving birth to ART-exposed children, scientists have expressed concern about neurological effects caused by these drugs that can be passed on to developing fetuses. The CNS plasticity that results from the critical periods of development could potentially make it especially vulnerable to neurotoxicity because of some of the components of ART, such as protease inhibitors. There have been preliminary clinical reports and studies that have tried to investigate the effects of in utero exposure on neurodevelopmental outcomes with acute and delayed effects. The interest in ART treatment's effect on the CNS has encouraged further studies on the crossroads of maternal HIV treatment and neonatal neuroprotection, and therefore this is a fascinating area of study with significant social implications (Celsi et al., 2017).

Definition of the Central Nervous System (CNS)

The CNS is the primary signaling hub of the body, consisting of the brain and the spinal cord. This intricate system is responsible for integration and processing of sensory information to enable responses to internal and external stimulation. With its integration of many bodily processes, the CNS is indispensable to the achievement of homeostasis and permitting complex behavior. The brain, constituting the central structure in the CNS, comprises several regions that govern functions ranging from motor to cognition, with the spinal cord branching out from the brain as a conduit for nerve impulses from the brain to the peripheral nervous system. All of these structures form an extremely specialized network required for survival and function, which highlights the urgency of CNS health and its associated disorders. The building blocks of the central nervous system are cells referred to as neurons, and every neuron is a conduit for electrical impulses. Neurons convey information across synapses, which is crucial in the CNS. In addition, glial cells serve a supportive function by keeping the environment from which neurons operate in good health, supplying them with nutrients, and helping repair nervous tissue if it is damaged.

The interplay between neuronal activity and glial support is essential to the optimal functioning of the CNS. It has been shown that dysfunction in these cellular interactions can contribute to a wide range of neurological disorders, so it is important to understand their roles in CNS health in-depth. It is crucial to realize how these cellular dynamics influence CNS function as a whole, particularly with the increase in neurodegenerative diseases of aging and oxidative stress (Chen et al., 2020). Recent studies have also established the significance of mitochondrial health in the integrity of the central nervous system. Mitochondria, the cellular organelles responsible for energy generation, are essential for neuronal function and metabolism, and mitochondrial dysfunction can have extensive implications for CNS functions. In specific, research in various model organisms, including zebrafish, has revealed the interaction of mitochondrial proteins and CNS development. This research has shown an association of mitochondrial dysfunction with neuroinflammation and apoptotic pathways, leading to visual impairment and neurodegenerative diseases (Martín-Jiménez et al., 2018). Furthermore, research into neuroprotective agents , such as Klotho that enhance mitochondrial activity offers hopeful therapeutic possibilities for interrupting myelin disorders. As knowledge of mitochondrial processes further advances, so too do the implications for treatment and prevention of CNS disorders (Figure 6.1).

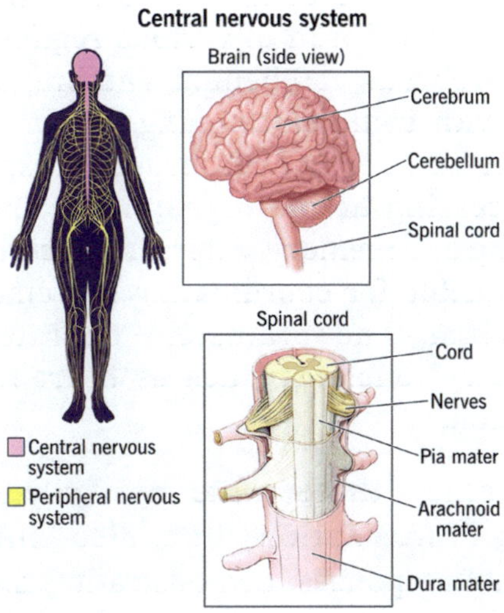

Figure 6.1. Central nervous system (CNS).

Source: https://my.clevelandclinic.org/-/scassets/images/org/health/articles/central-nervous-system.

Importance of the Central Nervous System (CNS) in Human Physiology

The CNS of a human being is the primary communication network of the body, making the overall physiology and behavior possible. The CNS encompasses the brain and spinal cord, and it analyzes sensory information and controls the activities of the body, enabling individuals to respond to changing circumstances. At the core of this regulatory mechanism is integration of the complex neural pathways, controlling voluntary and involuntary action. For instance, it regulates external stimulation and sends commands to other organs to reach homeostasis. Its interdisciplinarity with the endocrine system is another instance of its physiological importance as it regulates hormones that regulate metabolism, growth, and stress.

Therefore, the complexity of CNSs has to be understood to realize how it regulates not just the bodily functions but also emotional and psychological well-being. Moreover, the function of the central nervous system extends beyond mere coordination to also encompass its important role in mental health and control over emotions. Since the neural networks associated with emotions are found to make major contributions to psychological reactions to stimuli,. Based on models , such as the three circle model of emotion that describes affect regulation dimensions, it becomes possible to comprehend how the CNS influences mental health via physiologic processes. The model focuses on how feelings have the ability to affect behavioral reactions and impact treatments for mental health.

Since the earliest and most important function of the CNS is mediating between states of feeling and body responses, any alteration in neural function has wide-reaching implications for psychological health. The dynamic between CNS function and mental health is additional rationale to pursue a search for knowledge of these dynamics in clinical and research environments (Maratos et al., 2016). Attachment theory also describes the role of the central nervous system in managing stress and its ultimate impact on physical health. The attachment behavioral system has close association with physiological responses that influence an individual's capacity to handle stressors. Research on individual differences in attachment modalities can be helpful in determining the extent to which various emotional regulation systems impact the CNS's functioning. For instance, those who are securely attached are expected to have more resilient responses to stress, thus promoting better health and better physiological regulation. Also, the interplay between attachment, stress, and CNS activity illustrates the utility of biologically feasible models in the treatment of the relationships between psychological processes and chronic diseases in an integrated manner. As viewed in more recent studies, it is through describing such relationships that doors are opened to new mental health interventions respecting the intricate interplay between the central nervous system and their implications on global health (Robles & Kane, 2014) (Figure 6.2).

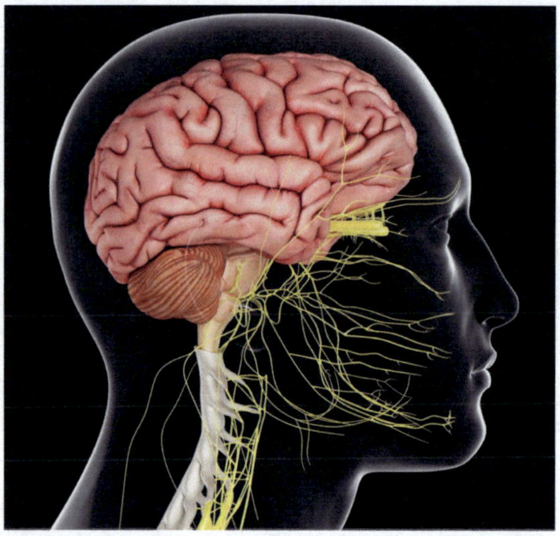

Figure 6.2. Central Nervous System (CNS) in Human Physiology.

Source: https://www.verywellmind.com/thmb/CoPq8udVEWA_4xEEqTv-dFBiksk=/1500x0/filters:no_upscale():max_bytes(150000):strip_icc()/brain_spinal_cord-57fe96b15f9b5805c26d5072.jpg.

6.1. Anatomy of the Central Nervous System (CNS)

Learning Outcome

1. Describe the major components: brain and spinal cord;
2. Emphasize the structure of the brain: lobes and regions;
3. Define the protective layers: meninges and cerebrospinal fluid.

The structure of the central nervous system (CNS) is a complex structure composed predominantly of the brain and spinal cord and serves as the control center of the body. The brain, composed of various regions , such as the cerebrum, cerebellum, and brainstem, is tasked with complex thinking, motor activity, and homeostasis. The cerebrum is responsible for processing at the higher level, including reasoning and memory, whereas the cerebellum is responsible for coordinating movement and equilibrium. The brainstem operates vital involuntary functions, such as heart rate and respiration.

Together, these units not only control sensory information but also integrate emotional responses, demonstrating the CNS's vast versatility and accommodation. There are protective coverings around the CNS, including the meninges, which consist of three layers: dura mater, arachnoid mater, and pia mater. The membranes shield the brain and spinal cord from harm and also provide a supportive environment through which cerebrospinal fluid (CSF) circulates. This fluid acts to cushion the CNS and maintain intracranial pressure. Furthermore, the blood-brain barrier (BBB) offers an additional layer of protection by selectively permeating substances from the blood into the brain so that neural tissue is isolated from potentially disorganizing agents. These anatomical features make clear the highly developed protective mechanisms of the CNS necessary to preserve neural integrity and function as a whole. Criticically, the contrasts between the central nervous system and the peripheral nervous system (PNS) underscore the significance of glial cells in neuronal health. The PNS is much more capable of regeneration, mostly due to the unique characteristics of its glial cell types, such as Schwann cells and olfactory ensheathing cells. These cells allow nerve damage recovery via clearance of debris and provision of required growth factors, which identifies their putative function in therapeutic recovery with CNS damage. Understanding these glial mechanisms is important in designing new treatments that take advantage of the regenerative power of PNS glia to offer CNS afflictions and promote recovery (Barton et al., 2017). Development in anatomical modeling, particularly in three-dimensional reconstructions, brings about the possibility of improved surgical interventions and biomechanical evaluations, resulting in an improved understanding of complex neural structures (Audenaert et al., 2010) (Figure 6.3).

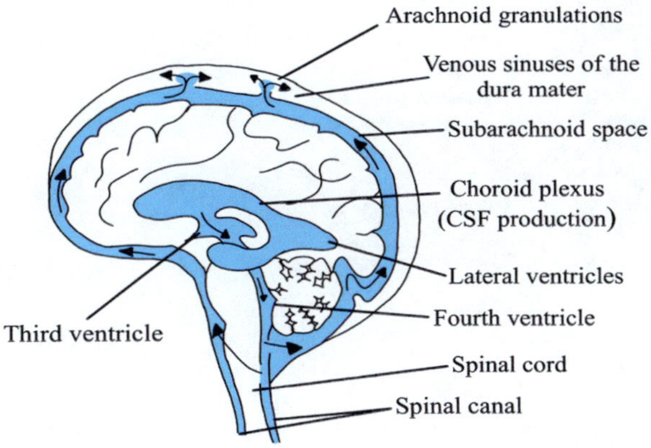

Figure 6.3. Cerebrospinal fluid (CSF).

Source: Czarniak N, Kamińska J, Matowicka-Karna J, Koper-Lenkiewicz OM. Cerebrospinal Fluid–Basic Concepts Review. Biomedicines. 2023; 11(5):1461. https://doi.org/10.3390/biomedicines11051461

6.1.1. Major Components: Brain and Spinal Cord

The CNS consists of two major components: the brain and the spinal cord, both of which are critical in assisting the body's functioning. The brain serves as the command center to control coordinating sensory input, decision-making, and emotional control, and the spinal cord is the primary pathway for information being relayed between the brain and the rest of the body. This complex relationship enables reaction to stimuli and coordinating voluntary and involuntary movement. Sensory information received from peripheral nerves is processed by the brain and produced as a response, relayed via the spinal cord. Therefore, grasping the structural and functional hierarchy of these components is essential to demystifying the CNS's complexities and its role in human health, especially in neurologic disorders and trauma. The brains complex structure features separate parts, each offering specialized functions essential for behavioral and physiological control. The cerebral cortex, which handles advanced cognitive processes, is crucial in processing sensory information and facilitating advanced decision-making. Conversely, the brainstem regulates elementary autonomic functions , such as breathing and heart rate. These areas are connected through an enormous association of neurons that permit communication among various parts of the brain and the spinal cord. Additionally, increasing research targets the brain's ability to be plastic, its capability to reorganize and modify following injury. Research has shown that neurobiologically informed interventions may enhance rehabilitation from neurological disabilities, thereby discerning the brain's remarkable resilience and the importance of ongoing research into therapeutic interventions (Edgerton et al., 2016). As far as the spinal cord is concerned, it acts both as the function of sensory as well as has motor functions while acting in a crucial role of also being a pathway of communication between the brain and the peripheral nervous system. The spinal cord contains segments corresponding to different parts of the body and can thus be used for motor signal localization and sensory input localization. There is also recent evidence towards spinal cord recovery following injury. Evidence now demonstrates that interventions , such as neuroprotective therapy and synaptic connection manipulation are able to enhance motor function considerably, undermining longstanding assumptions of the fixedness of neurological recovery (Adler et al., 2016). Understanding these functions not only enhances our knowledge regarding the CNS but also underscores the importance of an interdisciplinary therapeutic plan for improving patient outcomes with spinal cord injury as well as other CNS-associated disorders (Figure 6.4).

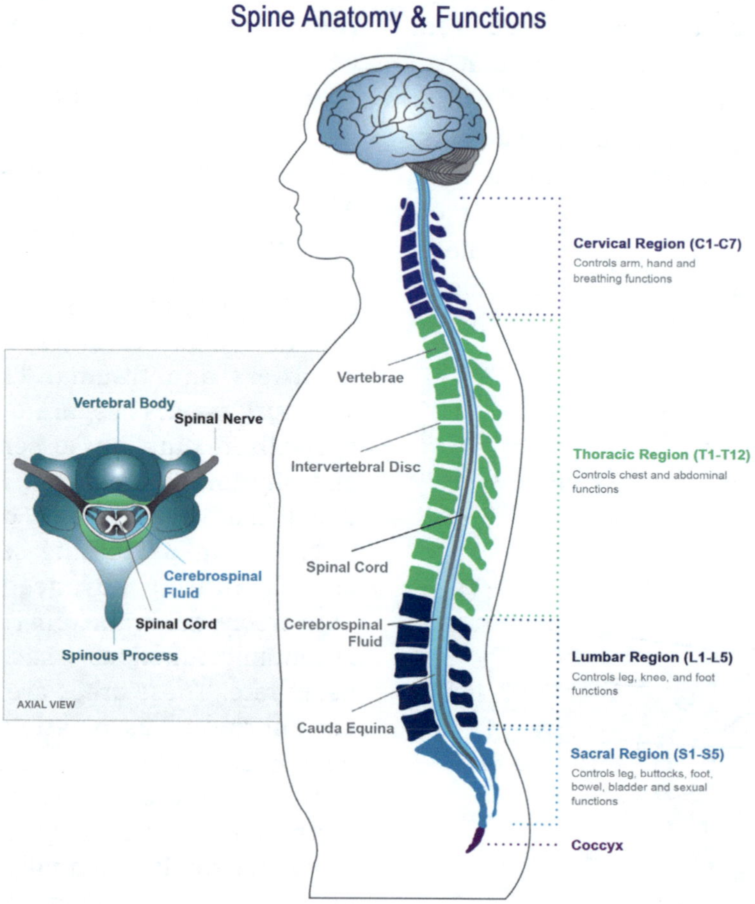

Figure 6.4. Brain and spinal cord.

Source: https://www.cancer.gov/rare-brain-spine-tumor/sites/g/files/xnrzdm226/files/styles/cgov_article/public/cgov_infographic/2020-01/Spine-Functions-infographic.gif?itok=hnqGQrMz.

6.1.2. Structure of the Brain: Lobes and Regions

The structure of the brain is divided in a complex manner into numerous lobes and areas, each having its own set of functions that all contribute to the general functions of the central nervous system. Broadly categorized, the brain is divided into the frontal, parietal, temporal, and occipital lobes. The frontal lobe, at the front part of the brain, is the area for executive function , such as decision-making, problem-solving, and emotional regulation. It also houses the primary motor cortex, with direct access to voluntary movements. The parietal lobe, conversely, processes sensory inputs in relation to touch and sense of space. The temporal lobe plays a crucial role in auditory interpretation and construction of memory. The occipital lobe at the posterior aspect of the brain is the center for processing visual information, emphasizing the specialized function of these cortical areas in the modular structure of the brain (Padovani, 2016). Understanding the modular structure of brain areas is essential in examining how various cognitive functions and physiological conditions are interconnected. Each lobe is connected to the others, forming networks that are attributed to complex processing functions, as well as sharing special functionalities. Research indicates that interactions are predictive of a community structure among functional brain networks, whereby clusters of regions collaborate towards the achievement of some results. For instance, network dynamics indicate significant alterations under consciousness states, particularly following anesthetic induction, to manifest the plasticity of brain modularity. As demonstrated by anesthetic effect evidence, the waking state involves the increased activity of large clusters in parietal and frontal regions, the direct opposite of the anesthetized states' disturbed connectivity patterns (Padovani, 2016). Hence, understanding these modular structures not only accounts for brain function but also informs neuroscientific inquiry into consciousness. Other than the primary lobes, several other regions constitute the complex functions of the brain. For example, the limbic system, consisting of structures like the amygdala and hippocampus, has an important function in emotion and memory. Basal ganglia also regulate movement and procedural learning, and the cerebellum provides coordination and balance. Each one of these regions possesses characteristic patterns of neurons and synaptic circuits that increase its specialized role. Recent studies employing advanced imaging techniques have indicated these contacts, thus providing additional evidence for the existence of modular organization in the structure of the brain. Ultimately, the discovery of interaction amongst a number of lobes and subdivisions will give hints regarding their combined influences on behavior, cognitive functioning, and overall neural transmission in the central nervous system (Figure 6.5).

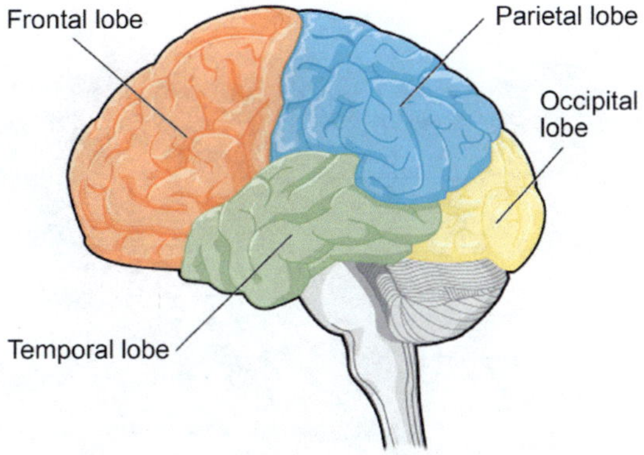

Figure 6.5. Lobes of the brain.

Source: https://s3-us-west-2.amazonaws.com/courses-images-archive-read-only/wp-content/uploads/sites/902/2015/02/23224600/CNX_Psych_03_04_Lobes.jpg.

6.1.3. Protective Layers: Meninges and Cerebrospinal Fluid

The CNS is well protected by several coverings, particularly the meninges and CSF. The meninges comprise three distinct layers—the dura mater, arachnoid mater, and pia mater—of which they perform significant protective and supportive roles. The outermost layer is the dura mater, a thick, tough membrane that provides a robust protection against physical trauma. Below it is the arachnoid mater, a web-like layer which facilitates the flow of CSF and its subarachnoid space. Finally, the pia mater closely enfolds the surface of the brain, providing a delicate barrier which aids in the transport of chemicals to neural tissues. These layers act as a whole to create an environment that is conducive to proper CNS functioning, effectively shield it from external mechanical stress and infectious pathogens.

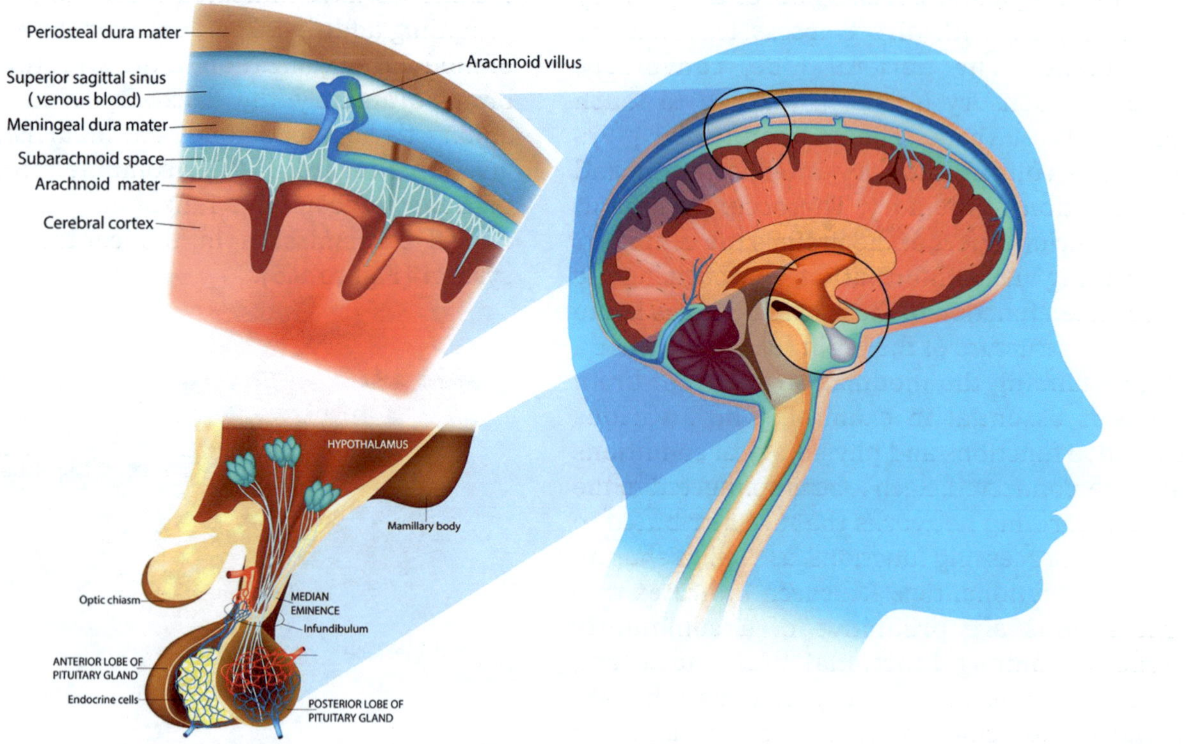

Figure 6.6. Meninges: Function and layers, and health problems.

Source: https://www.thoughtco.com/thmb/_bBUyGHg1YlzRqCVdsricau77Tc=/1500x0/filters:no_upscale():max_bytes(150000):strip_icc()/anatomy-of-the-brain--meninges--hypothalamus-and-anterior-pituitary--1134486874-240d1e77d3364d5b8572be4b44a43666.jpg.

Cerebrospinal fluid plays an important role in the protection and optimal functioning of the CNS. CSF travels through the subarachnoid space and ventricular system of the brain and has the function of cushioning the delicate CNS structures. This clear, colorless liquid serves not only as a shock absorber, cushioning the impact of trauma, but also facilitates the removal of metabolic products of metabolism from the brain. CSF also assists with maintaining intracranial pressure and provides buoyancy, so the net weight of the brain is reduced and it does not sag under its own weight. This dynamic fluid space is essential in facilitating homeostasis of the CNS, so that the unbroken flow of neural impulses is not interrupted and general neurological well-being is preserved. The relationship between meninges and cerebrospinal fluid is particularly vital in neurological disease. Recent studies have demonstrated the formation of tertiary lymphoid organs (TLOs) in the meninges of patients with multiple sclerosis (MS) (Mitsdoerffer et al., 2016). These pathological organs promote disease development by enabling autoreactive cell function, emphasizing the meningeal contribution to immune function. Furthermore, the historical analysis of the blood-brain and blood-CSF barriers demonstrates how modern neuroscience has evolved to comprehend such protective coverings (Butt et al., 2011). As research continues to reveal the complexity of the meninges and CSF, the implications for the treatment of neurological diseases become increasingly evident, necessitating further investigation of their roles in health and disease (Figure 6.6).

Test Your Knowledge

1. How is the brain structurally divided, and what are the main functions of the cerebrum, cerebellum, and brainstem?
2. What is the role of the spinal cord in CNS function, and how is it anatomically organized?

6.2. Functions of the Central Nervous System (CNS)

Learning Outcome

1. Explain the processing of sensory information;
2. Explain the coordination of motor functions;
3. Explain the regulation of homeostasis.

The CNS performs a set of crucial functions critical to the entire human body's functioning. In the first place, the CNS is responsible for the processing of sensory information from the body and the environment. Through complex neural pathways, the brain interprets data from multiple sensory organs in order to allow people to respond suitably to stimulation. For instance, visual data is interpreted in the occipital lobe, and auditory signals are interpreted in the temporal lobe. This not only makes perception easier but also gives information about motor functions, a sign of the interrelation between sensation and action. Understanding human processes serves as the basis for broader human considerations of the CNS contributions to behavior and control of physiology, emphasizing its role as the body's command center of various body functions. In addition to processing sensory data, the CNS plays a critical role in maintaining homeostasis in the body. Homeostasis is the state when the body is in equilibrium required to maintain a state of optimal physiological regulation. Hypothalamus, a CNS structure, is particularly important since it regulates important functions of the body , such as temperature, hunger, and hydration levels. Through information collection and processing from within, the CNS is able to generate appropriate responses, e.g., triggering thirst when dehydrated or regulating the body temperature based on environmental changes. Further, the CNS is also responsible for controlling the autonomic nervous system, which governs involuntary body functions like heart rate and digestion. The delicate balance so obtained by the CNS is vital for human health, as interference leads to a host of metabolic and cardiovascular diseases, showing the importance of its regulatory mechanism (Carnevale et al., 2017). Apart from its regulatory role, CNS also facilitates higher cognitive processes like learning, memory, and decision-making. The intricate neural network in the brain facilitates cognitive flexibility that allows a person to modify behavior based on experience. Neuroplasticity, or the capacity of the brains to reorganize itself through the creation of new neural connections, is the foundation of learning and memory. As individuals acquire new information or learn skills, the CNS organizes brain regions that process this information to influence future decision-making and behavior. Furthermore, cognitive processes are very intermixed with emotional processing because regions like the limbic system in association with the prefrontal cortex organize responses to situations. Thus, the CNS is not merely a reflexive system; it performs a pivotal role in higher-order functions that make up human experience and behavior, indicating its wide reach in the field of mental and emotional well-being (Buchner & Heisenberg, 2009) (Figure 6.7).

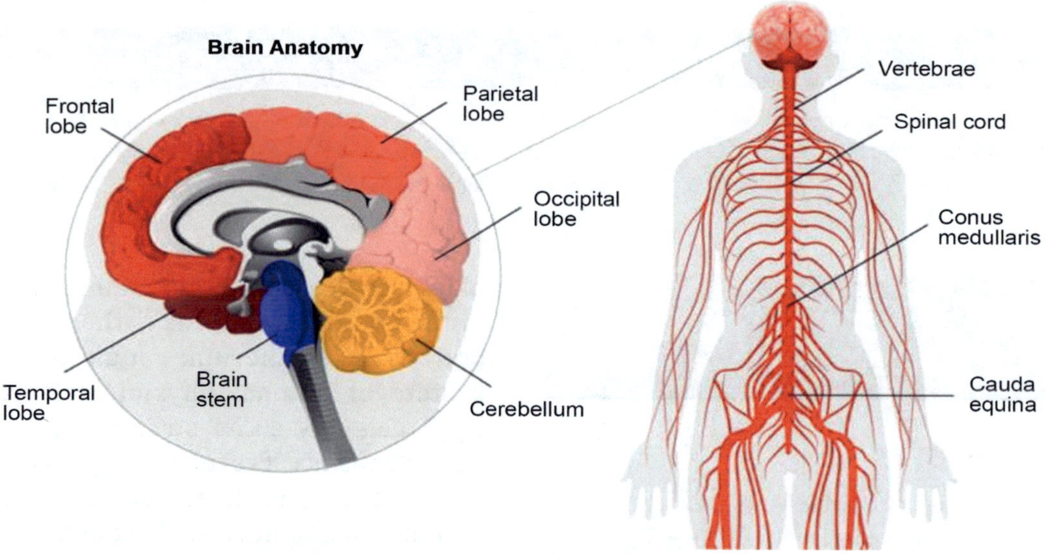

Figure 6.7. Functions of the central nervous system (CNS).

Source: https://dims.healthgrades.com/dims3/MMH/787163f/2147483647/strip/true/crop/1024x575+0+0/resize/800x449!/quality/75/?url=https%3A%2F%2Fucmscdn.healthgrades.com%2Ff3%2F83%2F54b0ad24a071b5a98d7d180c1938%2F178649-hg-central-nervous-system-body-1296x728-1-1-1024x575.jpg.

6.2.1. Processing Sensory Information

Sensory processing of information is a critical CNS function which enables the organism to act efficiently in the environment. Sensory receptors in the external and internal world detect the stimulus and convey it as neural information to various regions of the brain for processing. This intricate process requires precise coordination of neurons, particularly within the dorsal hindbrain and spinal cord, which are in charge of receiving and transmitting sensory input. The way these regions deal with the sensory perception ultimately accounts for the intricacies involved with sensory-motor output, which is crucial to maintain homeostasis and respond to the environment. The integration of different neural pathways ensures that information from the senses is processed efficiently as well as coupled with motor command for a proper response. The central nervous system also relies on a high-level network of neuronal circuits for adaptive processing of sensory information. When there is sensory conflict, as occurs for instance during balance and motion activities, the CNS must employ an internal model referenced control strategy. This framework allows body spatial orientation to be estimated and active body motion to be controlled. There have been experiments that have provided a nonlinear conflict averaging model for considering the way in which the sensory signals, particularly those that are implicated in motion sickness, are converted and blended to yield appropriate behavioral outputs. The dynamic mechanism underlying them highlights the role of sensory conflict signals in movement control and sensory-motor adaptation in allowing free motion response to meet requirements of the environment. This adaptability is vital to existence and general well-being since it enables organisms to apply themselves to complex functions in precision. Also, the diverse mechanisms controlling sensory processing reflect a multistranded developmental history between populations of neurons in the CNS. Experiments have confirmed that the mechanisms generating neuronal diversity in the dorsal spinal cord and hindbrain exhibit shared patterns of specification and innervation.

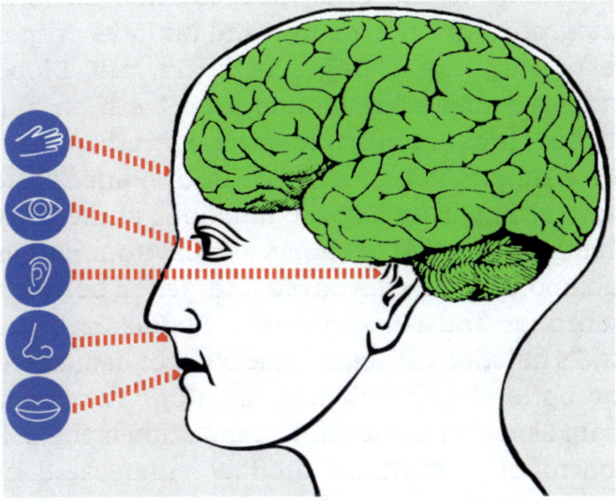

Figure 6.8. Processing sensory information.

Source: https://d3gms0sggi16d7.cloudfront.net/sas/55629/issue-group-I18n/9I5Rzb.png.

Knowledge of these developmental processes sheds light on the encoding processes for sensory modalities , such as mechanosensation and pain under both health and neuropathy. By examining the cellular and molecular mechanisms that control these processes, scientists anticipate gaining insights into the complexity of sensory perception and its impact on human health. These research studies not only further our understanding of rudimentary physiological function but also pave the way for the development of therapeutic approaches in the treatment of sensory disorders, and it therefore becomes necessary to learn more about the processing of sensory information and its application in medical and clinical settings (Birchmeier et al., 2017) (Figure 6.8).

6.2.2. Coordination of Motor Functions

Coordination of motor function in the CNS plays the fundamental role in facilitating complex bodily movements, emphasizing the intricate co-function of various neural structures. The brain, more so the motor cortex, coordinates planning, control, and execution of voluntary movement by issuing commands to the spinal cord and peripheral nervous system. This sensory feedback relay is significant since it serves in the modulation of motor commands accordingly. In addition, the cerebellum and the basal ganglia are significant in coordinating motor function through fine-tuning and modulating movements in a manner that allows precision and stability to be achieved. Pathologies in these pathways may lead to movement disorders, and this highlights the importance of functional motor coordination in the maintenance of overall functional capacity. Parkinsons disease (PD) is a paradigmatic illustration of the consequences of impaired motor function coordination, primarily due to the degeneration of dopamine-secreting neurons of the midbrain. The neurodegenerative disorder specifically targets the basal ganglia, producing insufficient motor control, tremor, rigidity, and bradykinesia. The consequences of such incapacitations serve to underscore the importance of the role played by dopamine in facilitating smooth and coordinated motor function. Physicians typically find it difficult to adequately assess the motor capabilities of PD patients; thus, techniques , such as the development of mobile applications for dynamic testing are being utilized. The applications assist in the quantitative assessment of motor function in terms of parameters , such as spiral deviation and pen pressure, which can offer useful information regarding the severity of the disease and allow for informed treatment decisions. As such, the coordination of motor functions can become something important to know not just in order to help relieve PD but also in order to measure more general motor-related disorders.

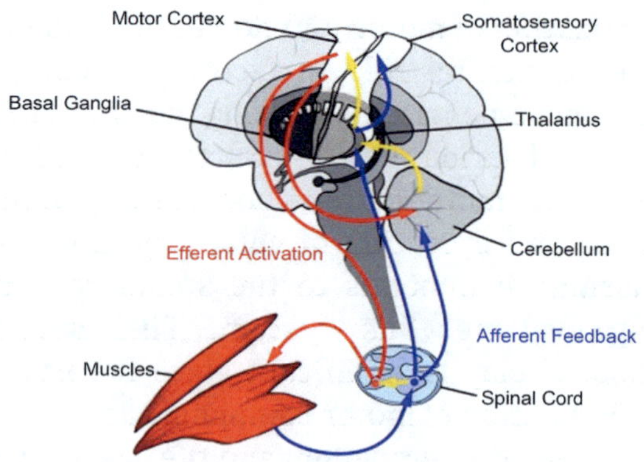

Figure 6.9. Motor coordination.

Source: https://ars.els-cdn.com/content/image/1-s2.0-S1571064523000775-gr001.jpg.

Recent studies have shown that environmental toxins, like formaldehyde, likewise have a decisive influence on the functioning condition of the CNS, especially in children. Studies have shown that changes in formaldehyde excretion were linked to cognitive and sensorimotor performance, the interaction between environmental exposure and motor coordination. The children who had greater exposure to formaldehyde exhibited lower sensorimotor coordination and CNS function. The study emphasizes the importance of environmental protection in healthy neurodevelopment. It suggests that extrinsic influences could disrupt not just the motor activities dependent on the CNS but also cognitive processes to perform activities of daily life and to learn. Thus, both biological and environmental factors affecting the CNS need to be addressed through an integrative approach for developing the best motor coordination in various populations (Figure 6.9).

6.2.3. Regulation of Homeostasis

CNS is the central part of homeostatic control, governing a number of important physiological functions necessary for survival. Coordination of the sensory inputs and motor outputs is the most significant manner in which CNS fulfills its regulatory functions. Sensory receptors found throughout the body continuously supply information about internal and external conditions to the CNS. As a counter, the CNS integrates this information and initiates proper responses, e.g., changes in heart rate, blood pressure, and body temperature, with an aim to develop equilibrium. The hypothalamus, for example, is a central organ of homeostatic control, ensuring that the functions of the body change as a result of changes in environment or metabolism. This advanced interaction between neuronal and sensory input emphasizes the CNS's function in securing the balance demanded for optimal physiological function. The other main aspect of homeostatic regulation is the CSF control of interstitial fluid flow within the CNS. CSF provides essential mechanical support as well as the transport of nutrients while buoying up the brain and spinal cord. According to more recent studies, the relationships between CSF pressure and intraocular pressure are essential for homeostatic stability of the optic nerve and emphasize the role of CSF in proper neural health (Fern Gández et al., 2021). The loss of dynamics of cerebrospinal fluid can lead to pathological changes, such as glaucomatous injury, so it is crucial that homeostatic control mechanisms be sustained. This activity illustrates how effective control of body fluids is exerted by the CNS's regulation of CSF to maintain not only structural integrity but also functional homeostasis in the central nervous system. The autonomic nervous system (ANS), a significant branch of the CNS, assists in the regulation of homeostasis too through regulation of involuntary physiological functions. The interaction between the sympathetic and parasympathetic outflows demonstrates how the ANS coordinates responses to metabolic demand and energy homeostasis. Overfeeding has been shown to disrupt this balance by enhancing sympathetic tone and parasympathetic activity with consequences for energy substrate homeostasis (Prins et al., 1996). This shift is an expression of the intricate feed-forward loops between sensory afferents and effector pathways in the CNS, affecting metabolic regulation overall. By understanding the mechanisms by which the autonomic nervous system interacts with changes in nutritional status, we are coming to realize its contribution toward maintaining homeostatic balance and the potential effects of dysregulation in illnesses , such as obesity and metabolic disease (Figure 6.10).

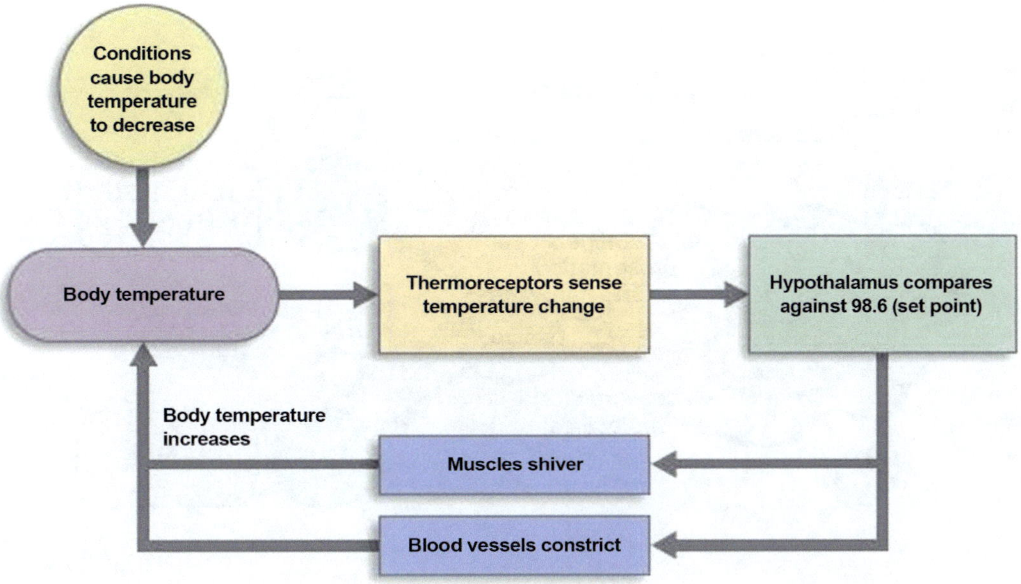

Figure 6.10. Homeostatic regulation across organ systems.

Source: https://s3-us-west-2.amazonaws.com/courses-images-archive-read-only/wp-content/uploads/sites/167/2014/11/20062419/feedback_lowtemp.jpg.

Test Your Knowledge

1. What is the main function of the central nervous system?
2. What part of the CNS controls voluntary muscle movements?

6.3. Neurons and Neurotransmission

Learning Outcome

1. Explain the structure and neurons and types of
2. Define the process of neurotransmission
3. Explain how neurotransmitters play a role in communication

The intricate interaction between neurons and neurotransmission is the main foundation of the central nervous system's operation. Neurons, the brain and spinal cord building block cells, communicate information through electrical signals and chemical messengers. The process begins with the generation of action potentials, which extend along the axon to synaptic terminals. Upon reaching these terminals, neurotransmitters are released into the synaptic cleft. These chemical messengers bind to certain receptor sites on adjacent neurons, enabling information to be passed. This quick and efficient process reinstates the role of neurons in regulating various body processes, from reflexes to higher mental functions.

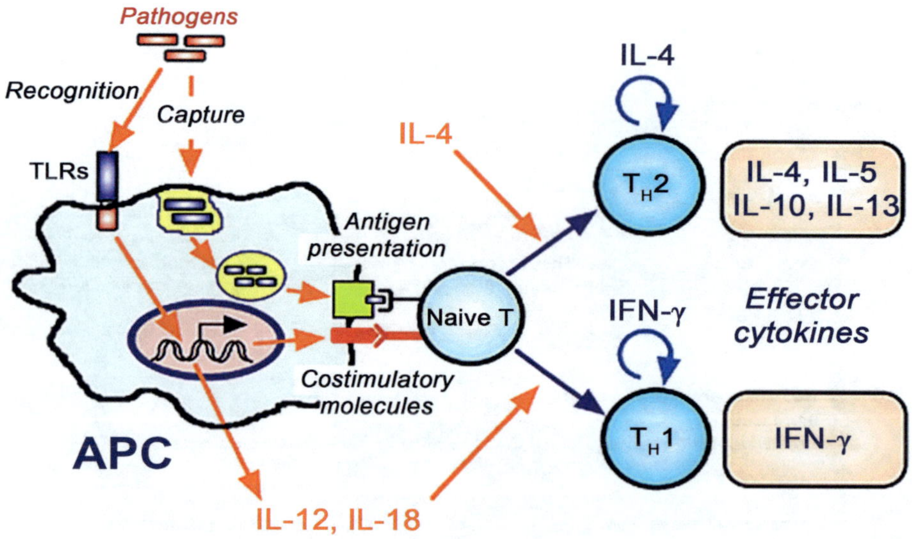

Figure 6.11. Toll-like receptors.

Source: https://media.springernature.com/full/springer-static/image/art%3A10.1038%2F90609/MediaObjects/41590_2001_Article_BFni0801_675_Fig1_HTML.gif.

It is therefore essential to understand the dynamics of neurotransmission if one is to appreciate how the central nervous system acquires sensory input and integrates behavioral output. The role of neurotransmitters is more than just the process of communication among neurons; they play significant roles in the regulation of neuronal activity and homeostasis. Different neurotransmitters, such as dopamine, serotonin, and acetylcholine, are associated with different functions of the body. For instance, dopamine is important in mood, reward, and motor control; its impairment is associated with conditions , such as Parkinsons disease and schizophrenia. Similar to dopamine, serotonin also affects mood, sleep, and appetite, highlighting the delicate balance required for efficient neurotransmission. Abnormalities in neurotransmitter signaling can lead to neurotoxicity, such as with some chemicals disrupting neural function and possibly leading to enduring deficits. Neurotransmitter-neural health interaction is therefore a primary area of research in neuroscience because it sheds light on the etiologies of various neurodegenerative and psychiatric disorders (Brust et al., 2014). Recent studies have illuminated the complexities of neurotransmitter mechanisms, with a special focus on inflammation. Toll-like receptors (TLRs), and TLR4 in particular, have been implicated in influencing neuronal survival and neurotransmission in the enteric nervous system (ENS). TLR4 deficiency has been associated with massive alterations in the ENS, triggering gliosis and reducing the population of essential $nNOS^+$ neurons. This change not only disrupts cholinergic excitatory neurotransmission but also enhances inhibitory neurotransmission, leading to altered gastrointestinal motility. These findings underscore the intricate relationship between immune signaling and neurotransmission and suggest that modulation of neurotransmitter function can be affected by systemic states of inflammation. Therefore, understanding how TLR4 and other signaling pathways speak with neurons provides more information about gastrointestinal diseases and their neural etiology (Giulivi et al., 2017) (Figure 6.11).

6.3.1. Structure and Types of Neurons

The CNS is essentially composed of neurons, which may be classified according to structure and function. Neurons are generally divided into three main categories: sensory neurons, motor neurons, and interneurons. Sensory neurons, which are located in the peripheral nervous system, transmit impulses from sensory receptors to the CNS so that stimuli , such as light, sound, and touch can be sensed. Motor neurons, which transmit impulses from the CNS to glands and muscles, enable movement and reflexes. Interneurons function as middlemen in the CNS, processing information and facilitating higher-order cognitive processes and complex reflexes. This three-way structure of neurons points to their unique roles of maintaining the sophisticated networks of communication that constitute the CNS and eventually influencing behavior and bodily responses. Neurons are extremely heterogeneous in their forms, being tailored to carry out their unique roles. Usually, each neuron consists of three significant parts: the soma or cell body, dendrites, and an axon. The soma houses the nucleus and organelles to maintain the cell and permit metabolic functions to occur. The dendrites branch off from the soma and possess numerous synaptic relations that receive signals from other neurons. By this branching, there is extensive connectivity and integration of signals. The axon, however, is the output channel, carrying electrical impulses out from the soma to the target cells. Axon length and the sheaths of myelination can significantly vary among types, influencing the conduction speed of the signals. The structural difference among types of neurons makes it easier for them to perform their respective functions in the CNS. A knowledge of the distribution of neuron types across the CNS also serves to heighten our understanding of their function. Recent research has highlighted a really diverse range of neuronal morphology across various regions of the brain, including the olfactory bulbs, the cerebral cortex, and the cerebellum. For example, studies have shown that these areas are populated by neurons that express specific markers, and these can shed light on their functional aspects. Of particular interest is the occurrence of some glycosphingolipids, such as Gb3, in numerous types of neurons in the CNS, indicative of the complex interaction between molecular signals and neuronal processes

(Abbott et al., 2010). This complexity in neuronal structure and markers depicts the specialized functions that have been assigned to neurons in various parts of the CNS, yielding overall neural network function and behavior (Buchner & Heisenberg, 2009). This information is valuable in the construction of our understanding of the CNS and its associated disorders (Figure 6.12).

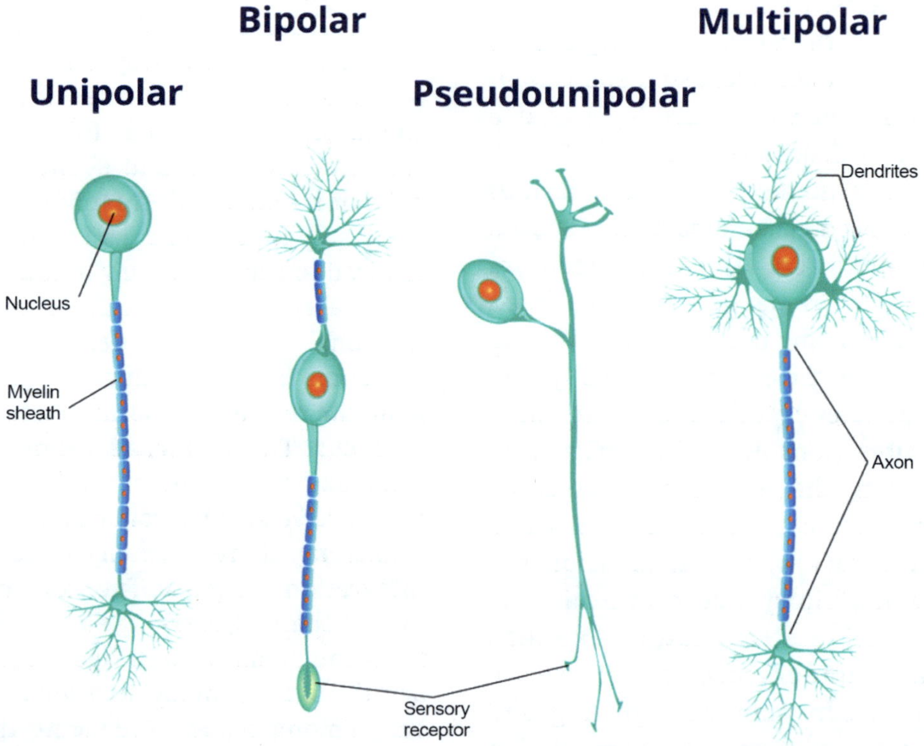

Figure 6.12. The neuron: external structure and classification.

Source: https://interactivebiology.com/wp-content/uploads/2021/09/Types-of-Neurons.png.

6.3.2. Mechanism of Neurotransmission

The intricate mechanism of neurotransmission is at the center of the physiology of the CNS. Neurotransmission is, in essence, a process by which signal molecules, known as neurotransmitters, are released from neurons to communicate with other neurons and target cells. As the action potential travels down a neuron, it triggers the opening of voltage-gated calcium channels at the axon terminal. The influx of calcium ions leads to the fusion of synaptic vesicles containing neurotransmitters with the presynaptic membrane, releasing them into the synaptic cleft. This synaptic transmission is not one-way; it activates complex cascades of signals in the postsynaptic neuron, which activate a chain of receptors and second-messenger systems that ultimately control or influence neuronal excitability and synaptic plasticity. Neurotransmission mechanisms are thus important to as basic processes as reflexes and as complex processes as learning and memory in the CNS. The chemical composition of the neurotransmitters involved in signaling in the CNS is intricate and depends upon their functions and interactions. The traditional neurotransmitters acetylcholine, dopamine, and glutamate coexist with purinergic neurotransmitter molecules , such as adenosine triphosphate (ATP). The concept of purinergic cotransmission has also been identified, highlighting the complexity of neurotransmission. Released together with other neurotransmitters, ATP is a cotransmitter in various neural circuits, enhancing synaptic modulation. Such co-release can change the efficacy of neurotransmission depending on whether the state of the nervous system is physiological or pathological, as different concentrations or ratios of neurotransmitters can lead to alterations in synaptic responses. As discussed, ATP is released with noradrenaline or glutamate, and the versatile role for short- and long-term signaling indicates the significance of understanding how such interactions impact neuronal communication (Burnstock, 2025). The current fascination with purinergic mechanisms of neurotransmission heralds a paradigm shift in the understanding of how neurons talk to each other and how this affects CNS disorders. Science has revealed that ATP is not only a neurotransmitter but also an autonomic modulator within the peripheral and central nervous systems, unveiling its multifaceted role throughout pathologies. For instance, developmental alterations in purinergic signaling pathways have been associated with states of neurodegeneration and neuropathic pain. The cotransmission dynamics in such cases may be the cause of maladaptive neural responses. In addition, coupling of neurons and glial cells is now increasingly viewed as having a central role in modulating the effects mediated by ATP in the CNS and influencing conditions like trauma and ischemia. This reaffirms the importance of understanding mechanisms of purinergic neurotransmission and their implications in brain health and disease (Burnstock, 2009) (Figure 6.13).

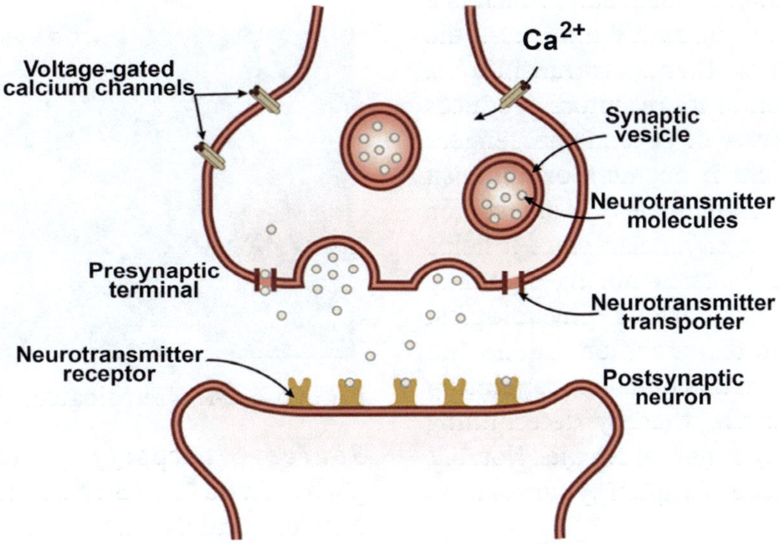

Figure 6.13. Neurotransmission.

Source: https://www.genetex.com/upload/media/research/neuro/Neurotransmission/Neurotransmission_header.jpg.

6.3.3. Role of Neurotransmitters in Communication

The intricate interconnectivity of neurotransmitter communication is the core of CNS function. Neurotransmitters are biochemic molecules that are charged with the transmission of signals between neurons such that the myriad functions of the CNS are carried out in a seamless manner. Among these molecules, nitric oxide (NO) has been a fascinating exception that has a very significant function in evolution. NO is a strange neurotransmitter that contributes to different neural activities by controlling synaptic efficacy and neuronal excitability. Its mode of action is particularly impressive; NO acts through receptor proteins to signal a cascade of cellular processes by way of cGMP generation, which magnifies even weak signals. Such flexibility not only denotes its evolutionary success but also underscores its vital contribution to neural communication and plasticity in facilitating learning and memory mechanisms in the brain, essential to adaptive behavior in response to external stimuli (Garthwaite, 2008). Another significant neurotransmitter in synaptic communication is adenosine, which is a neuromodulator that significantly influences the sensitivity of neurons to other neurotransmitters. Adenosine stimulation of its receptors produces alterations in the levels of second messengers within neurons that either augment or diminish excitatory responses based on the type of receptor. This modulatory role is significant since it helps the CNS obtain homeostasis during signaling processes, reacting to various physiological and pathological states. Further, adenosine affects synaptic transmission by regulating neurotransmitter release, thereby determining the general excitability of neural circuits. Notably, adenosine activity can be disrupted by substances , such as alcohol, which compromises the operation of adenosine-transporting nucleoside transporters, illustrating the delicate relationship between neurotransmitter systems and peripheral factors (Diamond et al., 1997). Awareness of the role of neurotransmitters in central nervous system communication highlights the complexity of neural interaction and dependence on chemical communication. Both nitric oxide and adenosine demonstrate distinct but complementary ways by which neurotransmitters may modulate not only synaptic transmission but also more spread-out neural circuits. While nitric oxide acts rapidly to control synaptic efficacy, for instance, adenosines modulatory effect assists to refine neuronal excitability and plasticity. The convergence of these signaling pathways enables the CNS to adapt to challenges, learn, and store memory, hence improving the organisms ability to navigate its environment effectively. Continued research on these neurotransmitter systems has the potential to elucidate more about the fundamental processes that regulate neural function and what they imply for the comprehension of neurological disorders (Figure 6.14).

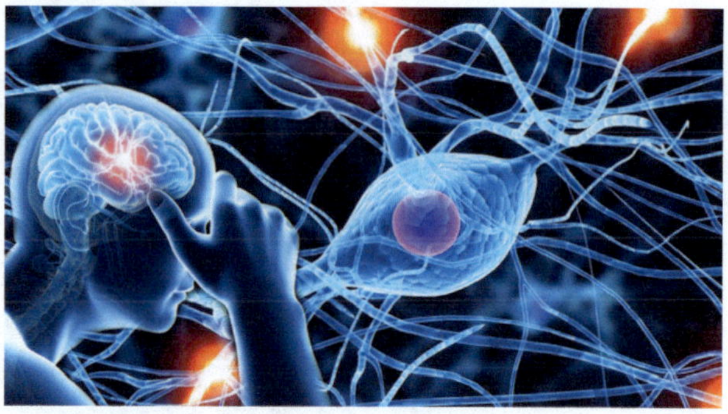

Figure 6.14. Neurological disorders.

Source: https://dphhs.mt.gov/assets/publichealth/SchoolHealth/Photos/Neurologicaldisordersbrain.jpg.

Test Your Knowledge

1. What receives incoming signals?
2. What is a synapse?

6.4. Central Nervous System (CNS) Disorders

Learning Outcome

1. Enumerate the common disorders: Alzheimer's, Parkinson's, and multiple sclerosis
2. Explain the etiology and risk factors of CNS disorders
3. Enumerate the impact of CNS disorders on daily life

Having just a detailed background of the etiology and effects on neurological functions is enough for someone to comprehend CNS disorders. Alzheimer's disease, multiple sclerosis, and Parkinson's disease are among the most prevalent diseases, highlighting the imperative for therapeutic options immediately. The rising tide of cognitive impairment with age means that risk factors associated with these diseases are critical to the understanding of their onset. More specifically, the novel concept of the microbiota-gut-brain axis has emerged as a consideration for cognitive health as well as for neurodegenerative disease. With the aging of the world population, the resultant rise in cognitive impairment highlights the need to explore these interconnected pathways to develop preventive interventions and new treatments. The understanding of these risk factors is key in addressing disorders pervasive impact on individuals and society as a whole. Gut microbiota and their metabolites have also attracted interest based on recent evidence, placing focus on a different perspective of how they affect the development and progression of CNS disorders.

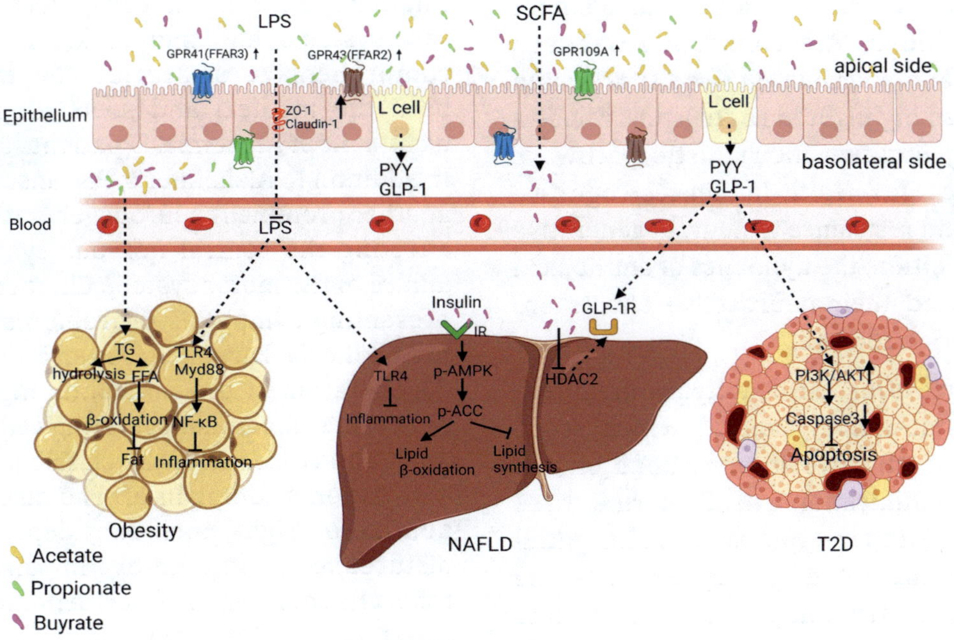

Figure 6.15. Short-chain fatty acids (SCFAs) in diseases.

Source: https://media.springernature.com/lw1200/springer-static/image/art%3A10.1186%2Fs12964-023-01219-9/MediaObjects/12964_2023_1219_Fig4_HTML.png.

Scientists have developed significant alterations in short-chain fatty acids (SCFAs) in patients with conditions like autism spectrum disorder, multiple sclerosis, and Parkinson's disease. Their metabolites might interact with the central nervous system through various pathways, emphasizing their possible role in modulating neurological health.

In particular, dysregulation of this microbiome and the resultant secondary alterations in microbial production of metabolites can promote neuroinflammation and cognitive dysfunction. Analysis of these bacterial metabolites is useful in assessing how they contribute to brain disease, because putative therapeutic interventions might leverage such findings to reverse the increasing incidence of CNS disorders and their effects on quality of life.

The significance of the microbiota-gut-brain axis holds promise for novel diagnostic and therapeutic modalities in the management of CNS conditions. The connection between neurohealth and microbial-derived short-chain fatty acids was highlighted in stringent reviews as providing putative mechanistic pathways through which gut health influences cognitive functioning and resistance to neurodegenerative disease. In addition, the dynamics of amino acid metabolites and their neuroactive effects are related to CNS disorders.

An example is histone deacetylase inhibition and immunomodulatory effect, which could yield leads for effective interventions on the gut-brain communication axis. Exploring these associations at deeper levels can yield insightful information that not only may enhance the effectiveness of treatment but also initiate preventative action in a population grappling with increasing neurological disorders in an ageing population (Tran & Mohajeri, 2021; Connell et al., 2022) (Figure 6.15).

6.4.1. Common Disorders: Alzheimer's, Parkinson's, And Multiple Sclerosis

The CNS is severely impacted by a number of neurodegenerative diseases, including Alzheimer's disease, Parkinson's disease, and multiple sclerosis. Alzheimer's disease is the most common form of dementia, and it is the gradual loss of cognitive and memory function that results from the accumulation of amyloid plaques and tau tangles in the brain. Alzheimer's primarily influences older individuals and leads to severe impairment of daily functioning, causing increasing demands for care. There is stress on the necessity of unraveling the mechanisms underlying Alzheimer's, since the pursuit of effective treatments continues to challenge medical science. The multi-dimensional character of this condition affects not only individuals afflicted directly by it but also places tremendous emotional and financial burden on caregivers and health care systems, and thus makes it obvious that comprehensive strategies for treatment of both the medical and social implications of treatment of Alzheimer's patients are called for. In addition to Alzheimer's, Parkinson's disease is another prominent neurodegenerative condition affecting the central nervous system through failure of the motor system. Characterized by its presenting symptoms of tremor, stiffness, and bradykinesia, Parkinson's is an aftermath of the degeneration of the substantia nigra region of the brain's dopamine-secreting cells. Dopamine depletion comes with the classic motor deficits that patients complain of. The disease also has non-motor signs, including depression, sleep disturbances, and cognitive impairment, which reflect its comprehensive presentation. Symptom relief is the treatment goal, usually using pharmacological interventions in the guise of dopamine replacement therapies. Nonetheless, more recent studies have begun exploring the role of physical activity as an adjunct therapy, with some of them showing exercise to be able to reduce some of Parkinson's motor and cognitive impairments by offering improved neuroprotection and recovery processes in the central nervous system (Arbat-Plana et al., 2017). MS offers yet another perspective for understanding the complexity of central nervous system disorders. This autoimmune disorder is triggered by demyelination of the nerve cells and leads to an autoimmune disorder with an enormous array of neurological disturbances ranging from physical disability to mental dysfunctions. The pathogenesis of MS is a complex interplay of environmental and hereditary factors that together are the cause for the body's own immune system attacking its own myelin sheath. As the disease progresses, patients experience phases of deterioration of neurological symptoms, indicating the unpredictable nature of MS. Current therapies aim at the modulation of immune response and symptom management without producing a cure. Preeminent, new research suggests the potential added value of exercise not only as management of MS symptoms but also to enhance the overall life quality of MS patients, suggesting a protective overlap between lifestyle intervention and neuroprotection in central nervous system illnesses (Arbat-Plana et al., 2017) (Figure 6.16).

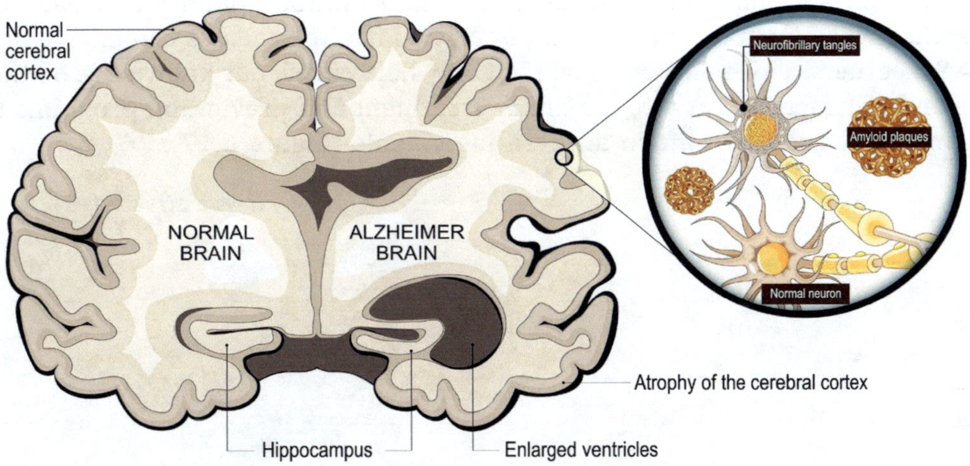

Figure 6.16. Alzheimer's disease.

Source: https://www.news-medical.net/images/Article_Images/ImageForArticle_25209_17252931864138889.jpg.

6.4.2. Causes and Risk Factors of Central Nervous System (CNS) Disorders

The cause of CNS conditions is multifactorial because it is an interaction of complex genetic, environmental, and lifestyle factors. Genetic predispositions would potentially play a crucial role in the risk of individuals having CNS conditions, with certain genes being associated with certain conditions , such as Parkinson's disease and multiple sclerosis. Environmental factors like toxins and pathogen exposure could also trigger or exacerbate these conditions. For example, it has been shown through studies that stressful life events tend to favor the emergence of neurodegenerative diseases, focusing on the contribution of psychosocial stressors to brain health. Estrine & DeLisle (2006) emphasize the necessity of understanding the comprehensive interplay between these stressors and biological processes. Also, lifestyle habits, including physical activity and diet, have been found to affect CNS health, and in turn, the risk of developing related disorders throughout one's lifetime. Besides genetic and environmental factors, socioeconomic status plays a major role in the risk involved with CNS disorders. Studies have shown that those belonging to lower socio-economic strata tend to experience barriers in accessing health care services, and hence may experience delayed diagnosis and treatment. Delayed diagnosis and treatment may result in poorer outcomes and higher rates of disorders because initial symptoms are not properly managed. For instance, one celiac disease study revealed that socio-economic determinants can also act as effect modifiers when managing chronic diseases, with lower education groups having the potential to utilize healthcare resources less efficiently. Canova et al (2016) demonstrate the relationship between economic welfare, level of education, and health outcomes and how crucial that public health interventions for CNS disorders must deal with these inequalities. The combined impact of these factors emphasizes the significance of early intervention as well as preventive services in neutralizing the threat presented by CNS disorders. Public health programs based on educational outreach can promote awareness of the early warning signs of CNS disorders, thus facilitating early intervention. Stress reduction interventions and promoting healthy lifestyle practices can also contribute to both physical and mental well-being. Thus, multidisciplinary approaches combining genetic research, environmental surveys, and population health schemes can enable an integrative analysis of CNS disorders. These strategies will not only help enrich our knowledge on the etiological determinants and risk factors, but also maximize treatment and prevention programs towards the final goal of improved quality of life in affected individuals (Figure 6.17).

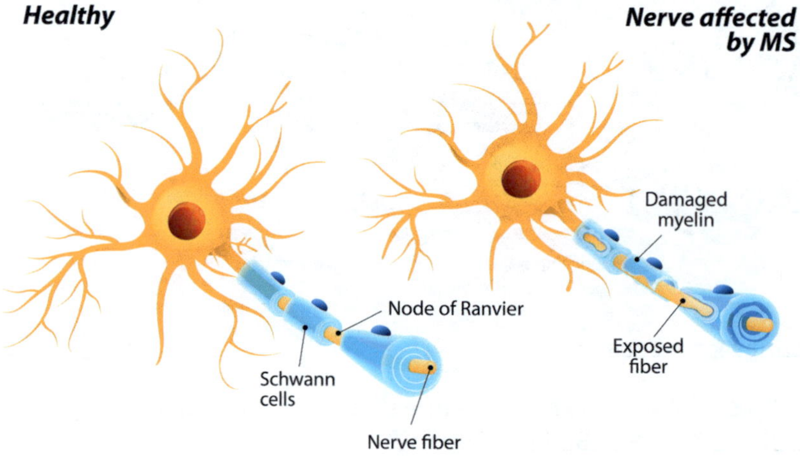

Figure 6.17. Multiple sclerosis.

Source: https://s3.amazonaws.com/content.stockpr.com/zyversa/files/pages/pipeline/about-multiple-sclerosis/MultipleSclerosis.jpg.

6.4.3. Impact of Central Nervous System (CNS) Disorders on Daily Life

The effect of CNS disorders on daily life is extensive and far-reaching, touching people on an individual and societal level. MS is a disorder that illustrates the complexity of problems people experience as they cope with their daily activities and social interactions. Typical impairments cited are mobility problems, cognitive impairment, and pain, which extensively interfere with individual and work functions. MS patients typically develop limitations in self-care, domestic activities, and activities in the community that increasingly impair their quality of life. The incapacities of these diseases could induce increased caregiver dependency, interfering with interpersonal relationships and placing a psychological burden on patients as well as support systems. These problems require a multi-level comprehension of how CNS diseases in various forms influence daily functioning and, consequently, introduce a high level of support. Moreover, psychosocial factors to a large extent define the severity of the influence CNS diseases exert on daily life. Since the patient is struggling with symptoms such as fatigue, depression, and cognitive impairment, his overall well-being can become seriously compromised. This psychological load not only impacts their ability to function in everyday life but also their resilience. Individuals may struggle to maintain employment, leading to financial insecurity, which in turn exacerbates stress and isolation. Moreover, the stigma related to neurological conditions may deter individuals from seeking social support, leading to a cycle of isolation and mental load. The intricacy of addressing these psychosocial factors underscores the necessity for integrative healthcare interventions that take into consideration physical and psychological needs in order to promote an overall better support system for affected groups. Finally, not only do CNS disorders have individual implications, but they also on family structures and society at large. Caregivers are more likely to experience greater burdens and emotional stress in managing their ill family members with activities of daily living, healthcare management, and emotional support. This added expense can cause care burnout and frustration, straining familial relationships. Furthermore, the economic effects of CNS disorders are significant as victims require special care or modifications to their living arrangements, which incur an additional economic cost on medical systems and families. Accepting the cascading impact of CNS disorders on family members and society generally is the key to an inclusive consideration of the resources and policy changes needed to treat impacted parties. Healthcare systems can become more closely matched to the needs of families facing the challenges of CNS disorders by addressing these systemic issues, and in the process, promote more general well-being for all involved.

Test Your Knowledge

1. What are the major symptoms and causes of multiple sclerosis, and how does it affect the central nervous system?
2. How does Parkinson's disease interfere with movement, and how do changes appear in the brain's dopamine system?

6.5. Diagnostic Techniques

Learning Outcome

1. Describe the imaging procedures: MRI and CT scans;
2. Define the electrophysiological procedures: EEG and EMG;
3. Describe neuropsychological assessments.

Good diagnostic procedures play a key role in understanding and treating CNS disorders. More sophisticated imaging modalities , such as magnetic resonance imaging (MRI) and computed tomography (CT) scans are typically reserved to image structural pathology. MRI, with its improved soft tissue contrast, is particularly valuable for detection of lesions, tumors, and inflammatory conditions not visible on CT scans. Moreover, functional imaging modalities like positron emission tomography (PET) and functional MRI (fMRI) allow for real-time assessment of cerebral function by the clinician, giving insight into patterns of metabolic activity and blood flow within the brain.

Functional tests of this type can detect pathological findings in relation to various CNS disorders, enhancing diagnostic specificity and informing the management plan. Aside from imaging tests, electrophysiological assessments also play an important role in the diagnosis of CNS disorders. Techniques , such as electroencephalography (EEG) provide valuable information about electrical brain activity and allow the identification of abnormal patterns of activity associated with diseases , such as epilepsy and other neurological conditions. Furthermore, evoked potentials, which are the brain's electrical reaction to sensory stimulation, can help diagnose demyelinating illness , such as multiple sclerosis by identifying conduction delay. The correlation with neurophysiological features and clinical presentations enhances the diagnostic utility of these methods, as in the case of illnesses like Stiff Person Spectrum Disorders (SPSD), where abnormal neurophysiological findings reflect the hyperexcitability of the CNS that characterizes the disease (Balint et al., 2025). These testing modalities have to be combined to achieve a comprehensive understanding of CNS pathologies. A multidisciplinary approach, combining imaging and electrophysiological methods, not only aids in the accurate diagnosis of disorders but also examines their mechanism. For instance, functional measures made by electrophysiological means can account for the relationship between symptomatic findings and neurophysiological abnormalities, eventually leading to diagnostic accuracy and therapeutic maneuvers. In SPSD, recent research focuses on the importance of explaining the autoimmune basis of the condition as well as the localization of primary abnormalities in the CNS (Balint et al., 2025). Advances in such diagnostic modalities in the future are poised to improve patient outcomes by enabling more individualized and targeted treatment approaches (Figure 6.18).

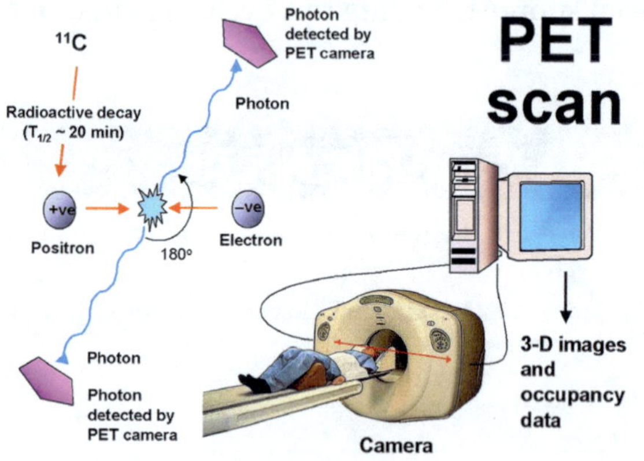

Figure 6.18. Positron emission tomography (PET).

Source: https://i.pinimg.com/originals/49/78/30/4978309a12bd0bbca3dc98326bf99a27.jpg.

6.5.1. Imaging Techniques: Magnetic Resonance Imaging (MRI) and Computed Tomography (CT) Scans

The advent of imaging technologies , such as MRI and CT scans has revolutionized the diagnosis of CNS disorders as well as treatment planning. MRI employs strong magnetic fields and radio waves to generate detailed images of the spinal cord and brain, making it an indispensable machine in diagnosing soft tissue status. In contrast to CT scans, which involve ionizing radiation, MRI gives a non-invasive way of viewing the complex CNS structures with better contrast resolution. This is particularly useful in identifying abnormalities , such as tumors, stroke, and neurological disorders, where the tissue characteristics are important for medical intervention. The accurate anatomical visualization of MRI has been shown to significantly improve patient outcomes by providing correct diagnoses and customized treatment planning. CT scans, however, use X-rays to generate cross-sectional images of the body, which are fast and effective in determining acute abnormalities like hemorrhage or fracture in cranial bones and are particularly useful in emergencies. CT scanning is generally the first test of choice for head injury, because it can rapidly identify life-threatening issues that must be managed urgently. Moreover, technical advances in CT, such as high-resolution computed tomography (HRCT), have enhanced the specificity of findings for neurological diseases. For instance, studies have established the importance of HRCT when evaluating candidates for cochlear implantation, and its role in identifying inner ear and brain pathology that can dictate surgical outcomes (Aimoni et al., 2015). Such a role emphasizes the diversified applications of CT imaging in CNS diagnosis. MRI and CT scans have roles apart from mere imaging, with prognostic features being implicated in certain neurological diseases. Studies have indicated that some neuroimaging results can reliably forecast outcomes in patients, particularly when the conditions involved are infections like tuberculous meningitis (TBM). In a study involving 100 TBM-diagnosed patients, MRI showed abnormal findings in 88.5% of them, which enabled early diagnosis and prognosis (Ahmed et al., 2016). MRI enabled the identification of important features, such as infarcts and tuberculomas, which can be employed to aid treatment planning and potential mortality risk. Thus, employing these advanced imaging modalities not only aids in the diagnosis of central nervous system disease but also assists in achieving an overall insight into disease evolution, ultimately culminating in improved quality care for patients.

6.5.2. Electrophysiological Methods: Electroencephalography (EEG) and Electromyography (EMG)

Electrophysiological methods, namely EEG and EMG, are essential means for examining the central nervous system's functioning. EEG measures electrical brain activity by monitoring the voltage changes produced by neuronal activity, which produces data regarding brain states, cognitive processes, and affective states. The non-invasive procedure provides temporal resolution so that scientists can track dynamic changes as a function of time. For instance, EEG has been central in studies of the impact of various stimuli on brain activity, such as the impact of caffeine on neuronal excitability and cognitive process, as seen in a number of electrophysiological research (Carvalho et al., 2010). EEG facilitates understanding of the causes of disorders like epilepsy, sleep, and even mood disorders by identifying patterns in brainwave activity. Contrarily, EMG is concentrated on the recording of electrical activity in skeletal muscles and is therefore key for the evaluation of motor neuron function as well as neuromuscular transmission. Through the quantification of the electrical signal generated by muscle fibers when contracting, EMG can diagnose motor neuron diseases and measure muscle recovery in rehabilitative settings. Recent studies have found the relationship between muscle function and brain activity, showing the interaction between the central nervous system and the response of the muscles. For example, changes in motor neuron excitability can influence muscle fiber resistance in tasks, further pointing to the interaction between central nervous functions and peripheral muscle function (Carvalho et al., 2010).

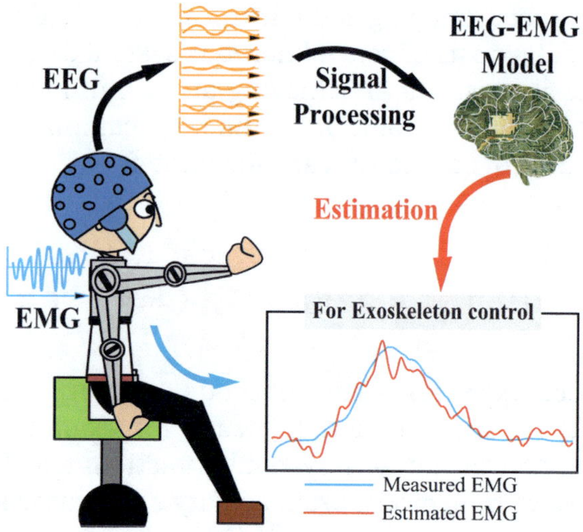

Figure 6.19. Electrophysiological methods, particularly electroencephalography (EEG) and electromyography (EMG).

Source: Liang H, Yu Y, Mochida M, Liu C, Ueda N, Li P, Zhu C. EEG-Based EMG Estimation of Shoulder Joint for the Power Augmentation System of Upper Limbs. Symmetry. 2020; 12(11):1851. https://doi.org/10.3390/sym12111851

EMG techniques have developed to include high-density surface electrodes, which yield more-resolution spatial representations of muscle activation patterns during various activities. In addition, EEG as well as EMG procedures can be combined in an attempt to investigate the nervous system response to various stimuli during different stages of sleep. As illustrated by research on nociceptive stimulation during sleep, autonomic nervous system activity elicited by EEG-identified cortical arousal speaks to complex interactions among brain function and physiological response. These interactions reiterate the significance of electrophysiological methods to clarify how cognitive and motor functioning is regulated under varying levels of consciousness. By combining both EEG and EMG, researchers have a complete picture of the coordination between neural and muscular systems, ultimately leading to the understanding of how the central nervous system coordinates behavior and physiological response in healthy and clinical populations (Figure 6.19).

6.5.3. Neuropsychological Assessments

Neuropsychological examinations are of fundamental utility in the assessment of cognitive functioning, particularly in disorders of the central nervous system. They utilize a number of standard tests to measure cognition on multiple dimensions including memory, attention, language, and executive functions. Neuropsychological examinations provide critical data on the characteristics of cognitive impairments in neurological disorders, for example, Alzheimer's disease and traumatic brain injury. Considering the brain's richness and complexity as well as its functions, these tests may need multiple methodologies to be combined so as to measure the entire range of cognitive impairments. For instance, as it has been pointed out in the development of the Neuro-Psychological Testing Ontology (NPT), test data classification and labelling offer a deeper insight and enable researchers to compare outcome across different studies, thus facilitating better diagnosis and treatment planning within clinical settings (Cox et al., 2012). Furthermore, neuropsychological tests usage is particularly relevant when handling specific populations, such as those affected by post-concussion syndrome (PCS). There is evidence that most PCS patients are capable of developing long-term cognitive and balance impairments long after the initial injury. For example, studies have been able to pinpoint that such patients have difficulty with balance control as indicated by increased medial-lateral center of pressure (COP) excursion during functional activities, which directly affects their susceptibility to future injuries. Such findings emphasize the importance of neuropsychological screening not only to detect cognitive impairments but also for the formulation of rehabilitation programs tailored to individual needs (Cinelli et al., 2017).

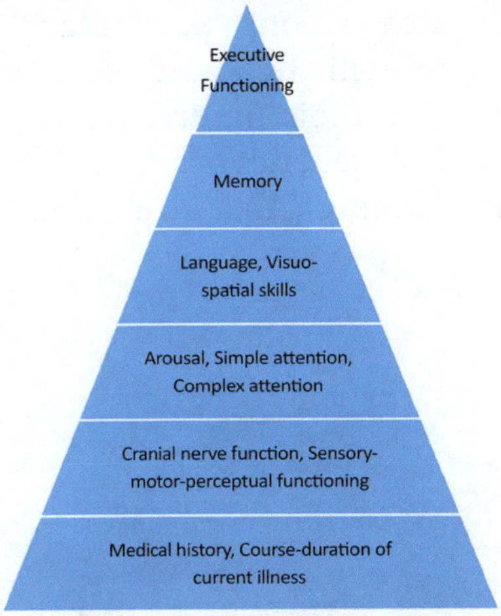

Figure 6.20. Neuropsychological assessments.

Source: https://m4.healio.com/~/media/journals/psycann/2016/2_february/10_3928_00485713_20151229_01/fig1.jpg.

Detection of specific cognitive impairments enables clinicians to formulate special interventions that enable the recovery process and enhance the quality of life of individuals with such impairments. Since the role played by neuropsychological tests is critical, their findings have a significant effect on the management of conditions that are attributed to the central nervous system.

They not only play a role in the diagnostic process but also act as crucial tools in determining disease progression and treatment efficacy. With advancements in our understanding about neurological disorders, the use of neuropsychological tests in clinical evaluation will become increasingly significant. The ongoing development of ontologies, such as the Neurological Disease Ontology (ND) and NPT, illustrates a commitment to furthering clinical models and enhancing neuropsychological test accuracy. Through the establishment of bridges between cognitive testing and a variety of neurological diseases, researchers and clinicians will be better equipped to address the complex challenges posed by central nervous system diseases (Cox et al., 2012) (Figure 6.20).

Test Your Knowledge

1. What type of scanning is commonly used to view brain structures in detail?
2. Which test measures electrical brain activity?

6.6. Treatment and Management

Learning Outcome

1. Describe the pharmacological management of the central nervous system (CNS);
2. Define the rehabilitation therapy of the central nervous system (CNS);
3. Understand the emerging research and experimental management for the central nervous system (CNS).

In the treatment and management of CNS diseases, several aspects of the approach are at times most important. Due to the variety and severity of conditions in the CNS, treatments must be personalized to handle individual patient requirements, with consideration for age, overall health, and the type of disorder. For instance, neurologic disturbances can have a strong impact on development in children, so there must be extensive familiarity with the ways treatment approaches will affect normal neural development. In the instance of vascular malformations , such as brain arteriovenous malformation, good management can decrease risks that come with these conditions. Children who have such lesions, particularly those of high-flow type, will often have severe challenges to manage, and their natural history and risk factors based on genetics are crucial for effective treatment planning (Abla et al., 2020).

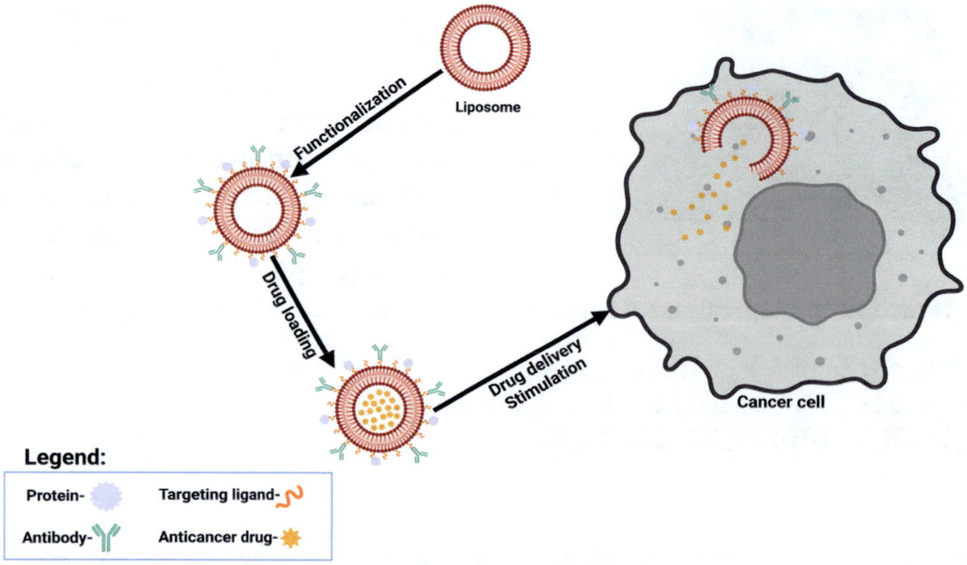

Figure 6.21. Nanoparticle strategies for treating central nervous system (CNS) disorders.

Source: Toader C, Dumitru AV, Eva L, Serban M, Covache-Busuioc R-A, Ciurea AV. Nanoparticle Strategies for Treating CNS Disorders: A Comprehensive Review of Drug Delivery and Theranostic Applications. International Journal of Molecular Sciences. 2024; 25(24):13302. https://doi.org/10.3390/ijms252413302

Treatment of metastatic conditions that involve the CNS, such as angiosarcoma, is especially demanding. These tumors are extremely aggressive by nature, and hence premature intervention is warranted. A case report of a patient with brain metastasis due to primary cardiac angiosarcoma shows the importance of surgical management, particularly gross total resection of the metastasis. The systemic disease is managed in an adjuvant role post-resection using chemotherapy, which is a tried and tested treatment modality in CNS oncology. Most importantly, vigorous follow-up is essential in such cases, due to the great likelihood of repeat metastasis and the intricacy of development of these tumors (Ducis et al., 2017). These treatments address not only the care of the initial threat posed by the tumor but also the provision of the patient with a maximum quality of life in the long term. In conclusion, use of several types of treatment, surgery, chemotherapy, and radiation, combined is paramount in the case of CNS therapy. Management guidelines should be kept flexible to the dynamic characteristics of the disease as evidenced by new research and patient response to treatment. With the advances of genomics revealing the mechanisms of CNS tumors, new targeted therapies might soon complement conventional treatments in further improving treatment outcomes. The future of CNS treatment thus does not solely lie in well-established practices but also in new strategies that utilize genetic knowledge to provide more individualized care options, ultimately improving outcomes for patients with broad-spectrum CNS disorders (Ducis et al., 2017) (Figure 6.21).

6.6.1. Pharmacological Treatments

The pharmacological context of CNS disorders treatment is broad and diversified and underscores the necessity of individualized therapy. Among them, triptans are a leading treatment for the alleviation of migraine. As a primary treatment for severe-to-moderate headache, triptans like eletriptan are selective 5-HT1B/1D receptor agonists that decrease vascular inflammation and pain through vasoconstriction of dilated cerebral vessels. Recent studies affirm the effectiveness, safety, and tolerability of eletriptan, particularly in cardiovascular-risk factor-positive patients with no history of coronary artery disease. Such specificity can substantially enhance the quality of life for migraineurs, demonstrating that drug therapy is tailor-made to patient profiles and fresh clinical data (Capi et al., 2016). Although pharmacologic treatments like triptans are essential in management of acute pain within CNS disorders, other agents are more important in chronic pain management within neurological rehabilitation models. A systematic review highlights the importance of psychological therapies in conjunction with traditional drug therapy in maximizing pain control. Interventions , such as Cognitive-Behavioral Therapy and mindfulness-based interventions have been demonstrated to reduce the level of pain in a wide range of neurological diseases, from fibromyalgia through to Central Post-Stroke pain. This comprehensive approach highlights the necessity to add psychological technique to ensure that treatment is tailored to a patient's multifaceted experience of pain. By addressing both the psychological and physiological components, such integrative care not only optimizes pain relief but also facilitates improved functional recovery (Agostini et al., 2016). Furthermore, interactions between pharmacological and psychological interventions raise significant questions regarding optimal strategies in neurorehabilitation. Pharmacological agents not only need to be selected in terms of efficacy but also based on potential interactions and patient-specific characteristics, e.g., triptans and the CYP3A4 enzyme as the site of their metabolism. Similarly, synchronizing the pharmacotherapy with the psychological therapies can optimize the beneficial effects. For instance, multidisciplinary treatment wherein such choices as eletriptan are paired with psychological interventions can not only alleviate temporary symptoms but also pay long-term dividends by improving coping abilities.

Ultimately, by establishing an interdisciplinary setting, health care professionals are better able to manage complex CNS disorders, providing integrated and effective care for their patients (Agostini et al., 2016) (Figure 6.22).

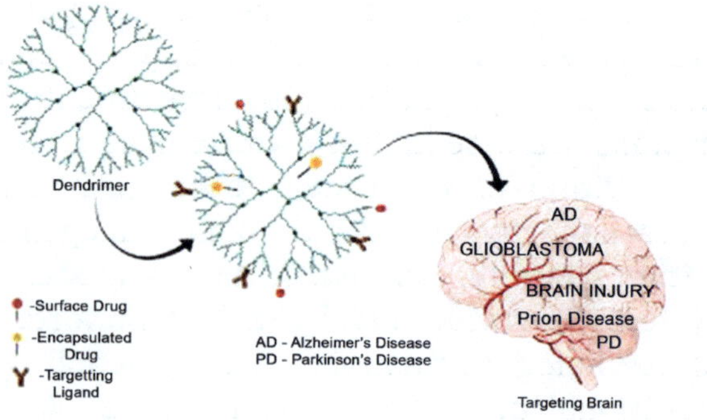

Figure 6.22. Dendrimers in the context of targeting central nervous system (CNS) disorders.

Source: https://ars.els-cdn.com/content/image/1-s2.0-S1773224722003847-ga1.jpg.

6.6.2. Rehabilitation Therapies

Rehabilitation therapies play a critical role in recovery following central nervous system trauma, such as strokes or traumatic brain injury. Rehabilitation therapies aim to restore lost motor functions, cognitive function, and quality of life through organized and evidence-based therapies. Physical therapy, occupational therapy, and speech-language pathology are all integral components that provide for the diverse needs of patients navigating the complexities of neurological impairment. Each of these modalities employs individually tailored exercises and techniques that push the limits of neuroplasticity, the brain's capacity to reorganize itself, and increase functional autonomy. Effectiveness of such therapies is normally enhanced when they are combined and carried out in a multidisciplinary manner, thus providing the patient with an intensive care that fully addresses their varied rehabilitation needs. Myofascial release therapy is an essential type of treatment in the array of rehabilitation modalities for central nervous system disorder patients. This soft tissue intervention attends to fascia, a sophisticated network of connective tissue enveloping and supporting muscles and organs. It has only been in recent years that myofascial release has been found to not only relieve pain but also promote stability and increase range of motion, which is significant in rehabilitation for patients with neurological disease recovery.

Therapists can facilitate more efficient movement patterns and functional results by attending to myofascial health. As Hetherington (2019) makes clear, greater clinical attention to the active role of fascia in the body underscores the need for continued study and incorporation of myofascial techniques into rehabilitation regimes, as these have the potential to be an important part of the patient's recovery and optimal physical functioning. Supplementing traditional rehabilitation treatments, acupuncture provides a unique and time-honored technique that is now becoming appreciated as part of modern medical practice. It is the art of penetrating needles into chosen acupoints along the body's principal meridians, which are presumed to be related to the nervous system and influence other physiological functioning. Though it has been around for centuries, its mechanisms by which acupuncture influences the body are not yet understood. However, fMRI research has indicated that acupuncture has specific effects on central nervous system processing that have profound implications for the functioning of the brain. In its application of ancient methods to current neuroanatomic understanding, as in Dorsher (2009), acupuncture is an effective adjuvant therapy for the rehabilitation of central nervous system disorders and can contribute to the therapeutic arsenal presented to clinicians and enhance patient outcomes (Figure 6.23).

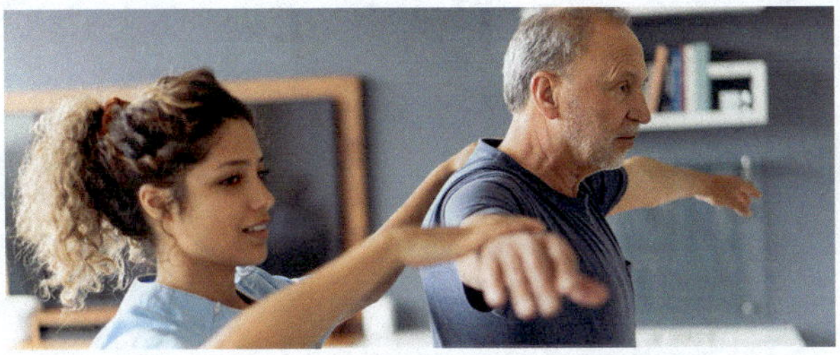

Figure 6.23. Rehabilitation therapy.

Source: https://southportseniorliving.com/wp-content/uploads/7ab0faf0-sps_aug_blog_2a.jpg.

6.6.3. Emerging Research and Experimental Treatments

Recent research on the area of the CNS is more and more attracted to new therapies that benefit from the interplay between technology and biology. A main point of such initiatives is the design of the JENTIL® Collection, which brings together the latest sensory technologies with the art of perfumery. This cross-disciplinary research aims to create a unique therapeutic setting where apparel not only serves functional purposes but also contributes to emotional welfare through odors. Through incorporating fragrances of well-being in fabrics, researchers are studying how such clothes induce positive psychological responses, thus fighting mental wellness problems associated with the stresses of living that often get fueled further by day-to-day living. The integral approach emphasizes the potential of multisensory design to transform clothing into tools for enhancing self-awareness and confidence, particularly in individuals suffering from depressive disorders, ushering in a new pattern of wearable therapy treatment (Tillotson, 2008). Another very promising avenue in CNS disorder therapy is the Klotho gene and its intriguing neuroprotective potential. Characterized as a master regulator of mitochondrial homeostasis, Klotho is a co-receptor that plays a critical role in fibrous growth factor action, perhaps in the regeneration of myelin. Dysregulation of Klotho pathways has been implicated in neuroinflammation and oxidative stress leading to various neurodegenerative diseases affecting myelin sheath integrity. The quest for therapies that enhance Klotho expression is a paradigm shift, tackling not just symptom management but also the induction of endogenous repair processes. This paradigm shift can change outcomes for patients suffering from diseases that currently have no effective treatment options available, captioning the urgency and potential that includes Klotho-related research in the CNS (Chen et al., 2020). With constant research now showing the complexities of the central nervous system, experimental treatments based on such knowledge promise much in the future of patients. Novel treatments, such as the synergy between Klotho-stimulating compounds and new sensory technologies, show the ongoing revelation in comprehending CNS disorders. Both projects demonstrate the potential to bring together diverse disciplines, ranging from fashion and art to molecular biology, to produce not just healing, but profound changes in patient quality of life. As continued understanding of how these novel treatments are functioning comes to light, the scientific community holds out promise for the potential for effective treatments of previously untreatable conditions. Hence, the use of interdisciplinarity in research methods appears essential in advancing the horizon of CNS research and increasing therapeutic advantages among patients dealing with several neurological conditions (Tillotson, 2008; Chen et al., 2020).

Test Your Knowledge

1. What are the most common types of medications used to treat seizures in epilepsy?
2. How can physical therapy benefit patients with CNS diseases , such as stroke?

SUMMARY

The investigation of the CNS reveals that its fundamental contribution is more than just coordination of bodily functions but extends to encompass crucial functions like intellectual functions, emotions, and motor functions. Knowing the complex mechanisms of the CNS has a profound impact on treatment modalities for many disorders. The statistics reflect a growing tendency toward implementation of novel therapeutic interventions , such as, for instance, respiratory muscle training (RMT) that has been proven to enhance the quality of life of patients suffering from internal and CNS disorders. Research suggests that participants in RMT not only have enhanced exercise capacity but also increased respiratory function, as measured through parameters like maximal inspiratory pressure (MIP) and forced vital capacity (FVC), thus shedding light on possible avenues for specialized rehabilitation (Baldan et al., 2022).

Also, the inclusion of technology in treatment methods sheds light on a critical transition within neurological rehabilitation. Functional electrical stimulation vs. ankle foot orthoses contrasts the promising advancement in devices applied in rehabilitation for impairments resulting from central nervous system impairment. Both interventions exhibit similar improvements in walking speed, thereby unfolding their capability to improve ambulation in non-progressive CNS-diagnosed patients like stroke and cerebral palsy. With ongoing research, the ongoing evaluation of these modalities will continue to shed light on mechanisms for functional recovery and mechanisms involved and propose that the integration of the above methods will enhance the therapeutic outcome in a person's daily life (Hollands et al., 2017).

Ultimately, the importance of understanding the Central Nervous System is propagated to the development of personalized and effective therapeutic modalities. This serves to emphasize the importance of continued empirical research to further refine interventions according to individual patient need. With ongoing review of current studies, such as the impact of RMT and the value of assistive technology, their practice application and long-term implications must be considered. The insight gained from such studies not only promises to open the door to better treatment protocols but also provokes a deeper, more holistic appreciation of patient care as it applies to the complex interplay of CNS disorders. Ensuring that future studies work to address the broader implications of such discoveries will be essential to advancing our approach to CNS-related health concerns.

The CNS serves as the body's central command center, coordinating sensory information and response. The essential aspect to keep in mind is the intricate interaction between CNS and peripheral systems to facilitate a proper communication process within the body. The CNS consists of the brain and spinal cord, both of which provide vital functions in information processing and motor functions. Neurotechnology advances, like cochlear implants, are perfect examples of how electronics can be interfaced with the nervous system to greatly expand our knowledge of sensory output and input. As highlighted in the recent literature, not only do these interfaces enhance medicinal utilization, but they also provide opportunities for non-medicinal utilization, transforming patient interaction with their environments and treatments available (Ward et al., 2000). This exciting area of neuro-electronic technology brings into focus the need for ethical consideration of its applications. The second essential function of the CNS is its involvement in cognitive processes , such as decision-making and free will. Various brain structures and neurochemical processes are involved in how individuals experience decisions and make them. The complex character of these functions reflects the subtle interaction between deep and superficial subcortical and cortical structures, bearing witness to the complexity of CNS. The dopaminergic input into reward behaviors bears witness to the neurobiology-experience interlink, influencing motivation and action plans. Specifically, studies employing brain imaging techniques like Single Photon Emission Computer Tomography offer evidence regarding decision-making processes among subjects with neurological conditions like Parkinson's disease (Georgiev et al., 2025). Such study of cognitive neuroscience does thus advance our understanding of the CNS in physiological as well as psychological contexts, unlocking the profound influence of brain activity on human behavior. Lastly, the study of CNS-technology interfaces provokes some fundamental questions about future innovations along with ethical dilemmas. The ethical dilemma involves the boundary between therapeutic treatments and improvements, in addition to the anticipated social impacts through neurotechnology. With development still ahead, there is a greater need to confront public perceptions and ethics over using the technologies, particularly for enhancements beyond medicine. The discussion of such matters is crucial to informing prudent use and deployment, such that gains are channeled to benefit society as a whole without compromising rights or freedom of individuals. The study defined in the literature identifies areas of future research as being of prime importance, with urgency placed on continuous investigation into the means by which burgeoning technologies can be harmoniously applied to healthcare without undermining personal freedom or aggravating pre-existing inequalities (Ward, 2000). Lastly, these dialogues are an integral part of understanding the evolving function of the Central Nervous System in our lives.

KEY TERMS FROM THIS CHAPTER

- Blood-Brain Barrier
- Brainstem
- Cerebellum
- Cerebrum
- Glial Cells
- Hypothalamus
- Meninges
- Neurons
- Spinal Cord
- Brain
- Central Nervous System
- Cerebrospinal Fluid (CSF)
- Corpus Callosum
- Gray Matter
- Medulla Oblongata
- Midbrain
- Pons
- Synaptic Transmission

CRITICAL THINKING QUESTIONS

1. **Which of the following structures is part of the central nervous system?**
   a. Spinal nerves
   b. Cranial nerves
   c. Brain
   d. Autonomic ganglia
2. **What is the primary function of the spinal cord in the CNS?**
   a. Digestive regulation
   b. Reflex actions and signal transmission
   c. Hormone production
   d. Blood filtration
3. **Which part of the brain is responsible for coordinating voluntary muscle movements and maintaining balance?**
   a. Cerebrum
   b. Medulla oblongata
   c. Hypothalamus
   d. Cerebellum
4. **The blood-brain barrier primarily functions to:**
   a. Allow free passage of all substances into the brain
   b. Protect the brain against poisonous chemicals in the blood
   c. Regulate oxygen in the brain
   d. Initiate nerve impulses
5. **Which lobe of the brain interprets visual information?**
   a. Frontal lobe
   b. Temporal lobe
   c. Parietal lobe
   d. Occipital lobe

Short Answer Questions

1. What are the two main divisions of the autonomic nervous system?
2. Which division of the ANS regulates "fight or flight" responses?
3. Name the neurotransmitter released by the parasympathetic nervous system at the target organ.
4. What is the primary function of the sympathetic nervous system?
5. Which area of the brain regulates autonomic functions?
6. Explain the physiological effects of sympathetic stimulation on organs.
7. Explain the role played by the parasympathetic nervous system in regulating digestive processes.
8. Explain the pathway of autonomic nerve fibers from the CNS to target organs.
9. Compare neurotransmitters and receptors employed in the sympathetic and parasympathetic nervous systems.
10. Explain the role played by autonomic reflexes in the regulation of blood pressure.

Answers to Critical Thinking Questions

1. (c); 2. (b); 3. (d); 4. (b); 5. (d)

REFERENCES

1. Abbott, N., Bale, T., Brasher, B., Cimolai, N., Duvernoy, H., Fujii, M., Obata, F., et al. (2010). Distribution of Gb3 immunoreactivity in the mouse central nervous system. https://core.ac.uk/download/pdf/8443091.pdf (accessed on 16th June 2025).
2. Abla, A. A., Braunstein, S., Cooke, D. L., Fullerton, H., et al. (2020). High-flow vascular malformations in children. https://core.ac.uk/download/322311021.pdf (accessed on 16th June 2025).
3. Acosta-Cabronero, A., Bach, M., Baliki, M., Barad, M., Bengtsson, S., Chen, R., et al. (2017). Complex regional pain syndrome: The matter of white matter? https://core.ac.uk/download/147689584.pdf (accessed on 16th June 2025).
4. Adler, N. S., Coronel, M. F., de Nicola, A. F., Gonzalez, D., et al. (2016). Temporal changes in the expression of the translocator protein TSPO and the steroidogenic enzyme 5α-reductase in the dorsal spinal cord of animals with neuropathic pain: Effects of progesterone administration. https://core.ac.uk/download/159292394.pdf (accessed on 16th June 2025).
5. Agostini, M., Alfonsi, E., Aloisi, A. M., Alvisi, F., et al. (2016). Psychological treatments and psychotherapies in the neurorehabilitation of pain: Evidences and recommendations from the Italian consensus conference on pain in neurorehabilitation. https://core.ac.uk/download/54538696.pdf (accessed on 16th June 2025).
6. Ahmed, S., Badshah, M., Khattak, I., Nabi, G., et al. (2016). Neuroradiology in tuberculous meningitis: Diagnostic significance and prognostic value. https://core.ac.uk/download/47264784.pdf (accessed on 16th June 2025).
7. Aimoni, C., Busi, M., Calzolari, F., Castiglione, A., et al. (2015). Cochlear implant outcomes and genetic mutations in children with ear and brain anomalies. https://core.ac.uk/download/53523126.pdf (accessed on 16th June 2025).
8. Robles, T. F., & Kane, H. S. (2014). The attachment system and physiology in adulthood: normative processes, individual differences, and implications for health. *Journal of personality*, *82*(6), 515–527. https://doi.org/10.1111/jopy.12052https://core.ac.uk/download/294625964.pdf (accessed on 16th June 2025).
9. Alingh Prins, A., Scheurink, A., Steffens, A. B., et al. (1996). Overfeeding, autonomic regulation and metabolic consequences. https://core.ac.uk/download/pdf/12942087.pdf (accessed on 16th June 2025).
10. Martín-Jiménez, R., Faccenda, D., Allen, E. *et al.* Reduction of the ATPase inhibitory factor 1 (IF_1) leads to visual impairment in vertebrates. *Cell Death Dis* **9**, 669 (2018). https://doi.org/10.1038/s41419-018-0578-x (accessed on 16th June 2025).
11. Arbat-Plana, A., Cobianchi, S., López-Álvarez, V. M., Navarro, X., et al. (2017). Neuroprotective effects of exercise treatments after injury: The dual role of neurotrophic factors. https://core.ac.uk/download/324189726.pdf (accessed on 16th June 2025).
12. Audenaert, E., Mahieu, P., Pattyn, C., Van Hoof, T., et al. (2010). Soft tissue structure modelling for use in orthopedic applications and musculoskeletal biomechanics. https://core.ac.uk/download/55761253.pdf (accessed on 16th June 2025).
13. Baharav, A., Bastuji, H., Bentley, A., Blasi, C., Boly, M., Bonnet, M., et al. (2011). Autonomic pain responses during sleep: A study of heart rate variability. https://core.ac.uk/download/55758223.pdf (accessed on 16th June 2025).

14. Baldan, F., Cacciante, L., Federico, S., Pregnolato, G., Rutkowska, A., Rutkowski, S., & Turolla, A. (2022). The use of respiratory muscle training in patients with pulmonary dysfunction, internal diseases or central nervous system disorders: A systematic review with meta-analysis. https://core.ac.uk/download/554066152.pdf (accessed on 16th June 2025).

15. Balint, B., Bhatia, K. P., Latorre, A., Moura, D., et al. (2025). Neurophysiological insights into the pathophysiology of stiff-person spectrum disorders. https://core.ac.uk/download/636780814.pdf (accessed on 16th June 2025).

16. Barton, M. J., Clarke, M., Ekberg, J., St. John, J. A., et al. (2017). The glia response after peripheral nerve injury: A comparison between Schwann cells and olfactory ensheathing cells and their uses for neural regenerative therapies. https://core.ac.uk/download/196605084.pdf (accessed on 16th June 2025).

17. Bernabeu, M., Hernandez-San-Miguel, J., Marnetoft, S. U., Martinell-Gispert-Sauch, E., et al. (2010). Rehabilitation for multiple sclerosis in adults (I); Impairment and impact on functioning and quality of life: An overview. https://riunet.upv.es/bitstream/10251/103163/3/Part%201%20VANCOUVER%20FINAL%20v2%2019.6.12.pdf (accessed on 16th June 2025).

18. Birchmeier, C., Hernandez-Miranda, L. R., & Müller, T. (2017). The dorsal spinal cord and hindbrain: From developmental mechanisms to functional circuits. https://core.ac.uk/download/300325565.pdf (accessed on 16th June 2025).

19. Brust, V., Creeley, C., Feldman, S., Grandjean, P., Herken, H., Panzica, G., Parent, M., et al. (2014). Neurotoxicity. https://core.ac.uk/download/286729125.pdf (accessed on 16th June 2025).

20. Buchner, E., & Heisenberg, M. (2009). Neurofly 2008 Abstracts: The 12th European Drosophila Neurobiology Conference, 6–10 September 2008, Wuerzburg, Germany. https://core.ac.uk/download/4881258.pdf (accessed on 16th June 2025).

21. Burnstock, G. (2009). Purinergic signaling: Past, present and future. https://core.ac.uk/download/1670991.pdf (accessed on 16th June 2025).

22. Burnstock, G. (2025). Purinergic cotransmission. https://core.ac.uk/download/pdf/8443838.pdf (accessed on 16th June 2025).

23. Buter, R. K., Noyons, E. C. M., Schwechheimer, H., van Raan, A. F. J., et al. (2000). The role of Europe in world-wide science and technology: Monitoring and evaluation in a context of global competition. https://core.ac.uk/download/15993103.pdf (accessed on 16th June 2025).

24. Butt, A., Gregory, A., Krogh, A., Vein, A. A., Holdorff, B., Russel, B., Crone, C., et al. (2011). Fluids and barriers of the CNS: A historical viewpoint. https://core.ac.uk/download/pdf/8527362.pdf (accessed on 16th June 2025).

25. Canova, C., Pitter, G., Ludvigsson, J. F., Romor, P., Zanier, L., Zanotti, R., & Simonato, L. (2016). Risks of hospitalization and drug consumption in children and young adults with diagnosed celiac disease and the role of maternal education: a population-based matched birth cohort study. *BMC gastroenterology*, *16*, 1. https://doi.org/10.1186/s12876-015-0415-y (accessed on 16th June 2025).

26. Capi, M., Curto, M., De Andrés, F., Gentile, M., et al. (2016). Eletriptan in the management of acute migraine: An update on the evidence for efficacy, safety, and consistent response. https://core.ac.uk/download/74319151.pdf (accessed on 16th June 2025).

27. Carnevale, D., Lembo, G., Lori, A., Perrotta, M., et al. (2017). The spleen: A hub connecting

nervous and immune systems in cardiovascular and metabolic diseases. https://core.ac.uk/download/98347401.pdf (accessed on 16th June 2025).

28. Carvalho, M., Marcelino, E., & Mendonça, A. de. (2010). Electrophysiological studies in healthy subjects involving caffeine. https://core.ac.uk/download/12426132.pdf (accessed on 16th June 2025).

29. Celsi, F., Coelho, A. V. C., Crovella, S., Tricarico, D., et al. (2017). Antiretroviral treatment in HIV-1-positive mothers: Neurological implications in virus-free children. https://core.ac.uk/download/84676059.pdf (accessed on 16th June 2025).

30. Chen, X., Faller, D. V., Glavas, I. P., Harpp, D. N., et al. (2020). Klotho pathways, myelination disorders, neurodegenerative diseases, and epigenetic drugs. https://core.ac.uk/download/322973341.pdf (accessed on 16th June 2025).

31. Childre, D., & McCraty, R. (2002). The Appreciative Heart: The Psychophysiology of Positive Emotions and Optimal Functioning. https://core.ac.uk/download/71342518.pdf (accessed on 16th June 2025).

32. Cinelli, M. E., Kalmar, J. M., Kaster, M., et al. (2017). Task-dependent modulation of cortical excitability and balance control in individuals with post-concussion syndrome. https://core.ac.uk/download/143689897.pdf (accessed on 16th June 2025).

33. Connell, E., Le Gall, G., Pontifex, M. G., Sami, S., Cryan, J. F., Clarke, G., Müller, M., et al. (2022). Microbial-derived metabolites as a risk factor of age-related cognitive decline and dementia. Molecular Neurodegeneration, 17. https://doi.org/10.1186/s13024-022-00548-6 (accessed on 16th June 2025).

34. Cox, A. P., Diehl, A. D., Duncan, W., Jensen, L. J., et al. (2012). Ontologies for the study of neurological disease. https://core.ac.uk/download/131216214.pdf (accessed on 16th June 2025).

35. Diamond, I., Dohrman, D., & Gordon, A. (1997). The role of the neuromodulator adenosine in alcohol's actions. https://core.ac.uk/download/323079180.pdf (accessed on 16th June 2025).

36. Dircksen, H., Hansson, B., Harzsch, S., Kirchhoff, C., et al. (2020). Functional morphology of the primary olfactory centers in the brain of the hermit crab Coenobita clypeatus (Anomala, Coenobitidae).

37. Dorsher, P. (2009). The neuroanatomic basis of the acupuncture principal meridians. https://core.ac.uk/download/pdf/288827.pdf (accessed on 16th June 2025).

38. Ducis, K., Lin, C. T., Tranmer, B., Tucker, A., et al. (2017). Metastatic cardiac angiosarcoma to the lung, spine, and brain: A case report and review of the literature. https://core.ac.uk/download/129148849.pdf (accessed on 16th June 2025).

39. Edgerton, V. R., Krucoff, M. O., Rahimpour, S., Slutzky, M. W., et al. (2016). Enhancing nervous system recovery through neurobiologist, neural interface training, and neurorehabilitation. https://core.ac.uk/download/323078214.pdf (accessed on 16th June 2025).

40. Judith Estrine, Lisa DeLisle. "Stress: Putting the Brain Back Into Medicine" International Longevity Center-USA, 2006, doi: https://core.ac.uk/download/71356692.pdf(accessed on 16th June 2025).

41. Fernández, J. G., Marfany i Nadal, G., & Mirra, S. (2021). Under pressure: Cerebrospinal fluid contribution to the physiological homeostasis of the eye. https://core.ac.uk/download/427407814.pdf (accessed on 16th June 2025).

42. Garthwaite, J. (2008). Concepts of neural nitric oxide-mediated transmission. https://core.ac.uk/download/pdf/8234693.pdf (accessed on 16th June 2025).

43. Georgiev, D., Gregoric-Kramberger, M., & Pirtosek, Z. (2025). Decision making and the brain: Neurologists' view. https://core.ac.uk/download/pdf/6481489.pdf (accessed on 16th June 2025).

44. Giulivi, C., Napoli, E., Galuppini, F., Orso, G., Marsilio, I., Lante, I., et al. (2017). Toll-like receptor 4 modulates small intestine neuromuscular function through nitrergic and purinergic pathways. https://core.ac.uk/download/84923513.pdf (accessed on 16th June 2025).

45. Hetherington, C. S. (2019). Myofascial Release. https://core.ac.uk/download/289198166.pdf (accessed on 16th June 2025).

46. Hollands, K. L., Kenney, L. P., Onmanee, P., Prenton, B., et al. (2017). Functional electrical stimulation and ankle foot orthoses provide equivalent therapeutic effects on foot drop: A meta-analysis providing direction for future research. https://core.ac.uk/download/110588624.pdf (accessed on 16th June 2025).

47. Kalafati, M., Kakarountas, A., & Chroni, E. (2022). Testing of motor coordination in degenerative neurological diseases. Healthcare, 10. https://www.semanticscholar.org/paper/3add329402f8d2fb2ef23d47ed01b173b5973888 (accessed on 16th June 2025).

48. Maratos, F. A., McEwan, K., Richardson, M., Sheffield, D., et al. (2016). Joy and calm: How an evolutionary functional model of affect regulation informs positive emotions in nature. https://core.ac.uk/download/46171420.pdf (accessed on 16th June 2025).

49. Mitsdoerffer, M., & Peters, A. (2016). Tertiary lymphoid organs in central nervous system autoimmunity. https://core.ac.uk/download/210651370.pdf (accessed on 16th June 2025).

50. Oman, C. M. (2025). A heuristic mathematical model for the dynamics of sensory conflict and motion sickness. https://core.ac.uk/download/pdf/42853676.pdf (accessed on 16th June 2025).

51. Padovani, E. C. (2016). Characterization of the community structure of large-scale functional brain networks during ketamine-medetomidine anesthetic induction. http://arxiv.org/abs/1606.04719 (accessed on 16th June 2025).

52. Rukavishnikov, V., Efimova, N., Mylnikova, I., & Zhurba, O. (2019). Assessment of the impact of admissible concentrations of formaldehyde on the functional state of the central nervous system in adolescents. Hygiene and Sanitation. https://www.semanticscholar.org/paper/63a0a31083a88ab44ba0374e25a7e83686b3ff0f (accessed on 16th June 2025).

53. Tillotson, J. (2008). JENTIL: Responsive clothing that promotes an 'holistic approach to fashion as a new vehicle to treat psychological conditions. http://ualresearchonline.arts.ac.uk/4907/1/Tillotson_Scent_IFFTI2008_doc_.pdf (accessed on 16th June 2025).

54. Tran, S. M. S., & Mohajeri, M. H. (2021). The role of gut bacterial metabolites in brain development, aging and disease. Nutrients, 13, 732–732. https://doi.org/10.3390/nu13030732 (accessed on 16th June 2025).

55. Ward, J. A. (2000). Neuro-electronic technology in medicine and beyond. https://core.ac.uk/download/70097.pdf (accessed on 16th June 2025).

SPECIAL SENSES PHYSIOLOGY

7

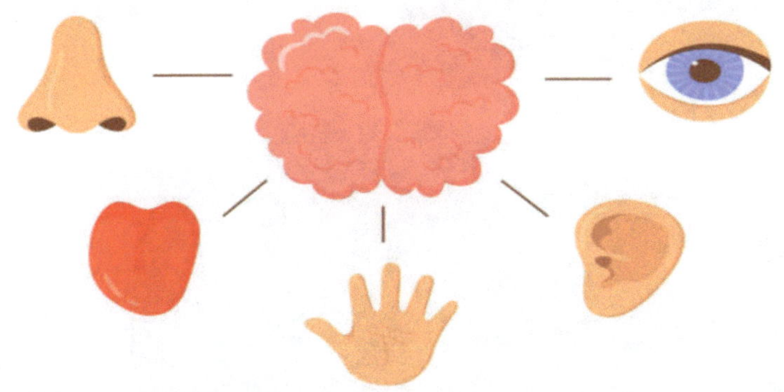

LEARNING OBJECTIVES

After studying this chapter, you will be able to:

1. Describe the anatomy of the eye;
2. Describe the physiology of vision;
3. Describe the anatomy of the ear;
4. Concentrate on the physiology of hearing;
5. Study the anatomy of the olfactory system;
6. Assess the physiology of smell.

Introduction

The special senses physiology is an intricate science that is concerned with how humans perceive their environment. Sensory modality topics , such as vision, hearing, taste, smell, and touch provide insight into the pathophysiology of sense processing. The ability to interpret what is entering the environment is crucial for survival and communication, and hence familiarity with this physiological process is required. Various sensory receptors, implanted in specialized organs, transduce external stimuli to neural signals that are perceived by the brain to form a complex sense. Through understanding these mechanisms, scientists are able to appreciate more how sensory information constructs its behaviors and influences neural functions, which in turn underscores the significance of special senses physiology in both health and disease. Understanding the physiological underpinnings of the special senses also illustrates the complexity of neural interactions. The sensory pathways are not merely simple conduits but are complex pathways of neurons that interact and consolidate sensory information. For instance, vision operates not only by direct photoreceptor input but by integrating contextual information processed in higher-order areas of the brain. Moreover, neuroplasticity, which is the ability of the nervous system to reorganize structurally and functionally due to environmental changes, introduces a further complexity between action, perception, and sensory input.

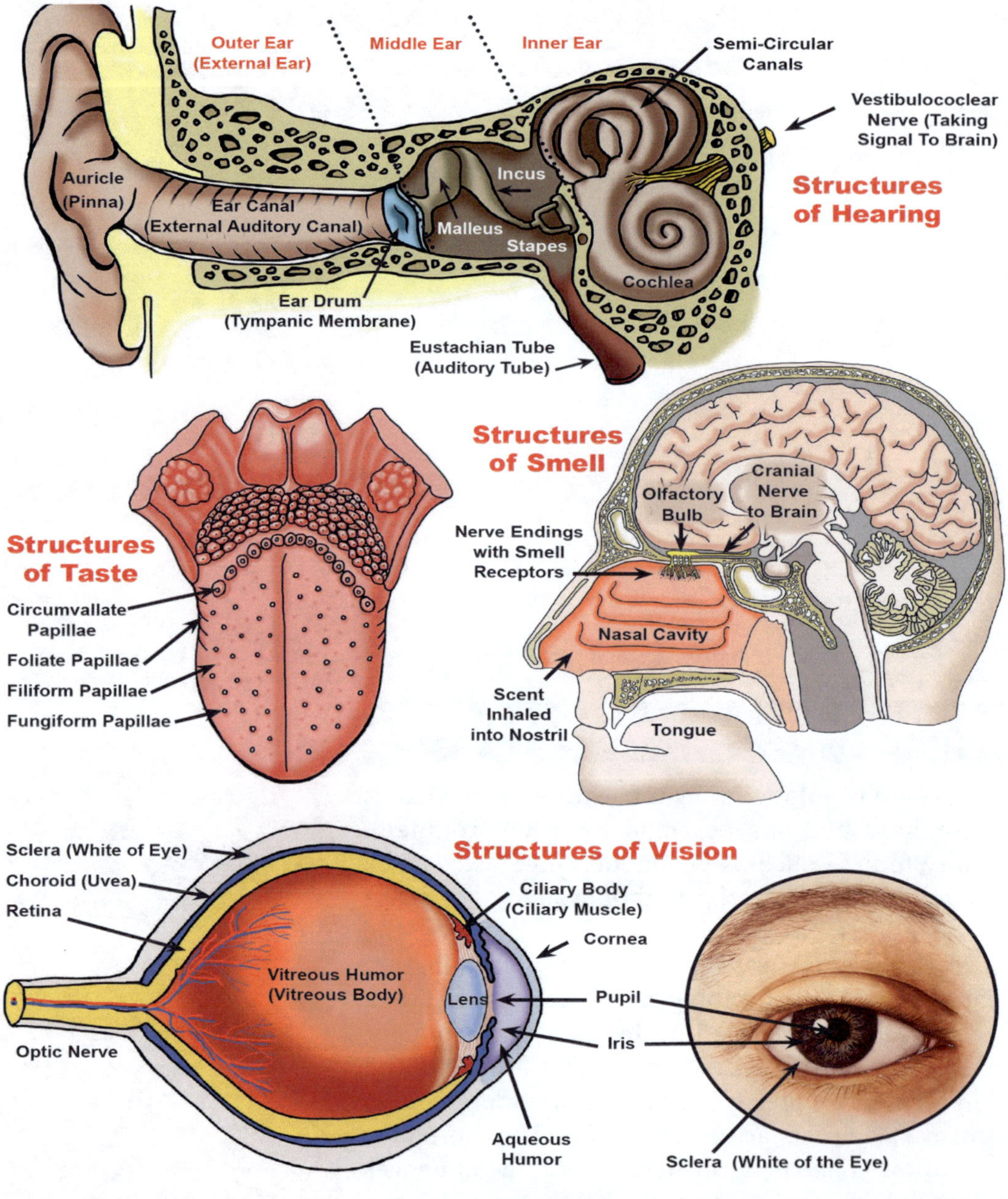

Figure 7.1. Special senses.

Source: https://www.exploringnature.org/graphics/biomedical_illustration/special_senses_poster2.jpg.

Thus, studying special senses physiology provides more insight into how the sensory systems may influence cognitive processes and behavioral adaptations. Research in this field can also provide access to technology development, particularly in the advancement of high fidelity systems imitating or supplementing sensory experience, as suggested by infusion of human capability in technological facilitation (Mair et al., 2007). Physiology of special senses is increasingly being taught by computational simulations that simulate real biological systems, particularly by the use of Artificial Neural Networks (ANNs). These models attempt to simulate the growth and functioning of human neurons through comparisons between natural and artificial systems. They contribute to more than simply our understanding of sensory processing; they also provide new areas of research in robotics and artificial intelligence. The decentralized nature of these models, similar to that of real nervous systems, illustrates the possibility of self-organization and adaptability under artificial conditions (Adami et al., 1998). As special senses physiology evolves, the use of interdisciplinary methods will enhance our knowledge of sensory processes as well as facilitate synergy among neuroscience, technology, and cognitive science. This convergence would enable revolutionary uses that would enhance the sensory experiences of humans and fix sensory dysfunctions (Figure 7.1).

Definition of Special Senses

Definition of special senses involves the physiological mechanisms through which organisms perceive and decipher sensory inputs from their environment. The conventional classification enumerates five primary special senses: vision, hearing, taste, smell, and touch. All of these senses rely upon specialized sensory cells and organs to transduce specific kinds of external stimuli into nerve impulses, which the brain interprets. Vision, for instance, relies upon the intricate anatomy of the eye, such as the cornea, lens, and retina, that work together to convert light waves into visual information. Similarly, noises are transduced to mechanical and electrical signals in the inner ear, proving the specificity and complexity of sensory experience. The distinct pathways and centers of each sense prove the advanced coordination required for humans to navigate the world effectively and meaningfully. Special senses operate more subtly to show the interdependence of sensory modalities and their shared contribution to human experience. Perception of urban places as evidenced by interconnectivity shows this as the settings engage several senses simultaneously, creating richness of experience. Urban walking, as a case in point, is not as much visual interaction with building forms but as well as audio experiences as are defined by ambient sounds of traffic and social engagement. This cross-sensory experience structures an individual's perception of space; as noted in the analysis of urban design, scale and sensory range strongly inform the manner in which individuals experience their world (Lucas et al., 2008). Every sense has a unique function to create the overall effect, and it thus follows that one can only understand special senses through an appreciation of their interlocking influences and interactions. In addition, technological innovations increasingly blur historical sensory borders, broadening the scope of special senses. Advances in virtual reality and telepresence demonstrate how sensory perceptions in human beings are simulated and controlled, allowing interactive immersion in remote environments (Mair et al., 2007). This increases the dynamic essence of senses as they adapt to evolving technologies, posing the challenge to human perception in the future. With these technologies being firmly implanted in day-to-day existence, not only should one study the biological foundation of special senses but also the potential transformations they will experience as a result of enhanced technological development. The research on special senses is thus a dynamic field, with the interaction of biology, environment, and technology dictating the dynamic history of human sensory perception.

Importance of Special Senses in Human Physiology

Vision, hearing, taste, smell, and touch are special senses that are part of the integral human physiology that enables interaction with the environment to facilitate survival and enhance quality of life. All senses employ specific sensory receptors that convert outside stimuli to neural impulses interpretable by the brain. For instance, photoreceptors in the retina allow us to perceive by responding to light waves, whereas auditory receptors in the cochlea respond to sound waves, allowing us to hear. This system is an example of how sensory input helps determine behavioral responses and cognitive processes. Intermodality interdependence allows better understanding of the stimuli, reinforcing the critical function of special senses in reacting to complex environments, thus supporting their physiological relevance. Special senses also have a critical function in maintaining the equilibrium of homeostasis and overall body health. Sensory information directs significant physiological responses, such as reflex behavior to protect the body from damage. For example, the withdrawal reflex elicited by painful stimulation illustrates how sensory input provokes immediate motor response and thus prevents injury. In addition to simple reflexes, sensory integration is crucial to emotional and psychological health. The psychomotor theory proposes an active interrelationship of mental, motor, and sensory processes and that our perceptions directly shape behavior and states of mind. Thus, the interrelationship between special senses and cognitive function underscores their vital role not just in perception, but in the functioning of human physiology as a whole (TAN et al., 2007).

Another key aspect of special senses is the effect that they have on learning and adaptation, particularly to environmental stimulation.

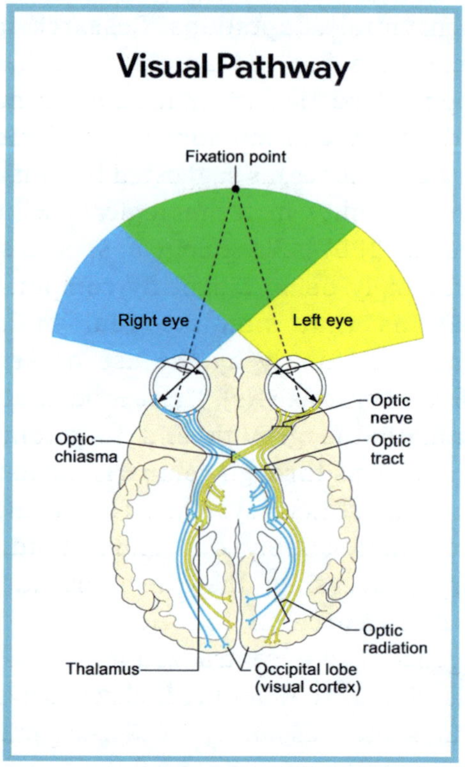

Figure 7.2. Special senses in human physiology.

Source: https://nurseslabs.com/wp-content/uploads/2017/06/Visual-Pathway-Special-Senses-Anatomy-and-Physiology.jpg.

Rising research underscores the capacity of the brain to be resilient, and this is enhanced by the learning from experience with varied sensory stimulation. Exposure to varied environments activates neurobiological processes that facilitate the creation of new neural networks, resulting in cognitive resilience and flexibility in working with emotions. This adaptive process is a significant part of coping with the challenges of life, as evidenced by adventure education and therapy programs utilizing outdoor challenges to activate sensory immersion. Through enhancement of sensory exploration, these interventions are able to consolidate psychosocial equilibrium and facilitate long-term mental health benefits. This connection between special senses and neuroplasticity informs the relevance of special senses, stressing their capacity to drive not only short-term perception but also long-term adaptation and resilience of the human body and mind (Allan et al., 2012) (Figure 7.2).

7.1. Anatomy of the Eye

Learning Outcome

1. Describe eyeball anatomy;
2. Highlight the role of retina;
3. Find out the role of the optic nerve.

The human eye is a highly developed organ whose most dominant function in special sense physiology, and particularly vision, is more than that of any other human organ. Essentially, the anatomy of the eye enables it to collect light and translate it into neural impulses that can be interpreted by the brain as visual images. The eye possesses a variety of crucial components that include the cornea, lens, retina, and optic nerve. The cornea, its transparent slope, is responsible for the eye's first refracting power of bending light so it is focused onto the retina. The lens further refracts this to allow objects to be viewed at various distances. The retina contains photoreceptor cells, rods and cones, which change light into electric currents. This intricate interplay of structures illustrates the sophistication of the eye's anatomical structure and its essential function in vision. Central to the function is its ability to adjust to varying light levels by means of mechanisms , such as the pupillary reflex. The iris, a muscle diaphragm surrounding the pupil, manages the intensity of light reaching the eye, constricting or dilating in response to the amount of ambient light. Additionally, the flexibility of the eyes also involves their ability to focus on objects at different distances through a process known as accommodation. It is where the ciliary muscles alter the shape of the lens to maintain sharpness as objects move toward or away from us. These active responses not only reflect the eye's great flexibility but also the vital role in exploring and interpreting the visual world. Cooperative functioning of these structures ensures maximum vision function, confirming the dependence of several aspects of the eye on each other. In addition, understanding eye structure is more than structure; it includes the paths traveled by visual information to the brain for interpretation.

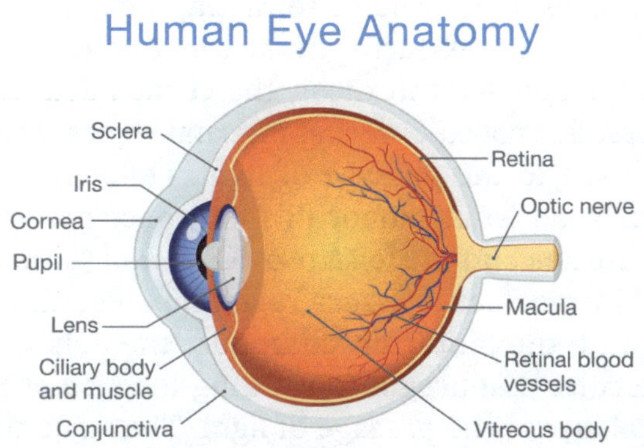

Figure 7.3. Eye Anatomy's effect on vision health.

Source: https://www.elmanretina.com/wp-content/uploads/shutterstock_657947488-1.jpg.

After phototransduction occurs in the retina, electrical stimuli travel through the optic nerve to the visual cortex of the brain. This neural process underlies the detection of patterns, color, and motion and eventually culminates in visual perception. Surprisingly, recent evidence has indicated that disruption of any part of this intricate system will lead to visual impairment or disease, emphasizing the critical status of each anatomical component. As we delve into the interactions between the anatomy of the eyes and their physiological processes, we gain a better understanding of the mechanisms involved in vision and how the integrity of anatomy is necessary for sight to be fully perceived. Delving into these topics can also yield novel interventions for visual impairments, demonstrating the relevance of anatomical data in practical applications (Sinha et al., 2016) (Figure 7.3).

7.1.1. Structure of the Eyeball

The eyeball is formed with a complex structure to accommodate the multiple functions of vision. At the center of the complicated system is the cornea, which is a transparent outer covering and plays a key role in refracting light coming into the eye. Measuring in the range of 435–501 micrometers in thickness, the cornea acts as a protective cover, covering internal structures in addition to the passage of light. Following the cornea, aqueous humor fills the space between the cornea and the lens, providing nourishment and intraocular pressure regulation. Positioned behind the anterior chamber, the iris is a muscular diaphragm controlling the size of the pupil, hence the passage of light. The structural variations among the parts of the eyeball, for example, the level of pigmentation in anterior and posterior iridal epithelium, are both protective and functional and enhance visual capacities (Akbalık et al., 2015). Aside from the anterior segment, the internal eyeball structure is the lens and vitreous humor, both of which are vital in light focusing to the retina. The lens, a soft bioconvex tissue, alters its shape through the exertions of the ciliary body in an effort to accommodate in order to enable the eye to see objects at varying distances. This adaptive interaction between the lens and the adjacent ciliary processes enables the creation of clear images on the retina, where photoreceptor cells convert light into neural signals. The vitreous humor, a gel that fills the posterior chamber, maintains the eye's shape and suspends the retina. The composition of such emphasizes the significance of the structural integrity of every component in preserving maximum vision function as well as demonstrates how much these elements rely on each other in the general physiology of special senses (Richart et al., 2025). In analyzing the structure of the eyeball, one cannot overlook the importance of the retina, a multilayered organ that is the critical medium between light and neural interpretation. The retina contains a myriad of cells, including rods and cones, which are the primary agents responsible for contrasting light and color perception. Structurally, the retina is built in layers with every layer possessing discrete roles in phototransduction and transmission of visual information to the brain via the optic nerve.

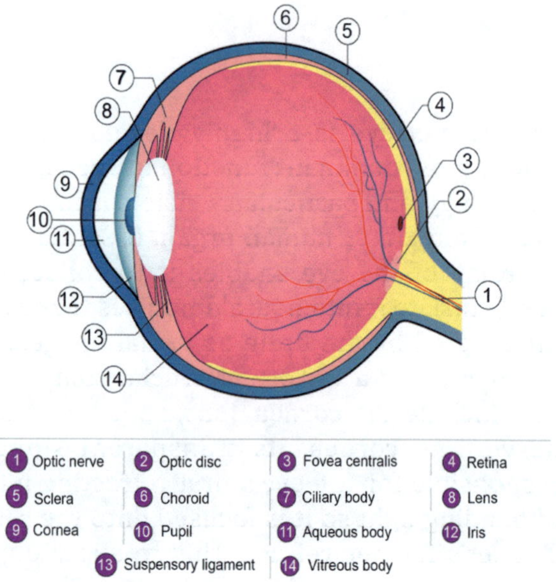

Figure 7.4. Structure-of-human-eye.

Source: https://cdn1.byjus.com/wp-content/uploads/2018/11/Structure-of-Human-Eye.png.

The retinal pigment epithelium also plays a vital role in providing retinal visual cells with nutrients and eliminating excess light to reduce glare, thereby maximizing the quality of vision. The several layers prove to be the result of evolutionary advancements that make vision more efficient. Realizing these intricate architectural designs of the eyeball not only explains physiological processes of seeing but also emphasizes vulnerability to visual disabilities in the event of damage to any of the components (Akbalık et al., 2015) (Figure 7.4).

7.1.2. Function of the Retina

The retina, an essential component of the eye's visual apparatus, is the light-sensitive tissue in the back of the eye, and its function is necessary to convert light to neural impulses. Composed of a variety of specialized cell types, including photoreceptor rods and cones, the retina begins the complex process of vision. Rods are predominantly sensitive to dim light and movement, while cones handle color vision and tasks that demand high acuity. The intricate structure of the cells allows the retina to capture a broad spectrum of light and transform it into electrical impulses that alert the brain. Without the ability of the retinas to transduce light, sight would never occur, highlighting its fundamental role in special senses physiology. Aside from its role in the process of light transduction, the retina is also key to enhancing contrast and edge detection, both of which are absolutely essential to visual sharpness. It uses a process named lateral inhibition, where associated retinal neurons inhibit each other's activity to clarify the visual image. This ability increases the perception of the light and dark areas so that shapes and depth are distinguishable. These abilities imply that the brain receives not only raw visual information but also processed information that helps interpret the environment better. The very complex operations of the retina illustrate its complex anatomy and emphasize how much it is a component of our understanding of vision processing within special senses physiology (Macpherson et al., 2010). Also, the health of the retinas is essential for having proper vision, and numerous diseases can influence their functioning significantly. Diseases , such as diabetic retinopathy, age-related macular degeneration, and retinal detachment can result in profound visual impairments. Understanding pathophysiological changes in the retina during such diseases is a stimulus for treatment and prevention. The advanced retinal imaging technologies available today enable better diagnostics and treatment, and hence, retinal physiology research is more pertinent. Finally, the complex mechanisms of the retina not only improve our perception of the world around us but also provide an important area of study in the physiology of special senses (Figure 7.5).

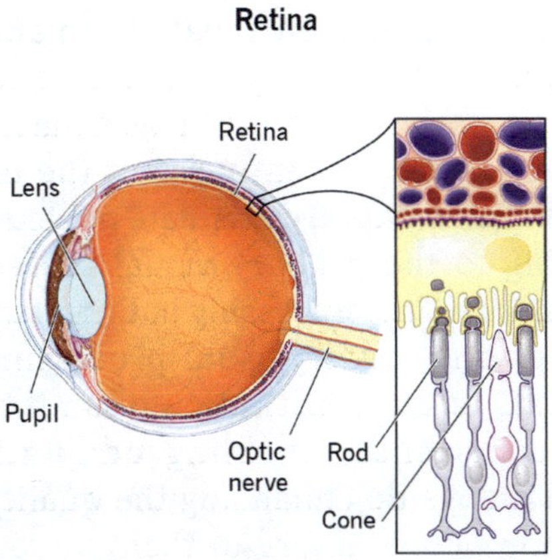

Figure 7.5. Retina of the eye.

Source: https://my.clevelandclinic.org/-/scassets/images/org/health/articles/22694-retina.

7.1.3. Role of the Optic Nerve

The optic nerve, alternatively referred to as cranial nerve II, is an important channel for visual information from the retina to the brain. It contains approximately 1.2 million axons originating from retinal ganglion cells. The axons form the intricate optic nerve structure that conveys the visual signal following initial phototransduction occurring in the photoreceptor cells of the retina. These photoreceptors, upon illumination, convert light stimuli into electrical impulses, and the impulses travel through the layers of the retina before finally converging into the optic nerve. This transmission of sensory information is also imperative for elementary visual processing and other reflexive and cognitive processes involving vision, thereby pointing to the optic nerve's vital function in visual perception and integration in the larger framework of sensory physiology. Once the optic nerve reaches the optic chiasm, there is an impressive decussation, whereby approximately half of the nerve fibers cross over to the opposite side. This anatomic structure is elementary as it enables visual information from both visual fields to be processed by both hemispheres of the brain. Such processing is crucial for three-dimensional vision and depth perception, which are parameters needed in locomoting through complex environments. This relay system consequently relays the impulses to the thalamic lateral geniculate nucleus before projecting to the primary visual cortex of the occipital lobe. The processing in these structures enables higher-order visual processing. Each stage adds to the constitution of an integrated visual experience, enabling adaptation for survival alongside enhancing the quality of life by making people aware of their surroundings in an efficient manner. The optic nerve is not independent; rather, it functions synergistically with other sensory systems as well as neural pathways. In particular, the integration of visual input with auditory and tactile perception increases an organism's ability to respond to its environment. For instance, cetaceans have exhibited sensory-system adaptations that facilitate their effectiveness at navigating and hunting in underwater environments, where the optics of light are significantly different from those of terrestrial environments. Their adapted neuroanatomy implies enhanced processing of spatial information, a feature common to many animals, as well as humans. With increasingly more research bringing to light the complexities of optic nerve function and the neuroanatomy-specific alterations within groups , such as cetaceans, gaps exist in our existing knowledge and highlight the need to study sensory physiology and conservation biology further, thereby enabling us to value the contribution of the optic nerves fully in the comprehension of sensory perception and adaptation, particularly as witnessed through different ecological niches (Gerussi et al., 2023).

Test Your Knowledge

1. What is the function of the cornea in the eye?
2. Which eye structure controls the amount of light entering the pupil?

7.2. Physiology of Vision

Learning Outcome

1. Explain the refraction of light;
2. Explain the process of phototransduction;
3. Find visual pathways to the brain.

The physiology of vision is crucial in the context of how humans perceive the world. Vision begins with the transduction of light by the eye as it is focused into a form by the cornea and lens onto the retina. It possesses a multi-layered structure made up of light receptor cells known as rods and cones, which are tasked with converting light into electrical signals. Rods are highly sensitive to light and enable one to see in darkness, while cones enable one to see colors and details in conditions of brightness. Not only do these specific elements complicate vision, but also how they interact and conjoin a unified perceptual experience. This type of multi-faceted conception contradicts the existence of one-dimensional simplification of categorization of senses, supporting a more complicated setup for sensory physiology, as argued in arguments over sensory modalities, which has the ability to provide an insight into an exploration of the physiology of vision (Macpherson et al., 2010). Once the photoreceptors within the retina have converted light into electrical impulses, the impulses are carried along the optic nerve to the brain. This results in a series of complex processes, primarily in the visual cortex, wherein interpretation of the visual stimulus takes place. Within this area, the brain integrates information regarding movement, color, and depth to synthesize a consistent representation of the visual environment. This process is not static; it is directed by past experience and contextual information, again displaying the dynamic nature of visual perception. As critics note, the binding of disparate dimensions, like representation and phenomenal character, illustrates the integrated work of numerous neurological processes that decide the way we perceive visual information (Macpherson et al., 2010). Thus, the physiology of vision is more than mere eye anatomy, and includes the intricate neuronal systems underlying perceptual awareness. Beyond mere light detection and processing mechanisms, the physiology of vision also extends into general issues in metrology related to how we measure and characterize visual stimuli. The Concept of Man as a Measuring Instrument demonstrates the significance of human observation in product, experience, and even general welfare measurement in society. Research initiatives, including those promoted by the European 'Measuring the Impossible' Network, examine measurement concerning human senses and extend through psychophysics into psychology. Such an interdisciplinary approach highlights the need to consider vision not as physiology alone but as a basic element of man's interface with the world. Such understanding permits innovation in measuring methodologies, ultimately to better quantify the significant role served by vision in a broad spectrum of applications, including safety and human performance in general (Figure 7.6).

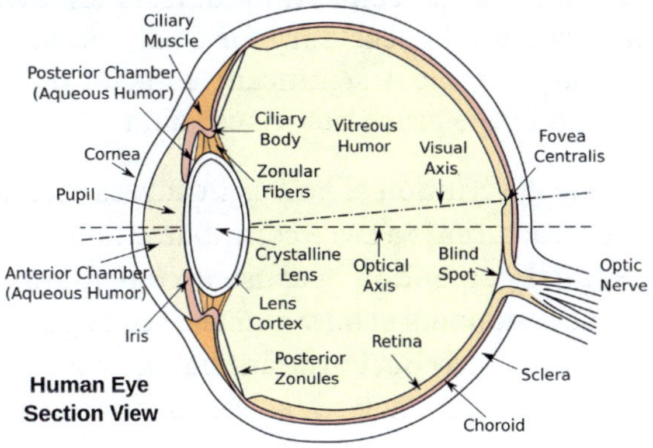

Figure 7.6. Eye anatomy and physiology.

Source: https://www.share4rare.org/sites/default/files/inline-images/Eyesection.svg_0.png.

7.2.1. Process of Light Refraction

Refraction of light is a very important process in the study of vision and how eyes perceive what is around them. Refraction occurs when light travels from different media, i.e., air into glass, and results in a change of its speed and direction. This bending of light enables the formation of images through the focusing of light rays on the retina to enable clear visual identification. The basic principles of light refraction trace back to early hypotheses imagined by such scholars as Ibn al-Haytham and Descartes, who laid the foundation for modern optics. Their findings reinforced the significance of geometric models in visual perception, underpinning the theory of a two-dimensional sensory core from which depth and spatial vision can be derived. Examination of refraction of light is therefore not merely a physical process but an intrinsic component of our cerebral processing of visual information. In special senses physiology, the refraction mechanism of light is directly related to the anatomical structures of the eye. Light is refracted predominantly by the cornea and lens and together with one another to focus light rays onto the retina. The cornea provides most of the eye's refractive power, while the lens adjusts for fine-tuning focus concerning objects far away. This structure is necessary for clear vision and is among the most significant contributors to how the brain processes visual data.

The description of how light curves through these structures is a large contributor to theories on spatial perception because it contributes to our understanding of how humans see depth and distance. As aptly put by the ancient philosophers, the interconnection between sensory experience and refraction of light forms the interconnection between the physical constitution of the eye and its sensory effects, illustrating the complex process of vision. More sophisticated studies on refraction of light have implications that transcend simple visual understanding, impacting sciences , such as astronaut hiring and retention standards for space exploration. Physiological demands of maintaining visual acuity under microgravity conditions require intense assessments of one's visual capacity, especially as they relate to refractive efficiencies. Research that investigates the demands placed upon performance under such circumstances has highlighted the importance of subtlety in visual perception as well as its dependence upon the precise refractive features of the eye.

In fact, the subtlety of light refraction can have direct impacts upon an astronaut's functional vision under adverse circumstances, as described in current literature on the topic. Highlighting the functional uses of light refraction thus places emphasis upon ongoing study in special senses physiology that further elucidates the interface between human biology and the challenges of space exploration (Figure 7.7).

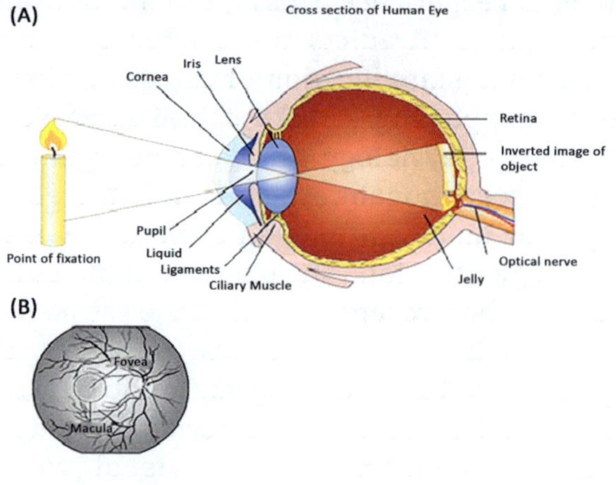

Figure 7.7. Summary of eye anatomy and the refraction process.

Source: https://www.researchgate.net/profile/J-Hejtmancik/publication/312002509/figure/fig1/AS:1176614993956865@1657538283850/A-Summary-of-eye-anatomy-and-the-refraction-process-The-light-refraction-trace-from.jpg.

7.2.2. Mechanism of Phototransduction

The phototransduction mechanism is a critical component of sensory physiology that enables organisms to perceive light and its changes. At the heart of phototransduction, particularly in the vertebrate retina, is the conversion of light stimuli into electrical responses so that vision can be perceived. This is triggered when photons are captured by the photopigments in the photoreceptor cells, i.e., rods and cones. The primary photopigment, rhodopsin in rods, is altered by a conformation when a photon is absorbed, with the activation of a G-protein termed transducin. Intracellular reaction cascade activation leads to the closure of cyclic guanosine monophosphate (cGMP) gated ion channels. The subsequent hyperpolarization of the photoreceptor cell is an important event, which allows the transfer of visual information to downstream retinal neurons to be processed further and interpreted by visual stimuli. As phototransduction proceeds, the role of cGMP becomes particularly pivotal. Under darkness, a rise in levels of cGMP that keeps ion channels in open conformation and allows the flow of sodium ions inside the cell, thus causing the depolarized condition. Exposure to light and activation of transducin causes activation of a phosphodiesterase enzyme and a rapid decline in levels of cGMP. This decline closes the sodium channels and induces further hyperpolarization of the cell membrane. The decreased polarization causes a decrease in the release of neurotransmitters from the synaptic terminals of the photoreceptors. The response is a signal relayed to the bipolar cells of the retina. Understanding these molecular events proves the complicated nature of sensory transduction and illustrates how small changes at the cellular level can produce profound consequences on overall sensory perception. Additionally, the progress of phototransduction mechanisms illustrates the significance of the process in different organisms. For example, studies on neofunctionalization and gene duplications have explained how environmental signals drive visual receptor adaptation in organisms. Particularly, research documented in Hamilton et al. (2012) indicates that gene duplications are also at the heart of sensory perception evolution to the point where it enhances the capacity of animals to detect and respond to copious amounts of visual stimulation. Such adaptations are especially observed in cases where large-sized visual pathways give rise to certain photoreceptor cell types, thereby giving rise to color vision and greater visual acuity. As these evolutionary progressions are explored, they do not merely reveal the biological complexity of phototransduction but also its significant role as a crossing point between the external world and sensory experience, ultimately dictating how organisms recognize and engage with their environment (Figure 7.8).

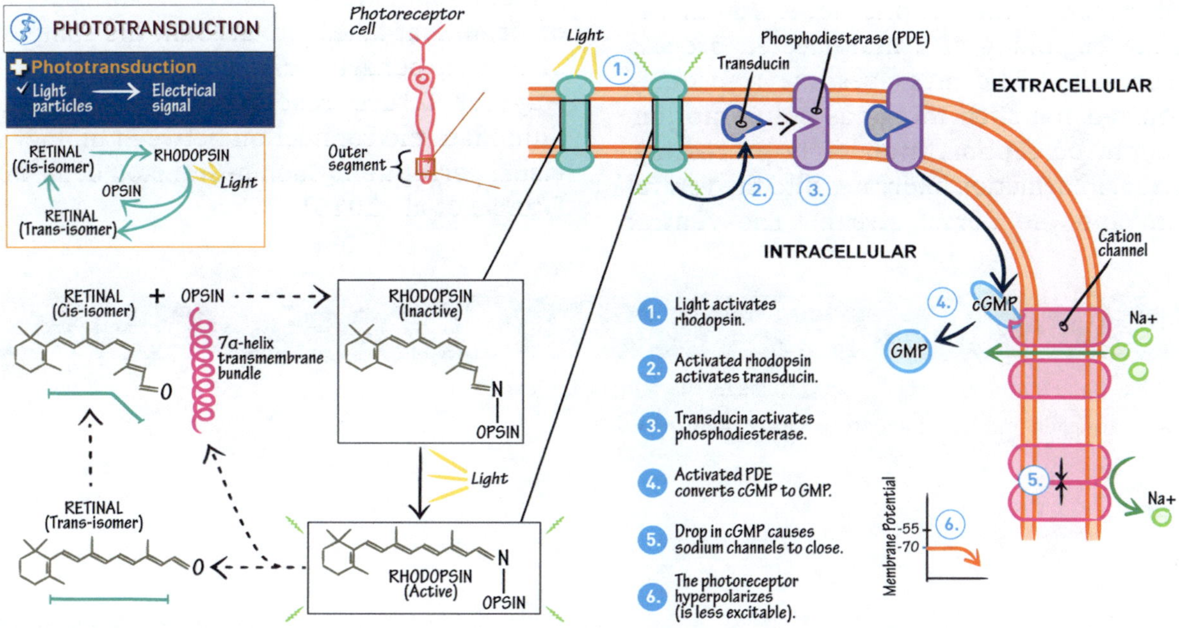

Figure 7.8. Phototransduction.

Source: https://d1j63owfs0b5j3.cloudfront.net/tutorial/finalImage/1303-1465334165119.png.

7.2.3. Visual Pathways to the Brain

The exploration of visual pathways to the brain is a fundamental component of the special senses physiology. Light enters the eye through the cornea and subsequently the lens, where it is refracted by the lens and onto the retina. The retina contains the photoreceptor rods and cones, which convert light energy into electrical impulses. These are transmitted through a retinal network of bipolar and ganglion cells to terminate in the formation of the optic nerve. The optic nerve is the primary channel of visual information, carrying impulses from the retina to the brain's visual centers. The path of these optical stimuli doesn't just end at the primary visual cortex but follows a complex route, including lateral geniculate nuclei and other cortical areas. This extended path is what processes visual stimuli and contributes to our understanding of visual perception and cognition. After the visual information has reached the lateral geniculate nucleus (LGN) of the thalamus, it is relayed to the primary visual cortex of the occipital lobe. But this is only the beginning of a multifaceted process of processing. The messages are rigorously scrutinized for such things as color, motion, and depth perception. After early processing, the visual information bifurcates into the ventral stream and the dorsal stream. The ventral stream, also known as the what pathway, plays a crucial role in object perception and naming, while the dorsal stream, or where pathway, makes significant contributions to awareness of space and locomotion. This dual processing allows individuals to navigate their world. Thus, the disruptions within these pathways, which take place in most neurological disorders, can elucidate the significance of these intricate visual pathways to normal visual performance. The binding of visual information within the brain not only allows perception but also facilitates higher cognitive functions. The interconnected nature of visual pathways facilitates the balance of sensory input with emotion and memory. Recent evidence indicates that brainstem nuclei are involved in regulating sensory information flow, influencing global excitability of cortical areas involved in visual processing. Disruption of this system can have a range of symptoms, as with migraines, where both visual disturbance and pain occur along common neural pathways. Through these interactions, scientists can design a more sophisticated model of the processing of vision that takes into account the complexity of human behavior and cognition, paving the way for future research that may further illuminate the connection between biology and visual perception (Cuomo-Granston et al., 2010; Francis et al., 2016).

Test Your Knowledge

1. What happens to light as it passes through the lens of the eye?
2. How do rods and cones (photoreceptor cells) help us see?

7.3. Anatomy of the Ear

Learning Outcome

1. Describe the structure of the outer, middle, and inner ear
2. Define the cochlea's function
3. Describe the function of the auditory nerve

The ear is a highly complex organ and is crucial to special sense physiology. It is especially important in hearing and balance. Its structure can be divided into three main parts: the outer ear, the middle ear, and the inner ear. The outer ear consists of the pinna and auditory canal, both of which are utilized to funnel sound waves onto the tympanic membrane, or eardrum. The membrane vibrates along with the sound and establishes a complex mechanical process. In essence, the outer ear is a sound catcher that amplifies frequencies that are crucial to effective auditory perception. As sound waves travel through the sound canal, they ultimately lead to the middle ear, where there are specialized bones referred to as the malleus, incus, and stapes, which transfer vibrations to the inner ear. Thus, the structural organization of the outer ears is pivotal to initial sound processing mechanisms within the context of ear anatomy. Progressing from the middle ear, the inner ear holds essential elements required for hearing and equilibrium. The cochlea, being a spiral fluid-filled structure, is responsible for converting the vibrations in the sound to neural signals. When the stapes works on the oval window, it produces waves in the cochlear fluid, which cause hair cells lining the basilar membrane to be stimulated.

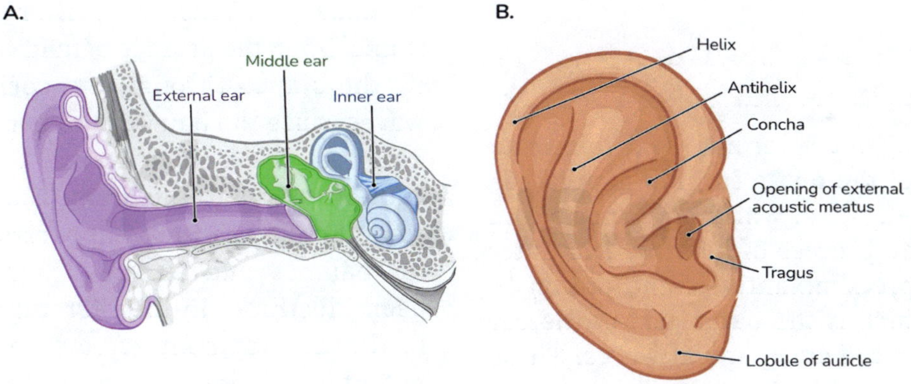

Figure 7.9. Anatomy of the external and middle ear.

Source: https://d16qt3wv6xm098.cloudfront.net/y43N1I6NTLegcYYjydmFgXENT1mPA1-C/_.png.

Mechanotransduction results in converting sound waves into electric signals, which are delivered to the auditory cortex by the auditory nerve. Additionally, the vestibular system of semicircular canals and otolith organs maintains the body's balance. This double function underlines the inner ears vital importance in our understanding of ear anatomy. Both auditory and vestibular operations are necessary for movement and interaction within our world, highlighting the intricate integration of sensory physiology. The anatomical structure of the ears and their physiological function possess an extremely interwoven relationship. For instance, any flaw in any ear part can seriously affect hearing and balance, demonstrating the ear's intricate structure. Conditions , such as conductive hearing loss which can be caused by issues in the outer or middle ear or sensorineural hearing loss, which affects the inner ear, demonstrate the importance of the health of every part. Moreover, familiarity with ear anatomy is crucial for the treatment development of most sound disorders since treatment typically targets specific ear structures. With the progress in medical technology , such as cochlear implants, new treatments have been invented to treat individuals with severe deafness and thus the direct implication of anatomical facts in practice. In a way, the ear structure is a testament to the intricacy of human physiology and serves to underscore the significance of each structure within the equilibrium of the senses and hearing (Figure 7.9).

7.3.1. Structure of the Outer, Middle, and Inner Ear

Human anatomy of the ear may be divided into three divisions: the outer ear, the middle ear, and the inner ear, all of which have specialized functions in the process of hearing. The outer ear consists predominantly of the pinna, or the auricle, which is the outer part of the ear responsible for collecting sound waves. These sound waves travel through the external auditory canal and ultimately to the tympanic membrane, or eardrum, which separates the outer ear from the middle ear. This structure not only receives sound vibrations but also directs them to the next point of sound processing. The outer ear's highly developed structure, its folds and curves, is used to enhance its ability to amplify sound as well as localize sound, the platform for successful hearing in complex environments. Proceeding further inward, the middle ear contains three little but important bones, the ossicles: malleus, incus, and stapes. These bones function to transmit and condense the vibrations they receive from the tympanic membrane, carrying them in the form of mechanical energy before being handed over to the inner ear. The stapes, being the smallest of the ossicles, directly interfaces with the oval window, a membrane-covered opening onto the inner ear. This interface is necessary in order to transfer sound waves into fluid waves since the inner ear is filled with perilymph and endolymph. Also, the middle ear houses the Eustachian tube, which delivers equal pressure of air on each side of the tympanic membrane, necessary for optimal conduction of sound.

This space arrangement puts emphasis on the middle ear's role as a crucial link in the sound chain, where the energy forms are converted for efficient hearing. The inner ear is where sound waves get transformed into neural messages that the brain interprets as sound. It contains the cochlea, a spiral-shaped organ that contains hair cells, the sensory receptors for sound. Upon the passage of fluid waves produced by the stapes through the cochlea, the fluid waves cause the hair cells to bend, establishing a series of electrochemical signals via the auditory nerve to the brain. The inner ear also contains the vestibular apparatus, responsible for balance and spatial orientation. As has been illustrated in the literature, for instance, in the development of cochlear microphonic potentials, understanding how the physiology of the cochlea and its connected neural pathway functions is still the key to designing effective auditory devices and therapies (Lominchar et al., 2016). Overall, the integration of anatomical and physiological information from all three components of the ear is required to appreciate fully auditory perception and the complications of human hearing (Gerussi et al., 2023) (Figure 7.10).

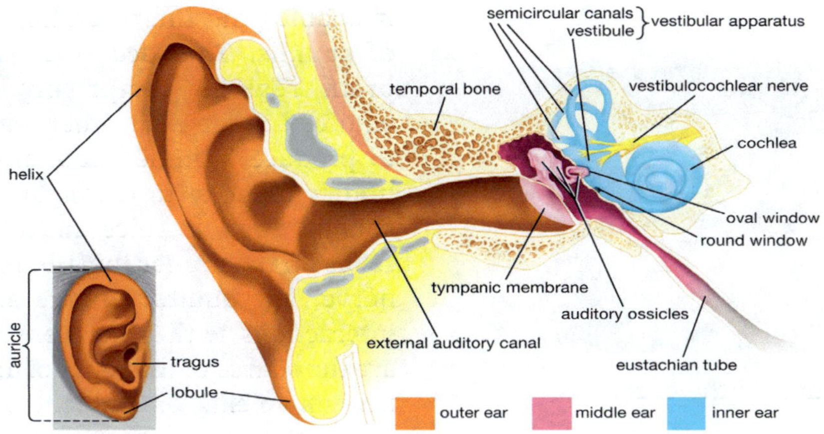

Figure 7.10. Structures-outer-ear.

Source: https://cdn.britannica.com/04/14304-050-1A5E3289/structures-outer-ear.jpg.

7.3.2. Function of the Cochlea

The cochlea plays a significant role in the auditory system to transform sound waves into electrical impulses that the brain can comprehend. This intricate spiral structure within the inner ear is filled with fluid and lined by specialized sensory hair cells that are responsible for hearing. Once the sound waves enter the cochlea via the oval window, they create pressure waves in the fluid and cause the basilar membrane to vibrate. The vibrations stimulate the hair cells, and the mechanical energy is converted into electrical signals. This rudimentary process is the initial step in sensory transduction, which allows sound information to travel through the auditory nerve to the central nervous system to be processed and eventually become the basis of our auditory perception. Aside from its role in transducing the sound signal, the cochlea is tightly coupled with feedback systems that optimize hearing capacity. The medial olivocochlear efferent system demonstrates this interaction in that it provides sound data modulation passing through the cochlea. Through synapsing with outer hair cells, these efferent neurons inhibit amplification provided by outer hair cells during sound processing. Such a system is particularly beneficial under noisy conditions, as it improves signal detection and discrimination. The efferent-activated cholinergic receptors, that is, the α9α10 receptor, are a vital part of the feedback system and show how the cochlea receives not only the sound but participates actively in the tuning of hearing (Elgoyhen et al., 2009). Additionally, the discriminative power of frequency and intensity of the cochlea supports its sensitivity and adaptability. Studies on species , such as Eigenmannia indicate that hearing systems can display impressive accuracy in detecting minuscule variations in pitch and volume, crucial for effective communication and sensing the environment. The structure of the cochleas allows for the detection of minute changes in pitch and volume, crucial in perceiving complex hearing situations. As indicated in Eigenmannia, the functional properties of the cochlea confirm its evolutionary status across a variety of species. These findings underline the cochlea's dual role in sensing diverse acoustic stimuli while interacting well with nervous system activity, thus explaining hearing as an interactive physiological process within the scope of special senses (Kaunzinger et al., 1991) (Figure 7.11).

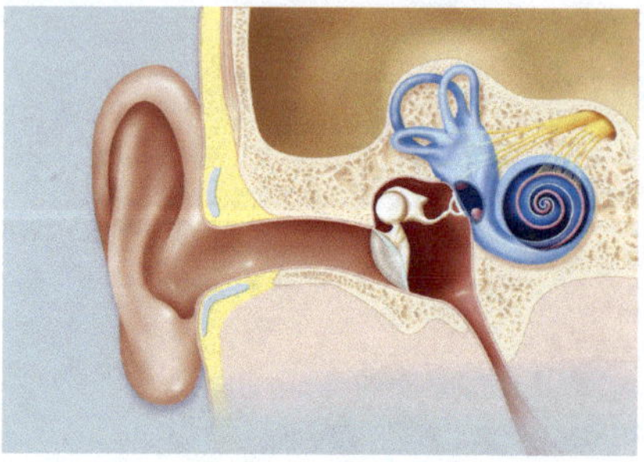

Figure 7.11. Function of the cochlea.

Source: https://www.verywellhealth.com/thmb/6OnyWVsqKiVNcF1pqKXzH3grmNA=/1500x0/filters:no_upscale():max_bytes(150000):strip_icc()/Ear-GettyImages-586038190-42999e6443b441d5876c5e3c5dd640cf.jpg.

7.3.3. Role of the Auditory Nerve

The auditory nerve plays a key role in hearing, serving as the primary conduit through which sound perception occurs and is delivered from the inner ear to the brain. Comprising bundles of nerve fibers, the auditory nerve is supplied with electrical impulses generated by hair cells within the cochlea due to stimulation by sound waves. All of these signals are types of auditory features like frequency, intensity, and duration, which are essential for hearing. Precision in such transmission is a priority; interference in any form leads to hearing loss or degradation of tones. Thus, the auditory nerve not only facilitates hearing but also ensures that this sense process is continuous, highlighting its significance in the overall physiology of special senses. The cochlear structure and the auditory nerve's mutual dependence underlines the intricacy of hearing. As the auditory nerve sends signals to the brain's auditory cortex, it enables the interpretation and localization of sounds. This occurs in an apparatus of brain regions comprising a synthesis of auditory input with other sensory modalities to produce a unified auditory landscape. The brain's capacity to distinguish among various sounds, such as voice and background noise, relies on the proper functioning of the auditory nerve. The auditory nerve also has complex interactions with other sensory tracts, which are the source of the sense of auditory feedback, i.e., for voicing or ambient perception. These interactions reveal the central role of this in the physiological organization of the special senses and demonstrate how it lies not just behind hearing but also fundamental behavioral and cognitive functions, with stress on the integrated nature of auditory perception within human experience. Further, studies of the functions of the auditory nerve provide deep insights into the complexities of neurophysiology. Studies of such disorders as auditory neuropathy, where the auditory nerve is damaged, have brought to light auditory processing disorders. Such disorders are able to illustrate the full scope of auditory nerve contribution, showing the impact interruption of normal auditory conduction can have on communication impairment. In broader contexts, knowledge of the auditory nerve can inform the development of interventions , such as cochlear implants to make hearing-impaired patients' quality of life easier. The physiological grounds, set forth by the intense interaction of sensory sensations, foreground the auditory nerves central role within the subject of special senses physiology. So broad a perspective underscores the continued need for studies and education related to hearing processes.

Test Your Knowledge

1. What are the three parts of the ear?
2. Which of the parts of the ear hold the ossicles (malleus, incus, and stapes)?

7.4. Physiology of Hearing

Learning Outcome

1. Name the transmission of the sound wave;
2. Explain the mechanism of sound perception;
3. Describe the pathways of sound to the brain.

The physiology of hearing encompasses a complex interaction of mechanisms and structures that allow the perception of sound. The sound waves travel through the air and are directed by the outer ear into the auditory canal and induce the vibration of the tympanic membrane. This vibration is conducted by the three little bones, the malleus, incus, and stapes, of the middle ear and produces a magnified sound and sends it to the inner ear. The inner ear's cochlea converts the mechanical vibrations into electrical signals with the assistance of hair cells, a critical sensory receptor in the organ of Corti. The transformation of sound from its mechanical form to an electrochemical stimulus is required for the auditory nerve to be able to pass information to the brain, and thus the understanding of these processes is indispensable in the study of the complicated mechanisms of the auditory apparatus. Other than the anatomical structures, the physiological mechanisms of hearing are interpretation and processing of sound by the brain. Once the cochlea transmits electrical impulses, they travel along the sensory pathways to brain regions, the most significant being the auditory cortex. This region is essential in differentiating between varied frequencies, intensities, and intricacy of sounds.

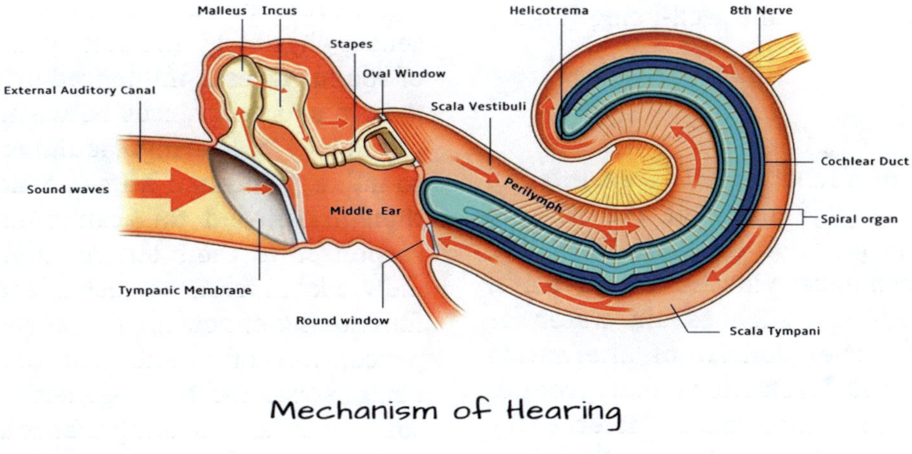

Figure 7.12. Physiology of hearing.

Source: https://www.entlecture.com/wp-content/uploads/2023/01/Dr-Rahul-Bagla-Mechanism-of-Hearing-2-2048x1319-1.jpg.

Further, the brain syntheses auditory input into sensory information from other modalities, which contributes to an integrated sense of the world. The process whereby the brain recognizes and analyzes such sounds has relevance not only to communication, but also to emotional existence and social relationships. And so, knowledge of such processes illuminates the central importance of hearing to human cognition and conduct. Disruptions in any portion of this auditory pathway, however, can lead to hearing disabilities, which are increasingly prevalent in modern society. These are exposure to abnormally loud noise, age, and certain medical conditions that may affect the complex mechanisms of the ear. For instance, prolonged exposure to high decibels results in noise-induced hearing loss affecting the functioning of the hair cells in sound detection. Similarly, age-related alterations in the cochlea result in presbycusis, a common form of hearing loss among the elderly. Research further suggests that the underlying physiological processes of hearing are crucial in grasping larger sensory physiology, as reflected in the interconnectedness of chemical senses, taste and smell, that, although quite generally thought to be separate, show the complex nature of perception as an overall experience (Smith et al., 2015). Also, the on-going advancements in hearing research further emphasize the significance of physiology of hearing to our sensory understanding and well-being (Figure 7.12).

7.4.1. Sound Wave Transmission

Transmission of sound waves is an integral part of hearing physiology, at the core of how organisms perceive their world. Sound waves are mechanical vibrations that travel through a medium , such as air, water, or solids. Sound waves consist of alternating compressions and rarefactions that produce pressure variations that can be detected by hearing systems. Well-defined properties , such as frequency and amplitude, corresponding to pitch and loudness, respectively, are transported by sound waves. The ability to detect these differences enables refined communication and perceptual perception of the environment, hence enhancing survival. An understanding of sound wave transmission mechanisms is required for comprehension of the broader physiological processes controlling the special senses and thus forming a platform for continuing research into processing and perception of sound. The process of transmission of the sound wave is made more complex by the anatomical and physiological mechanisms of hearing. Once the waves of sound reach the ear, they travel via the outer ear and into the middle ear, where they make the tympanic membrane oscillate. The mechanical movements that are triggered are then amplified by the ossicles, a system of three very small bones known as the malleus, incus, and stapes. This makes the sensitivity of the detection of sound such that the inner ears cochlea can transform the mechanical signals to electrical signals. Furthermore, the cochleas intricate fluid-filled compartments enable the process of sound frequency conversion and encoding into neural signals interpreted by the brain. The mechanism involved not only demonstrates the efficiency of sound wave transmission but also emphasizes the very highly integrated interaction between sensory function and anatomical structure, foregrounding the significance of auditory processing in special senses physiology. In addition, the transmission of sound waves is influenced by environmental factors and differences between people in the physiology of hearing. Mediums alter speed of sound; e.g., through water, sound travels faster than in air, and this can influence animals' responses to their environment. In addition, individual differences, such as ear shape or even functioning of hearing pathways, can influence perception of sound. All these variations demonstrate the heterogeneity of reception of sound waves, indicating that sound experience is not a mechanical phenomenon but one conditioned by biological and environmental frames as well. Sound perception possesses more than basic communication significance; it's also crucial for social interaction, space perception, and emotional response. Therefore, enhancing our understanding of sound wave transmission not only contributes to special sense physiology but also results in developing the curing of auditory disorders and improving auditory technologies.

7.4.2. Mechanism of Sound Perception

Sound perception is a complex process which begins with the interaction of the sound waves and the auditory system. When the sound waves come to the ear, they first travel through the external auditory canal, striking the tympanic membrane and vibrating it. This vibration is converted into mechanical energy by the ossicles, three little bones inside the middle ear, which intensify the sound. The stapes bone then translates the vibrations into the cochlea, a fluid structure in the inner ear. Here, the vibration results in displacement of hair cells along the basilar membrane and stimulates them. The stimulation initiates electrical impulses that are conveyed to the auditory cortex of the brain to facilitate conscious perception of sound. This advanced mechanism highlights the function of various sensory and anatomical structures acting together to show the multidimensional nature of hearing (Macpherson et al., 2010). Interestingly, sound information is processed not only in the cochlea but also involves higher-level processing in the brain. The auditory cortex of the brain processes various aspects of sound, such as pitch, loudness, and duration, which are crucial to process differences among various auditory stimuli. Localization, or the ability to tell from which direction a sound is coming based on both ears' sound input, is also involved in this processing. The brain employs interaural time differences and intensity variations to create a spatial representation of the immediate acoustic environment, in support of situational awareness. Furthermore, multimodal integration with other sensory modalities of auditory information allows for a global conception of the environment, as represented by models scaling to the complexity of multi-sensory processing. This underscores that the perception of sound is not a straightforward linear process but an intricate interaction of the peripheral and central nervous system components (Berglund et al., 2010). Finally, psychophysics research also helps to explain how humans perceive sound through the application of various measurement procedures, which are required to further the understanding of the auditory perception. Under initiatives like the Measuring the Impossible Network, studies focus on the relationship between sound characteristics and human perception, especially how body processes compare to subjective experience. A study of notions like measurement uncertainty and decision-making in audio-related phenomena provides significant information about the suitability of human perception under ultimate decision-making situations. The potential for innovation in metrological approaches to hearing perception affects not just the physiological assessment but also behavior and cognition. The application of multipurpose psychology, sociology, and other related methodologies allows the examination of sound perception to take a more integrated approach to knowing human interaction with sound beyond the boundaries of traditional disciplines (Berglund et al., 2010; Macpherson et al., 2010) (Figure 7.13).

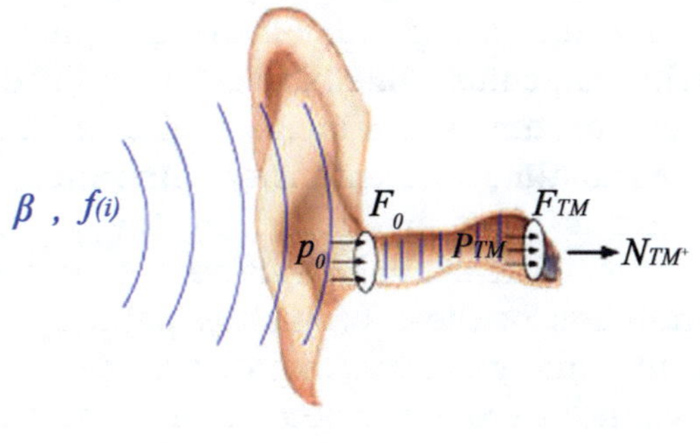

Figure 7.13. A simplified analytical model of sound propagation in the human ear.

Source: https://encrypted-tbn0.gstatic.com/images?q=tbn:ANd9GcRzOlUBaHRfMw_CPXQV_h7N_Famvl4d0kOEvw&s.

7.4.3. Auditory Pathways to the Brain

The auditory system is a complex series of pathways that allow for the perception of sound, which culminates in the transmission of vital information to the brain. The sound waves move through the outer ear, where they cause the tympanic membrane to vibrate. These vibrations are subsequently passed on by the ossicular chain—malleus, incus, and stapes—to the oval window of the cochlea. In the cochlea, fluid motion stimulates hair cells in the Organ of Corti, which convert mechanical energy to electrical energy. This is the beginning of auditory transduction, a process crucial for discrimination and localization of sound. These neural signals are transmitted via the nerve of hearing, or auditory nerve, and this data gets transmitted to the brainstem, where initial processing occurs, performing a basic function in hearing that will impact future higher cognitive functions. Once one is at the brainstem, one is still processed within various nuclei before getting as far up as the auditory cortex. The brainstem, which is a sophisticated area made up of multiple nuclei, is involved in the modulation of sensory input as well as the integration of sound information. The main nuclei of the auditory system are the cochlear nuclei, superior olivary complex, and inferior colliculus, which are engaged in sound localization, timing, and intensity discrimination. Interaural time and intensity differences are key at this point for identifying the origin of sounds so that spatial awareness may ensue. Dysfunction of these brainstem pathways can lead to auditory processing disorder, whereby one cannot decode the sounds or differentiate among different auditory inputs. The presence of these impairments therefore highlights the importance of the brainstem in the overall auditory experience and reaffirms its role in organizing our perceptual world within noisy auditory environments (Cuomo-Granston et al., 2010). The final stage in the processing of sound occurs in the auditory cortex, which is a region in the temporal lobe where higher-order complicated processing and interpretation of sound occur. It is at this region of the brain that further processing of the representation of sound occurs. The cortical network possesses remarkable plasticity, which renders it susceptible to auditory experience and learning, as evidenced by research that reveals how groups of neurons generalize sensory input to emphasize meaningful patterns (Hubel et al., 2012). Its flexibility is a significant feature in musicians and linguists, who utilize acutute auditory discrimination capacity extensively. Overall, the merging of auditory pathways from the cochlea to the auditory cortex underlines an elaborate interaction between peripheral sensory equipment and central neural processing to ultimately result in our ability to decipher and respond to our sound world with precision (Figure 7.14).

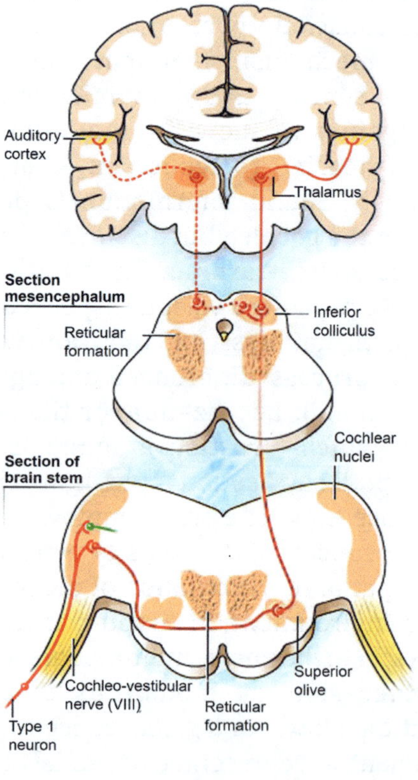

Figure 7.14. Auditory brain.

Source: https://www.cochlea.eu/wp-content/uploads/2024/11/en-voies-auditives-primaires.jpg.

Test Your Knowledge

1. What is the process by which the ear translates sound waves into electrical signals?
2. What is the role of the tympanic membrane (eardrum) in hearing?

7.5. Anatomy of the Olfactory System

Learning Outcome

1. Describe the nasal cavity structure;
2. Define olfactory receptors role;
3. Discuss olfactory bulb function.

The olfactory system, part of odor sensory processing, is initiated by the specialized receptor cells of the olfactory epithelium. The mucous layer that lines the top of the nasal cavity and is accountable for detecting odor molecules binds with olfactory receptors. These receptors are contained within cilia that extend into the air full of odor, triggering a succession of neural signals. Activated, olfactory sensory neurons transmit information through their axons, making up the olfactory nerve, which synapses onto the olfactory bulb directly. This direct path distinguishes the olfactory system from other senses, which tend to route signals through the thalamus en route to the cortex. Understanding the intricate organization and operation of the olfactory epithelium is crucial in learning how humans perceive and interpret a vast number of odors, an event tightly integrated with memory and emotion.

Following this initial processing within the olfactory bulb, the neural signals are relayed to other areas of the brain, including the primary olfactory cortex and the limbic system. The engagement of the limbic systems demonstrates the powerful link between smell and emotion, as smells have the ability to evoke strong memory and mood. Importantly, the olfactory bulb and cortical areas it projects to have a function not just in the detection of odors, but in the interpretation of their meaning in a specific context. The neuroanatomy of olfactory circuits makes such complexity possible, e.g., projections to the amygdala will determine the likelihood of odors to generate emotional reactions. Further investigation into these neurological corridors reveals the facile integration of sensory experience and cognition, as evidence of the olfactory systems ability to affect human behavior and experience. In addition, the olfactory system is highly plastic and adjusts to variations in environment and experience, representing a major focus area in neuroscience. Age, health status, and olfactory training are some factors that affect sensory perception, resulting in differences between people in terms of perception of smells. Such heterogeneity opens up the possibility of further investigation into the anatomical and physiological basis that regulates olfactory sensitivity and function. Researchers have begun to investigate ways in which alterations of the olfactory system can predict some neurological diseases, describing an important link between olfactory functioning and overall health. Through continued investigation of the anatomy of the olfactory system, researchers hope to uncover novel aspects in special senses physiology, potentially paving the way for novel diagnostic and therapeutic strategies for olfactory dysfunction-related disorders (Figure 7.15).

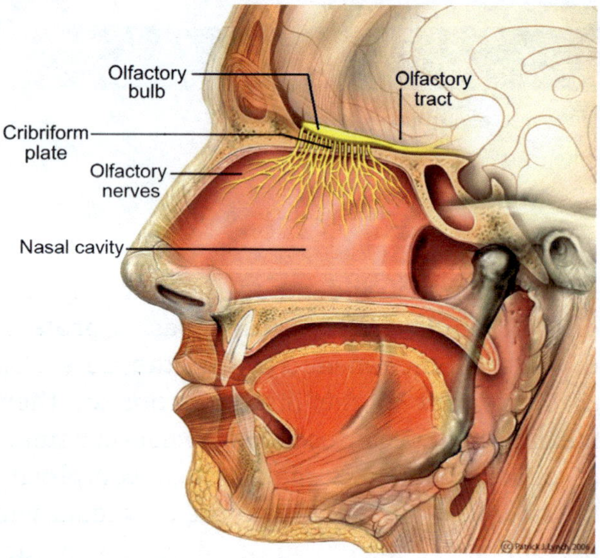

Figure 7.15. Olfactory system.

Source: https://upload.wikimedia.org/wikipedia/commons/3/34/Head_Olfactory_Nerve_Labeled.png.

7.5.1. Structure of the Nasal Cavity

The nasal cavity has a multifunctional role in special sense physiology, primarily olfaction and respiration. Its structure is also divided into three primary regions: the vestibular, respiratory, and olfactory regions. The vestibular region, located just inside the nostrils, is lined by coarse hairs known as vibrissae, which form a physical filter, permitting air passage while keeping particulate material of larger size. This initial filtration is crucial as it prepares the air for deeper penetration in the respiratory tract. The respiratory region, characterized by its extensive surface area covered with mucous membranes, helps in warming, humidifying, and further filtering of aerial matter. The intricate structure of these regions facilitates the nasal cavitys role in respiration and detection of odorants in airborne substances, demonstrating a close relationship between structure and physiology inherent to the overall sensory perception of the organism. Clearing the way for the olfactory region, the typical anatomy of the nasal cavity largely contributes to the sense of smell, essential for survival in the majority of species. The olfactory epithelium at the top of the nasal cavity contains the olfactory receptor neurons responsible for detecting odor molecules and transmitting the message to the brain. The structure of the nasal cavity promotes turbulent airflow that supports effective odorant deposition across this epithelium, thereby increasing the sensitivity of olfactory detection. Further, the structural arrangement of the nasal cavities includes conchae, which increase the surface area and create turbulence to enable effective odor sampling. This anatomical adaptation is found in many different species, as research has found numerous different adaptations that allow for olfactory ability, reflecting then the evolutionary pressures that influence sensory functions, especially those found in rich olfactory environments (0000-0002-0116-2736 et al., 2023). The functional consequences of nasal cavity anatomy go beyond mere olfactory perception, as respiratory health and resistance to disease are also affected. The nasal mucosas' ongoing mucous secretion not only catches airborne pathogens and particulates but also functions as the body's first line of defense against respiratory infections. This versatility emphasizes the significance of a properly organized nasal cavity in homeostasis. Furthermore, the appreciation of the subtleties of nasal anatomy can shed light on the pathways by which several respiratory disorders can act on both humans and animals. Recent studies examining the nasal anatomy of different species reveal a variation in the structure-function dynamic that can inform therapy for respiratory disorders (Chapman et al., 1965). Through investigation of the unique organization and physiological relevance of the nasal cavity, researchers can inform the ways this structure is employed for sensory perception as well as for the overall function of the respiratory system, offering insight into interspecies evolutionary adaptation mechanisms (Figure 7.16).

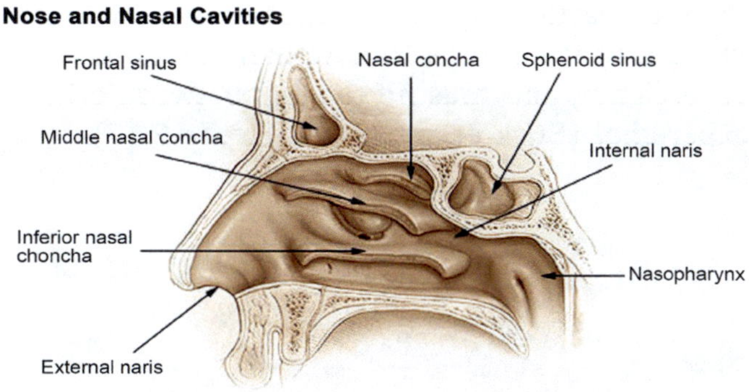

Figure 7.16. Structure of the nasal cavity.

Source: https://training.seer.cancer.gov/images/anatomy/respiratory/nose_nasal_cavities.jpg.

7.5.2. Function of Olfactory Receptors

The intricate functionality of olfactory receptors is pivotal to the comprehension of the mechanism of smell sense in the broad spectrum of special senses physiology. Olfactory receptors, positioned in the olfactory epithelium of the nasal cavity, are specialized proteins that bind with airborne particles to initiate the process of signal transduction. These receptors are highly heterogeneous, with humans possessing about 400 distinct olfactory receptor genes that can be used to detect a vast variety of odorants. Heterogeneity enables the detection of a wide variety of odors, not only required for flavor perception but also for detecting environmental stimuli important for survival. While the sensory process is intricate, the specific way in which olfactory receptors identify and respond to unique molecular shapes remains the subject of investigation, opening the question of the deeper meaning of olfactory processing to human cognition and behavior, as reflected in the research on the quantum mechanical nature of olfaction postulated by the latest theories (Buck et al., 2010). The function of olfactory receptors extends beyond simple smell sensing; they play critical emotional and memory processes. This sensory process is deeply rooted in the limbic system, the brain region responsible for emotions and memory creation. Upon engaging with odorant molecules, the resulting neural signals are transmitted to the olfactory bulb and subsequently passed on to regions of the brain , such as the amygdala and hippocampus. This channel explains the way in which certain odors can stimulate robust memories or feelings. The role that the olfactory receptors have on these neurological pathways underscores the wealth of multisensory experience, as smell is not an isolated process. It should be noted that the impressions derived from olfaction, combined with taste and touch, converge to build a global perception of flavor, once more indicating the intricate interaction between various modes of sensory input in human perception (Smith et al., 2015). Although traditionally relegated to a secondary status in contrast with vision and hearing, recent findings uphold the function of olfactory receptors within the philosophy of perception. It is evident that olfaction cannot be accounted for by models constructed for vision anymore but possesses a rich tapestry of sensory interdependencies. Perception of smell can provide objective information regarding the environment, showing that chemical senses possess interpretative meaning. In addition, the complexity of odorant receptor function subverts established paradigms in sensory perception to offer a clear show of hands that the receptors offer information not only into smell, but into the nature of perception as a multisensory process. Advances in smell research, or particularly the subtleties of how small molecules interact with intricate proteins, may shine a light on ways to new therapeutic treatments in other areas, such as pharmacology and neuroscience, and thus fill the gap between critical sensory processing and comprehensive human experience (Buck et al., 2010) (Figure 7.17).

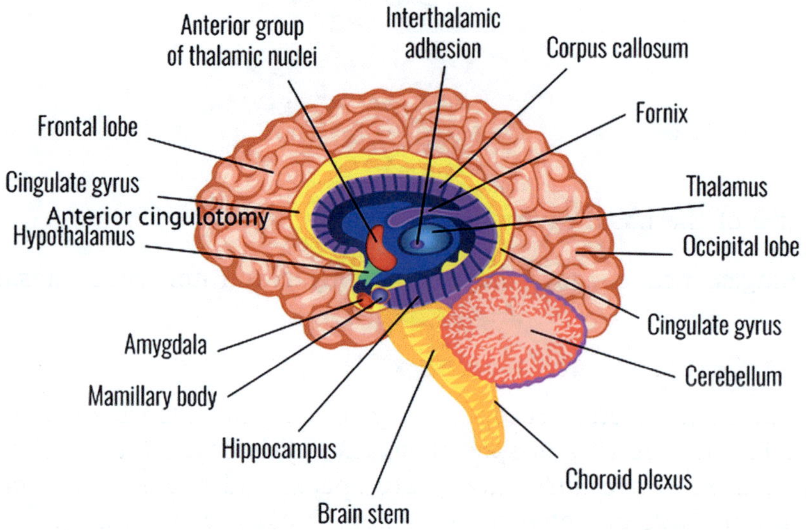

Figure 7.17. Limbic system.

Source: https://external-content.duckduckgo.com/iu/?u=https%3A%2F%2Fmood-disorders.co.uk%2Fimager%2Fnews%2F11245%2FThe-Limbic-System_2fbc6d6996738f03a243b9b0e2ef47dd.png&f=1&nofb=1&ipt=cafac286690daa62a447f5b57d266568fc6d6287638f4627124dc4909e4f7ffd.

7.5.3. Role of the Olfactory Bulb

The sense system component is the olfactory bulb and it is primarily responsible for the sense of smell. Located at the base of the brain, it is the first processing site for olfactory information received from the olfactory epithelium. The sensory neurons, which are stimulated by odorant molecules, transmit signals to the olfactory bulb, where the input information is processed through complex neural circuits. This initial processing is vital as it allows for discrimination among a vast array of odors and contributes to the identification and understanding of odors important in many behaviors like food selection and social interaction. The ability of the olfactory bulb to process and convey information to the central brain centers underscores its role not just in olfactory perception but also in regulating emotional reactions linked to odors. Beyond its sensory processing role, the olfactory bulb is also very engaged with neuroplasticity and regeneration, particularly concerning the olfactory epithelium. Research has established that olfactory sensory neurons can regenerate following injury, a process fundamental to the maintenance of olfactory function across an individual's lifetime. The fact that the olfactory epithelium can regenerate is made possible by the neurogenic niche of the olfactory bulb, which guarantees the generation of new neurons. Such a process becomes pertinent in the context of smell and taste dysfunction, which can have a critical influence on the general quality of life. Increased understanding of olfactory bulbs' role in such regenerative processes has led to therapy interventions targeting the restoration of olfactory function, validating its significance in physiological as well as clinical contexts (Enders et al., 1996). Further, recent studies have found that the olfactory bulb is not only central to smell perception but also exhibits overlap with other cognitive and emotional brain centers. This interaction provides the possibility for odors to be connected with memories and emotional responses, demonstrating the olfactory bulbs broader influence on human experience. For example, some odors have the ability to induce rich recollections or emotional responses, commonly known as the "Proustian phenomenon," an expression of how much our sense of smell is intertwined with personal experience and emotion. In this way, the olfactory bulb is a pivotal point of convergence of the sensory routes, linking biological perception with psychological sensation. Understanding its far-reaching function contributes to our knowledge of special senses physiology and emphasizes the olfactory bulbs function beyond mere sensory reception, and so an interesting but multifaceted discipline (Chapman et al., 1965).

Test Your Knowledge

1. Which structure of the nasal cavity contains the sensory receptors of smell?
2. In which structure do messages of smell pass to the brain?

7.6. Physiology of Smell

Learning Outcome

1. Describe the process of odor detection;
2. Define the mechanism of signal transduction for the olfactory signal;
3. Identify the olfactory pathways to the brain.

The physiology of smell, or olfaction, is critical for human experience and interaction with the world. This complex sensory process begins at the olfactory epithelium, a special tissue located in the nasal cavity. Here, the olfactory receptor neurons react to odorant molecules, and a chain of biochemical events ultimately leads to the perception of smell. These receptors are able to tell thousands of different odorants apart and relay this information to the olfactory bulb in the brain via their axons. The olfactory bulb then decodes these messages and sends them to other parts of the brain, like the limbic system, which handles emotion and memory. This direct link between odor and affect underscores the importance of olfaction in social interactions and everyday experiences, thereby making it a fascinating area of study for the discipline of sensory physiology. The integration of olfactory input with psychological and behavioral response emphasizes the function of smell beyond recognition. Studies have demonstrated that olfactory stimulation might regulate mood, enhance cognitive function, and even influence social behavior. For instance, certain odors are reported to evoke nostalgia or comfort, which can be worth their weight in gold in therapeutic settings. With the advancement of technology, applications of olfactory science have been extended to new horizons , such as olfactory Metrology, where the emphasis is on how subjective human judgement can be computed and measured (Berglund et al., 2010). This approach not only sheds light on the physiological basis of smell but also how such senses interact with mental and behavioral processes, further supporting the need for multidisciplinary research that provides bridge building between physiology, psychology, and even sociology. Innovative ventures are redefining the role of olfaction in health and wellbeing, assuming that smell is not merely an ancillary sense but a critical component in terms of quality of life improvement. The JENTIL® Collection, for instance, marries technology with perfumery to create apparel which responds to emotional states through embedded scents (Tillotson et al., 2008). This is an innovative approach that illustrates how scent experiences can be utilized to influence psychological well-being and emotional health. By examining the study of olfactory-driven Aroma-Chology, researchers are paving the way for creating methods to add aroma to clothing as an emotional coping tool, possibly establishing a new model for the perception and application of smell stimulation in therapy. This merging of sensory physiology and emotional health further underscores the interconnectedness of smell, behavior, and mental health, which encourages an integrated approach to human senses (Figure 7.18).

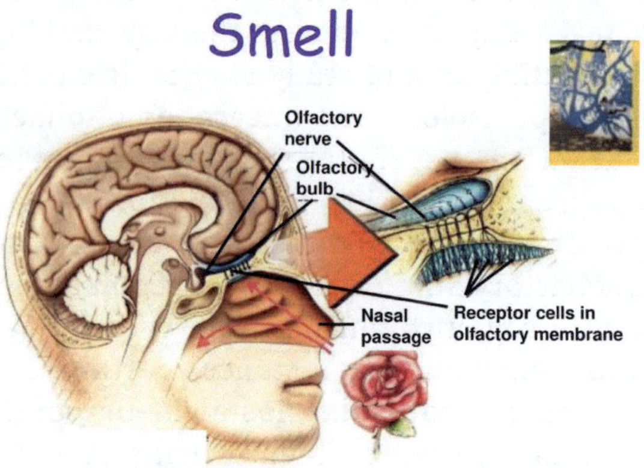

Figure 7.18. Sensation of smell.

Source: https://image3.slideserve.com/5698759/smell-l.jpg.

7.6.1. Process of Odor Detection

The sensation of odor detection begins with the breathing in of air that contains volatile chemical compounds. These molecules are detected by the olfactory epithelium, a specialized tissue that occurs in the nasal cavity. Olfactory receptor neurons are embedded in this epithelium that are responsible for the initial stages of olfactory processing. These olfactory receptor neurons each have cilia that extend into the nasal mucus, in which these receptors bind to specific odorant molecules. This binding triggers a series of biochemical reactions to depolarize the olfactory neurons. The generated electrical impulses are then transported by the axons of these neurons to the olfactory bulb, where initial integration and processing of smell information occur, forming the foundation of further neural pathways in odor detection. Once the impulses reach the olfactory bulb, they are structured and relayed to different primary brain regions, such as the olfactory cortex and the limbic system. This two-way process highlights the unique nature of olfaction, as it is directly connected to memory and emotional brain centers. The limbic system is particularly notable, as it is responsible for the behavioral and emotional responses to odors, which can evoke vivid memories or feelings. The identity and quality of the odors are also interpreted by the olfactory cortex. This complex processing enables subtle discrimination between various odors, which makes it possible for us to detect and respond to a wide range of odorants in the world around us, thereby highlighting the importance of olfaction in survival and social behavior. Beyond the detection of smell is the implication of odor detection of enhancing multimedia experiences using olfactory cues. Current developments in smell-enhanced applications demonstrate the potential in integrating immersive environments with scent for the improvement of user interaction and engagement. This development outlines the long-term applicability of smell research, particularly in neuroscience and technology. While there are issues in the development of effective olfactory displays, the initial findings of olfactions' role in multimodal experiences indicate significant potential for leading future technologies. Through the study of how odors are able to convey information or elicit emotional responses, researchers aim to broaden the knowledge of the complexity of the human sense perception, which may have breakthroughs in branding and virtual narrative, as suggested through advances of smell-enriched multimedia devices (Ademoye et al., 2010; Young et al., 2020).

7.6.2. Mechanism of Olfactory Signal Transduction

The mechanism of olfactory signal transduction is an interplay between dynamic molecular recognition and neural representation that is central to understanding special sense physiology. Olfactory receptors are signaling proteins on the cilia of olfactory sensory neurons. On odorant molecule binding, odorant receptors induce a conformational change activating a G-protein-coupled receptor cascade. This chain of events raises the levels of cyclic adenosine monophosphate (cAMP), which leads to opening of ion channels and thus depolarization of the sensory neuron. The electrical signal produced is subsequently relayed to the olfactory bulb, where further processing occurs. This process demonstrates how physical stimuli—odor molecules—are translated into neural signals for brain interpretation and demonstrates the intricate processes involved in olfactory processing. In spite of the familiar mechanisms of signal transduction in olfaction, the nature of why particular molecules elicit specific smells is not understood. Existing theories, including those suggesting a quantum mechanical basis for smell detection, add a level of complexity not seen in mainstream sensory science. Research indicates smaller molecules binding to large proteins in a way essential to smell perception but tantalizingly evasive in precise description. Others have argued that probing these interactions using new theoretical frameworks can be a source of insight into olfactory science, possibly reconfiguring such frameworks of sensory perception as presently understood. A grasp of these mechanisms is not only explanatory of the olfactory systems operation but potentially closes the circle of understanding to a wider set of physiological processes, including drug-receptor interactions that underlie therapeutic realization (Buck et al., 2010).

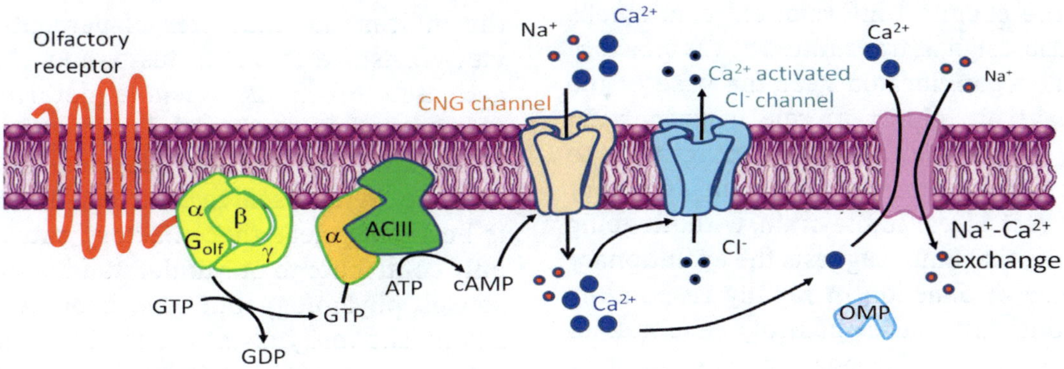

Figure 7.19. A schematic diagram of olfactory signal transduction.

Source: https://www.researchgate.net/profile/Jae-Koo-2/publication/233787858/figure/fig2/AS:669665458151434@1536672095403/A-schematic-diagram-of-olfactory-signal-transduction-Olfactory-signal-transduction.jpg.

In addition, advances in olfactory research have important potential ramifications for a variety of disciplines, from psychophysics to neurobiology. As researchers investigate the olfactory transduction process, they uncover promising lines of inquiry that may ultimately contribute to therapeutic treatment for olfactory dysfunction, disorders that have a profound impact on the quality of life. Interestingly, unraveling the mysteries of olfactory signal transduction also generates fascinating questions regarding the subjective character of smell. If the perception of an individual contributes significantly to olfactory experience, as supported by recent research, it challenges scientists to improve methods of measuring and comprehending olfactory signals objectively (Young et al., 2020). The research in olfactory transduction is, therefore, not only a way to grasp sensory physiology but also a basis for trailblazing research into perception and cognition (Figure 7.19).

7.6.3. Olfactory Pathways to the Brain

The olfactory system stands apart among the sensory modalities by virtue of its access to the brain. When odor molecules are inhaled, they bind to olfactory receptors in the nasal cavity, setting off a series of biochemical events. These olfactory receptors are specialized neurons that convert the chemical information from smells into electrical signals transmitted by the olfactory bulb. This organ, located near the base of the brain, plays an important role in processing olfactory information before sending it on to higher brain regions , such as the olfactory cortex. Direct access to the brain, without going through the thalamus, suggests the evolutionary importance of olfaction in rapidly responding to environmental cues, possibly essential to survival, such as odor perception of food or danger (Young et al., 2020). Following the initial sense of the odor stimuli, the olfactory bulb processes the incoming information and forwards this information to various parts of the brain for odor interpretation and emotional response. For example, input to the piriform cortex, necessary for the identification and discrimination of odors, is provided. Input is also provided to the amygdala and hippocampus, regions central to emotion and memory. Such connectivity forms the foundation of the ability of odors to evoke powerful memories or emotional reactions, often more potent than other senses. These channels demonstrate the integrative and sophisticated character of odor processing, which goes beyond detection and engages a range of cognitive processes and demonstrates how our sense of smell supports our experience of the world (Smith et al., 2015). Olfactory system, while being highly valuable in sensory perception, has been immensely underemphasized when it comes to sensory modalities. In contrast to visual or auditory systems, often given prominence in academic treatments, olfactory systems have traditionally been relegated to secondary or even peripheral status. Recent research contradicts this assertion, maintaining that the chemical senses, of which olfaction is one, are pivotal to a deeper appreciation of the multimodal character of perception. This view insists that smell, taste, and chemically activated touch as a whole determine our sensory experience and flavor perceptions, highlighting the interdependence of the sensory modality. With research evolving, increasingly it is becoming clear that olfactory pathways not only contribute to our understanding of special senses physiology but also provide us with significant insights into the multidimensional process of perception (Young et al., 2020).

Test Your Knowledge

1. How are odor molecules activating olfactory receptors?
2. What occurs when an olfactory receptor neuron is stimulated?

SUMMARY

The physiology of the special senses illuminates the intricate mechanisms of human perception and interaction with the environment. This interplay of sensory stimulation and neural processing forms the basis of cognitive function, facilitating adaptation and survival of the organism. As shown throughout this essay, the physiological features of each sensory system provide unique insight into how sensory information is converted to perceivable experience. This crossover of physiological function and perceptual consequence not only testifies to the intricacies of the sensory systems but also to the stunning adaptability of the human brain in interpreting and responding to diverse stimuli. An understanding of these systems thus forms a foundation upon which further investigation can be based, particularly in neurophysiological situations, where the nuances of sensory perception remain to be unraveled. Moreover, the intersection of physiology and psychology in research on special senses only serves to prove the intricacy of human experience that is defined by sensory capability. Fundamental principles around mythmaking show how mythological narratives can reflect anatomical and physiological features, for instance, cultural depictions of vampires in literature, where physiology brings together elements like speed and power, thereby defining perceptions of reality. As the analysis of the Twilight Saga's Breaking Dawn brings out, the integration of scientific understanding with fictional accounts enriches both fields. Examining how mythical accounts fit sensory abilities provides profound insights into the enduring power of physiology on cultural narratives and the human self. Such intersections require closer examination of how myths affect cultural understanding of sensory experience and meaning. Finally, progressive knowledge in sensory physiology contributes greatly to various fields like psychology, neuroscience, and even technology. Neuronal network research has recently proved mechanisms that show learning and prediction capabilities in sensory systems, and this agrees with the discoveries of the brain's complex processing processes. The development of models like the Inductive Conceptual Network explains the process of complexity in classifying and generalizing sensory inputs as it occurs in biological processes in humans. By addressing the biological plausibility of such models directly, future studies have the potential to deepen our insight into sensory interactions and their implications for human cognition. The union of the knowledge gained via both biological and psychological routes to special senses physiology thus provides avenues for new paradigms in sensory research, clinical practice, and creative arts and also potential pathways to curing sensory processing disorders.

In the study of special senses physiology, it is important to realize the intricate mechanisms by which sensory information is processed by the brain. The special senses of vision, hearing, taste, smell, and touch are mediated by distinct sensory organs that transduce external stimuli into neural signals. The signals are transmitted to the brain, where processing occurs, so perception and response can be enabled. It is also important to know the processing centers and pathways involved, as they can illuminate the conditions that affect sensory function, as represented in most studies. For example, work on the critical properties of the brain implies that it is near a second-order phase transition state, allowing flexibility as well as stability in behavior, which indicates the usefulness of neural plasticity in sensory processing (Buonocore et al., 2008). Furthermore, the brainstem possesses an inaugural role of confluence of sensory input from cranial structures and special senses. It consists of numerous nuclei that are responsible for governing basic body functions as well as being important sites for afferent sensory input. Modulation of sensory tracts within the brainstem not only affects the transmission of information to the higher centers of the cortex but also implications in the pathophysiology of diseases , such as migraine. Specifically, dysfunction of these pathways has been associated with neurovascular symptoms that have implications for the evolutionary and physiological significance of this structure for sensory perception. Remarkably, the inter-sensory interconnectedness is exemplified in the co-morbidity of migraine and motion sickness, which share common neuroanatomical pathways (Cuomo-Granston et al., 2010). Investigating the interface between sensory physiology and neurological disorders reveals a complex interface feeding back into clinical and theoretical accounts. Underlying is recognition that disturbances in the senses have complex implications with impacts on wellbeing in general. As illustrated by studies of motion sickness and migraine, the function of neurotransmitters and neural pathways shows how disturbances in sensory processing can lead to over-sensitivity to specific stimuli. By integrating study findings, we can learn about the processes of sensory states and their broader relevance to health. Thus, a cohesive understanding of special sense physiological specifics emphasizes their relevance not just in day-to-day phenomena but also in clinical presentations of sensory impairment (Cuomo-Granston et al., 2010).

KEY TERMS FROM THIS CHAPTER

- Auditory Pathway
- Cones
- Equilibrium
- Hearing
- Olfactory Receptors
- Organ of Corti
- Retina
- Semicircular Canals
- Special Senses
- Vestibular System
- Cochlea
- Cranial Nerves
- Gustation (Taste)
- Olfaction (Smell)
- Optic Nerve
- Photoreceptors
- Rods
- Sensory Transduction
- Taste Buds
- Vision

CRITICAL THINKING QUESTIONS

1. **Which structure of the eye converges light onto the retina?**
   a. Iris
   b. Lens
   c. Cornea
   d. Optic nerve
2. **The organ of Corti that is used for hearing can be located in which ear structure?**
   a. Outer ear
   b. Middle ear
   c. Cochlea
   d. Semicircular canals
3. **Which cranial nerve is most linked with the sense of smell?**
   a. Optic nerve (CN II)
   b. Olfactory nerve (CN I)
   c. Facial nerve (CN VII)
   d. Glossopharyngeal nerve (CN IX)
4. **Which photoreceptor is used for color vision?**
   a. Rods
   b. Cones
   c. Bipolar cells
   d. Ganglion cells
5. **Which special sense is primarily controlled by the vestibular apparatus of the inner ear?**
   a. Taste
   b. Vision
   c. Balance
   d. Hearing

Short Answer Questions

1. What photoreceptors are responsible for night vision?
2. What is the function of the cochlea in the ear?
3. Which cranial nerve is responsible for the sense of smell?
4. What is the function of the Eustachian tube?
5. Explain the physiology of taste sensation and the function of the taste buds.
6. Explain the olfactory pathway and mechanism of odor detection.
7. Compare the structure and function of rods and cones of the retina.
8. Explain how sound waves are converted to electrical signals in the cochlea.

Answers to Critical Thinking Questions

1. (b); 2. (c); 3. (b); 4. (b); 5. (c)

REFERENCES

1. Nellis, M. E., Spinella, P. C., Tucci, M., Stanworth, S. J., Steiner, M. E., Cushing, M. M., Davis, P. J., Karam, O., & Pediatric Acute Lung Injury and Sepsis Investigators (PALISI) network, Pediatric Critical Care Blood Research Network (BloodNet), and the P3T Investigators† (2020). Effect of platelet storage duration on clinical outcomes and incremental platelet change in critically ill children. *Transfusion*, *60*(12), 2849–2858. https://doi.org/10.1111/trf.16094(accessed on 16th June 2025).
2. Abu Kasim, N. H., Alabsi, A. M., Haque, N., Rahman, N. A., et al. (2014). Hypoxic culture conditions as a solution for mesenchymal stem cell based regenerative therapy. https://core.ac.uk/download/30437779.pdf (accessed on 16th June 2025).
3. Adams, R., Ahmed, S., Anbalagan, M., Annunziata, M., Antonyak, M., Bain, G., Barbarulo, A., et al. (2013). JNK signaling in cancer: In need of new, smarter therapeutic targets. https://core.ac.uk/download/29139231.pdf (accessed on 16th June 2025).
4. Agas, D., Douni, E., Marchetti, L., & Sabbieti, M. G. (2015). The unbearable lightness of bone marrow homeostasis. https://core.ac.uk/download/54653580.pdf (accessed on 16th June 2025).
5. Aidun, C. K., Clausen, J. R., Liu, Z., Rao, A., et al. (2019). A unified analysis of nano-to-microscale particle dispersion in tubular blood flow. http://arxiv.org/abs/1905.11202 (accessed on 16th June 2025).
6. Robles, T. F., & Kane, H. S. (2014). The attachment system and physiology in adulthood: normative processes, individual differences, and implications for health. *Journal of personality*, *82*(6), 515–527. https://doi.org/10.1111/jopy.12052Allen, J., & Kyriacou, P. A. (2024). Advances in basic and applied research in photoplethysmography. https://core.ac.uk/download/610735098.pdf (accessed on 16th June 2025).
7. Alleva, E., Angiulli, E., Cioni, C., Malavasi, V., et al. (2017). Variation in environmental parameters in research and aquaculture: Effects on behavior, physiology and cell biology of teleost fish. https://core.ac.uk/download/153366757.pdf (accessed on 16th June 2025).
8. Altman, P. L., & Fisher, K. D. (1986). *Research Opportunities in Nutrition and Metabolism in Space*. https://core.ac.uk/download/pdf/10458014.pdf (accessed on 16th June 2025).
9. Andersen, M., Benevenga, N., Berlin, J., Beynon, R., Bier, D., Blagoev, B., Brakebusch, C., et al. (2008). Silac mouse for quantitative proteomics uncovers kindlin-3 as an essential factor for red blood cell function. https://core.ac.uk/download/18492217.pdf (accessed on 16th June 2025).
10. Arun, P. R., K. V., Rajashree, P., Venkatakrishna, M. K. S., & Vinushree, V. (2024). Understanding of Pranavaha Sroto Moola in the purview of modern physiology. https://core.ac.uk/download/617189952.pdf (accessed on 16th June 2025).
11. Ballarino, M., Fatica, A., & Morlando, M. (2015). Long non-coding RNAs: New players in hematopoiesis and leukemia. https://core.ac.uk/download/54520197.pdf (accessed on 16th June 2025).
12. Balola, A. H. A., Bartolmäs, T., Mayer, B., Salama, A., et al. (2019). Sub lytic terminal complement components induce eryptosis in autoimmune hemolytic anemia related to IgM autoantibodies. https://core.ac.uk/download/286567997.pdf (accessed on 16th June 2025).

13. Baum, H., Brochet, J. P., Buhagiar, G., Charilaou, A., et al. (2012). The EC4 European syllabus for post-graduate training in clinical chemistry and laboratory medicine: Version 4-2012. https://core.ac.uk/download/227992301.pdf (accessed on 16th June 2025).

14. Bicer, S., Clark, Y., Devine, R. D., Jing, X., et al. (2015). Losartan treatment attenuates tumor-induced myocardial dysfunction. https://core.ac.uk/download/213059445.pdf (accessed on 16th June 2025).

15. Bich, L., Moreau, J. F., & Pradeu, T. (2019). Understanding multicellularity: The functional organization of the intercellular space. https://core.ac.uk/download/228134961.pdf (accessed on 16th June 2025).

16. Birch, R. E., Peppiatt-Wildman, C. M., Schwiebert, E. M., Wildman, S. S., et al. (2013). Emerging key roles for P2X receptors in the kidney. https://core.ac.uk/download/30711999.pdf (accessed on 16th June 2025).

17. Brenes, A., Hettyey, A., Kelber, A., Kistler, A., Reppert, A. K., Davis, A. K., Brenes-Soto, A., et al. (2017). Coloration in amphibians as a reflection of nutritional status: The case of tree frogs in Costa Rica. https://core.ac.uk/download/91292641.pdf (accessed on 16th June 2025).

18. Brown, R. L., & Clarke, T. B. (2016). The regulation of host defenses to infection by the microbiota. https://core.ac.uk/download/77016328.pdf (accessed on 16th June 2025).

19. Brownlee, I., & Seal, C. J. (2015). Whole-grain foods and chronic disease: Evidence from epidemiological and intervention studies. https://core.ac.uk/download/287613637.pdf (accessed on 16th June 2025).

20. Buta, A., Danciu, C., Ognean, L., Spătariu, A., et al. (2019). Controversies regarding compatibility in Xeno transfusion with blood from dog to cat (Review). https://core.ac.uk/download/267071041.pdf (accessed on 16th June 2025).

21. Cala, P. M., & Maldonado, H. M. (1994). pH regulatory Na/H exchange by *Amphiuma* red blood cells. https://core.ac.uk/download/323069890.pdf (accessed on 16th June 2025).

22. Cavarretta, E., Dal Sasso, E., Forte, M., Frati, G., et al. (2017). The light and shadow of senescence and inflammation in cardiovascular pathology and regenerative medicine. https://core.ac.uk/download/141694265.pdf (accessed on 16th June 2025).

23. Cerliani, M. B., Gili, J. A., Klein, G., Pavicic, M., et al. (2015). Association between *PER3* length polymorphism and onco-hematological diseases and its influence on patient's functionality. https://core.ac.uk/download/153567200.pdf (accessed on 16th June 2025).

24. Chan, Y. Y., Kurzrock, E. A., Osborn, S. L., Sandlin, R. D., et al. (2017). The current use of stem cells in bladder tissue regeneration and bioengineering. https://core.ac.uk/download/323068966.pdf (accessed on 16th June 2025).

25. Chollet, M. E., Harrison, S. P., Lauritzen, K. H., Roman, M., et al. (2023). iPSC-derived liver organoids and inherited bleeding disorders: Potential and future perspectives. https://core.ac.uk/download/614769142.pdf (accessed on 16th June 2025).

26. Christie, D. A., Tansey, E. M., & Zallen, D. T. (2004). The Rhesus factor and disease prevention. https://core.ac.uk/download/30696199.pdf (accessed on 16th June 2025).

27. Claramunt Lozano, A., Gavaldá Esteve, C., & Sarrión Pérez, M. G. (2011). Dental management in patients with hemostasis alteration. https://core.ac.uk/download/71058980.pdf (accessed on 16th June 2025).

28. Collado-Boira, E., Hernando, B., Martínez-Navarro, I., Panizo, N., et al. (2019). Cardiac damage biomarkers and heart rate variability following a 118-km mountain race: Relationship with performance and recovery. https://core.ac.uk/download/232116702.pdf (accessed on 16th June 2025).

29. Compernolle, V., Feys, H., & Six, K. (2020). Platelet biochemistry and morphology after cryopreservation. https://core.ac.uk/download/287941861.pdf (accessed on 16th June 2025).

30. Crispin, A. (2017). HSCB, a co-chaperone in mitochondrial iron-sulfur cluster biogenesis, is a novel candidate gene for congenital sideroblastic anemia. https://open.bu.edu/bitstream/2144/26669/5/Crispin_bu_0017N_13280.pdf (accessed on 16th June 2025).

31. Ellis-Lepard, K. (2018). Does hydration impact memory: A systematic review. https://core.ac.uk/download/215462394.pdf (accessed on 16th June 2025).

32. Garshnek, V., Hooke, L. R., Radtke, M., Rowe, J., et al. (2025). *USSR Space Life Sciences Digest*, issue 3. https://core.ac.uk/download/pdf/42842161.pdf (accessed on 16th June 2025).

33. Garshnek, V., Hooke, L. R., Rowe, J., & Teeter, R., et al. (2025). *USSR Space Life Sciences Digest*, issue 31. https://core.ac.uk/download/pdf/42816647.pdf (accessed on 16th June 2025).

34. Helm, B., & Martinez-Bakker, M. (2015). The influence of biological rhythms on host–parasite interactions. https://core.ac.uk/download/42361213.pdf (accessed on 16th June 2025).

35. Herms, J., Kretzschmar, H. A., & Vassallo, N. (2004). The molecular pathology of prion diseases. https://core.ac.uk/download/46601891.pdf (accessed on 16th June 2025).

36. Heusner, W. W., & Vanhuss, W. D. (1979). Space flight research relevant to health, physical education, and recreation: With particular reference to Skylab's life science experiments. https://core.ac.uk/download/pdf/10345816.pdf (accessed on 16th June 2025).

37. Holtby, R. J., Jahr, J. S., & Roghani, K. (2014). Effects of hemoglobin-based oxygen carriers on blood coagulation. https://core.ac.uk/download/323078517.pdf (accessed on 16th June 2025).

38. Hooke, L. R., & Teeter, R. (2025). *USSR Space Life Sciences Digest. Index to Issues 1–4*. https://core.ac.uk/download/pdf/42841024.pdf (accessed on 16th June 2025).

39. Hurst, R. A. (2014). The effects and differences of sprint interval training, endurance training and the training types combined on physiological parameters and exercise performance. https://core.ac.uk/download/29841767.pdf (accessed on 16th June 2025).

40. Hutchins, B. R., Brown, J., Buchwald, D., Clarke, D., D., D., et al. (2015). Descartes, corpuscles and reductionism: Mechanism and systems in Descartes' physiology. https://core.ac.uk/download/147061302.pdf (accessed on 16th June 2025).

41. Ibañez, A. E., Larsen, K. E., Montalti, D., Najle, R., et al. (2015). Hematology, biochemistry and serum protein analyses of Antarctic and non-Antarctic skuas. https://core.ac.uk/download/161267705.pdf (accessed on 16th June 2025).

42. Li, S. C., Li, Z., Ran, Q., Wu, Y., et al. (2018). The differentiation balance of bone marrow mesenchymal stem cells is crucial to hematopoiesis. https://core.ac.uk/download/323062656.pdf (accessed on 16th June 2025).

43. Oliveira, S. de, & Saldanha, C. (2010). An overview about erythrocyte membrane. https://core.ac.uk/download/12426151.pdf (accessed on 16th June 2025).

44. Pal, R., Chatterjee, P. K., Chatterjee, P., Vinodini, N. A., PrasannaMithra, S., Banerjee, S., Suman, V. B., et al. (2014). Polycystic ovary syndrome, blood group & diet: A correlative study in South Indian females. https://core.ac.uk/download/pdf/27151617.pdf (accessed on 16th June 2025).

45. Pimienta, M., Edderkaoui, M., Wang, R., & Pandol, S. (2017). The potential for circulating tumor cells in pancreatic cancer management. https://core.ac.uk/download/323077820.pdf (accessed on 16th June 2025).

46. Prasad, N. K., Dubey, S., & Tripathi, R. (2023). A critical review on *Samana Vayu* apropos regulation of gastrointestinal tract. https://core.ac.uk/download/617189551.pdf (accessed on 16th June 2025).

47. Rawling, B. (2012). Providing the gift of life: Canadian medical practitioners and the treatment of shock on the battlefield. https://core.ac.uk/download/143686944.pdf (accessed on 16th June 2025).

48. Ross, A. P., & Zarbalis, K. S. (2014). The emerging roles of ribosome biogenesis in craniofacial development. https://core.ac.uk/download/323070204.pdf (accessed on 16th June 2025).

49. Rowe, J., Stone, L. R., & Teeter, R. (2025). *USSR Space Life Sciences Digest*, issue 30. https://core.ac.uk/download/pdf/42817408.pdf (accessed on 16th June 2025).

50. Stotts, N. A., & Wong, V. K. (2003). Physiology and prevention of heel ulcers: The state of science. https://core.ac.uk/download/70426031.pdf (accessed on 16th June 2025).

51. The Boston University Photonics Center. (2015). *The Boston University Photonics Center Annual Report 2014–2015*. https://open.bu.edu/bitstream/2144/29753/1/Photonics-Center-Annual-Report-2015-final.pdf (accessed on 16th June 2025).

52. Torday J. S. (2015). Homeostasis as the Mechanism of Evolution. *Biology*, *4*(3), 573–590. https://doi.org/10.3390/biology4030573(accessed on 16th June 2025).

BLOOD PHYSIOLOGY

8

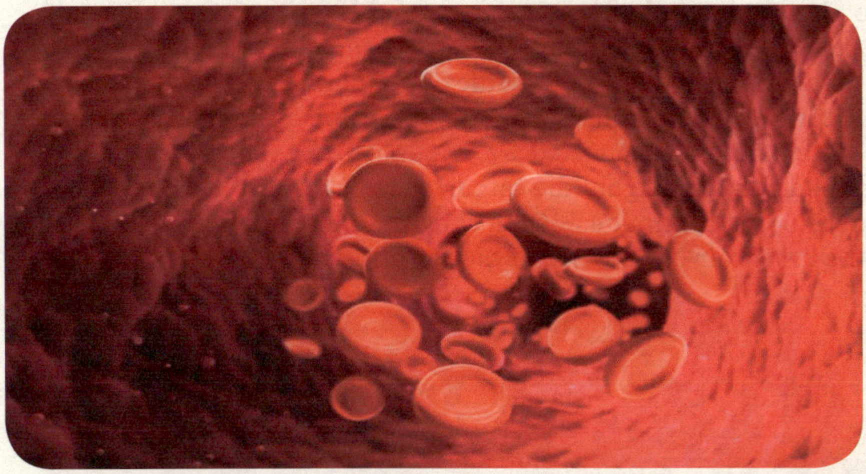

LEARNING OBJECTIVES

After studying this chapter, you will be able to:

1. Describe the structure of blood;
2. Describe the roles played by blood;
3. Describe the hematopoiesis;
4. Highlight the blood disorders;
5. Learn blood typing and transfusion;
6. Evaluate the advancements in blood research.

Introduction

Blood physiology is a vital area of study within the broader field of human biology in the sense that it tries to determine the complex functions and properties of blood. Central to this inquiry is the understanding of the circulation of blood in the body, the distribution of essential nutrients and oxygen to cells, and concurrently, the elimination of by-products. Blood contains a number of distinct components, i.e., red blood cells, white blood cells, platelets, and plasma, each with distinct but complementary functions. Red blood cells, for instance, carry oxygen using hemoglobin, while plasma offers a transport mechanism for nutrients, hormones, and proteins. Understanding these factors and their individual functions gives tremendous understanding of how blood physiology is capable of maintaining homeostasis, particularly in response to physiological stressors or pathophysiologic disease states that would compromise normal circulation or oxygen delivery. Additionally, blood physiology exists in intimate association with other body physiologic systems, clearly illustrating its importance to general well-being. The cardiovascular system, for example, works synergistically with the blood to regulate the pressure of blood and achieve optimal circulation. Changes in blood volume and viscosity also have a direct impact on cardiovascular function, overall body health. Space biology has had much to take these correlations into account; research has underscored the significance of hematology in addressing altering loads of gravity that become apparent during space travel. The reactions observed in astronauts illustrate the degree to which blood physiology is influenced by external forces, with a dynamic interaction between blood components and the outside world. Thus, having a thorough understanding of blood physiology is not merely a scholarly objective, but a vital component in the learning of human resilience and health in different conditions, such as in space flight. In clinical and health contexts, innovations in studies of blood physiology have created significant implications on medical practice, particularly in hematology and transfusion medicine. Current knowledge about blood constituents and their functions allows for the refinement of diagnostic techniques and therapeutic intervention aimed at treating blood disorders , such as anemia or clotting deficiency. Furthermore, studies of the immunology of blood teach one about how various blood cells can be used to enhance immune reaction against infections or even neoplasms. Current research in hematology, supported by evidence from sources with an orientation towards space biology and medicine, highlights the importance of blood physiology in informing interventions for health. By developing continuously in this direction, we not just enhance clinical results but also contribute to the reservoir of knowledge that informs future research and medical advancements (Figure 8.1).

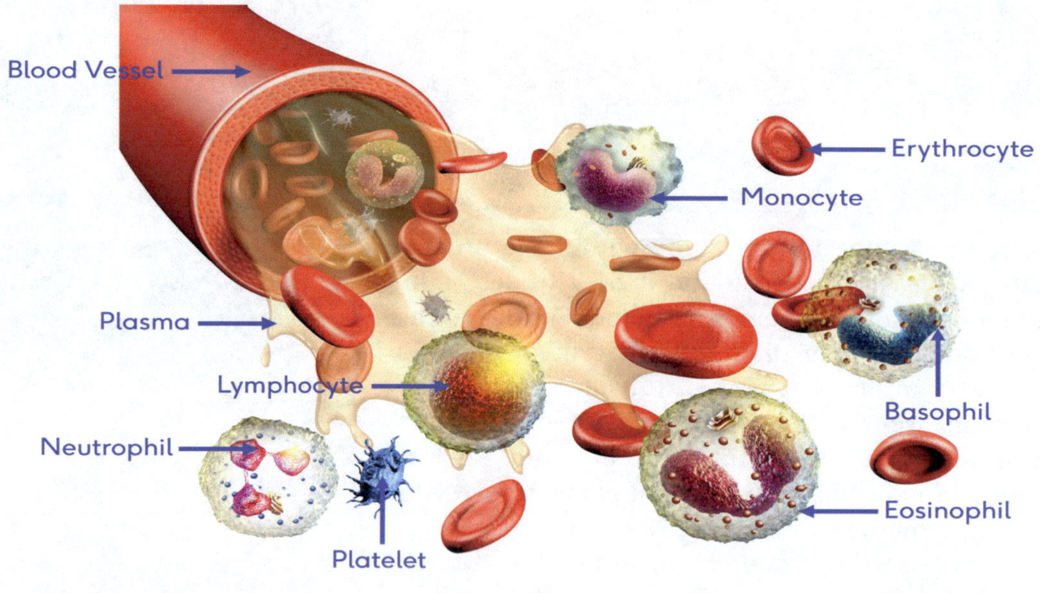

Figure 8.1. Blood physiology.

Source: https://www.physio-pedia.com/images/thumb/5/55/Blood_with_description.png/1000px-Blood_with_description.png.

Definition and Importance of Blood

Blood is a connective tissue within the human body and is primarily composed of plasma, red blood cells, white blood cells, and platelets. Its fundamental role is to carry essential materials, including oxygen and nutrients, to the tissues and eliminate metabolic waste products. The blend is intricate, and through it, various physiological processes are capable of functioning efficiently, maintaining homeostasis. For instance, erythrocytes are the red blood cells that transport hemoglobin, a protein charged with the responsibility of binding oxygen and delivering it to tissues. White blood cells are also integral to the immune system, serving to defend the body against infection and foreign invaders. The fine balance of these cellular constituents is a quintessential example of the varied definition of blood and serves to underscore its integral place in keeping us alive. Aside from its transport roles, blood controls various essential physiological parameters. Its most important role is thermoregulation, which ensures the body's core temperature is kept at an optimal level. Heat produced by metabolic processes in cells is dissipated through blood circulation all over the body, thus allowing homeostasis even under changing environmental conditions. Blood is also crucial in keeping pH levels and osmotic pressures in check, which are important for cellular function. As stated, blood volume and circulation are totally reliant on body levels of hydration, linking the function of water to blood physiology. Proper hydration is what keeps blood volume intact, enhancing circulation and enabling all organ systems to achieve correct oxygenation and nutrients, hence identifying the connection between these vital factors and the general role of blood in physiological health (Ellis-Lepard et al., 2018). Finally, the function of blood extends beyond transportation and regulation; it is also of particular importance in other repair processes, most significantly where injury is concerned. When damaged tissue is injured, platelets aggregate to form a clot, which is known as hemostasis, and stops blood loss in excess while allowing future healing. Additionally, blood plasma carries many proteins, such as clotting factors that aid in this process and contribute to the healing of broken tissues. The ability of blood to regenerate highlights its importance in recovery and overall health. Recent research emphasizes the importance of quality composition and circulation of blood towards mitigating the risk of lifestyle-related diseases, with a new, suggested enhanced comprehension of blood physiology potentially translating to new fronts in therapy (Brownlee et al., 2015). Such multi-faceted appreciation of blood solidifies its irreplaceable role as both transport medium and dynamic partner in the body's healing processes.

Overview of Blood Components

The composition of blood is intricate and vital to its different physiological functions. Blood is predominantly constituted by plasma and formed elements, namely red blood cells, white blood cells, and platelets. Plasma, which constitutes about 55% of the volume of blood, is a yellowish-colored liquid with a high concentration of protein, nutrient, hormone, and waste. It is the medium of carriage of these contents within the body. The plasma proteins , such as albumin, globulins, and fibrinogen play critical roles in osmotic pressure maintenance, immune function, and clotting. Understanding this structure organization and how it functions is crucial to realizing the manner in which the blood behaves as an aggregate to ensure homeostasis in the body. Red blood cells (RBCs) are the most abundant blood constituent and are pivotal in oxygen and carbon dioxide transport. Biconcave cells, in their mature state, with no nuclei or organelles have a large surface area-to-volume ratio, enabling them to maximize gas exchange. Hemoglobin in RBCs captures oxygen in lungs and distributes it in tissues. New studies have elucidated the intricacy of the erythrocytes cellular membrane, showing evidence of the expression of a variety of adhesion molecules to mediate interactions with other cell types, e.g., endothelial cells. These findings suggest that erythrocytes play functions beyond the mere transportation of oxygen, and there are possible effects on the understanding of their functions in pathological mechanisms , such as inflammation and thrombosis (Oliveira et al., 2010). Platelets or thrombocytes are another crucial component of blood, with their primary function being hemostasis—prevention and cessation of bleeding. With injury to blood vessels, platelets adhere to the site and become activated, which results in the release of chemical messengers that pull other platelets and form a tight clot. In addition to their role in clotting, platelets have emerged as dynamic participants in immune responses and repair processes. Their interactions with other blood constituents further emphasize the sophistication of blood physiology. This intricate dance among blood constituents highlights the imperative for cooperation of function in order to promote physiological equilibrium, any derangement threatening disastrous consequences like hemorrhage or thrombotic disease (Bich et al., 2019) (Figure 8.2).

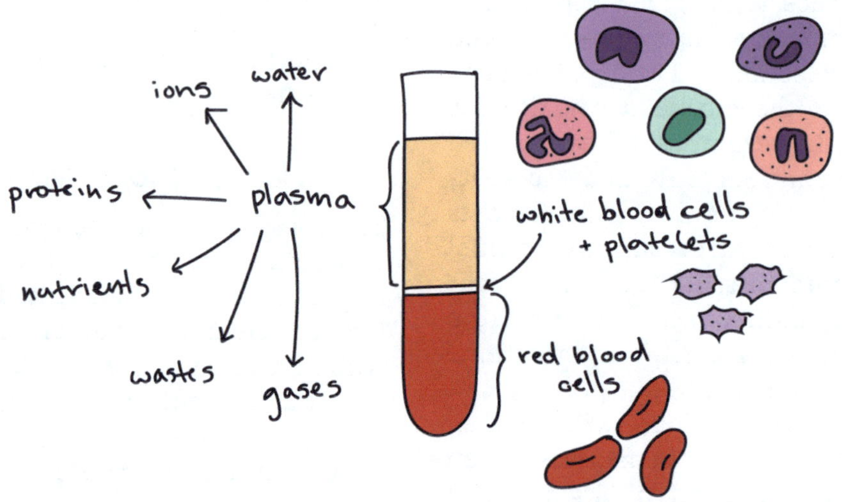

Figure 8.2. Components of blood.

Source: https://cdn.kastatic.org/ka-perseus-images/8b58582c697c7bc7cc83755edbb599218f8164fe.png.

Purpose of Studying Blood Physiology

Physiology of blood is a central pillar in learning human disease and health. It encompasses the study of blood components, such as red blood cells, white blood cells, plasma, and platelets, each with singular yet interdependent functions in maintaining homeostasis. A detailed understanding of blood physiology enables health care professionals to diagnose and manage a long list of disorders, from anemia to disorders of coagulation. In addition, understanding the physiological responses of blood can provide insights into mechanisms behind systemic responses to stressors, whether physiological, such as exercise, or pathological, such as infection. For instance, information from experiencing the reaction of blood with alterations in the degree of physical activity is very effective in enhancing patient care practices, particularly in the framework of rehabilitative procedures, affirming the central role that blood physiology occupies in the practice of medicine and in clinical investigation

(Heusner et al., 1979). In addition, blood physiology plays a critical role in the practice of sports medicine and exercise science. Blood work parameter analysis can provide useful information regarding an athlete's metabolic condition and overall cardiovascular wellness. Some biomarkers, such as cardiac troponins and B-type natriuretic peptides, have been shown to be correlated with exertion levels and recovery needs following endurance exercise.

As an example, a recent study depicted the remarkable alterations in biomarkers of cardiac damage and heart rate variability following a mountain ultramarathon, highlighting the importance of understanding these parameters for tailored training and recovery protocols (Martínez-Navarro et al., 2019). The findings from such physiological assessment not only help maximize physical performance but also enhance recovery protocols so that athletes are able to recover efficiently between contests. Finally, the uses of blood physiology extend beyond the context of medicine, reaching out to populations , such as public health and epidemiology. Comparing the blood parameters within various populations can establish the trends of hematological health and potential disease epidemics and recommend prevention strategies. For instance, knowledge of how the elements in blood respond to environmental changes , such as altitude or weather, can inform general health programs based on populations. In addition, ongoing research into blood physiology can lead to new breakthroughs in modalities of treatment, particularly for conditions associated with blood disorders. Through a deep understanding of blood physiology, health practitioners and researchers can contribute towards better health outcomes, which highlights the fundamental role that this area of study has towards individual patient care and population health management (Figure 8.3).

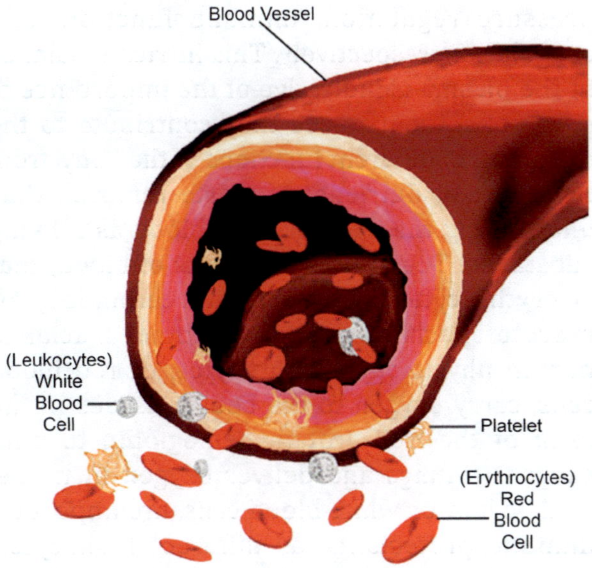

Figure 8.3. Purpose of studying blood physiology.

Source: https://www.vhlab.umn.edu/atlas/physiology-tutorial/graphics/blood.jpg.

8.1. Composition of Blood

Learning Outcome

1. Define the plasma: the liquid matrix;
2. Highlight cellular constituents: red blood cells, white blood cells, and platelets;
3. Investigate electrolytes and proteins in blood.

Blood composition is a complicated subject that requires an understanding of various components which work in unison to sustain physiological processes. Blood is composed predominantly of plasma, which occupies about 55% of its content, and formed elements, including red blood cells, white blood cells, and platelets. Plasma is itself a sophisticated liquid containing water, electrolytes, proteins, hormones, and waste materials, allowing for an environment necessary for transport and biochemical processes. Of great importance are proteins , such as albumin, globulins, and fibrinogen, with essential roles in osmotic pressure regulation, immune function, and coagulation, respectively. This intricate balance in the plasma is indicative of the importance of such constituents since they contribute to the execution of different functions of the body, from transport of nutrients to waste removal, thus underlining the dynamism of blood as a living substance. The formed elements of blood, that is, erythrocytes, leukocytes, and thrombocytes, execute special and vital functions crucial to human physiology. Erythrocytes, or red blood cells, carry oxygen to the body's tissues in the form of the iron-protein hemoglobin to bind oxygen in lungs and deliver oxygen in tissue. Leukocytes, or white blood cells, are important immune protectants, as different leukocytes, such as lymphocytes and neutrophils, specialize in infection and disease combat. Platelets, or thrombocytes, are involved in hemostasis because they aggregate at the point of injury and facilitate clotting. The interaction among the formed elements shows how the blood not only functions in transportation and regulation but is also an essential line of defense against invasion by pathogens, once again demonstrating the intricacy of blood composition. An understanding of blood composition extends beyond individual components to encompass how these elements work within the larger scheme of physiology. Systemic circulation, for instance, relies on the efficient circulation of blood within the cardiovascular system and has an influence on processes throughout the body, such as thermoregulation and pH regulation. An integrated understanding of blood physiology must also take into consideration the homeostatic regulation that maintains it. In further pursuit of this objective, studies on the composition of blood have also explained relationships between organ function and blood parameters, as seen in research linking hemostatic factors to underlying illness. As is indicated in research like the one summarized in NASA's USSR Space Life Sciences Digest, the study of blood and its components continues to progress, providing critical data on the interrelatedness of blood physiology with the overall biological systems, affirming its central role in life support (Garshnek et al., 1980) (Figure 8.4).

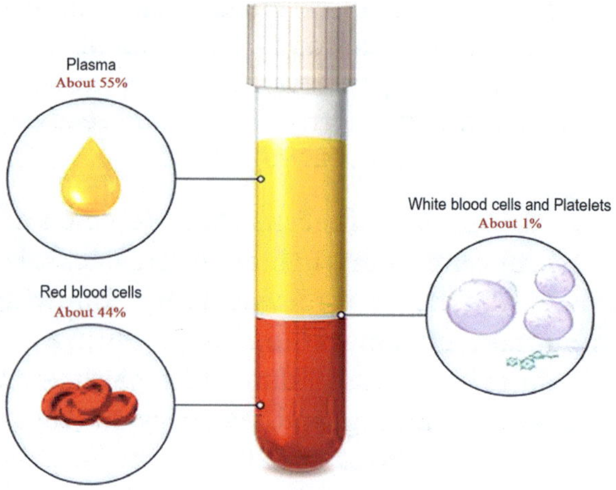

Figure 8.4. Composition of blood.

Source: https://www.hematology.org/-/media/hematology/images/patients/blood-composition.png?la=en&h=501&w=872&hash=04A91A7CB1617CEB0595141AA9C10955.

8.1.1. Plasma: The Liquid Matrix

Plasma structure, also known as the liquid matrix of blood, plays a significant role in the maintenance of homeostasis and the continuation of various physiological processes. Composed primarily of water that accounts for approximately 90% of plasma volume, plasma serves as a solvent for various solutes like electrolytes, nutrients, hormones, and waste products. Plasma proteins , such as albumin, globulins, and fibrinogen also contribute to colloidal osmotic pressure, facilitating transport of materials through the circulatory system. This intricate mixture not only helps in the exchange of gases and nutrients but also in maintaining blood pressure and volume. Therefore, it is important to learn about the plasma dynamics in order to understand the overall blood physiology, particularly given correlations with composition and disease states. The regulatory functions of the plasma are particularly emphasized in reference to hemostasis and immune response. Plasma contains a variety of proteins crucial for immune processes, including immunoglobulins and coagulation factors. The existence of the proteins enables plasma to effectively react to damage and infection. For instance, the coagulation cascade initiated by the plasma proteins is a fundamental process that prevents excessive blood loss following vascular injury. Also, plasma constituent alterations, such as occur in inflammatory processes, demonstrate its adaptive reactions to physiological injury. These alterations exert an immense impact on the functional potential of circulating immune cells and platelets, reflecting plasma's status as an active component of blood physiology with a proactive role in the body's defense responses. As a result of novel therapeutic uses, plasma constituent manipulation is being investigated more and more in clinical research. For example, the use of cryopreserved platelets is a significant advancement in blood storage and transfusion protocols. Platelets are maintained by cryopreservation techniques, improved by the discovery of dimethylsulfoxide as a cryoprotectant, and can be stored for extended periods while retaining some function. Remaining challenges include, among others, elucidation of how cryopreservation affects platelet morphology and function. Evidence is present that cryopreserved platelets can acquire a procoagulant phenotype, and significance to their use in trauma contexts where rapid hemostatic activity is of prime concern. But clinical heterogeneity of use requires greater investigation, underlining the complex interaction between plasma constituents and their role in health and disease (Bicer et al., 2015; Compernolle et al., 2020) (Figure 8.5).

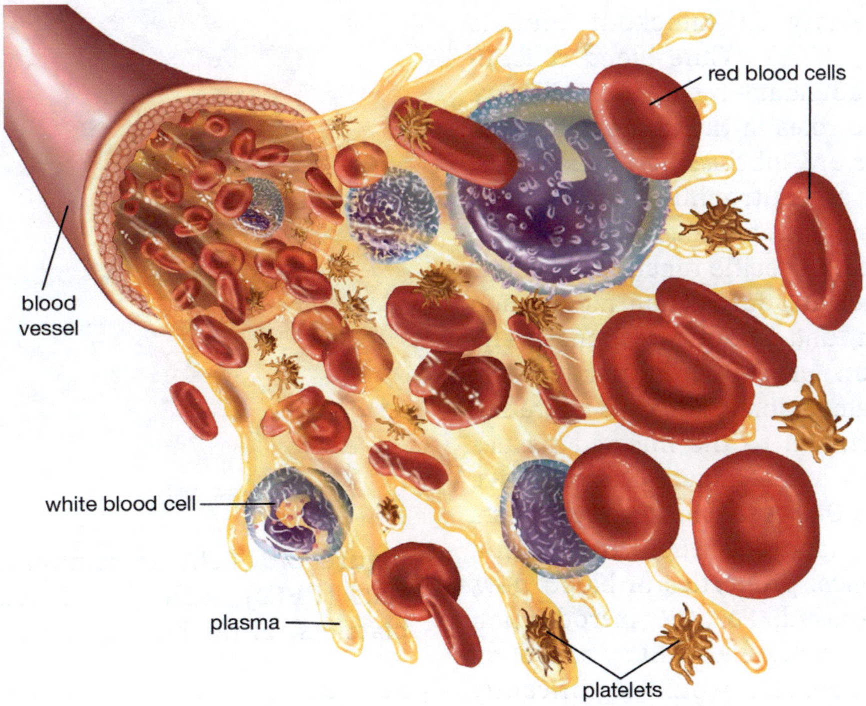

Figure 8.5. Blood-components-blood-cells-platelets-plasma-white.

Source: https://cdn.britannica.com/71/91871-050-30DCD54D/Blood-components-blood-cells-platelets-plasma-white.jpg.

8.1.2. Cellular Components: Red Blood Cells (RBCs), White Blood Cells (WBCs), and Platelets

The cellular components of blood are primarily composed of RBCs, WBCs, and platelets, each having special but synergistic roles in the maintenance of overall physiological integrity. Red blood cells, as biconcave disks, are tasked with the transport of oxygen from the lungs to peripheral tissues and return transport of carbon dioxide to the lungs. The unique structure of RBCs offers an extensive surface area for gas exchange and the absence of organelles leaves space for more hemoglobin content, adding to their ability to carry oxygen. It is necessary to comprehend how RBCs work, particularly how abnormalities within their structure lead to pathologies in the efficiency of oxygen transport, as highlighted by research that employs methods , such as SILAC to investigate red blood cell membrane integrity in knockout models (Andersen et al., 2008). White blood cells, in contrast to the abundant red blood cells, are crucial protective roles in the immune system. These leukocytes are subclassified into several subtypes , such as neutrophils, lymphocytes, monocytes, eosinophils, and basophils, each of which is assigned a specific function , such as pathogen detection and destruction, modulation of inflammation, and allergic response. The migratory action of WBCs is particularly significant in inflammation where their migration from the bloodstream to the infected tissues gives information to the innate and adaptive immune function. One of the interesting aspects of leukocyte transport is their interaction with the rheological properties of blood flow, which are size-based. For the introduction of microscale particles like RBCs, based on research, their behavior would significantly vary due to effects of margination under the influence of red blood cell concentration and dynamics in blood flow (Aidun et al., 2019). Platelets, or thrombocytes, are the blood's smallest cellular elements and are of central importance in hemostasis, the development of a blood clot. Platelets adhere to the site of injury of a vessel, rapidly becoming activated and aggregating to form a temporary plug that prevents over-bleeding. This platelet aggregation not only arrests the bleeding but also initiates the cascade of reactions leading to the formation of a stable fibrin clot. Furthermore, platelets are not mere inert particles; they release various growth factors and cytokines that allow repair of tissue and modulation of inflammation. Their functional efficiency is crucial in various physiological and pathological states, where platelet number or function changes can lead to thrombotic disease or haemorrhagic disorders, emphasizing their significance in the physiology of the blood (Figure 8.6).

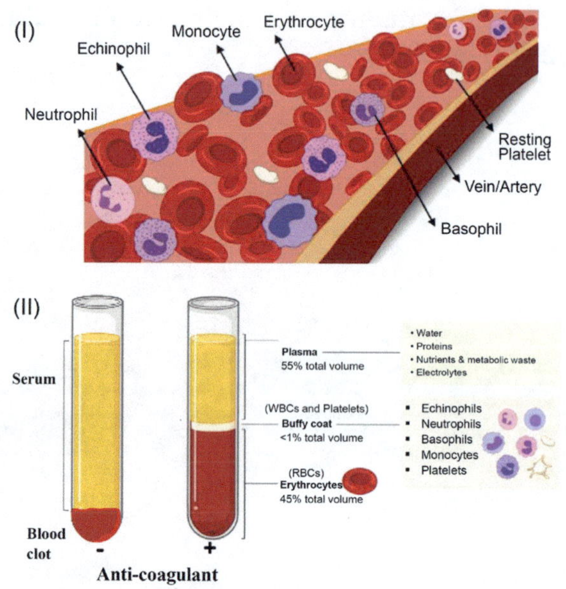

Figure 8.6. Cellular components (Red blood cells (RBCs), white blood cells (WBCs), and platelets) of the human blood.

Source: https://www.researchgate.net/profile/Anusuya-Pal/publication/369134181/figure/fig3/AS:11431281163602270@1685594398452/I-Cellular-components-RBCs-WBCs-and-platelets-of-the-human-blood-transported.png.

8.1.3. Electrolytes and Proteins in Blood

Electrolytes are essential for attaining blood homeostasis, influencing many physiological processes significantly. These cations, such as sodium, potassium, calcium, and chloride, are essential in fluid balance regulation, transmission, and muscle contraction of nerve impulses. Concentration of blood electrolytes is tightly controlled through dietary and renal mechanisms, e.g., sodium is crucial in maintaining blood pressure and volume high, while potassium is extremely crucial for normal cardiac function. Electrolyte imbalances lead to acute conditions like hypertension or arrhythmias. An awareness of electrolyte dynamics is hence indispensable when it comes to comprehending larger blood physiology, i.e., in terms of how these ions contribute to the overall physiological balance and reaction to physiological stressors of the body as well as ensure critical functions at their optimal levels of operation. Blood proteins, which are predominantly found in plasma, perform diverse and critical functions irreplaceable for overall health. The most prominent blood proteins are albumin, globulins, and fibrinogen, each performing an osmotic balancing function, immune function, and coagulation, respectively. The most abundant plasma protein is albumin, which is responsible for maintaining oncotic pressure as well as the transport of numerous substances like hormones, vitamins, and medication. Globulins are an important part of immune function that are made up of antibodies that recognize and disable pathogens. Understanding the relationship between protein concentration and bodily response is also provided through research that compares how proteins respond to different biological conditions. For example, protein concentration changes can reflect nutritional or health issues, and their importance has been indicated in blood physiology as well as in the general assessment of health, based on various physiological studies (Brenes et al., 2017). The multifaceted interaction among electrolytes and proteins enhances blood's capacity to respond against metabolic changes and external stimuli. For instance, the albumin binding with electrolytes influences their distribution and activity. The albumins binding capacity can determine the overall availability of electrolytes and thereby influence physiological effects. Additionally, some of the conditions that cause electrolyte derangement may lead to consequential alterations in protein synthesis or degradation with the generation of feedback loops that require close monitoring in the clinical environment. Studies , such as those conducted by LSRO for nutritional requirements in space, or for the study of amphibian coloration in physiological terms, demonstrates the interconnectedness of proteins, electrolytes, and overall metabolic needs (Altman et al., 1986). These relationships are not only explored to advance our understanding of blood physiology but also help in clinical practice aimed at maintaining good overall health and preventing disorders resulting from imbalance in blood composition.

Test Your Knowledge

1. What are the key constituents of blood?
2. Which cells of the blood transport oxygen?

8.2. Functions of Blood

Learning Outcome

1. Explain the transport of gas, nutrients, and waste;
2. Define body temperature regulation and pH control;
3. Explain immune response and defense mechanisms.

Blood has a variety of vital functions to perform within the human body, each of which contributes toward making a basic contribution towards homeostasis and health. Primarily, blood is the primary medium of transport that carries oxygen from the lungs to tissue and carbon dioxide from tissue to the lungs to be expelled. This transport is required for cellular respiration, which enables cells to generate energy. Blood carries nutrients from the digestive system to various body cells while, simultaneously, removing metabolic waste products and thereby maintaining a stable internal environment. The efficiency of this transport system indicates the vital role that blood plays in sustaining life since any slight disruption leads to severe physiological effects, which emphasizes the intricacy of bloods roles in terms of tissue health and metabolic efficiency. Equally important, blood participates in body heat regulation, pH equilibration, and fluid balance. Its temperature regulatory function is achieved through its ability to absorb and distribute heat within the body. For example, when there are alterations in body temperatures outside, blood vessels dilate or constrict to release or retain heat as required. In addition, blood is an important mechanism in acid-base balance where buffer constituents in plasma neutralize surplus bases or acids to keep optimal pH levels of body fluids. This regulatory role is particularly significant within the dynamic physiological environment where homeostasis is continuously challenged by metabolic activities or environmental stresses. These roles demonstrate how blood not only functions as a transport fluid but indeed is an active component in the establishment of physiological equilibrium. In addition to transport and regulatory roles, blood also plays a crucial role within the immune system, helping to resist infection and healing wounds. The blood elements, i.e., the white blood cells, are destined to play a key role in the detection and destruction of the foreign invaders, complementing the body's immune system directly. All of the leukocytes, i.e., neutrophils and lymphocytes, work in conjunction to recognize and respond to infections, underlining the sophisticated nature of the immune defense machinery. Specifically, blood is crucial to hemostasis; its clots close wounds and stop excessive bleeding due to a broad range of sophisticated biochemical processes. The equilibrium of its immune and clotting functions reveals the extent of sophistication of the body of blood as a guardian of bodily integrity and wellness, and therefore how applicable a topic it is to study in blood physiology (Garshnek et al., 1980; Rowe et al., 2025) (Figure 8.7).

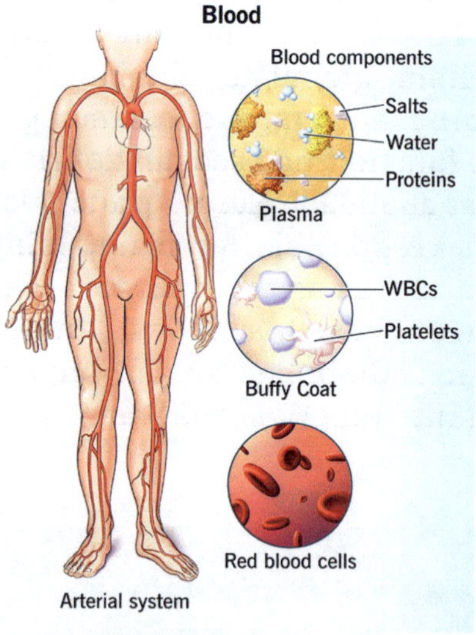

Figure 8.7. Functions of blood.

Source: https://my.clevelandclinic.org/-/scassets/images/org/health/articles/24836-blood.

8.2.1. Transportation of Gases, Nutrients, and Waste

Transport of waste products, nutrients, and gases is a critical function of blood physiology that ensures homeostasis and overall body wellness. The blood provides the primary medium of oxygen (O_2) transportation from alveoli in the lungs to tissues along with the removal of the metabolic waste carbon dioxide (CO_2). The role of the circulatory and respiratory systems is incorporated with this one, so that successful exchange of these gases occurs at the alveolar-capillary interface in the lungs and is determined by a number of factors, i.e., partial pressures and oxygen-hemoglobin affinity. According to Pranavaha Srotas, the body channels which are anatomical and functional and comprise of the heart and vessels correspondingly have an essential role to play in explaining how gases travel and get exchanged. Hence, better understanding of this transporting mechanism is most significant in the context of physiological equilibrium (Arun et al., 2024). Nutrient transport is another of the essential roles of blood physiology that involves the ingestion of essential elements from the gastrointestinal tract and their transport to cells throughout the body. After the digestion of food, nutrients can become absorbed into the bloodstream through the capillaries of the intestines, such as glucose, fatty acids, and amino acids. This process is best identified with the function of Samana Vayu, that of facilitating digestion and absorption of nutrients as described in Ayurvedic texts (Prasad et al., 2023). The absorbed nutrients, after being in the blood, are delivered to tissues where they utilize them in energy production, growth, and repair. The circulatory and gastrointestinal systems must coordinate in order for life to be sustained, emphasizing the significance of effective delivery of nutrients and the consequences of any hindrance of this function on overall health. Removal of waste is another crucial function that is performed by blood, namely transportation of metabolic wastes to excretory organs for elimination. The blood removes waste materials of cellular metabolism and transports them to organs , such as the kidneys, liver, and lungs. The kidneys remove urea and excess salts from the blood, and the liver metabolizes drugs to be excreted and detoxifies toxic substances. This waste removal demonstrates the co-dependency of various systems in the body; the expulsion of CO2 and removal of urea, for instance, are not singular actions but part of a similar reaction to maintain the body's internal equilibrium. Understanding how blood helps eliminate waste is important as any interference with this process can lead to toxic accumulation and severe health issues (Arun et al., 2024) (Figure 8.8).

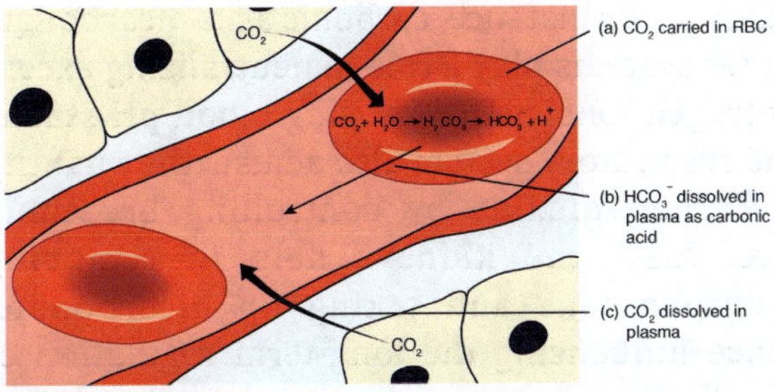

Figure 8.8. Transport of gases.

Source: https://open.oregonstate.education/app/uploads/sites/157/2021/02/2325_Carbon_Dioxide_Transport.jpg.

8.2.2. Regulation of Body Temperature and pH

Regulation of body temperature and pH is required to establish homeostasis within a biological system, especially with regard to blood physiology. Temperature changes can negatively influence enzymatic reactions that are necessary for metabolic functions. In humans, normal body temperature is strictly maintained at 37 degrees Celsius. This regulation is brought about by means of thermoregulation , such as vasodilation, where vessels widen to unload heat, and sweating, which allows body heat to be lost through evaporative cooling. These body responses not only maintain enzymatic processes at their optimum but also maintain cellular structures intact, thus endorsing health and functionality as a whole. In addition, the subtle interrelation between temperature regulation and other body systems justifies the necessity for maintaining homeostasis in accordance with environmental changes influencing body functions. Regulation of blood pH is also important because the acceptable range between 7.35 and 7.45 should not be violated, as any alteration may produce severenceffects on the body's physiology. The blood pH is controlled through buffer systems, respiration, and by kidney function, which act in combination to counteract changes in acid-base balance. For instance, carbonic acid-bicarbonate buffer systems play a role in neutralizing excess hydrogen ions, hence keeping blood pH stable. The respiratory system also adjusts the quantity of carbon dioxide by controlling breathing rate. Also, the kidneys help in removing hydrogen ions and taking up bicarbonate, hence influencing the long-term regulation of pH. These processes are fundamental to blood physiology since derangements in the control of pH can lead to acidosis or alkalosis, which have clinical significance far into the future. In discussing how temperature control is linked with pH balance, it is evident that these factors are dependent on each other in terms of homeostasis. Changes in body temperature over time may impact metabolic functions, which can, in turn, impact acid-base balance. For example, heightened metabolic states usually translate to the generation of more acids and hence lower pH levels. This exchange alludes to the need for an efficient homeostatic system, controlled by a complex network of dynamic processes set to keep physiological parameters at an optimal level. As mentioned, perceptions of homeostasis shed light on its operation throughout developmental time points, with particular stress on versatility and robustness in keeping homeostasis in the face of environmental stress. The understanding gained from research within these regulating processes is significant not only for the field of blood physiology but also for understanding broader biological responses to environmental change, reflective of the complexity of life (Alleva et al., 2017; Torday, 2015) (Figure 8.9).

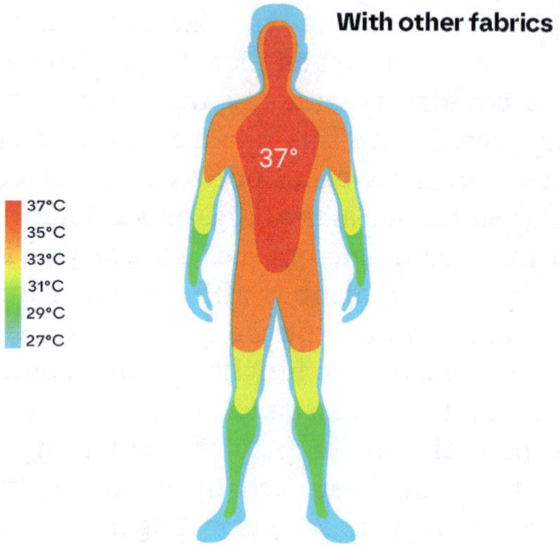

Figure 8.9. Regulation of body temperature and pH.

Source: https://news.six2.com/content/uploads/body-temperature-without-SIXS.png.

8.2.3. Immune Response and Defense Mechanisms

The immune response is a complex interaction of biological mechanisms that function to protect the body from pathogens, such as parasites, bacteria, and viruses. The defense is both innate and adaptive, both of which are crucial in the maintenance of homeostasis. Innate immunity is the first line of defense, using physical barriers , such as the skin and mucous membranes, along with immune cells , such as neutrophils and macrophages, to identify and kill intruders rapidly. Adaptive immunity, however, with its specific response to specific pathogens, involves lymphocyte activation, T cells, and B cells. Importantly, recent research points to the interaction between these forms of immunity and biological rhythms, demonstrating that the effectiveness of immune functions may be changed with circadian and seasonal rhythms, suggesting an adaptive relationship which requires further examination in host-pathogen dynamics (Helm et al., 2015). The microbiota, comprising a rich diversity of microorganisms dwelling in the human body, plays a significant role in modulating immune responses. It is this intricate relationship that begins in infancy and persists life long, having a constant regulatory influence on the immune system. Evidence points to the fact that the microbiota not just contributes to growing a healthy immune system by immunizing it against disease but also acts as a defense shield against pathogenic microbes by competing for available nutrients and utilizing mechanisms of immune signaling. These interactions can have significant effects on the host's susceptibility to infection and inflammation. The impact of the microbiota extends beyond the gastrointestinal tract, demonstrating the interconnectedness of various organ systems and highlighting how such microbial communities shape immune defenses against non-intestinal pathogens (Brown et al., 2016). Further, understanding the mechanisms through which immunity is tailored by the immune system against varied stimuli, including those that arise from the microbiota, is critical in the development of therapeutic interventions. Balance in the regulation of the immune system is a critical component in achieving an optimal response; hyperactive immunity leads to autoimmune disease, and hypoactive immunity might predispose individuals to a greater susceptibility to infections. Studies of the role of pattern recognition receptors (PRRs), which can perceive microbial components, are vital for understanding such mechanisms. What has been achieved through such studies will potentially lead to improved treatment for immune disease and infection, hence keeping research on this subject is important. By the interplay of knowledge of biological rhythms, microbiota, and immune mechanisms, scientists pave the way for novel thoughts on how to enhance immune health and disease resistance (Brown et al., 2016).

Test Your Knowledge

1. Why is blood involved in the transportation of gases like oxygen and carbon dioxide?
2. What is the role of blood in defense against infections?

8.3. Hematopoiesis

Learning Outcome

1. Describe the process of blood cell formation;
2. Define bone marrow and stem cell functions;
3. Describe the determinants of hematopoiesis.

Hematopoiesis, the formation of blood cells, occurs in the bone marrow and is a highly controlled process that is required to provide adequate numbers of erythrocytes, leukocytes, and platelets. Hematopoietic stem cells (HSCs) are the stem cells that contribute to all types of blood cells and go through a multi-step differentiation process that relies both on intrinsic genetic determinants and microenvironment. Agents , such as cytokines and cell-to-cell interactions within the bone marrow characterize hematopoietic niches, which are critical for support and survival of HSCs. The role of bone marrow mesenchymal stem cells (BMSCs) is particularly intriguing, as they not only constitute part of the structural component of the marrow but also modulate hematopoiesis by undergoing differentiation. Because BMSCs play such a crucial role in initiating this process, their impact on HSC homeostasis is key to maintaining hematopoietic health and mechanisms of recovery in times of stress (Li et al., 2018). As more and more research is being done, the role of long non-coding RNAs (lncRNAs) in hematopoiesis also came into the spotlight, acting as regulators of gene expression along the course of differentiation pathways of blood cells. These lncRNAs operate at every stage, acting against transcription, splicing, and ultimate translation of messenger RNA, thereby influencing the HSC fate. Misregulation of lncRNAs has been discovered to be implicated in various blood-related disorders, including leukemia, pointing towards their double role of ensuring normal hematopoiesis as well as disease states. Through the comprehension of mechanisms through which lncRNAs exert their effect, researchers begin to unravel the intricate dance of gene regulation in hematopoiesis. With this not-so-new field of study, the potential of lncRNA therapy is exemplified, having the potential for new answers in correcting cancer-induced hematopoietic disorders (Ballarino et al., 2015). In hematopoietic recovery, particularly after treatments , such as bone marrow transplantation, BMSC differentiation homeostasis is essential. Particular stress conditions, including chemotherapy and aging, will induce imbalance and, therefore, lead to an abnormal ability of replenishment for blood cell populations. Research suggests that a balance in this differentiation must be sustained for successful transplantation-induced hematopoietic recovery. In cases of stress, when BMSC differentiation becomes asymmetric, it may hinder the restoration of normal hematopoiesis and result in complications like anemia or infection due to decreased leukocyte count. Thus, therapeutic measures to regulate BMSC behavior and their microenvironment can facilitate improved recovery results in patients undergoing hematopoietic setbacks. As our understanding of these processes deepens, it offers promising avenues for developing treatments geared towards optimizing blood physiology (Li et al., 2018) (Figure 8.10).

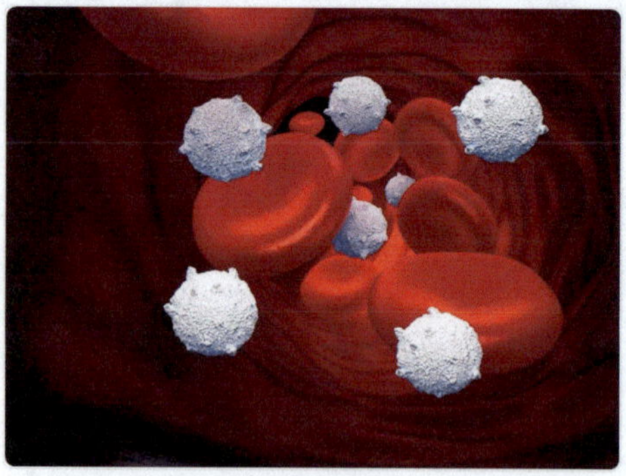

Figure 8.10. Hematopoietic stem cells (HSCs).

Source: https://www.news-medical.net/image-handler/picture/2019/1/By_decade3d_-_anatomy_online.jpg.

8.3.1. Process of Blood Cell Formation

Blood cell formation, a process known as hematopoiesis, occurs primarily in the bone marrow but can also take place in the liver and spleen during fetal development. Hematopoiesis entails the differentiation of HSCs into a number of different blood cell lineages, such as red blood cells (RBCs), white blood cells (WBCs), and platelets. This complex process is controlled by a group of growth factors and cytokines, which allow the production of blood cells to be sensitive to the body's requirements. For instance, erythropoietin plays a crucial role in RBC formation through HSC activation as a result of blood oxygen levels decreased. Their synchrony in proliferation and differentiation guarantees not just the presence of adequate blood cells but also the optimal immune response and efficient oxygen transport across the body, which confirms the relevance of hematopoiesis in overall blood physiology.

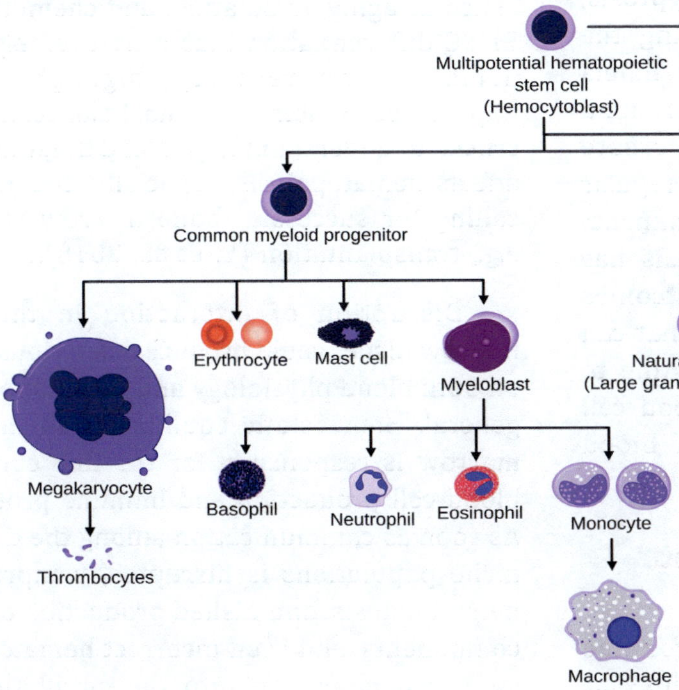

Figure 8.11. Process of blood cell formation.

Source: https://upload.wikimedia.org/wikipedia/commons/f/f0/Hematopoiesis_simple.svg.

At maturity, blood cells undergo significant morphological and functional transformations geared to their specific functions. For red blood cells, that implies the loss of nucleus and organelles for maximum oxygen delivery. For white blood cells, they differentiate into various subtypes , such as lymphocytes, neutrophils, and monocytes, each designed to combat various pathogens and immune stimuli. The process of erythropoiesis that produces red blood cells has stages , such as proerythroblast, erythroblast, and reticulocyte prior to maturity. These stages are crucial as they contribute to the cells' functionality, e.g., production of hemoglobin in RBCs, thereby impacting oxygen delivery. In addition, the intricate signaling networks governing these processes highlight the complexity and efficiency of blood cell formation in maintaining homeostatic equilibrium in the circulatory system, whose vital role can be seen from overall physiology. In addition, the modulation of blood cell formation is regulated by several pathological conditions, which can adversely affect hematopoiesis. For instance, anemias and leukemias can disrupt normal hematopoiesis, leading to decreased functional production of blood cells or cell proliferation in cancer. Existing data have confirmed the role of autoreactive antibodies in such disease conditions as AIHA, which cause eryptosis, programmed death of RBCs, enhancing the deficiency of these life-threatening cells (Balola et al., 2019). It is essential to comprehend these regulatory mechanisms to create therapy interventions that rehabilitate regular hematopoiesis. Understanding the determinants of normal and abnormal hematopoiesis has the potential to improve clinical outcomes and develop new treatment regimens that can treat blood disorders with effect, pointing to the ongoing relevance to studying blood cell development as part of the field of blood physiology (Figure 8.11).

8.3.2. Role of Bone Marrow and Stem Cells

Bone marrow is a critical organ for the maintenance of normal blood physiology as the primary location of hematopoiesis where various blood cells are produced. It is associated with stem cells, namely HSCs, that reside within specialized microenvironments known as niches. There are two principal niches, the endosteal niche at the bone-mar-row junction, and the vascular niche alongside blood vessels. In these niches, interactions between HSCs and other cell occupants, such as osteoblasts and mesenchymal stem cells, allow for the appropriate regulation and maintenance of hematopoiesis. Worthy of note is the complexity of such microhabitats, with cellular signaling and balance of various molecules of signaling being crucially important in supporting nutrient and physiological function of both immune and blood systems (Agas et al., 2015). BMSCs are another essential component of the bone marrow microenvironment, having a pivotal role in supporting hematopoiesis. Such cells are able to differentiate into more than one lineage, thus generating the supportive stroma for HSCs and regulating their function within the hematopoietic niches. Moreover, BMSC differentiation is required to maintain the balance of blood cell output under fluctuating physiological and disease states. In conditions , such as aging, irradiation, and chemotherapy, BMSC differentiation bias can adversely affect hematopoietic recovery, highlighting the importance of their functional balance. It is thus crucial to understand how BMSC differentiation affects hematopoiesis, especially in conditions calling for successful bone marrow recovery, e.g., transplantation (Li et al., 2018).

Disruption of interaction in the bone marrow niches could produce deleterious effects on both blood physiology and hematopoiesis in general. Homeostatic equilibrium in the bone marrow is responsible for the fine control of blood cell production and immune protection. As soon as communication among the different niche populations is disrupted, compromised hematopoiesis, diminished production of blood components, and even incorrect hematopoietic stem cell migration into the circulation can result. This interdependence reflects the degree to which structural and functional integrity of the bone marrow environment is critical in maintaining healthy blood physiology. While ongoing research continues to clarify these connections, what is increasingly clear is that enhancing our understanding of the bone marrows role will be essential in designing therapeutic strategies towards the control of hematologic disease (Agas et al., 2015) (Figure 8.12).

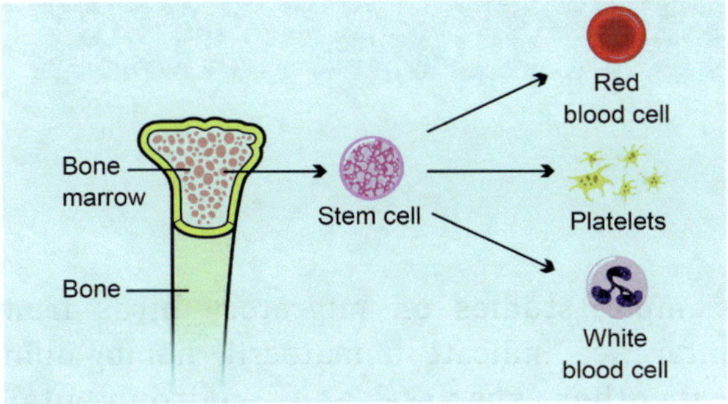

Figure 8.12. Stem cell bone marrow.

Source: https://www.stemcellcareindia.com/wp-content/uploads/2023/08/Bone-Marrow-Stem-Cell-480x270.jpg.

8.3.3. Factors Influencing Hematopoiesis

Hematopoiesis, or the production of blood cells, is regulated by a number of intrinsic and extrinsic factors that modulate and enhance it. Among these, growth factors and cytokines hold a key role. The signaling molecules help in the proliferation and differentiation of HSCs into various lineages of blood cells like leukocytes, erythrocytes, and platelets. These include key cytokines , such as erythropoietin (EPO), granulocyte-colony stimulating factor (G-CSF), and thrombopoietin (TPO) that are tasked with the facilitation of the survival and maturation of some progenitor cells. Disruption in these factors can lead to hematological disorders that are indicative of their significant role in hematopoiesis.

Besides, the interaction among various cells within the bone marrow microenvironment ensures optimal conditions for hematopoiesis, and hence an in-depth understanding of such factors would be valuable from the aspect of advancing treatment for blood diseases. The mesenchymal stem cells (MSCs) within bone marrow have also been identified as significant regulators of hematopoiesis. These cells also contribute to the formation of hematopoietic niches that provide essential support and signals to HSCs, thus affecting their maintenance and differentiation. Differentiation status of BMSCs can significantly influence hematopoietic function. In response to stress conditions , such as aging or chemotherapy, altered BMSC differentiation can result in an insufficient hematopoietic niche, ultimately leading to incompetent blood cell replenishment. Recent literature reveals that the equilibrium in BMSC differentiation is crucial to facilitate optimal hematopoietic recovery after occurrences like bone marrow transplantation. Therefore, an understanding of the dynamics of BMSC behavior under varied conditions is critical in formulating strategies to augment hematopoietic function and recovery (Li et al., 2018). The regulation of hematopoiesis is further complicated by the involvement of long non-coding RNAs (lncRNAs), which play significant roles in modulating gene expression at various phases of hematopoietic cell development. The molecules are implicated in the regulation of target gene expression, which influences critical events like blood cell precursor differentiation and proliferation. Recent studies have established that the misregulation of lncRNA can be linked with hematological malignancies, such as leukemia, and therefore be useful as biomarkers or therapeutic targets. These findings display the intricate web of hematopoietic regulation where lncRNAs take central molecular roles. As continued research continues to expose the complex interrelation of various genetic and extrinsic determinants, it is increasingly apparent that the full explanation of these determinants is essential to the advancement of hematological science and to the formulation of improved therapeutic interventions in hematologic disorders (Ballarino et al., 2015).

Test Your Knowledge

1. Hematopoiesis is what, and where does it primarily occur in adults?
2. What stem cell gives rise to all types of blood cells?

8.4. Blood Disorders

Learning Outcome

1. Identify the anemia: types and causes;
2. Define the leukemia and other blood cancers;
3. Describe the coagulation disorders and hemophilia.

The diagnosis of blood disorders is at the heart of the understanding of blood physiology because they exert great influence on the structure and function of blood. Blood disorders comprise a range of medical conditions, including anemia, hemophilia, and the leukemias, each of which is characterized by blood component pathology in the red blood cells, white blood cells, or platelets. For instance, anemia is characterized by a deficiency of red blood cells or hemoglobin, thereby impairing oxygen delivery to tissues, hence impairing physiological processes. In addition, hemophilia involves a disruption of blood coagulation due to genetic disturbances a resulting in excessive bleeding and complications in surgical procedures.

Knowledge of such conditions is valuable in terms of contributing immensely to preventive and therapeutic interventions with the aim of enhancing patient outcomes alongside overall blood physiology. Physiological consequences of blood disorders can also be appreciated from the impact they have on hematological parameters, which are critical indicators of health. Various determinants , such as age and nutritional status have been observed to influence these hematological parameters among various populations, even extending to wildlife. For example, studies on migratory birds from Antarctica indicate hematocrit, hemoglobin, and other species- and environmental-related variations in biochemical markers for adaptations and species life histories (Ibañez et al., 2015). These observations demonstrate the richness of blood physiology under different situations and the significance of establishing baseline values of physiology.

It is through these disparities that researchers are better able to understand more completely the pathophysiology of blood disease and how it relates both to human as well as avian biology. Additionally, studies of blood disease can have even broader implications for the understanding of physiological adaptation as well as evolutionary biology. Blood, as a transport medium for essential nutrients and gases, functions under strict controls. Disease can disinterrupt these processes and propagate broader effects on the organism. For example, shifts in blood protein fractions, as observed with various bird species, reflect the delicate balance that must exist in order to be capable of homeostasis (Ibañez et al., 2015).

It is additionally necessary to translate physiological information on environmental loads and life history traits since they are capable of influencing consequences to health. To understand the interplay between blood physiology and disorders finally unravels our concept of systemic health and guides clinical interventions in managing these complex diseases successfully (Figure 8.13).

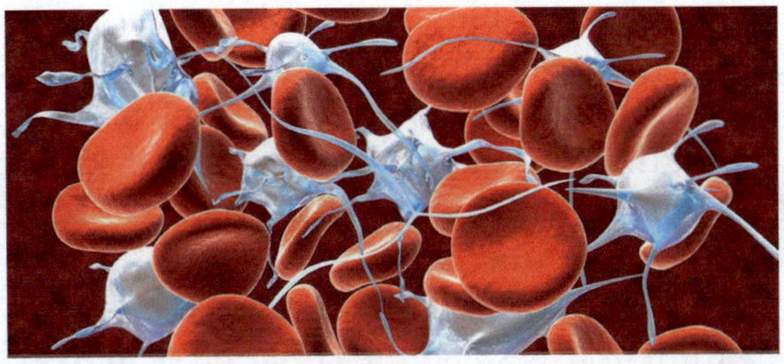

Figure 8.13. Blood disorders.

Source: https://s3-us-west-2.amazonaws.com/utsw-patientcare-web-production/original_images/GettyImages-188057859-1600x732.jpg.

8.4.1. Anemia: Types and Causes

Anemia is a multifactorial disorder in the blood that is marked by deficiency in RBCs or hemoglobin with concomitant compromise in oxygen delivery to tissues. This disorder can be classified into different types based on etiology, pathophysiology, and associated clinical presentation. Iron-deficiency anemia, for instance, is caused by insufficient iron levels, which impacts the synthesis of hemoglobin and leads to the symptoms of anemia, pallor, and breathlessness. Anemia of chronic disease occurs in patients with chronic infectious or inflammatory diseases, where the primary process of the disease interferes with erythropoiesis. It is crucial to recognize these distinctions in order to implement the appropriate diagnostic and treatment strategies and detect the systemic influence of anemia on overall health and well-being. Another extremely important classification of anemia is morphological red blood cell categorization. Microcytic anemia, like iron-deficiency anemia, has RBCs that are smaller than usual, whereas macrocytic anemia, usually due to vitamin B_{12} or folate deficiency, is characterized by red cells that are larger than usual. Normocytic anemia has RBCs that are of normal size but arises from different conditions, including acute blood loss or renal disease, in which there is impaired production of erythropoietin. The physiologic adaptation to anemia is also a function of the type, i.e., the augmentation of cardiac output in order to prevent failure of oxygen delivery that is bound to trigger with time compensatory mechanisms which will exacerbate other cardiovascular diseases.

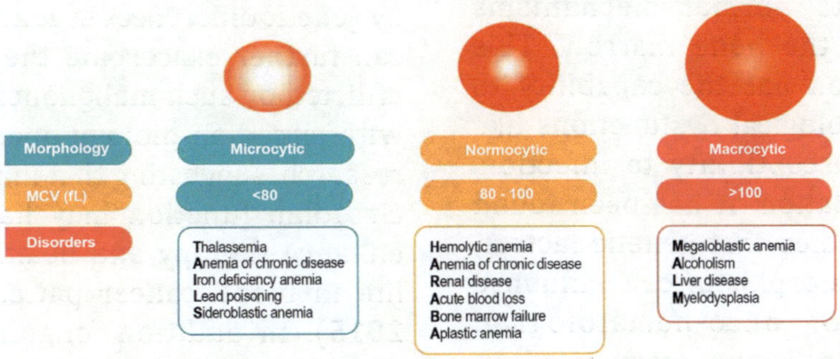

Figure 8.14. Morphological-classification-of-anemia.

Source: https://myhematology.com/wp-content/uploads/2023/11/Morphological-classification-of-anemia-1.jpg.

From the study of morphological classification, we know the vital significance of systemic oxygenation by RBCs and the body's adaptive mechanisms. In addition, congenital anemias, such as congenital sideroblastic anemias (CSAs) and Diamond-Blackfan anemia (DBA), illustrate the large effect genetic etiologies can have on hematological health. CSAs are caused by inherited heme biosynthesis or mitochondrial iron-sulfur cluster assembly defects, resulting in pathological iron accumulation in erythroid precursors. These defects manifest as abnormal erythropoiesis and can be accompanied by various clinical issues, such as growth retardation and susceptibility to iron overload. DBA, with its selective failure of erythropoiesis, also points to the complexities of anemia resulting from genetic defects. It is certain that such particular etiologies, like the role of key proteins like HSCB in erythropoiesis, need to be made clear to formulation of targeted interventions for effective management of anemias. The interaction of genetic information with clinical practice is the attempt to improve patient care and quality of life for patients suffering from such conditions (Ross et al., 2014; Crispin et al., 2017) (Figure 8.14).

8.4.2. Leukemia and Other Blood Cancers

The complex nature of leukemia and other blood cancers demonstrates their extreme impact in the field of blood physiology. Leukemia, through its unchecked proliferation of abnormal white blood cells, disrupts normal mechanisms of hematopoiesis in the bone marrow. This abnormal proliferation has the capability to lead to various physiological dysfunctions like anemia, increased susceptibility to infection, and inefficient coagulation. It has been found through scientific studies that genetic factors, i.e., PER3 gene polymorphism, can influence the development of onco-hematological disorders. These conditions were used in a study involving 125 patients, and it was proven that certain genotypes were associated with high risk for lymphoblastic myeloblastic leukemia, and it showed the connection between genetic predisposition and leukemia pathogenesis (Cerliani et al., 2015). Through these connections, we can maximize early detection and prevention strategies and, in turn, improve our management of leukemia in the larger context of blood physiology. The role of signaling pathways in blood cancers is crucial to the development of targeted therapies. Among these pathways, the c-Jun N-terminal kinases (JNKs) have played pivotal roles in tumor growth promotion and repression, primarily in hematological malignancies. Constitutive activation of JNK signaling could be responsible for the uncontrolled proliferation of cancer cells in blood cancers, reflecting its bivalent role in tumor biology (Adams et al., 2013). Besides, JNKs offer a unique therapeutic target; however, the challenge of determining which isoforms to inhibit derives from the fact that they play opposing functions in different tumor microenvironments. New small molecule inhibitors are in line to target specifically these proteins; however, their effect on normal physiological processes and possible toxicity are concerns. Overcoming such adversity is of paramount significance in maximizing therapeutic efficacy and minimizing collateral damage to normal blood physiology. Synergy among environmental factors, genetic predisposition, and signaling pathways provides a rich matrix for leukemia and other malignancies of the blood. Studies have shown that disruptions in circadian rhythm, as dictated by genetic differences in genes like the PER3 gene, can further exacerbate the condition of those afflicted by such malignancies. This association with circadian biology opens new avenues for research, suggesting that maintenance of typical circadian function may have the capacity to enhance therapy and health-related quality of life in blood cancer patients (Cerliani et al., 2015). In addition, ongoing development of JNK inhibitors makes clear the significance of drug strategies which are optimized with regard to both cancer and normal cellular contexts. As studies increasingly unravel these complex interactions, the integration of genetic, environmental, and physiological factors will be at the heart of the creation of novel diagnostic and therapeutic approaches in leukemia and blood diseases (Figure 8.15).

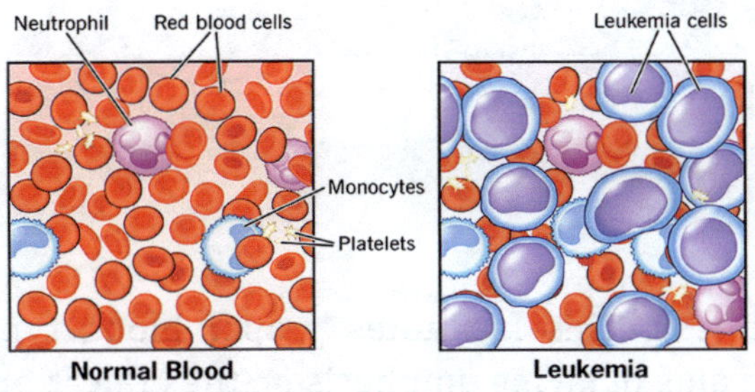

Figure 8.15. Leukemia: Symptoms, signs, causes.

Source: https://my.clevelandclinic.org/-/scassets/images/org/health/articles/4365-leukemia.

8.4.3. Coagulation Disorders and Hemophilia

The intricate mechanism of hemostasis is critical to the integrity of the circulatory system, where its failure can lead to extensive coagulation disorders, including hemophilia. Hemophilia is a hereditary disease where certain clotting factors are either deficient or lacking, most often Factor VIII in Hemophilia A and Factor IX in Hemophilia B. Such deficiencies hinder the body's capacity to create stable clots in the blood, causing excessive bleeding even from a slight wound. Understanding of the pathophysiology underlying hemophilia is important, as it highlights both the clinical relevance for the affected patients and the potential for treatment pathways.

Notably, advances in genetic therapy have been paralleled by new approaches based on emerging technologies like CRISPR, which seem to hold great promise for enhancing the management of these disorders and for improved clinical outcomes in the future. In addition to this, the pathophysiology of coagulation disorders requires a strong understanding of hemostatic mechanisms that manage clotting. Proper diagnosis and treatment of patients with such disorders require full examination, especially in procedures that are accompanied by bleeding risk, such as dental procedures. The necessity of taking a complete medical history is essential to avoid potential bleeding complications. This proactive approach can help health professionals in placing effective preventive measures in place, thus limiting the incidence of adverse outcomes. The combination of knowledge around inherited conditions , such as Von Willebrand disease, Hemophilia A, and Hemophilia B, raises the importance of including clinical expertise with a deep understanding of the biological mechanisms of hemostasis, particularly in the context of the impact of drugs on platelet function and coagulation in general.

Modern advances in biomedical science provide fascinating opportunities for the modeling of coagulation disorders and for therapeutic intervention targeting. Traditional *in vitro* models are limited, as they do not replicate the sophisticated *in vivo* human biological environment. The recent development of induced pluripotent stem cell technology presents a groundbreaking answer, allowing patient-specific liver organoids to be generated. These organoids mimic the cellular architecture and physiological properties of human liver tissue, essential for the production of coagulation factors. Coupled with the advancements in the gene editing tools, such as the CRISPR/Cas9 system, researchers can possibly correct the genetic mutations responsible for coagulation disorders.

These advances, in addition to enhancing our appreciation of disease mechanisms, also set the stage for developing cell-based therapies aimed at potentially dramatically improving the quality of life for patients with hemophilia and other disorders of coagulation, eventually revolutionizing treatment paradigms in blood physiology.

Test Your Knowledge

1. What is anemia, and how does it affect oxygen delivery in the body?
2. Which blood disorder includes uncontrolled bleeding due to the lack of clotting factors?

8.5. Blood Typing and Transfusion

Learning Outcome

1. Describe the ABO and Rh blood group systems;
2. Express the importance of compatibility in transfusion;
3. Describe risks and reactions to blood transfusion.

The procedures of blood typing and transfusion hold utmost importance in blood physiology and exert a profound impact on clinical practice and patient management. Blood typing, or the categorization of a person's blood group based on the presence of specific antigens and antibodies, is essential to transfusion safety. Most commonly employed are the ABO and Rh systems because incompatibility can lead to perilous hemolytic reactions, which are potentially fatal.

Correct blood typing, not only enabling successful transfusions, is also part of prenatal care and organ transplantation. Well-crafted protocols and rigorous testing protocols ensure proper results, ultimately ensuring patient safety and reducing the incidence of side effects during surgical procedures. Clinical understanding of blood typing extends beyond transfusion compatibility; it is a comprehensive understanding of how blood components behave in the human body. The experts who provide services in laboratory medicine are greatly contributing to this line of work since their expertise allows them to utilize diagnostic tests for screening blood group antibodies and antigens. This facilitates proper blood typing and aids in laying emphasis on the education of laboratory procedures. On top of that, continued advancements in laboratory medicine, especially in fields , such as hematology and immunology, aid in laying emphasis on standardized and quality practice. These advances not only enhance the efficacy of blood transfusions and hematologic disorder treatment but also align with the overall healthcare regulations for optimal patient outcomes (Baum et al., 2012). The implications for transfusion medicine extend even to patient prognosis and the regulation of treatment, particularly in critical care settings. As transfusions may be lifesaving for patients with trauma, surgery, or chronic disease, knowledge of the physiological response of the body to transfusions is important.

This helps predict possible complications that may arise, such as transfusion-related acute lung injury and allergic reactions. Greater understanding of such side effects is achieved through clinical experience and scientific research, and more effective methods of reduction in risk and observation of the patient ensue. In fact, emerging research and development in transfusion practices suggest a shift towards more personalized practices, which can potentially reduce unnecessary procedures and enhance patient recovery. Sharing and pooling of such information between the medical community is necessary, as it ensures continuous enhancement in transfusion practices and patient safety at large (Herms et al., 2004) (Figure 8.16).

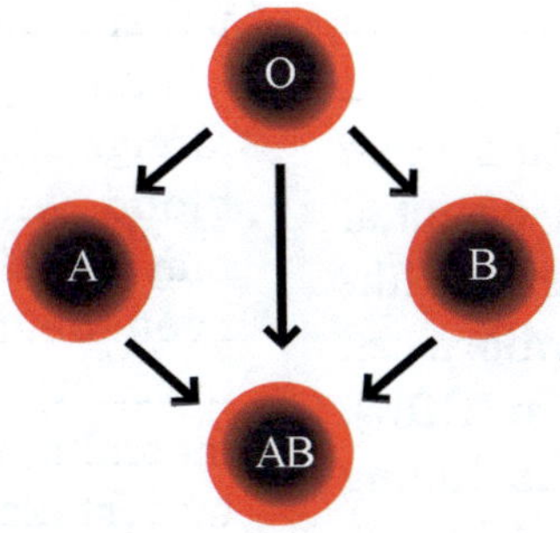

Figure 8.16. Blood typing and blood transfusion.

Source: https://s3-us-west-2.amazonaws.com/courses-images/wp-content/uploads/sites/2868/2019/04/30115504/blood-Compatiblity-Capture.png.

8.5.1. ABO and Rh Blood Group Systems

Understanding of the ABO and Rh blood group systems is essential to understand the complexities of human blood physiology. The ABO system, which classifies blood into four main groups—A, B, AB, and O—is founded upon the presence or absence of certain antigens on the surface of red blood cells. Compatibility for transfusion and transplantations is determined by the presence or absence of these antigens. Type A has A antigens, type B has B antigens, and AB and O individuals both have A and B antigens, respectively, none.

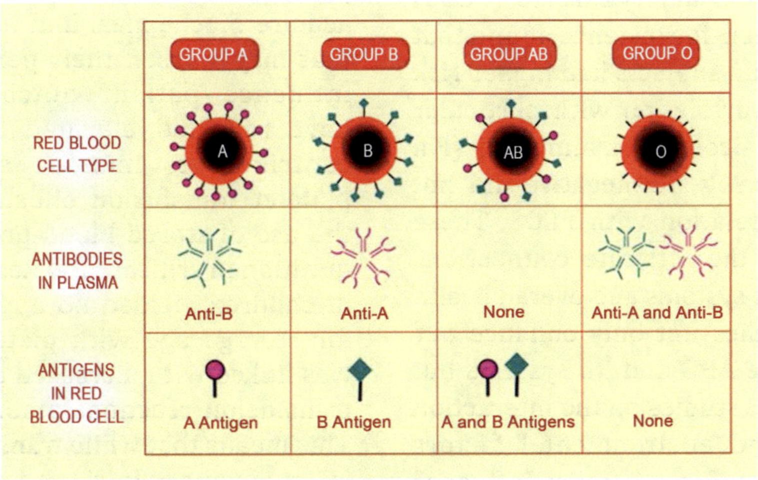

Figure 8.17. ABO-blood-group-system.

Source: https://cdn1.byjus.com/wp-content/uploads/2017/10/ABO-blood-group-system.jpg.

This system highlights the importance of immune response in the practice of medicine, since incompatible transfusions can cause severe adverse effects, including hemolytic transfusion reactions that are potentially fatal. Therefore, knowledge of these blood types not only benefits in a clinical capacity but also increases our understanding of genetics and heredity. The Rh blood group system is also mainly characterized by the presence of the Rh factor, in this case, the D antigen. Those who carry this antigen are termed Rh-positive, and those who do not carry this antigen are termed Rh-negative. The significance of the Rh system was particularly clear in relation to prenatal care, since Rh incompatibility between an Rh-negative mother and an Rh-positive newborn can lead to hemolytic disease of the newborn (HDN). HDN can lead to serious health issues, including jaundice, anemia, and in extreme cases, stillbirth. The achievement of the medical profession in developing preventatives, such as the administration of Rh immunoglobulin (RhoGAM) to mothers at risk, highlights the significance of the interaction of blood group systems in maintaining maternal-fetal health. It not only prevents HDN but also reflects the advancement made in knowing blood physiology. There have been recent investigations into clinical uses of blood groups other than transfusion needs, such as investigating correlations between ABO blood group and some health disorders. A study of polycystic ovary syndrome (PCOS) in South Indian women, for instance, found that O positive blood group subjects had higher risk of this disorder in correlation with particular dietary habits and alcohol consumption (Pal et al., 2014). Conversely, Rh-negative did not show a notable correlation with PCOS. These findings emphasize the intricate connections between blood group systems and overall health outcomes. Such studies not only enhance our understanding of the ABO and Rh systems but also necessitate more studies on the interaction between genetic and environmental factors within the blood physiology that may influence future medical practices and preventive interventions (Figure 8.17).

8.5.2. Importance of Compatibility in Transfusions

The significance of blood compatibility cannot be overstated because incompatibility will result in severe immune reactions, endangering patient safety and treatment efficacy. The human immune system is perfectly capable of detecting foreign antigens, and transfusion of incompatible blood will trigger hemolytic reactions that may result in acute kidney injury, shock, or even death. This serves to underscore the necessity for rigorous blood typing and cross-matching before any transfusion process being undertaken. Cats, for instance, in veterinary medicine have pre-existing alloantibodies which can induce untoward effects with even minor mismatches. Heterologous blood transfusions have been investigated in cats, with some mild hemolysis occurring in very anemic patients, but care should be taken since anaphylactic shock may result with multiple exposure. Thus, the evaluation of compatibility is essential not only to enhance transfusion outcomes but also to ensure patient safety (Buta et al., 2019). Secondly, the storage life of blood products is also a critical aspect of transfusion compatibility and efficiency. As blood components, i.e., platelet concentrates, when they grow old, they acquire biochemical and functional alterations that may worsen their performance and even influence patient outcomes. Experiments have revealed elevated storage periods to contribute to immune system failure and platelet transfusion effectiveness, challenging the use of stored blood products for extended duration in critical care. Research from critically ill children yielded no appreciable correlation for storage age with platelet increments but was linked with increased occurrence of febrile transfusion reactions among fresher platelets. This means that while transfusion compatibility is important, clinicians must also investigate the storage environment of blood products when determining the safety and efficacy of these products (Nellis et al., 2020). The need for compatible blood and the complexity of patient needs and diversity of blood groups mean that ongoing research and evolution in transfusion medicine are needed. Technological improvements, such as synthetic blood products and advanced blood screening technologies, can potentially expand compatibility and reduce risk with transfusions. Additionally, application of personalized medicine to transfusion therapy might allow individualized tailoring of blood components to patient-specific profiles, reducing adverse reactions even more. With advances in the physiology of blood, the resolution of compatibility issues will be essential to improving transfusion therapy. Lastly, the prioritization of compatibility not only ensures the safe transfusion of blood products but enhances general patient care in human and veterinary medicine, hence highlighting the critical role of transfusion compatibility in any therapy (Figure 8.18).

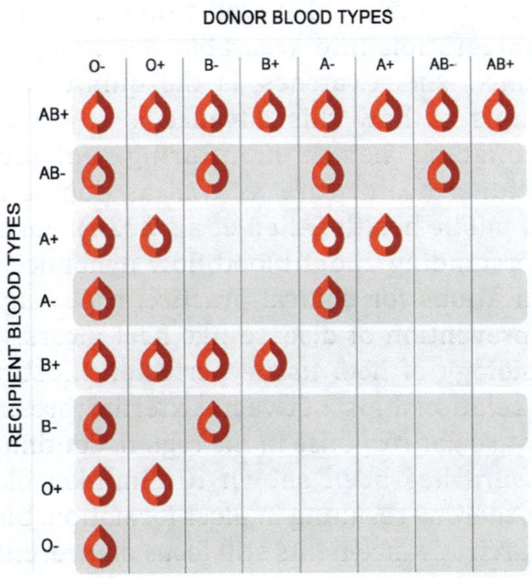

Figure 8.18. Blood type compatibility.

Source: https://www.blood.ca/sites/default/files/DonorRecipient-Chart_1.jpeg.

8.5.3. Risks and Reactions Associated with Blood Transfusions

The transfusion of blood transfusions, while often life-saving, is not devoid of significant risks and reactions that need to be considered carefully. Perhaps the most critical issue is immune risk, including hemolytic transfusion reactions. These occur as a result of the immune system of the recipient recognizing the transfused blood as foreign and lysing the red blood cells. Such reactions can lead to extremely severe complications, including acute renal failure and shock, radically altering the clinical course of transfusion. Additionally, blood group compatibility is another factor that significantly helps lessen such risks. Advances in transfusion medicine continue to center on refining compatibility testing to help lower the incidence of adverse immune reactions, which also present themselves in multiple forms, such as fever, rash, and anaphylaxis. In the end, it is the conscientiousness of the healthcare providers that is required to control these built-in risks of blood transfusions. Apart from immune reactions, transfusions can also transfer pathogenic organisms to the recipient's circulatory system, fostering utmost fear in blood transfusion schemes. Although stringent screening procedures have dramatically reduced the incidence of transfusion-transmitted infections (TTIs), transmission risks for virus, bacteria, and parasites still exist. Since 80% of the population resides in areas where fresh blood products are unavailable, other resuscitation techniques, such as Hemoglobin-based oxygen carriers (HBOCs), are gaining traction. These novel solutions attempt to mimic the oxygen-carrying ability of the red blood cell with less likelihood of infection. However, many problems still persist with HBOCs, including coagulopathy and complications, pointing toward the need for further studies to optimize these substitutes and ensure safer transfusions in clinical practice (Holtby et al., 2014). Furthermore, transfusion-related acute lung injury (TRALI) awareness is also vital based on the fact that it is still underreported and can be profound. TRALI is an immune-mediated process that results in acute respiratory distress and can cause severe morbidity and mortality in recipients of transfusion. TRALI has a propensity to occur due to the presence of antibodies in the donor plasma, aimed against white blood cells of the recipient, resulting in capillary leakage and pulmonary edema. As the medical community is still attempting to decipher the complexities involved in TRALI, identification of its signs and symptoms becomes necessary for timely intervention. Protocols for minimizing donor exposure and selection of donors are being more advanced in order to counteract this risk. The unity of nursing observation, patient history, and modifying transfusion protocols is all crucial in managing potential adverse effects and thus making the transfusion of blood a necessary component of modern medicine practice while safeguarding patient health (Rawling et al., 2012).

Test Your Knowledge

1. What are the four main blood types of the ABO system?
2. Why is blood type matching necessary prior to transfusion?

8.6. Advances in Blood Research

Learning Outcome

1. Describe the advances made in blood diagnostic and testing;
2. Define stem cell therapy and regenerative medicine;
3. Evaluate the future trends in blood physiology research.

The recent advances in blood research have greatly assisted in the understanding of peripheral vascular physiology, particularly through the application of new methodologies like photoplethysmography (PPG). The non-invasive optical method has received much attention in studying changes in blood volume of microvascular beds in tissues. The presence of published papers on PPG re-establishes its significance across applications from cardiovascular measurement to the monitoring of the body's vital signs , such as heart rate and blood pressure. As researchers explore correlations between the PPG pulse morphology and other physiological factors, knowledge on vascular disease, aging, and overall cardiovascular well-being is evolving. Its integration into wearable technology, for instance, smartwatches, is the quintessential example of how this advance is to be used for ongoing health monitoring, enhancing individual health care as well as population-level public health (Allen et al., 2024). Further, understanding about blood flow dynamics has implications for clinical practice, especially in the prevention of disease like heel ulcers. The physiology of heel tissue perfusion illustrates key relationships between external pressure and vascular response in the region. Continuous pressure has been shown to diminish blood flow, thereby resulting in ulcer formation. Blood research advancements still focus on preventive interventions on removing external pressure and enhancing local circulation. By fully grasping how pressure affects heel perfusion, clinicians can use more effective interventions to avert skin breakdown in vulnerable groups, ultimately enhancing patient care outcomes. Through such research, not only is the relevance of vascular physiology in real-life practice brought to the fore, but the support base of the fundamental principles on which preventive care rests is also enhanced (Stotts et al., 2003). Together with these advancements, the ongoing innovation in machine learning algorithms is bound to further revolutionize blood research. The convergence of PPG data and artificial intelligence is going to make health monitoring systems even more accurate, allowing for real-time analysis of various physiological parameters. This blending of technology and physiological study is going to enhance the diagnosis of ailments , such as arrhythmias and vascular diseases at an early stage. As researchers seek to push the boundaries of wearable technology, the ability to derive actionable insights from continuous data could potentially lead to individualized health interventions in the future. These technologies not only emphasize blood physiology's role in exposing health statuses but also have encouraging potential for cardiovascular disease prevention and control through continuous proactive monitoring of health (Allen et al., 2024) (Figure 8.19).

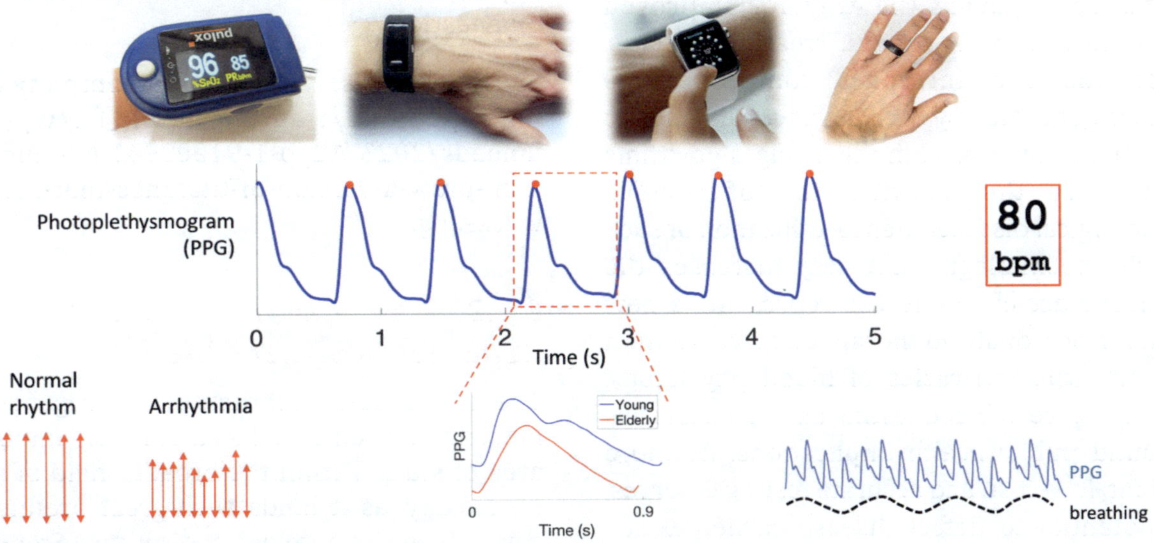

Figure 8.19. Understanding photoplethysmography.

Source: https://peterhcharlton.github.io/project/understanding-ppg/featured.png.

8.6.1. Innovations in Blood Testing and Diagnostics

The science of blood testing and diagnosis has witnessed phenomenal growth, greatly enhancing the speed and accuracy of medical evaluations. Traditional practices, which used to depend on long lab processes and delayed reports, are being supplemented or substituted with cutting-edge technologies , such as microfluidics and point-of-care testing platforms. These technologies allow rapid analysis of blood samples, lightening the load on patients and medical professionals. For instance, the development of hand-held diagnostic platforms facilitates easy access for healthcare workers to receive immediate results, allowing them to make prompt decisions and administer treatment promptly. These advancements are particularly vital in life-threatening situations, where every minute counts. Also, these technologies not only promote efficiency but expand access to diagnostic services to cover gaps in healthcare, especially in remote or underserved areas. This diagnostic revolution in the world of blood diagnostics is revolutionizing patient care procedures and outcomes across the globe. Moreover, the integration of advanced imaging techniques and artificial intelligence is revolutionizing the diagnostic landscape. The development of biophotonics, for example, takes advantage of the interaction between light and biological tissues to achieve real-time blood parameter analysis. The Boston University Photonics Center has been leading the way in such developments, with applications ranging from monitoring chemotherapy for the individual to producing tunable optical metamaterials.

These advancements allow for easier visualization and examination of blood components, paving the way for improved diagnosis and personalized treatment plans. Physicians can interpret comprehensive datasets generated by such advanced diagnostic equipment using machine learning algorithms to improve the identification of various hematological diseases. Hence, utilization of such superior technologies not only increases the diagnostic accuracy but also represents a new dawn for personalized therapeutic intervention reflecting the intricacies of blood physiology. Every advance in blood testing and diagnosis has profound public health implications. As more efficient, low-cost, and accurate testing emerges, the potential to detect disease earlier exists, critical for conditions like diabetes, anemia, and much cancer. By promoting a preventive approach to health care, these advances result in better patient outcomes and reduced healthcare costs over time. Moreover, enhanced access to advanced test technologies, supported by institutions , such as the Boston University Photonics Center, can lead to population-scale screening programs, eventually improving health of the population. Innovations in data analytics also fuel gathering of high-quality health records, allowing continuous monitoring of blood markers that can predict disease progression or treatment response. As a result, the future of blood diagnostics is not only concerned with technology advancement but also a paradigm shift towards preventative care (Figure 8.20).

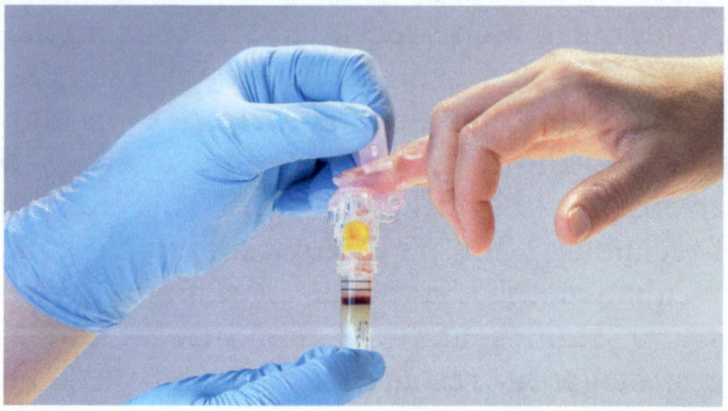

Figure 8.20. Innovations in blood testing and diagnostics.

Source: https://images.fastcompany.com/image/upload/f_auto,q_auto,c_fit/wp-cms/uploads/2023/12/p-1-91002941-bd-launches-mini-draw-a-version-of-theranos-that-actually-works.jpg.

8.6.2. Stem Cell Therapy and Regenerative Medicine

The field of stem cell therapy and regenerative medicine has emerged as a uniquely important area of study within the broader field of blood physiology, as it holds such great promise for curing many hematological disorders. Stem cells, as characterized by their ability to differentiate into several cell types and proliferate, represent a unique solution to repairing defective tissue and restoring blood function. This innovation is particularly important in the management of such diseases as anemia, leukemia, and peripheral vascular disease, where standard therapies may fall short. Recent studies point to the potential of MSCs as an important ingredient in regenerative therapies, both for their immunosuppressive properties and ability to regenerate hematopoietic compartments, thereby aiding in restoration of robust blood physiology through enhanced tissue repair and regeneration (Kasim et al., 2014). However, even with the seeming therapeutic potential of MSCs in regenerative medicine, there are a number of challenges that must be addressed in making them optimally clinically effective. Most prominently, these have included poor growth kinetics, early senescence, and genetic instability during *in vitro* culture as significant obstacles to successful MSC therapy. Further, such environmental conditions as oxygen levels in which such cells are grown also significantly affect their functionality and long-term viability. Studies have indicated that reproduction of the hypoxic microenvironment typical of the stem cell niche can significantly enhance MSC growth and multipotency, thus improving their application in regenerative medicine. This is one area that emphasizes the need to optimize culture techniques in order to realize the full regenerative potential of the stem cells for use in treatments for the blood (Kasim et al., 2014). In addition, the intersection between senescence and aging has additional challenges in the application of stem cell therapy to the physiology of the blood. Aging disrupts the functioning of cardiovascular systems and affects the integrity of endogenous and exogenous reservoirs of stem cells, leading to decreased regenerative capacities. Atherosclerosis and heart failure become more pronounced with increasing age, and scientists are investigating the molecular pathways that result in such age-related pathologies. Regenerative medicine, on the horizon now, promises that senescence-targeted interventions may activate rejuvenation of aging cardiovascular tissue and restore normal blood physiology. By investigating the mechanisms of aging on stem cell function, researchers are opening the door to new therapies that would reverse the effects of aging on blood health, setting a new frontier in cardiovascular therapies (Figure 8.21).

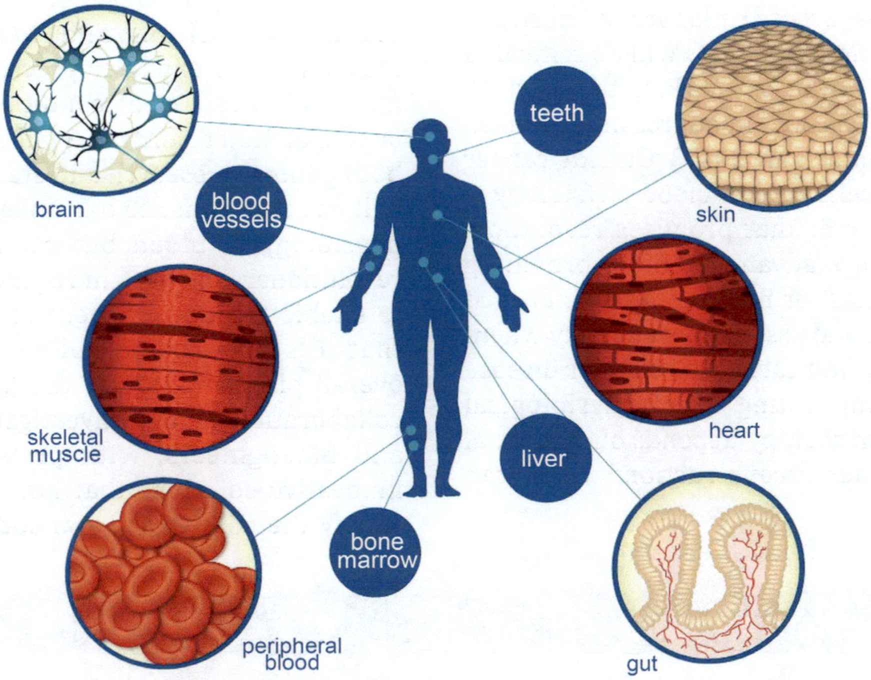

Figure 8.21. Types of stem cells in regenerative medicine.

Source: https://services.brieflands.com/cdn/serve/313ea/7e2f02a8f7e48282d8cff8e729c3840ddb87f889/jssc-1-3-28471-g002-preview.png.

8.6.3. Future Directions in Blood Physiology Research

With the progression of blood physiology, future studies are increasingly fascinated with integrating more recent diagnostic techniques, particularly those with circulating tumor cells (CTCs). Liquid biopsies' capability to detect CTCs also become a game changer in the early detection of cancer, particularly pancreatic cancer, an highly malignant neoplasm. Tumor biopsies were heretofore laborious from the access and invasive standpoints. Existing techniques for CTC detection provide critical genomic information regarding tumor nature, which can enhance early diagnosis, prognosis, and therapy. This can revolutionize the interface of blood physiology and oncology, allowing treatment to become more tailored and improving outcomes for patients. As the science advances, inter-specialty collaboration between hematologists and oncologists will be critical to maximize these advances, marking the need for cross-specialty research in addressing complex diseases (Pimienta et al., 2017). Outside cancer research, stem cells' role in blood physiology is yet another frontier that promises revolution. Stem cell biology advancement is providing new opportunities for new therapies aimed at restoring organs and tissues, most notably where reconstruction is indicated, e.g., bladder disease and cancer complicating usual physiological function. Current therapy depends on intestinal tissue for bladder reconstruction, which can have undesirable metabolic effects as well as long-term consequences. With the application of stem cells in tissue bioengineering, researchers anticipate safer and more reliable alternatives. This shift from traditional to regenerative methods has vast implications not only for clinical interventions but also for the understanding of the underlying principles of blood physiology with regard to tissue regeneration and repair. Research in these avenues can potentially create revolutionary advances in theoretical as well as applied research in blood physiology (Chan et al., 2017). The intersection of genomics, hematology, and stem cell biology is encouraging a multidisciplinary approach that can revolutionize treatment models for various blood diseases. Current research will be aimed at applying genomic technologies with hematology to take apart the complexity of most blood diseases. Understanding how genetic variations affect blood composition and behavior enables researchers to engineer precise therapies that more effectively treat conditions like anemias or coagulation disorders. Synthesizing data from both genomic research and stem cell utilization will not only enhance our understanding of the physiology of blood but could also usher in revolutionary changes in regenerative medicine to enable the development of new treatments that restore normal blood function. The overall plan emphasizes the need for ongoing collaboration among investigators, physicians, and bioengineers, with preference given to innovative solutions that have the capacity to satisfy the complexity of blood physiology.

Test Your Knowledge

1. How is stem cell technology applied to the treatment of blood diseases , such as leukemia?
2. What are synthetic blood substitutes, and what do they seek to overcome?

SUMMARY

When considering the intricacies of blood physiology, it becomes clear that the control of blood pH and volume is pivotal in the sustenance of homeostasis in the body. The study of the Na/H exchanger in Amphiuma red blood cells identifies the complex mechanism by which pH is maintained in relation to cellular conditions. That is, when intracellular pH declines, the Na/H exchanger responds to reestablish balance, effectively until a predetermined set point is reached. This adaptive response underscores the need for fine control mechanisms within the physiological processes underlying our knowledge of blood dynamics. Thus, physiological responses are not unpredictable; they are latent responses intended to adapt to varied levels of stressors on blood biochemistry and therefore overall well-being (Cala et al., 1994). Additionally, the blending of varied training paradigms , such as Sprint Interval Training (SIT) with conventional Endurance Training (ET) presents a significant implication for cardiovascular well-being and blood physiology. Current evidence has shown how short bursts of high-intensity training can induce increases in significant parameters , such as resting heart rate, blood pressure, and VO2max. This synergy of training protocols shows that adjustments in blood physiology can be maximized using time-effective protocols that blend the endurance-building attribute of ET with the intensity of SIT. The consequent physiological adaptations not only improve performance but also yield better health advantages, further underlining the relevance of exploring new exercise paradigms in blood physiology research (Hurst et al., 2014). In conclusion, the findings of blood physiology studies attest to an integrated model of how multiple physiological mechanisms collaborate to preserve life. The restoration of blood pH and volume by cellular processes illustrates the creativity of the bodys adaptive attempts to reach equilibrium. Simultaneously, the identification of new training techniques , such as SIT offers promising areas for optimal cardiovascular fitness and overall health. Together, these results reaffirm the necessity of continued research into blood physiology, since it is translated into functional techniques intended to optimize sports performance and improve health parameters in different populations. Future research should focus on determining further connections among exercise regimens and blood regulation processes and thus expanding our knowledge in this vital field.

Total comprehension of blood physiology encompasses a number of aspects including hematopoiesis, hemostasis, and regulation of blood flow. Hematopoiesis is the development of blood cells, primarily occurring within the bone marrow. This complex process is crucial to maintaining proper physiological function, as it offers an ongoing supply of red blood cells, white blood cells, and platelets. Moreover, these constituents represent individual functions that are of vital significance to oxygen carriage, immune protection, and clotting mechanisms, respectively. Perturbation of hematopoiesis may result in disease states , such as anemia or leukopenia, making it vital to disease and health. These diseases are a good illustration of why blood physiology is relevant since they directly impact general body functions and individual health outcomes. Hemostasis is also a significant aspect of blood physiology, meaning a sequence of complex mechanisms that guarantee the prevention of blood loss after vascular injury. It is a multifactorial system comprising vascular spasm, platelet plug, and the coagulation cascade, all acting together to yield a stable clot. Activation of clotting factors and subsequent formation of the fibrin mesh are mechanisms of securing the initial platelet plug. Additionally, regulation of hemostasis is also equally significant because more than what is needed clotting or less than what is needed clotting will result in serious complications in the nature of thrombosis or uncontrolled bleeding. Understanding of hemostatic mechanisms' dynamics does not just elucidate our knowledge of blood physiology but also makes clinical practice in the treatment of bleeding disorders and thrombotic disease more significant, with its relevance to current medical paradigms. The regulation of blood flow is also central to renal function and overall fluid management in renal physiology. The kidneys rely on proper blood flow to effectively filter out waste material and regulate electrolyte balance, processes that are highly dependent on renal blood flow dynamics. Experiments with P2X receptors, in particular P2X1R, indicate their regulation of renal blood flow and vascular tone, which implies a complex interrelation between purinergic signaling and kidney function. Enhanced understanding on P2X receptors, and especially their implication in both physiological and pathological process, may prove instrumental in guiding renal health and disease management. In this way, the enhanced knowledge is not only instrumental in illustrating the blood physiology's complexity but also in provoking ongoing research within the determination of such correlations, and consequently the creation of new therapeutic avenues (Birch et al., 2013; Robles & Kane, 2014).

KEY TERMS FROM THIS CHAPTER

- Antibodies
- Blood Types
- Carbon Dioxide Transport
- Erythropoiesis
- Hematocrit
- Hemostasis
- Oxygen Transport
- Plasma
- Prothrombin
- Blood Clotting
- Blood Viscosity
- Circulatory Function
- Fibrinogen
- Hemoglobin
- Immune Response
- pH Balance
- Platelets
- Red Blood Cells

CRITICAL THINKING QUESTIONS

1. **What is the primary function of red blood cells?**
   a. Immune defense
   b. Blood clotting
   c. Transport of oxygen
   d. Hormone secretion
2. **Which of the following proteins leads to blood clotting?**
   a. Albumin
   b. Globulin
   c. Hemoglobin
   d. Fibrinogen
3. **What is the normal pH range of human blood?**
   a. 6.5–6.8
   b. 7.0–7.3
   c. 7.35–7.45
   d. 7.5–7.8
4. **What hormone stimulates the production of red blood cells?**
   a. Insulin
   b. Erythropoietin
   c. Thyroxine
   d. Cortisol
5. **Which of the white blood cells is most prevalent in normal blood?**
   a. Lymphocyte
   b. Monocyte
   c. Basophil
   d. Neutrophil

Short Answer Questions

1. What are the main components of blood?
2. List the most prevalent plasma protein.
3. How long does a red blood cell usually last?
4. What cells are accountable for immunity?
5. What is normal blood pH?
6. Explain plasma protein functions and regulation.
7. Describe the oxygen-carrying capacity of hemoglobin and the factors affecting oxygen binding.
8. Describe the function of the liver in maintaining blood composition.

Answers to Critical Thinking Questions

1. (c); 2. (d); 3. (c); 4. (b); 5. (d)

REFERENCES

1. Nellis, M. E., Spinella, P. C., Tucci, M., Stanworth, S. J., Steiner, M. E., Cushing, M. M., Davis, P. J., Karam, O., & Pediatric Acute Lung Injury and Sepsis Investigators (PALISI) network, Pediatric Critical Care Blood Research Network (BloodNet), and the P3T Investigators† (2020). Effect of platelet storage duration on clinical outcomes and incremental platelet change in critically ill children. *Transfusion*, *60*(12), 2849–2858. https://doi.org/10.1111/trf.16094 (accessed on 16th June 2025).
2. Abu Kasim, N. H., Alabsi, A. M., Haque, N., Rahman, N. A., et al. (2014). Hypoxic culture conditions as a solution for mesenchymal stem cell based regenerative therapy. https://core.ac.uk/download/30437779.pdf (accessed on 16th June 2025).
3. Adams, R., Ahmed, S., Anbalagan, M., Annunziata, M., Antonyak, M., Bain, G., Barbarulo, A., et al. (2013). JNK signaling in cancer: In need of new, smarter therapeutic targets. https://core.ac.uk/download/29139231.pdf (accessed on 16th June 2025).
4. Agas, D., Douni, E., Marchetti, L., & Sabbieti, M. G. (2015). The unbearable lightness of bone marrow homeostasis. https://core.ac.uk/download/54653580.pdf (accessed on 16th June 2025).
5. Aidun, C. K., Clausen, J. R., Liu, Z., Rao, A., et al. (2019). A unified analysis of nano-to-microscale particle dispersion in tubular blood flow. http://arxiv.org/abs/1905.11202 (accessed on 16th June 2025).
6. Ainsworth, M., Avitsur, R., Baumeister, R., Beedie, C., Biomarker Definitions Working Group, Bolger, N., Bowlby, J., et al. (2014). The attachment system and physiology in adulthood: Normative processes, individual differences, and implications for health. https://core.ac.uk/download/294625964.pdf Robles, T. F., & Kane, H. S. (2014). The attachment system and physiology in adulthood: normative processes, individual differences, and implications for health. *Journal of personality*, *82*(6), 515–527. https://doi.org/10.1111/jopy.12052 (accessed on 16th June 2025).
7. Allen, J., & Kyriacou, P. A. (2024). Advances in basic and applied research in photoplethysmography. https://core.ac.uk/download/610735098.pdf (accessed on 16th June 2025).
8. Alleva, E., Angiulli, E., Cioni, C., Malavasi, V., et al. (2017). Variation in environmental parameters in research and aquaculture: Effects on behavior, physiology and cell biology of teleost fish. https://core.ac.uk/download/153366757.pdf (accessed on 16th June 2025).
9. Altman, P. L., & Fisher, K. D. (1986). *Research Opportunities in Nutrition and Metabolism in Space*. https://core.ac.uk/download/pdf/10458014.pdf (accessed on 16th June 2025).
10. Andersen, M., Benevenga, N., Berlin, J., Beynon, R., Bier, D., Blagoev, B., Brakebusch, C., et al. (2008). Silac mouse for quantitative proteomics uncovers kindlin-3 as an essential factor for red blood cell function. https://core.ac.uk/download/18492217.pdf (accessed on 16th June 2025).
11. Arun, P. R., K. V., Rajashree, P., Venkatakrishna, M. K. S., & Vinushree, V. (2024). Understanding of Pranavaha Sroto Moola in the purview of modern physiology. https://core.ac.uk/download/617189952.pdf (accessed on 16th June 2025).
12. Ballarino, M., Fatica, A., & Morlando, M. (2015). Long non-coding RNAs: New players in hematopoiesis and leukemia. https://core.ac.uk/download/54520197.pdf (accessed on 16th June 2025).

13. Balola, A. H. A., Bartolmäs, T., Mayer, B., Salama, A., et al. (2019). Sub lytic terminal complement components induce eryptosis in autoimmune hemolytic anemia related to IgM autoantibodies. https://core.ac.uk/download/286567997.pdf (accessed on 16th June 2025).
14. Baum, H., Brochet, J. P., Buhagiar, G., Charilaou, A., et al. (2012). The EC4 European syllabus for post-graduate training in clinical chemistry and laboratory medicine: Version 4-2012. https://core.ac.uk/download/227992301.pdf (accessed on 16th June 2025).
15. Bicer, S., Clark, Y., Devine, R. D., Jing, X., et al. (2015). Losartan treatment attenuates tumor-induced myocardial dysfunction. https://core.ac.uk/download/213059445.pdf (accessed on 16th June 2025).
16. Bich, L., Moreau, J. F., & Pradeu, T. (2019). Understanding multicellularity: The functional organization of the intercellular space. https://core.ac.uk/download/228134961.pdf (accessed on 16th June 2025).
17. Birch, R. E., Peppiatt-Wildman, C. M., Schwiebert, E. M., Wildman, S. S., et al. (2013). Emerging key roles for P2X receptors in the kidney. https://core.ac.uk/download/30711999.pdf (accessed on 16th June 2025).
18. Brenes, A., Hettyey, A., Kelber, A., Kistler, A., Reppert, A. K., Davis, A. K., Brenes-Soto, A., et al. (2017). Coloration in amphibians as a reflection of nutritional status: The case of tree frogs in Costa Rica. https://core.ac.uk/download/91292641.pdf (accessed on 16th June 2025).
19. Brown, R. L., & Clarke, T. B. (2016). The regulation of host defenses to infection by the microbiota. https://core.ac.uk/download/77016328.pdf (accessed on 16th June 2025).
20. Brownlee, I., & Seal, C. J. (2015). Whole-grain foods and chronic disease: Evidence from epidemiological and intervention studies. https://core.ac.uk/download/287613637.pdf (accessed on 16th June 2025).
21. Buta, A., Danciu, C., Ognean, L., Spătariu, A., et al. (2019). Controversies regarding compatibility in Xeno transfusion with blood from dog to cat (Review). https://core.ac.uk/download/267071041.pdf (accessed on 16th June 2025).
22. Cala, P. M., & Maldonado, H. M. (1994). pH regulatory Na/H exchange by *Amphiuma* red blood cells. https://core.ac.uk/download/323069890.pdf (accessed on 16th June 2025).
23. Cavarretta, E., Dal Sasso, E., Forte, M., Frati, G., et al. (2017). The light and shadow of senescence and inflammation in cardiovascular pathology and regenerative medicine. https://core.ac.uk/download/141694265.pdf (accessed on 16th June 2025).
24. Cerliani, M. B., Gili, J. A., Klein, G., Pavicic, M., et al. (2015). Association between *PER3* length polymorphism and onco-hematological diseases and its influence on patient's functionality. https://core.ac.uk/download/153567200.pdf (accessed on 16th June 2025).
25. Chan, Y. Y., Kurzrock, E. A., Osborn, S. L., Sandlin, R. D., et al. (2017). The current use of stem cells in bladder tissue regeneration and bioengineering. https://core.ac.uk/download/323068966.pdf (accessed on 16th June 2025).
26. Chollet, M. E., Harrison, S. P., Lauritzen, K. H., Roman, M., et al. (2023). iPSC-derived liver organoids and inherited bleeding disorders: Potential and future perspectives. https://core.ac.uk/download/614769142.pdf (accessed on 16th June 2025).
27. Christie, D. A., Tansey, E. M., & Zallen, D. T. (2004). The Rhesus factor and disease prevention. https://core.ac.uk/download/30696199.pdf (accessed on 16th June 2025).

28. Claramunt Lozano, A., Gavaldá Esteve, C., & Sarrión Pérez, M. G. (2011). Dental management in patients with hemostasis alteration. https://core.ac.uk/download/71058980.pdf (accessed on 16th June 2025).

29. Martínez-Navarro, I., Sánchez-Gómez, J. M., Collado-Boira, E. J., Hernando, B., Panizo, N., & Hernando, C. (2019). Cardiac Damage Biomarkers and Heart Rate Variability Following a 118-Km Mountain Race: Relationship with Performance and Recovery. *Journal of sports science & medicine, 18*(4), 615–622.(accessed on 16th June 2025).

30. Compernolle, V., Feys, H., & Six, K. (2020). Platelet biochemistry and morphology after cryopreservation. https://core.ac.uk/download/287941861.pdf (accessed on 16th June 2025).

31. Crispin, A. (2017). HSCB, a co-chaperone in mitochondrial iron-sulfur cluster biogenesis, is a novel candidate gene for congenital sideroblastic anemia. https://open.bu.edu/bitstream/2144/26669/5/Crispin_bu_0017N_13280.pdf (accessed on 16th June 2025).

32. Ellis-Lepard, K. (2018). Does hydration impact memory: A systematic review. https://core.ac.uk/download/215462394.pdf (accessed on 16th June 2025).

33. Garshnek, V., Hooke, L. R., Radtke, M., Rowe, J., et al. (1980). *USSR Space Life Sciences Digest*, issue 3. ANNUAL SUMMARY 1980 Prepared under the direction of Gerald A. Soffen, Ph.D., Director Life Sciences Division National Aeronautics and Space Administration Washington, D.C. 20546 Contract NASW-3469(accessed on 16th June 2025).

34. Helm, B., & Martinez-Bakker, M. (2015). The influence of biological rhythms on host–parasite interactions. https://core.ac.uk/download/42361213.pdf (accessed on 16th June 2025).

35. Herms, J., Kretzschmar, H. A., & Vassallo, N. (2004). The molecular pathology of prion diseases. https://core.ac.uk/download/46601891.pdf (accessed on 16th June 2025).

36. Heusner, W. W., & Vanhuss, W. D. (1979). Space flight research relevant to health, physical education, and recreation: With particular reference to Skylab's life science experiments. https://core.ac.uk/download/pdf/10345816.pdf (accessed on 16th June 2025).

37. Holtby, R. J., Jahr, J. S., & Roghani, K. (2014). Effects of hemoglobin-based oxygen carriers on blood coagulation. https://core.ac.uk/download/323078517.pdf (accessed on 16th June 2025).

38. Hurst, R. A. (2014). The effects and differences of sprint interval training, endurance training and the training types combined on physiological parameters and exercise performance. https://core.ac.uk/download/29841767.pdf (accessed on 16th June 2025).

39. Hutchins, B. R., Brown, J., Buchwald, D., Clarke, D., D., D., et al. (2015). Descartes, corpuscles and reductionism: Mechanism and systems in Descartes' physiology. https://core.ac.uk/download/147061302.pdf (accessed on 16th June 2025).

40. Ibañez, A. E., Larsen, K. E., Montalti, D., Najle, R., et al. (2015). Hematology, biochemistry and serum protein analyses of Antarctic and non-Antarctic skuas. https://core.ac.uk/download/161267705.pdf (accessed on 16th June 2025).

41. Li, S. C., Li, Z., Ran, Q., Wu, Y., et al. (2018). The differentiation balance of bone marrow mesenchymal stem cells is crucial to hematopoiesis. https://core.ac.uk/download/323062656.pdf (accessed on 16th June 2025).

42. Oliveira, S. de, & Saldanha, C. (2010). An overview about erythrocyte membrane. https://core.ac.uk/download/12426151.pdf (accessed on 16th June 2025).

43. Pal, R., Chatterjee, P. K., Chatterjee, P., Vinodini, N. A., PrasannaMithra, S., Banerjee, S., Suman, V. B., et al. (2014). Polycystic ovary syndrome, blood group & diet: A correlative study in South Indian females. https://core.ac.uk/download/pdf/27151617.pdf (accessed on 16th June 2025).

44. Pimienta, M., Edderkaoui, M., Wang, R., & Pandol, S. (2017). The potential for circulating tumor cells in pancreatic cancer management. https://core.ac.uk/download/323077820.pdf (accessed on 16th June 2025).

45. Prasad, N. K., Dubey, S., & Tripathi, R. (2023). A critical review on *Samana Vayu* apropos regulation of gastrointestinal tract. https://core.ac.uk/download/617189551.pdf (accessed on 16th June 2025).

46. Rawling, B. (2012). Providing the gift of life: Canadian medical practitioners and the treatment of shock on the battlefield. https://core.ac.uk/download/143686944.pdf (accessed on 16th June 2025).

47. Ross, A. P., & Zarbalis, K. S. (2014). The emerging roles of ribosome biogenesis in craniofacial development. https://core.ac.uk/download/323070204.pdf (accessed on 16th June 2025).

48. Rowe, J., Stone, L. R., & Teeter, R. (2025). *USSR Space Life Sciences Digest*, issue 30. https://core.ac.uk/download/pdf/42817408.pdf (accessed on 16th June 2025).

49. Stotts, N. A., & Wong, V. K. (2003). Physiology and prevention of heel ulcers: The state of science. https://core.ac.uk/download/70426031.pdf (accessed on 16th June 2025).

50. The Boston University Photonics Center. (2015). *The Boston University Photonics Center Annual Report 2014–2015*. https://open.bu.edu/bitstream/2144/29753/1/Photonics-Center-Annual-Report-2015-final.pdf (accessed on 16th June 2025).

51. Torday J. S. (2015). Homeostasis as the Mechanism of Evolution. *Biology*, *4*(3), 573–590. https://doi.org/10.3390/biology4030573(accessed on 16th June 2025).

CARDIAC PHYSIOLOGY

9

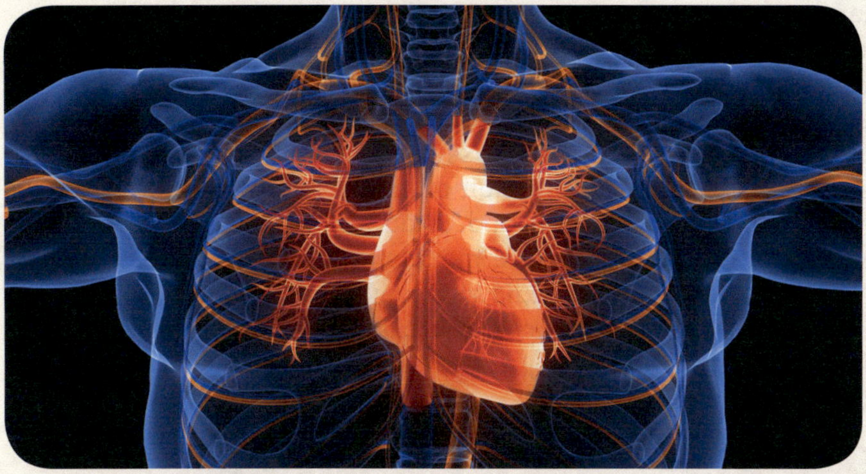

LEARNING OBJECTIVES

After studying this chapter, you will be able to:

1. Discuss the heart's anatomy;
2. Describe the conduction system of the heart;
3. Discuss the cardiac cycle;
4. Highlight cardiac output;
5. Learn heart rate regulation;
6. Evaluate the typical cardiac disorders.

Introduction

The field of cardiac physiology entails the examination of the heart's structure and function as well as its complex physiological mechanisms. Information on the anatomy of the heart is essential, given that various components , such as the myocardium, valves, and electrical conduction system work together to facilitate efficient blood circulation. The myocardium, which consists of special cardiac muscle cells, carries out the contractile activity of the heart. This vital function assists in the rhythmic pumping of blood, providing adequate perfusion to vital organs. The hearts' electrical system, controlled by pacemaker cells, initiates and regulates the heartbeat, ensuring synchrony and adaptation to changing physiological demands. By studying these intricate processes, researchers are able to gain an understanding of normal cardiac function and the pathophysiologic changes that have been made during illness, and utilize this information as a springboard for future investigation in conditions like myocardial infarction and heart failure. The process from a healthy cardiac state to one of dysfunction is often characterized by profound changes in cardiac remodeling. Pathologic molecular mechanisms play a role in the reorganization of the structure of the heart and cause cardiac dysfunction, especially after insults , such as myocardial infarction. Following injury, a cascade of signals evokes myocyte loss, hypertrophy, and fibrosis, eventually affecting the ability of the heart to contract and manage blood flow. Additionally, the remodeling phase can initially behave as a protective measure as a compensatory response. However, if inflammation is chronic or pressure overload becomes persistent, then it can significantly play a role in the onset of heart failure. It is necessary to understand such signaling pathways so that therapeutic interventions can be developed to avert the adverse effects of cardiac remodeling in the context of diseases like myocardial infarction and thus expect improved clinical outcomes by following targeted therapies (Angelini et al., 2017). Recent developments in cardiac imaging and computational modeling are ushering in the era of personalized therapy in the arena of cardiac physiology. Imaging modalities , such as echocardiography and cardiac magnetic resonance (CMR) imaging have become precious tools for quantifying myocardial damage and function following myocardial infarction. With the application of these imaging modalities, clinicians can derive detailed data sets, which are used to inform risk stratification and treatment planning. Moreover, advances in computational modeling of left ventricular (LV) dynamics offer better accuracy in the evaluation of biomechanical parameters , such as contractility and stiffness, which are critical to the understanding of patient-specific outcomes following acute myocardial injury. Translation of these models into clinical practice is also daunting, for example, through validation compared to known biomarkers and by making user-friendly software available. By overcoming these challenges, clinicians and researchers are able to develop a multidisciplinary framework that ultimately leads to better patient care and therapeutic outcomes (Berry et al., 2017) (Figure 9.1).

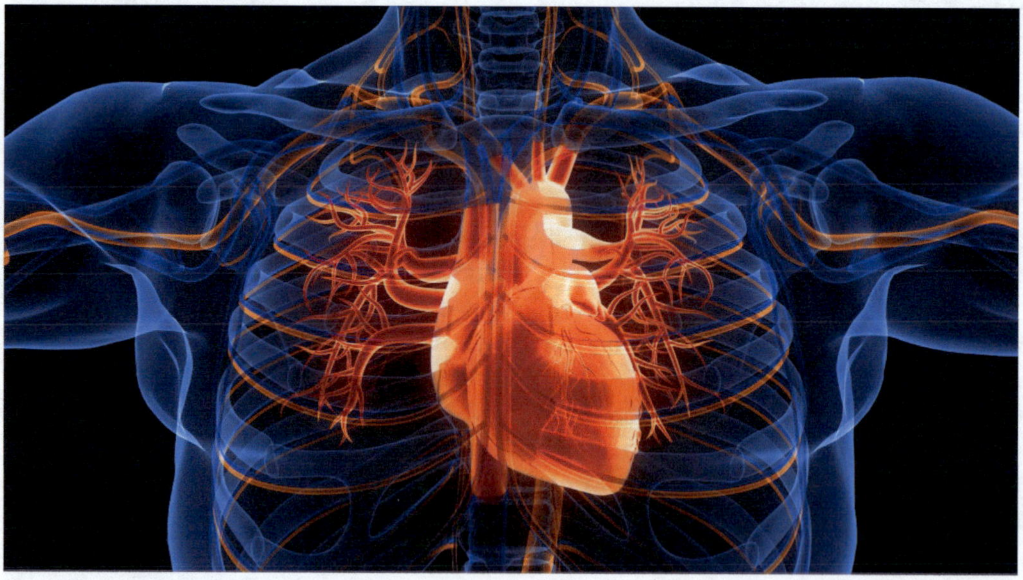

Figure 9.1. AHA vascular discovery.

Source: https://www.anesthesiaserviceswi.com/wp-content/uploads/2023/08/Heart-scaled.jpg.

Definition and Importance of Cardiac Physiology

Cardiac physiology must be understood in order to understand how the heart works and its central role in maintaining overall bodily health. Fundamentally, cardiac physiology entails the study of structure, heart function, and their controlling mechanisms for performance. It entails studies of electrical conduction, mechanical function, and effects of their various physiological and pathological states on cardiac function. Elucidation of these factors assists scientists and clinicians in establishing normal vs. abnormal cardiac function, which is crucial in the diagnosis and treatment of cardiovascular disease. Thus, cardiac physiology is more than description of anatomy; it is a component of human health that informs clinical interventions and ongoing medical research (Thierry et al., 2013). Cardiac physiology should not be overstated, particularly in a time when cardiovascular disease is on the rise.

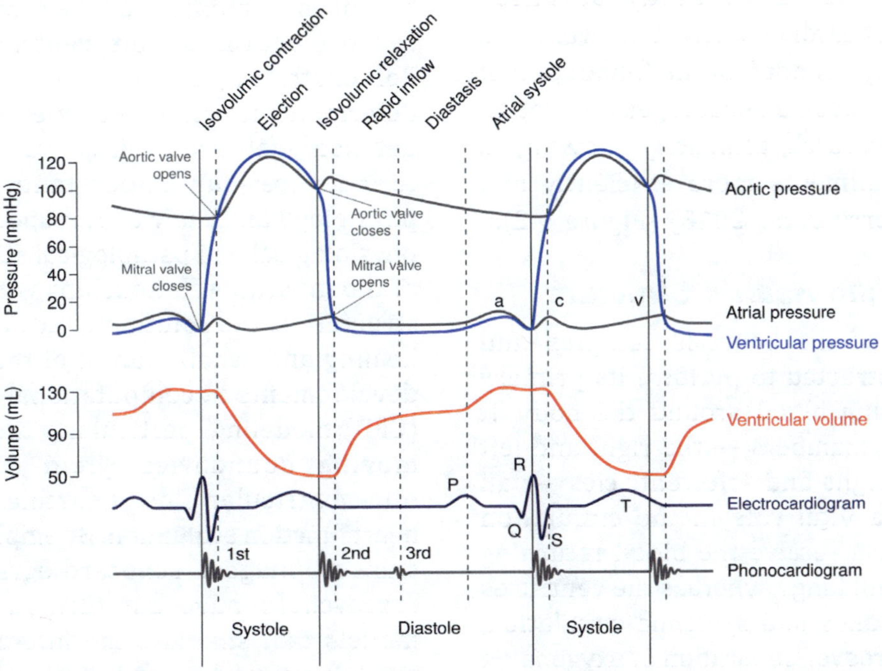

Figure 9.2. Importance of cardiac physiology.

Source: https://litfl.com/wp-content/uploads/2019/01/Wiggers-diagram.jpg.

A knowledge of cardiac physiology assists in understanding the impact of exercise, diet, and age on cardiovascular health. This understanding is crucial not only for health professionals but also for patients who wish to manage or prevent heart disease. In addition, the knowledge gleaned from cardiac physiology has a critical bearing on the development of therapeutic interventions. For instance, the data gathered from the investigation of the electrical activity of the heart have been instrumental in advanced techniques of arrhythmia control and surgical interventions like coronary artery bypass grafting. Hence, the relevance of cardiac physiology is not only theoretical research; it has a bearing on actual clinical outcome and management of patients (Diller et al.,

2009). Moreover, continued research in cardiac physiology continues to unveil new facets of heart function that demonstrate its malleability and complexity. Recent research has focused on the molecular and cellular processes of cardiac muscle cells and how they respond to various stressors and stimuli. Such questions are significant in that they may provide new insight into potential therapeutic targets for conditions like heart failure and hypertrophic cardiomyopathy. In addition, the integration of technology, such as cardiac imaging and bioengineering, has significantly advanced understanding of cardiac function *in vivo*. Thus, cardiac physiology is not just the foundation of clinical practice but also encourages innovation in biomedical research, ultimately allowing us to treat heart ailments more efficiently and effectively (Thierry et al., 2013) (Figure 9.2).

Overview of the Heart's Structure

The structure of the heart is complex and beautifully constructed to perform its primary function: pumping blood around the body. It consists of four chambers — the right and left atria, and the right and left ventricles — all of which play a vital role in the circulation process. The atria receive the blood returning from the body and lungs, whereas the ventricles eject it to the lungs and systemic circulation, respectively. Moreover, separation of oxygenated and deoxygenated blood is required for effective respiratory function and overall metabolism, reflecting the heart's role as an essential center to provide homeostasis. This optimized structure also permits transmission of the blood through four valves: the pulmonary, tricuspid, mitral, and aortic valves. These valves provide a mechanism for the one-way flow of blood to prevent backflow during the cardiac cycle, further providing effectiveness in cardiac action. In addition to its chambers and valves, the heart is encased in a covering organ known as the pericardium to enable frictionless gliding between contractions. The myocardium or heart muscle is made up of highly specialized cardiac muscle cells with the ability to generate and conduct electrical impulses, thereby enabling coordinated contractions. Between its inner lining endocardium and outer layer epicardium, the myocardium's structure plays a crucial role in the heart's mechanical properties. More recent computational models, as quoted in dynamic patient-specific model studies, further describe the stress and strain dynamics of the heart's structure under various conditions. Application of an immersed boundary/finite element method has been demonstrated to provide a realistic reconstruction of left ventricular anatomy, demonstrating the way in which structure determines function (Balay et al., 2014). Such detailed analyses are important as they assist to advance our understanding of cardiac physiology and the way it responds to different physiological and pathological states. Mimicking of the intricate relationships within the heart's structure is the solution to advancement in the healing and rehabilitation of the heart. Recent developments in computational fluid dynamics (CFD) modeling, particularly those concerning moving boundaries, yield data regarding intraventricular flow dynamics essential for heart function evaluation. By employing real-time transesophageal echocardiographic imaging, researchers have established sophisticated models that simulate the interaction between the left ventricle and mitral valve throughout the entire cardiac cycle (Bavo et al., 2016). Not only does this research extend knowledge of normal physiologic processes but also provides a valuable model for the identification of abnormal dynamics that pertain to disorders , such as mitral valve malfunction. In further advancing cardiac physiology through the addition of specialty models and imaging technology, the hope of improved patient-specific therapy ever grows, justifying an unequivocal understanding of heart anatomy.

Historical Context and Advancements in Cardiac Research

The evolution of cardiac research marks a path of milestones that have guided us to the current understanding of cardiac physiology. The initial efforts during the 19th century created the groundwork for contemporary cardiac research, progressing from rudimentary anatomical observations to more sophisticated physiological studies. Pioneer research papers by investigators , such as Willem Einthoven, who invented the electrocardiogram (ECG) in 1903, established a seminal tool for assessing heart function. This discovery showed the importance of electrical impulses in the functioning of the heart and enabled scientists to better describe various heart conditions. This early breakthrough not only advanced the discipline itself but went on to stimulate further study into mechanisms of heart disease and treatment modes and paved the way for more intricate research in the 20th and 21st centuries that has gone on to illuminate the complexities of cardiac health and pathology. The evolution of cardiac research has also placed emphasis on the role of technology in enhancing our understanding of heart function. With the evolution of advanced imaging modalities and biomarker analysis, researchers are now capable of examining the intricate dynamics that underlie cardiovascular disease.

One such instance is the use of vectorcardiography (VCG) that has identified differences in cardiac electrical activity between normal and STEMI-suffering populations. It has been shown by means of studies that planarity of vectorcardiographic QRS loops is able to separate healthy individuals from those suffering from acute cardiac diseases to a significant degree and thus illustrate the potential of novel technologies in diagnostics and planning for treatment (Goswami et al., 2017). This synergy of advances in technology with traditional cardiac physiology research is a significant step towards understanding the intricacies of hearts and addressing cardiometabolic disorders. In the recent years, the field has moved toward an integrated strategy where multi-omics data are employed to unravel the multifactorial etiology of cardiovascular diseases. Researchers are increasingly recognizing the importance of integrating various omics disciplines—, such as genomics, proteomics, and metabolomics—to elucidate the complex mechanisms of cardiac pathologies. The merging of such heterogeneous data types promises more understanding of cardiac function and disease progression, leading to improved biomarker development for improved diagnosis and treatment (Argano et al., 2019). The second contribution is that including gender-specific analysis shows expanding awareness of how psychosocial and biological influences influence cardiovascular health. As this convergence of diverse research strategies goes on, it holds great promise to advance cardiac physiology and further develop interventions based on the particular requirements of disparate patient populations (Figure 9.3).

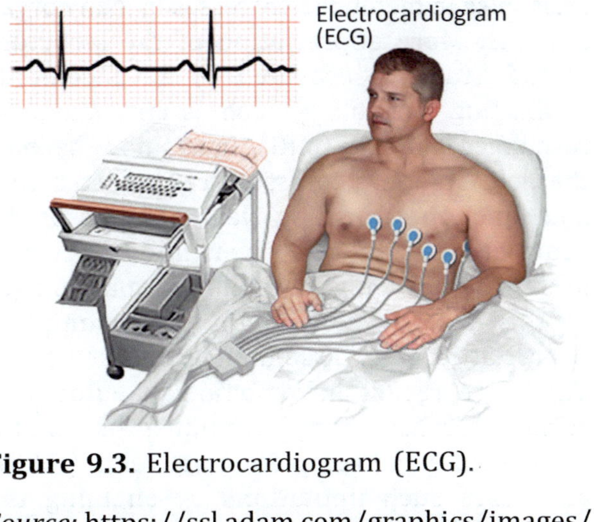

Figure 9.3. Electrocardiogram (ECG).

Source: https://ssl.adam.com/graphics/images/en/1135.jpg.

9.1. Anatomy of the Heart

Learning Outcome

1. Describe the heart's chambers: atria and ventricles;
2. Emphasize valves and function;
3. Comprehend the large blood vessels associated with the heart.

The cardiac anatomy is a vital subject in cardiac physiology due to the fact that it provides fundamental understanding of how the heart works under disease and healthy conditions. Structurally, the heart contains four chambers: two atria and two ventricles, which collaborate in order to facilitate blood circulation in the body. The right atrium collects systemic circulation deoxygenated blood, whereas the left atrium receives oxygenated blood from the lungs. The right ventricle then pumps the blood to the lungs to be oxygenated, and the left ventricle pumps oxygen-rich blood to the rest of the body. This intricate system of chambers, coupled with valves to prevent backflow, speaks to the heart's role as a strong muscular organ, critical in the service of homeostasis maintenance and assistance in metabolic processes in many organ systems. More appreciation of the structure of the hearts is provided by advancements in imaging technology, such as cine magnetic resonance imaging (MRI). It has now become the gold standard to assess cardiac structure and function, providing clear pictures of the heart architecture. However, traditional cine MRI provides only two-dimensional images of the heart, which might limit complete appreciation of its three-dimensional structure. The more recent introduction of automated surface reconstruction techniques like multi-class point cloud completion networks (PCCN) addresses such limitations by enabling the accurate three-dimensional cardiac anatomies to be reconstructed via sparse imaging data. These developments expand the horizons of cardiac research and enhance our ability for the evaluation of pathologies, and hence it becomes imperative to integrate continuously these advanced imaging methods into the study of cardiac physiology so as to depict the complexities of heart anatomy effectively (Banerjee et al., 2023). Further, comprehensive databases like the Cardiac Atlas Project (CAP) serve as a milestone in bridging the gap between cardiac anatomy and physiology by supplying big sets of cardiac imaging along with clinical data. CAP aims to build a structural and functional atlas of the heart through coordinated statistical analysis of various cardiac shapes and wall motions. By manipulating cardiac function in a range of populations, these collections of data are providing important insights into normal and diseased states of the heart. The integration of anatomy and physiological function is critical to the development of targeted therapeutic interventions for cardiac disorders. Hence, the convergence of advanced imaging techniques and comprehensive databases represents a grand stride in cardiac science, an era where accurate anatomical observations can lead to improved patient care and improved clinical outcomes (Kadish et al., 2011) (Figure 9.4).

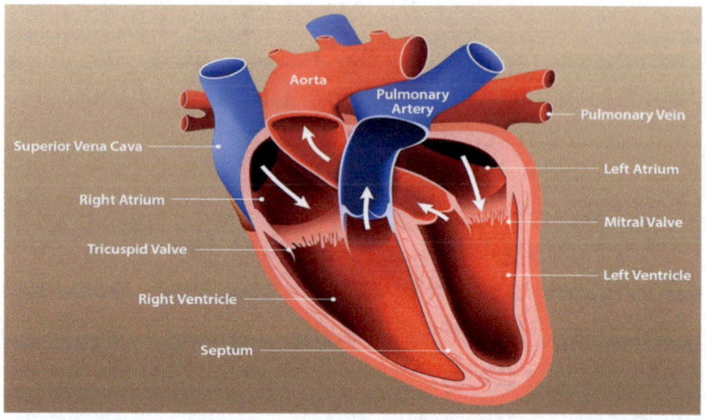

Figure 9.4. Heart anatomy.

Source: https://img.lb.wbmdstatic.com/vim/live/webmd/consumer_assets/site_images/article_thumbnails/BigBead/heart_anatomy_function_and_blood_circulation_bigbead/1800x1200_heart_anatomy_function_and_blood_circulation_bigbead.jpg.

9.1.1. Chambers of the Heart: Atria and Ventricles

The heart, which is a muscular organ located in the center of the circulatory system, is distinctly divided into four chambers: the right atrium, right ventricle, left atrium, and left ventricle. The two upper chambers are the atria and serve as receiving reservoirs for blood; the right atrium receives the deoxygenated blood returning from the body and the left atrium receives the oxygenated blood returning from the lungs. This division in anatomy is important for maintaining efficient blood flow and ensuring oxygenated and deoxygenated blood do not combine. The ventricles, the lower two of the chambers, are utilized to pump blood away from the heart. The deoxygenated blood is circulated by the right ventricle to the lungs for oxygenation, while the left ventricle is responsible for the circulation of oxygenated blood to the systemic circulation, thus being the key to sustaining life. Improved advances in cardiac modeling have revealed the complexity within the performance of the hearts, particularly among the atria and the ventricles. One of the early influential studies developed an integrated electromechanical model of the four-chambered heart that accurately captures the significant contribution of atrial contractions to overall cardiac function. The model shows that atrial function governs ventricular filling and related contractions and that omissions in atrial function result in poor descriptions of cardiac function. The simulation showed that a healthy cardiac function, as supported by pressure-volume loops and three-dimensional deformations, is dependent on the coordination of both the atrial and ventricular activities, emphasizing the key role that every chamber plays in cardiac physiology (Africa et al., 2022). Knowledge about the mechanical properties of heart tissues is essential in both clinical uses and basic physiological studies. Studies on mechanical characteristics of various heart chambers have determined that although the atria and ventricles share a common embryonic origin, their mechanical characteristics differ as they develop. For instance, investigations in an ovine model have shown that mechanical stiffness of the cardiac tissues varies significantly across the chambers, with ventricles generally containing greater strain energy storage than atria. These differences are associated with changes in collagen-to-myocyte ratios, which highlight the structural adaptation of cardiac tissues to their functional demands (Javani et al., 2016). These findings regarding the mechanical characteristics of each chamber further enhance the knowledge of cardiac physiology and may direct therapeutic interventions into various heart diseases (Figure 9.5).

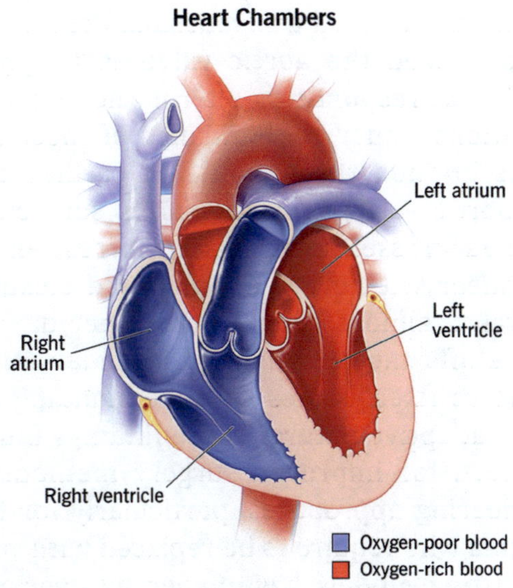

Figure 9.5. Chambers of the heart.

Source: https://my.clevelandclinic.org/-/scassets/images/org/health/articles/23074-heart-chambers.

9.1.2. Valves and Their Functions

The cardiac system relies almost entirely on valves to ensure the one-way movement of blood through the heart and circulatory machinery. The structures are strategically located at the junctions of inter-chambers and great blood vessels, for instance, the aortic and pulmonary valves. Every valve functions via a mechanical process that responds to pressure gradients formed in the course of the cardiac cycle. When the heart contracts, pressure is built up, leading to the opening of the valves, therefore allowing the blood to flow forward. On the other hand, when the heart relaxes, the reduction in pressure brings about the closure of the valves, thereby hindering the backward movement of the blood. This coordinated process is essential in the functioning of a proper circulatory system and in the supply of adequate oxygenated blood to the body, highlighting the vital function of heart valves within cardiac physiology. Recent studies indicate that heart valves, particularly the aortic valve, may be more than simple passive pathways for blood transmission. Research has characterized the aortic valve as a dynamic organ that responds to altering hemodynamic conditions under the guidance of mechanical forces applied throughout the cardiac cycle. The aortic valve, in particular, is subjected to elevated stresses under loading forces, bending, and shear with every opening and closure of the valve, almost 100,000 times per day. This view shifts the paradigm from understanding valves as fixed bodies to understanding their living, adaptive nature. These findings indicate the need for improved surgery methods and engineering approaches, particularly for those patients who require to be replaced with valves, as existing models have generally overlooked the complexity and durability of such basic components. Thus, the incorporation of tissue-engineered substitutes into the living cells could mimic the original functioning of heart valves (Bertazzo et al., 2014). In addition, the morphology and function of heart valves are inextricably linked with the overall mechanics of the heart, namely with respect to left ventricular (LV) morphology and its interaction with blood flow dynamics. Computational fluid dynamics (CFD) research has enabled the exploration of how the anatomical structures of trabeculae and papillary muscles affect the hemodynamic conditions of the LV. These geometries have the potential to alter intra-ventricular pressure drops and wall shear stress greatly, unveiling a rich interaction between cardiac geometry and valve function. Both detailed and smoothed LV endocardial geometries can be represented to illustrate that differences in anatomy have the potential to create different patterns of blood flow and influence total cardiac efficiency. Such findings emphasize the significance of considering accurate anatomical models in examining valve function and designing novel clinical approaches for the treatment of heart disease (Paun et al., 2018) (Figure 9.6).

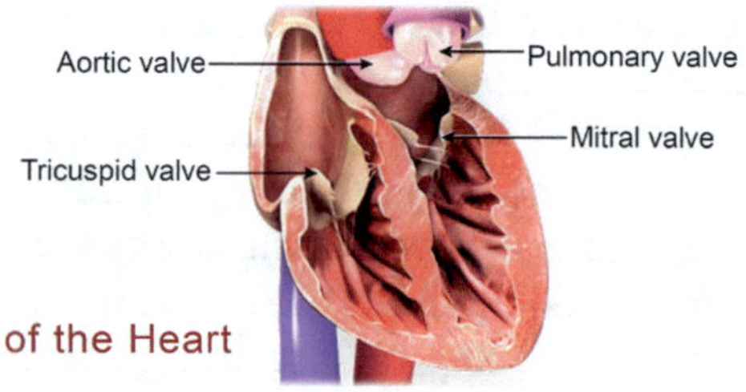

Figure 9.6. Heart valve problems and disease.

Source: https://www.heart.org/-/media/Images/Health-Topics/Heart-Valve-Problems-and-Disease/valves-of-the-heart-illustration.jpg?sc_lang=en.

9.1.3. Major Blood Vessels Associated with the Heart

The main blood vessels associated with the heart play a key role in obtaining hemodynamic stability and ensuring adequate circulation throughout the entire body. The largest artery, the aorta, emerges from the left ventricle and serves as the major pathway for oxygenated blood to systemic circulation. The elasticity and diameter of the vessels allow it to accept high-pressure blood flow while regulating the distribution of blood at the same time. Besides the aorta, the pulmonary artery, which bifurcates into the right and left pulmonary arteries, carries deoxygenated blood from the right ventricle to the lungs for their oxygenation. This double circulation system plays a vital role in meeting the metabolic demands of the body and serves to point out the importance of the major blood vessels to overall cardiac physiology, in which any aberration in their functioning can lead to monumental health problems. Veins also play a critical role in the circulatory system, completing the loop that allows blood to be returned to the heart. The superior and inferior vena cavae are the significant veins that are responsible for bringing oxygen-poor blood from the body back into the right atrium. As large components of the venous return system, they ensure that oxygen-depleted blood is brought back for reoxygenation. The functioning of these vessels is governed by various physiological factors like hydrostatic pressure and the action of gravity on blood flow. Particularly in the upright human posture, the intricate relationship between these blood vessels and the forces of gravity can influence cardiac output and venous return, demonstrating the dynamicity of cardiovascular physiology (Blomqvist et al.). Besides, the connection between the heart and corresponding blood vessels is not just that of transportation; they also exert metabolic influences that affect cardiac function. Recent investigations have cast light on the role of epicardial adipose tissue in cardiac physiology, highlighting its association with both normal and pathologic states of heart physiology (Agra et al., 2017). Since this tissue releases multiple bioactive factors, its close proximity to the coronary vessels suggests that it may have a regulatory effect on vascular inflammation and tone. It is important to understand how these large blood vessels communicate with the surrounding tissues, such as the epicardial fat, to develop specific therapeutic interventions for heart disease. This interdependence suggests that vascular optimization is a many-faceted process that needs to consider not only the physical characteristics of blood vessels, but also the metabolic requirements of the cardiac tissue it serves.

Test Your Knowledge

1. What are the four chambers of the heart?
2. Which blood vessels bring oxygen-depleted blood to the heart?

9.2. Electrical Conduction System

Learning Outcome

1. Explain the role of the sinoatrial (SA) node;
2. Define the path of electrical impulses around the heart;
3. Learn the importance of the atrioventricular (AV) node.

The heart's electrical conduction system is a complex network that ensures coordinated cardiac action. It consists of specialized cardiomyocytes that produce and transmit electrical impulses, thereby ensuring ventricular and atrial synchronized contraction. The center of this system is the sinoatrial (SA) node, atrioventricular (AV) node, bundle of His, and Purkinje fibers. Such an intricate structure facilitates quick conduction of electrical impulses to facilitate efficient circulation of blood in the cardiovascular system. Disruption of this network can lead to arrhythmias, syncope, or sudden cardiac death, and hence the importance of understanding the physiological and molecular processes of cardiac conduction (Bocchi et al., 2018). The most recent technological advances have provided us with an unprecedented understanding of the electrical conduction system and how it functions. For instance, development of optogenetic techniques now allows investigators to modulate and monitor cardiac electrical activity in real time. The techniques employ light to modulate the behavior of cells with high precision, creating new possibilities for interventions in cardiac pacing and defibrillation. A seminal study showed an all-optical platform with a built-in digital projector for imaging and provoking electrical activity in intact mouse hearts.

The device was able to restore normal conduction patterns after interruptions, a revolutionary cardiac manipulation and control over arrhythmia (Bocchi et al., 2018). The ability to observe cardiac rhythms with real-time intervention is a revolution in the field of cardiac physiology. Besides that, an understanding of cardiac conduction system development and regulation will also inform potential therapeutic interventions against arrhythmia. With the utilization of transgenic lines like the Tg(cmlc2:gCaMP)s878 zebrafish line, researchers were able to discern specific conduction developmental stages, involving cellular and anatomical changes important for the creation of a functional heart. Findings in epigenetic research, such as hemodynamic flow, provide an additional layer of understanding of how the conduction system adapts to physiological demand. New genetic screens have determined a number of conduction pathway mutations that provide new avenues for studying the genetic etiology of electrical system malfunction (Arnaout et al., 2008). The interdisciplinarity employing the genetic, optical mapping, and functional analyses offers the constant advancement in cardiac physiology research and its application to clinical outcome in terms of arrhythmias (Figure 9.7).

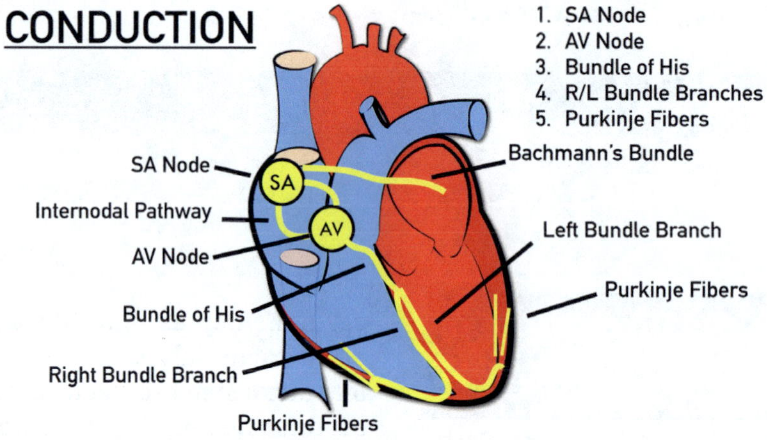

Figure 9.7. Electrical conduction system of the heart.

Source: https://images.squarespace-cdn.com/content/v1/5e48489da899cd09424943db/1601767512822-NA1VLQA4W9AM3A7Y2U8N/Austin.Kosier.43H.png.

9.2.1. Role of the Sinoatrial (SA) Node

The SA node is also referred to as the heart's natural pacemaker and plays a vital function in initiating as well as controlling the cardiac rhythm. Found in the right atrium, the SA node contains pacemaker cells uniquely programmed to discharge electrical impulses, regulating the number at which the heart beats. They radiate through the atria, making them contract, and thus lead to the ventricles filling up appropriately. This inbuilt ability to produce electrical activity is crucial in maintaining a stable heart rate and, consequently, any dysfunction of the SA node can lead to various arrhythmic states. It is essential to know the biophysiological mechanisms that control the SA node to appreciate the nuances of cardiac physiology and eliminate potential clinical implications of its dysfunction. At the heart of the SA node's pacemaking activity are the hyperpolarization-activated cyclic nucleotide-gated (HCN) channels, particularly the HCN4 isoform. The channels conduct the I-f current, which is a primary cause of spontaneous depolarization of pacemaker cells. The regulation of the heart rate by the interaction between HCN4 channels and intracellular cyclic adenosine monophosphate (cAMP) proves the SA sensitivity to autonomic nervous system control. Recent advances have shown that while HCN4 channels play a dominant role in heart rate control, their mechanisms diverge from those long supposed. The excitation process of the SA node is not only based on these currents but also on complex calcium dynamics and interaction with other ionic currents, revealing a more complex picture of the control of heart rates in healthy and disease conditions (Biel et al., 2022). Moreover, the role of sodium-calcium exchanger (NCX1) in relation to spontaneous calcium release events has been strongly underscored by SA node function studies. Through studies, it was reported that the absence of NCX1 can impair pacemaker function, thus highlighting its valuable contribution towards the SA node's overall functioning. In genetically modified mice studies, the absence of NCX1 caused the SA node to be unable to produce rhythmic depolarizations and ultimately reach a quiescent state but retain the capacity to participate in electrical coupling (Alber et al., 2013). This is aimed at emphasizing the intricate interdependence of ionic currents and cellular signal-transducing mechanisms in the SA node, again substantiating the argument that cardiac physiology is an amalgamation of intricate interdependency amongst various cellular mechanisms. Clarification of these dynamics is paramount in the establishment of therapeutic interventions aimed at the restoration of normal cardiac physiology in patients with arrhythmias secondary to SA node dysfunction (Figure 9.8).

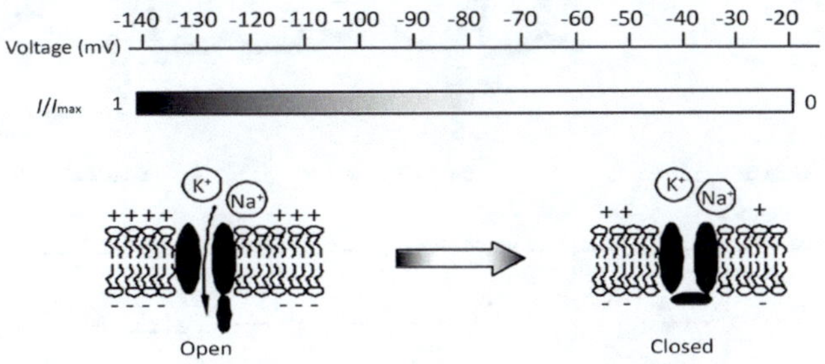

Figure 9.8. Hyperpolarization-activated cyclic nucleotide-gated (HCN).

Source: https://media.springernature.com/full/springer-static/image/art%3A10.1038%2Faps.2010.105/MediaObjects/41401_2010_Article_BFaps2010105_Fig1_HTML.jpg.

9.2.2. Pathway of Electrical Impulses Through the Heart

The heart operates using a highly organized system of electrical impulses governing cardiac rhythm and effective pumping of blood. Electrical impulse path begins at the SA node located in the right atrium. As the heart's normal pacemaker, the SA node generates spontaneous action potentials that result in atrial myocardial contraction. These impulses then travel through atrial walls, contracting both atria simultaneously and pushing blood into ventricles. Upon passing through the AV node, there is a critical delay that allows for the ventricles to fill with blood prior to them contracting. This carefully coordinated series of electrical transmission ensures proper circulation, emphasizing the importance of the heart's electrical system in overall cardiac physiology. Following the delay at the AV node, the electrical impulses are rapidly conveyed through the bundle of His, or the atrioventricular bundle. This bundle serves as a conduit to transmit impulses from the atria to the ventricles through specialized conduction fibers known as Purkinje fibers. The configuration of these fibers allows the electrical signals to propagate widely throughout the ventricular myocardium, facilitating a synchronized ventricular contraction. This fast conduction is crucial in the preservation of cardiac output and avoidance of arrhythmias, which can interfere with normal cardiac function. In addition, any blockage or retardation in the AV node, such as that encountered in research on acidosis, can cause prolonged conduction times or total block, highly affecting heart function and potentially leading to severe complications, including brady-arrhythmias (Burton et al., 2014).

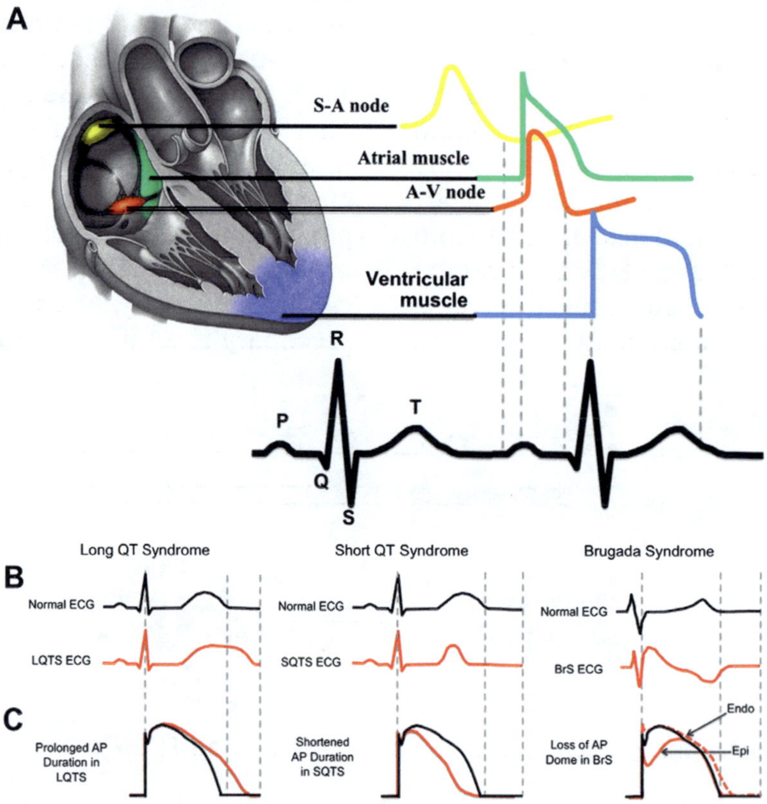

Figure 9.9. Electrical impulses through the heart.

Source: https://www.researchgate.net/profile/John-Giudicessi/publication/230894447/figure/fig2/AS:340527913422850@1458199589041/Electrical-activity-of-the-heart-in-health-and-disease-A-Schematic-representation-of.png.

Also, the mechanism of afterdepolarizations in cardiac electrical activity is informative regarding arrhythmogenesis. Afterdepolarizations appear following the first action potential and lead to potential extrasystoles or re-entrant circuits that cause arrhythmias. Computational models that model cardiac tissue response via simulation evidence suggest that the spatial characteristics of afterdepolarizations play important roles in their capacity to initiate these abnormal rhythms. If an afterdepolarization area exceeds a threshold value, the possibility of propagating extrasystoles is considerably raised. This emphasizes the dynamic mechanisms of electrical conduction within the heart, where directions for impulses become determined by internal or external factors, eventually on heart physiology and well-being (Clayton et al., 2009) (Figure 9.9).

9.2.3. Importance of the Atrioventricular (AV) Node

The AV node is one of the most important components of the heart's electrical conduction system, coordinating atrioventricular electrical signals. It is also a gate for the timing of the electrical stimuli from the atria to be synchronized in reaching the ventricles for proper contraction of the cardiac muscle. This coordination is particularly important during the cardiac cycle, where atrial contraction initiates ventricular contraction for adequate filling and maximal cardiac output. If the AV node fails to function properly, it can result in various arrhythmias, such as heart blocks, which disrupt regular rhythm and greatly hinder heart function. These interrupations highlight the AV nodes' vital role in not only sustaining rhythm but also cardiovascular health. Studies on the impact of acidosis on the AV node have revealed its performance limits in pathological conditions. Experiments show that hypercapnia can increase the time of conduction through the AV node, hence augmenting the chances of 2:1 AV nodal block and the occurrence of bradyarrhythmias. The increased delay is evidence of the susceptibility of the AV nodes to metabolic imbalances, which may aggravate underlying cardiac ailments. As the conditions worsen, the increased delay may result in complete AV nodal block, since this emphasizes the necessity of understanding the physiological as well as pathological conditions prone to influence AV node function. Overcoming such metabolic disturbances becomes necessary, since their correction may restore normal cardiac electrical activity, validating the pivotal position within the cardiac conducting system (Burton et al., 2014). Advances in electrophysiology have gone on to highlight further the complexity of the AV node, both anatomically and functionally. The success of interventions like radiofrequency ablation in the management of atrioventricular nodal reentrant tachycardias highlights just how deep the knowledge of the AV node has to be. Recent advances have given significant insight into the mechanism of atrioventricular transmission, facilitating closure of knowledge gaps in comprehending intrinsic conduction pathways. This information is not merely theoretical; it has a practical function in the treatment of arrhythmias, guiding therapeutic intervention, and directing the creation of targeted therapy. As research progresses, our understanding of the role of the AV nodes in cardiac physiology improves, promoting a more complete appreciation of heart disease and function (Anderson et al., 2001).

Test Your Knowledge

1. What structure is the heart's natural pacemaker?
2. How are Purkinje fibers and the bundle of His part of heart contractions?

9.3. Cardiac Cycle

Learning Outcome

1. Explain the cardiac cycle phases: diastole and systole;
2. Define heart sounds and their significance;
3. Explain the conditions regulating the cardiac cycle length.

The cardiac cycle is an advanced series of processes that makes it possible to efficiently pump blood into the body. It consists of two principal phases: diastole and systole. When the heart is in diastole, it relaxes so that the blood can fill up from the atria into the ventricles. This is a very critical process because it supplies the heart with an adequate volume of blood to be pumped during the subsequent systolic process. Systole then follows, in which there is contraction of the ventricular muscle, ejecting blood into the pulmonary artery and aorta. The regular functioning of the cardiac cycle is paramount in the process of achieving hemodynamic stability, and any alteration from this rhythm can result in various dysfunctions of the heart, and hence morbidities , such as heart failure, as highlighted in the present research on age- and drug-toxicity-related pathways (Ganeshan, 2019). On a molecular basis, cardiac cycle efficiency is disrupted by a multiplicity of factors, such as mitochondrial dysfunction, an important role in producing energy within cardiac cells. As the myocardium ages, physiological changes , such as cellular senescence will inhibit automaticity and contractility of the heart, and indirectly coordination necessary for an efficient cardiac cycle. In addition, some research has shown that there are some external factors , such as drugs, that may induce gene expression changes related to cardiac metabolism and function. For instance, cardiotoxic drugs have been reported to remodel oxidative phosphorylation pathways, thus causing the breakdown of the energy supply required for effective cardiac contraction (Cavarretta et al., 2017). Thus, the therapeutic interventions in these molecular targets are important to reverse the adverse effects on the cardiac cycle and general cardiac health. Advances in research identify the potential of new emerging therapies to enhance cardiac function, particularly in the contexts of aging and drug toxicity. Melatonin, a potent antioxidant hormone, has emerged as a prime candidate for cardioprotection. Studies reveal that melatonin possesses the capability to restore the metabolic abnormalities caused by other cardiotoxic drugs by halting the mitochondrial function and preserving cellular integrity.

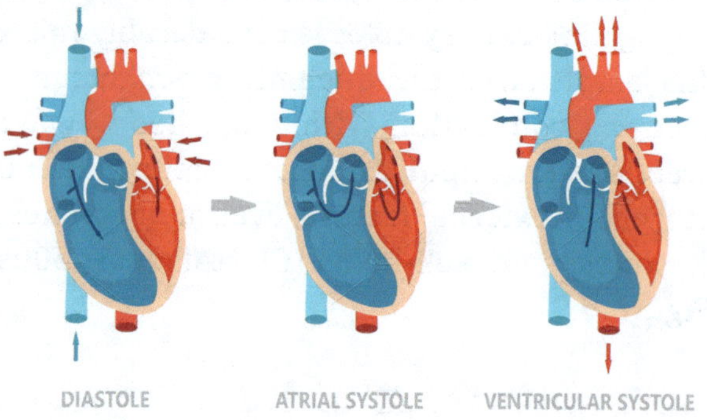

Figure 9.10. Phases of the cardiac cycle.

Source: https://tint.creativemarket.com/_Go3xhdXYQ2Kpf7Ltqk5hKjCNH5S3PNFEFmSwEEGzlA/width:3640/height:2410/gravity:nowe/rt:fill-down/el:1/preset:cm_watermark_ retina/czM6Ly9maWxlcy5jcmVhdGl2ZW1 hcmtldC5jb20vaW1hZ2VzL3NjcmVlbnNob3RzL3Byb2R1Y3RzLzEwNzAvMTA3MDY vMTA3MDY5MzMvaGVhcnRfZ290LTQyLTAxLW8uanBn.

Additionally, the fact that cellular senescence is a cause of cardiac dysfunction offers revolutionary strategies in regenerative medicine, bringing hope for heart rejuvenation therapy. With cardiovascular diseases continuing to rise with an aging population, focus on modulating the intricacies of the cardiac cycle remains at the forefront. Future research efforts have the potential to redefine therapy modalities to achieve maximum cardiac output and mitigate the burden of heart disease in an aging population (Cavarretta et al., 2017; Ganeshan, 2019) (Figure 9.10).

9.3.1. Phases of the Cardiac Cycle: Diastole and Systole

Two major phases of the cardiac cycle are diastole and systole, both of which are crucial in the efficient circulation of blood in the body. Diastole, which is the heart's resting phase, is when the heart ventricles become filled with blood returning from the body and lungs. Pressure at this point is reduced to the extent that AV valves open, allowing blood to flow by-pass from the atria to the ventricles. Meanwhile, aortic and pulmonary valves shut down to prevent backflow. This filling time is crucial because it has the duty of preparing ventricles for the next contraction, which has the duty of providing a perfect stroke volume and sufficient blood supply to systemic and pulmonary circulations, pillars to maintaining homeostasis in the human body. Systole is the contraction time of the cardiac cycle, when the ventricular muscles contract to pump the blood out of the heart. Increased intraventricular pressure causes closure of the AV valves to create the first heart sound and simultaneously opens the aortic and pulmonary valves. It has two critical phases: isovolumetric contraction and ventricular ejection. Ventricular volume does not change during isovolumetric contraction, but the pressure rises very quickly with contraction of the ventricles. Symmetrically, in return for this ventricular ejection, there occurs blood ejecting into the pulmonary artery and aorta. This extremely coordinated sequence of happenings provides a rhythmic and effective mechanism for blood distribution, crucial for the management of body needs throughout a range of activities from repose to intense exercise. Further, understanding the co-action between diastole and systole not only accounts for physiological function but also affects cognitive and affective processes involved with cardiac activity. Current studies highlight the fact that sensory perception can differ significantly during these two phases, and findings prove that the conscious perception of the stimuli is more robust during diastole compared to systole (Al et al., 2019). This confirms a sophisticated interrelation between cardiac rhythms and the functions of the mind, highlighting the influence of visceral feedback in conditioning mental and emotional states. These interactions illuminate the broader significance of cardiac physiology or how both internal bodily states and external stimuli influence human behavior and perception, further defining the body-mind interface (Anderson et al., 2015).

9.3.2. Heart Sounds and Their Significance

The significance of heart sounds in cardiac physiology extends beyond a mere aural observation; they are essential indicators of underlying cardiovascular illness. The heart produces characteristic sounds with its rhythmical contractions, which are primarily categorized as the first and second heart sounds (S1 and S2). They are largely generated because of the closure of atrioventricular and semilunar valves, respectively, and their characteristics can yield vital physiological information. For instance, alterations in the timing, duration, or degree of these heart sounds will usually indicate pathologic conditions , such as valvular heart disease or congestive heart failure. Moreover, the occurrence of additional sounds, i.e., murmurs, will indicate turbulent blood flow or structural abnormalities within the heart, pointing towards the importance of meticulous auscultation during clinical examination and constant monitoring of cardiac function. The evaluation of heart murmurs yields important insights into hemodynamic changes within the cardiovascular system. Since the physiological importance of systolic ejection murmurs was determined in studies to be differentiated, the impact of such murmurs can be important, particularly among groups exemplified by the boxer dog breed, whose cardiac states are similarly of interest to human cardiology. Murmurs, typically originating from turbulence caused by conditions like aortic stenosis, represent the dynamic status of blood flow and provide indications about the performance of the left ventricular outflow tract (LVOT) during systolic time. It has been found through research that the identification and grading of the murmurs require significant clinical experience, underlining the relationship between physiological examination and clinical experience in providing accurate diagnoses (Höglund et al., 2007).

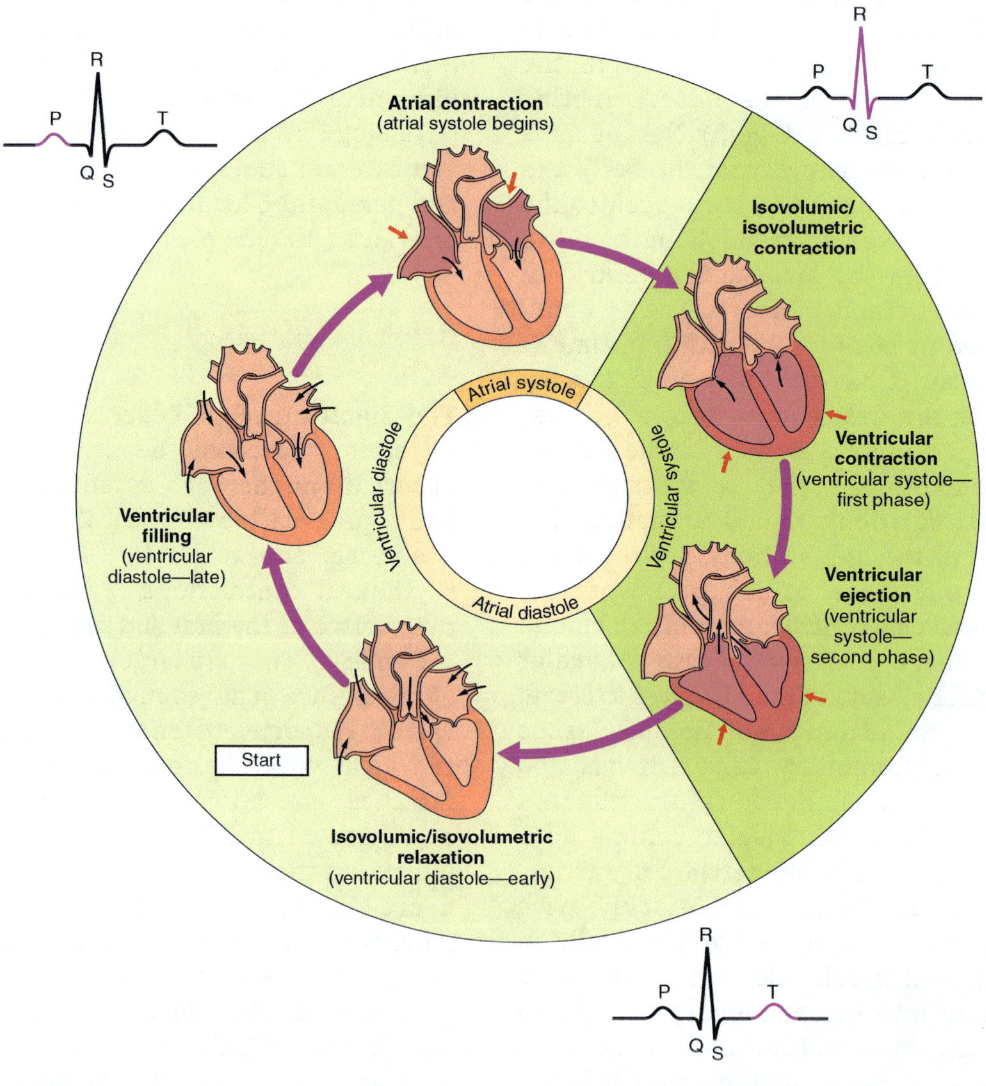

Figure 9.11. Heart sounds.

Source: https://d3uigcfkiiww0g.cloudfront.net/wordpress/blog/pics-en/uploads/Overview-of-the-Cardiac-Cycle.jpg.

Thus, cardiac murmurs not only signal the presence of potential pathologies but also highlight the requirement for knowledge of heart sounds in various contexts. Furthermore, the knowledge of heart sounds encompasses their application within sports populations, where separation of physiological responses and pathologic findings may be most challenging. The competitive stresses most commonly lead to cardiac remodeling that can be expressed as disease states, thereby interpreting heart sounds in the context of screening tests challenging. Here, cardiac screening programs aim to detect real dangers like sudden cardiac death without marking benign physiological changes. The relevance of assessing heart sounds in these groups is that they can detect abnormalities otherwise not detectable with less sensitive forms of diagnostic testing (Ingle et al., 2010). As such, distinguishing normal physiological processes from potential pathologies based upon heart sounds is essential to maintaining cardiovascular safety during sporting exercise as well as for enhancing the understanding of individual cardiac physiology (Figure 9.11).

9.3.3. Factors Influencing the Duration of the Cardiac Cycle

The duration of the cardiac cycle is influenced by a vast array of factors, primarily the autonomic nervous control of contractility and heart rate. The heart is innervated by sympathetic and parasympathetic fibers, which both modulate cardiac performance in response to physiological requirements. A sympathetic tone augmentation, for instance, augments the heart rate and reduces the systole and diastole durations, ultimately reducing the cardiac cycle as a whole. The stimulation of parasympathetic, via the vagus nerve, facilitates a reduced heart rate, augmenting the duration of the cardiac cycle. Other factors , such as preload and afterload in the cardiovascular system, play a significant role in this sense as well. Preload alterations affect ventricular filling and cardiac output, while changes in afterload affect the resistance the heart must work against to eject blood, contributing to the complexity of cardiac cycle length. Hormonal regulation contributes as well to the complexity in cardiac cycle duration. The hormones epinephrine and norepinephrine, released under stress or exercise, can substantially increase myocardial contractility and heart rate. This physiological response is significant in high-demanding situations where rapid circulation of oxygen and nutrients is critical. Regulation of the cardiac cycle length to such hormones exemplifies the cardiac adaptive characteristic. Besides, the concentration of electrolytes, most notably potassium, calcium, and sodium—similarly changes cardiac excitability and conduction, further changing heart rate and cycle length. It is essential to consider that the interaction of these hormonal and chemical factors with the inherent nature results in a highly controlled mechanism capable of adapting to physiological demands. Apart from these physiological factors, outside inputs , such as psychological pressure and physical exercise contribute significantly to the duration of the cardiac cycle. Research has proven that during mental stress, the heart can have variable PEP and CO responses, which complicate the interpretation of cardiac function (Czippelová et al., 2017). Sympathetic activation and exercise may synergistically give rise to complex patterns of arrhythmias or varying heart rates. For instance, during exercise or orthostatic stress, PEP can be an index of altering sympathetic activity, being modulated by alterations in preload and systemic vascular resistance (SVR). Monitoring these external variables is therefore essential to an adequate appreciation of cardiac physiology. As more research discloses the fine dynamics between the variables, the length of the cardiac cycle can progressively be positioned within both clinical and sports contexts (Borrione et al., 2017).

Test Your Knowledge

1. What are the two main phases of the cardiac cycle?
2. What heart sounds are associated with the closing valves in the cardiac cycle?

9.4. Cardiac Output

Learning Outcome

1. State the factors of cardiac output;
2. Define the determinants of cardiac output;
3. Describe the ways of measuring cardiac output.

Cardiac output measurement is critical in the knowledge of the ability of the heart to supply tissues of the body with oxygen and nutrients. Cardiac output, in terms of the volume of blood pumped out by the heart in a minute, relies on two components: stroke volume and heart rate. Heart rate, or beats per minute, is controlled by autonomic nervous system function, while stroke volume is determined by factors like preload, afterload, and myocardial contractility. Under patients with a normally functioning cardiovascular system, the system can compensate for cardiac output under varying physiological demands, such as exercise or rest.

Dysfunctions in these factors, however, result in conditions of inadequate perfusion, leading to systemic complications. Understanding the regulation of cardiac output is important for the diagnosis of cardiovascular disease and determining the efficacy of interventions for the optimization of cardiovascular health. Heat stress and exercise exert strong influences on cardiac output, and their combination presents unique challenges to cardiovascular homeostasis. During the performance of vigorous physical exercises, as during exposure to heat and humidity, demands for blood flow become bimodal. The circulatory system must supply working skeletal muscles and provide thermoregulation through cutaneous perfusion simultaneously, at the cost of diminished cardiac output and stroke volume, as already found in previous research. This stress upon the heart increases the risk of heat illness and decreases the capacity for endurance under prolonged effort.

The complexity of this physiological adaptation highlights the significance of understanding cardiovascular responses, particularly when exercise is conducted under heat stress. The effect warrants additional research into how chronic heat exposure may have lasting consequences for cardiovascular health, particularly in vulnerable populations. With recent advances in exercise physiology, high-intensity training has been shown to enhance cardiac output through a number of beneficial adaptations to the cardiovascular system. Engagement in regular high-intensity exercise promotes increased heart rate variability and stabilizes autonomic control of cardiac function, which are critical components of cardiac output.

For instance, studies indicate such training enhances left ventricular compliance and increases the arterial–cardiac baroreflex, thereby maximizing hemodynamic responses to activity. Furthermore, new modeling methods to describe cardiovascular regulation emphasize the interdependence of stroke volume and cardiac output. This inclusion emphasizes the efficacy of high-intensity exercise to enhance cardiovascular health and function in adults, particularly middle-aged adults. These adaptations validate exercise as a treatment intervention to reverse age-related declines in cardiac output and overall cardiovascular function, ultimately enhancing quality of life and reducing morbidity rates associated with heart disease (Figure 9.12).

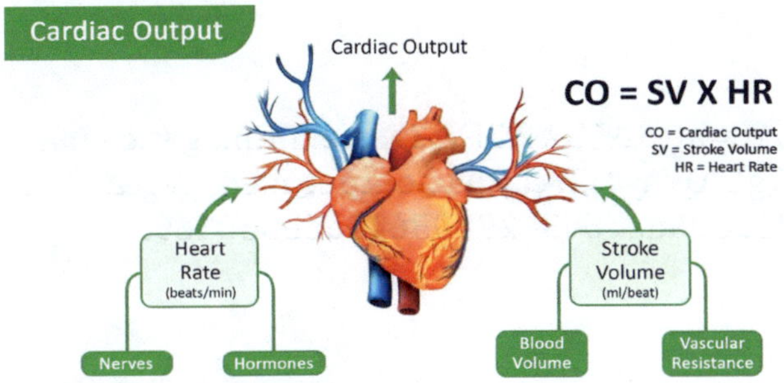

Figure 9.12. Cardiac output.

Source: https://external-content.duckduckgo.com/iu/?u=https%3A%2F%2Fmedia.geeksforgeeks.org%2Fwp-content%2Fuploads%2F20240305111106%2FCardiac-Output.webp&f=1&nofb=1&ipt=852b0b0526212568ed9fabe898fb277d1dc498e368e3022d438c619492a182d8.

9.4.1. Definition and Components of Cardiac Output

Cardiac output is a fundamental physiological measure that defines the efficacy of the heart as a pump, that is, the volume of blood that the heart ejects in a minute. Cardiac output is determined using two predominant components: stroke volume and heart rate. Stroke volume refers to the amount of blood that the left ventricle pushes out per beat, while heart rate describes the number of times a heartbeat occurs per minute. The relationship is provided by the equation: cardiac output = stroke volume × heart rate. Understanding these factors is crucial as alterations in either can have an immediate effect on overall cardiovascular health and function, setting parameters , such as tissue oxygen supply, cardiac burden, and total metabolic demand. Various factors can establish both stroke volume and heart rate and thus cardiac output. For instance, stroke volume can be established by preload, afterload, and contractility of the myocardium. Preload is the degree of elongation of the cardiac muscle fibers before contraction, which is defined by the venous return, while afterload is the resistance the ventricles must overcome to expel the blood. Contractility, a quality of the intrinsic ability of the cardiac muscle to contract, is also an important factor. Whereas heart rate modulation is made possible via autonomic nervous system actions, hormonal changes, and intrinsic cardiac mechanisms, hence enabling the quick modulation of cardiac output in response to changing physiological demands, e.g., exercise or quiet rest.

Furthermore, variation in ionic conductances may also be observed in ion channels and transporters that modulate cardiac excitation to control cardiac output regulation. Such conductances may differ within a population as a function of unequal patterns of cardiac gene expression, which lead to variation in stroke volume and heart rate. Variations in genetically heterogeneous populations, such as the Hybrid Mouse Diversity Panel, are revealed to explain specific adaptation patterns of conductance for maintaining a normal intracellular Ca2+ transient necessary for effective cardiac contraction (Karma et al., 2018). Such feedback control permits the heart to handle changing physiological conditions while keeping cardiac output optimal. Hence, an understanding of this complexity operates to accentuate the importance of integrative aspects presented in the cardiac physiology context, demonstrating the flexibility of the heart under different biological situations (Figure 9.13).

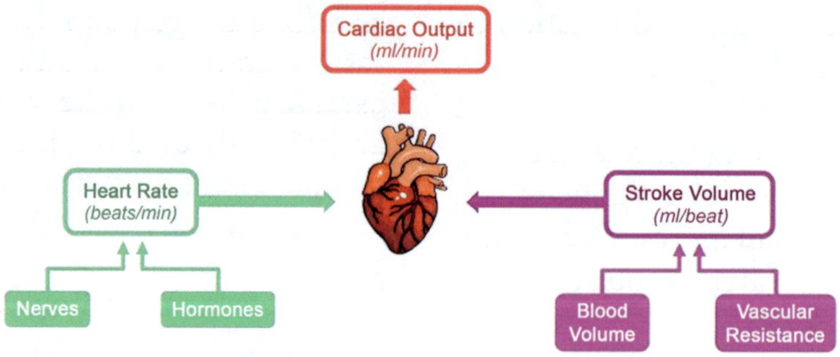

Figure 9.13. Components of cardiac output.

Source: https://external-content.duckduckgo.com/iu/?u=https%3A%2F%2Fsteemitimages.com%2FDQmYEWcBEuCxpMo7cGSkLA5vpGcFUGY2SeLcVAUVgLYQxAy%2Fcardiac-output_med.jpeg&f=1&nofb=1&ipt=ac70f74fd7a7687f5b6f532ad5a86447bed02890da7603429105643d6bb68169.

9.4.2. Factors Affecting Cardiac Output

The law of cardiac output is central to cardiovascular physiology studies, as it defines the volume of blood the heart ejects minute by minute. It has determinants that are multifaceted and include heart rate, stroke volume, and overall cardiovascular health. Heart rate, under the regulation of autonomic nervous system inputs as well as by hormones, is also a very important determinant; rising heart rate will typically increase cardiac output, provided the heart can sustain adequate contractility and filling pressures. However, too rapid heart rates can compromise cardiac efficiency and reduce stroke volume due to inadequate diastolic filling time. Hence, a delicate balance needs to be maintained in order to optimize cardiac output, highlighting the complexity of relationships involved in the cardiovascular control mechanisms regulating heart activity. Stroke volume, being the amount of blood pumped by the heart per beat, is equally crucial in determining cardiac output and is influenced by preload, afterload, and contractility. Preload is the original stretching of the cardiac myocytes, which relies on venous return and blood volume; a rise in preload will raise stroke volume by the Frank-Starling mechanism. A rise in afterload, because of hypertension or elevated vascular resistance, will, however, impede the heart from expelling the blood. In addition, contractility, meaning the intrinsic ability of the cardiac muscle to contract, can be augmented by sympathetic stimulation or pharmacologic agents that increase myocardial function. Studies combined, these show the dynamic nature of stroke volume and its pivotal role in controlling cardiac output, illustrating the need for precise physiological control. In addition, disease alterations in the cardiovascular system can dramatically disrupt the fine equilibrium that supports cardiac output. These consist of myocardial infarction, which triggers complex remodeling phenomena whereby the heart structurally and functionally changes to undermine its efficiency in circulation (Angelini et al., 2017). Myocardial infarction-induced chronic inflammation triggers a series of myocyte death, cardiac hypertrophy, and fibrosis that ultimately result in reduced cardiac output and the progression of heart failure (Angelini et al., 2017). These pathological events highlight the interaction between cardiac failure and compromised physiological parameters. The identification of these variables not only enables comprehension of cardiac physiology but also highlights the importance of early intervention in halting the development of adverse effects of cardiovascular disease, as demonstrated by altered therapeutic focus on increasing cardiac output in such participants (Figure 9.14).

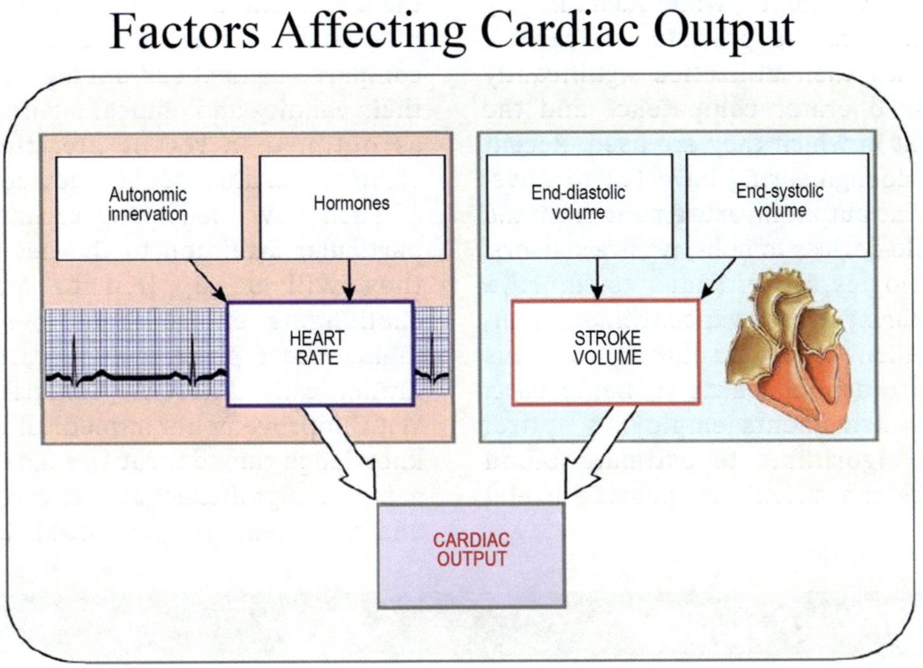

Figure 9.14. Factors affecting cardiac output.

Source: https://image.slidesharecdn.com/151heart-100401125821-phpapp01/95/heart-31-728.jpg?cb=1270126767.

9.4.3. Measurement Techniques for Cardiac Output

Measurement of cardiac output is at the heart of cardiovascular function measurement and cardiovascular disease diagnosis. Methods based on the Fick principle, which calculates cardiac output based on oxygen uptake and arterial-to-venous oxygen content differences, and thermodilution, which quantifies blood flow from temperature change, are used most commonly. Both methods have their own definite applications and drawbacks; one such application is that Ficks method is highly accurate but is based on approximated measurements of oxygen content, which may not always be feasible in the clinical setup. Thermodilution, on the other hand, is slightly less challenging to perform but may give erroneous information in patients with atypical circulation routes. The applicability of each technique could vary with patient conditions, and thus, there is a need for differentiated strategies to achieve accurate cardiac output measurement in varied clinical situations. Apart from conventional techniques, advanced imaging modalities have emerged as valuable tools for cardiac output measurement. Echocardiography, for example, uses ultrasound waves to produce images of the heart and assess blood flow, allowing for noninvasive measurement of cardiac output. Furthermore, improvements in Doppler ultrasound technology allow real-time measurement of the velocity of blood flow, further encouraging comprehension of cardiac function. Coupling these newer technologies with more traditional imaging strategies improves morphological and hemodynamic data regarding the heart. However, difficulties , such as the need for highly competent operators and the risk of variation in measurement must be addressed. Consequently, while such imaging modalities enhance the precision of cardiac output estimates, their utilization significantly depends upon operator competence and the clinical context in which they are used. Recent advances in bioengineering have led to novel means of cardiac output measurement, from the use of wearable devices to non-invasive sensors. These technologies are intended to improve cardiac monitoring access via continuous real-time measurement of cardiac output in various settings, from hospital wards to home care. For example, instruments employing optical sensors and algorithms to estimate blood flow dynamics can potentially provide useful information regarding cardiac function without the invasiveness of traditional approaches. Such innovations must, however, be extensively compared against current methods to ascertain their validity and clinical significance. Besides, as outlined in recent literature contrasting various cardiovascular devices, integration of such new measuring technologies entails particular attention to the new environments they will be applied to, particularly in challenging environments , such as space flight, where physiological reactions might be dramatically different (Ganiaris et al., 2025). With improvements in medical technology, the knowledge gained through such new techniques can be of significant value to cardiac physiology and treatment (Höglund et al., 2007).

Test Your Knowledge

1. What is cardiac output, and how is it calculated?
2. How do stroke volume and heart rate affect cardiac output?

9.5. Regulation of Heart Rate

Learning Outcome

1. Describe the autonomic nervous system role;
2. Define the hormonal regulation of heart rate;
3. Discuss the impact of physical exercise on heart rate.

Regulation of heart rate is a complex interaction of neural and hormonal influences necessary for cardiovascular homeostasis. Central to this regulation is the autonomic nervous system, which gains control via its sympathetic and parasympathetic branches. Although sympathetic activation is normally the cause of tachycardia through release of catecholamines, parasympathetic withdrawal, involving the vagus nerve as the primary mediating agent, is responsible for decreasing heart rate at rest. The responses are modified with dynamic exercise to allow for sufficient oxygenation of contracting muscles and optimal removal of metabolic waste products. Its effectiveness relies on various neural reflexes, such as the arterial baroreflex and chemoreflex, which report to alterations in blood pressure and blood chemistry, respectively, to make adjustments to heart rate accordingly (Crisafulli et al., 2014). Heart rate regulation is also significantly changed under disease conditions, particularly in heart failure. Heart failure (HF) not only complicates global cardiovascular function, but it also disturbs the fine balance of autonomic control. The disease entails complex alterations like structural and electrical remodeling, which impair the heart's ability to respond appropriately to autonomic signals. Cardiac dysfunction resulting from heart failure can lead to increased sympathetic drive and decreased vagal tone, ultimately worsening arrhythmias and other complications.

Understanding these regulatory mechanisms is significant, as they identify therapeutic directions. Existing evidence supports that modulation of the autonomic balance via interventions would improve cardiac function and relieve HF symptoms (Ganeshan, 2019). Moreover, existing evidence is such that compounds like melatonin, traditionally thought to be implicated in sleep regulation, may also have a cardioprotective role in the regulation of heart rate. Melatonin modulates cellular apoptosis and oxidative stress, indicating the potential of its use to treat drug-induced cardiac dysfunction and heart failure. In more precise terms, using *in vitro* models, it has been observed that melatonin can counteract the toxic actions of cardiotoxic agents like doxorubicin by acting on mitochondrial metabolism and gene expression specific to cardiac function. This indicates the interest in researching non-conventional regulators of the heart as potential adjuncts for treating heart failure. Through the utilization of the various mechanisms of heart rate control, both physiological and pharmacological, new therapies can emerge to move patient care in cardiovascular disease forward (Ganeshan, 2019) (Figure 9.15).

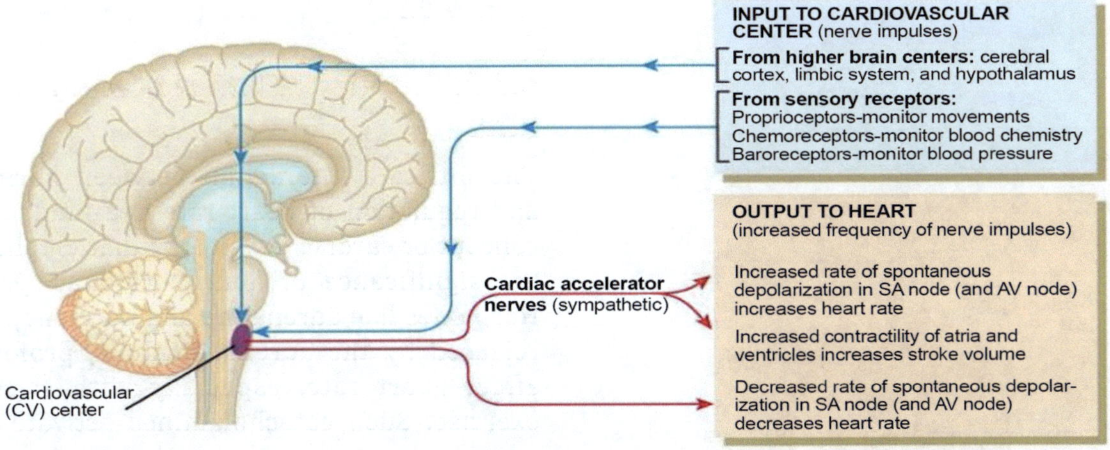

Figure 9.15. Regulation of heart rate.

Source: https://image1.slideserve.com/2088310/regulation-of-heart-rate1-l.jpg.

9.5.1. Role of the Autonomic Nervous System (ANS)

The ANS in cardiac physiology is paramount since it regulates heart rate, myocardial contractility, and vessel tone. This complex system is composed of two main branches: the sympathetic and parasympathetic nervous systems. The sympathetic branch is linked with fight-or-flight, boosting cardiac output by enhancing heart rate and contractility through the release of norepinephrine. The parasympathetic branch, mediated primarily through the vagus nerve, promotes a rest-and-digest state, lowering heart rate and myocardial oxygen demand. The interaction between these two branches allows for an appropriate physiological response to environmental stresses and metabolic needs in change, emphasizing the intricate regulatory impacts of the ANS on cardiac dynamics. Moreover, the mechanisms of signaling initiated by the ANS greatly influence the control of heart rate as well as cardiovascular health. Suppression of heart rate by G-protein action is an area that continues to be researched, and gaining insights into modulatory events. The involvement of several regulators of G-protein signaling is required in understanding how the ANS can modulate cardiac responses. Recent studies by global genetic deletion of inhibitory G protein alpha subunits have contributed basic insight into central and peripheral roles in heart rate regulation, emphasizing the close association between the ANS and cardiac physiology. Greater insight into this network not only pushes the science of cardiology forward but also illuminates possible therapeutic targets for arrhythmia and other cardiovascular disease treatment (Ang et al., 2012). The relationship between respiration and the autonomic nervous system also works to illustrate its intricacy and significance in cardiac physiology.

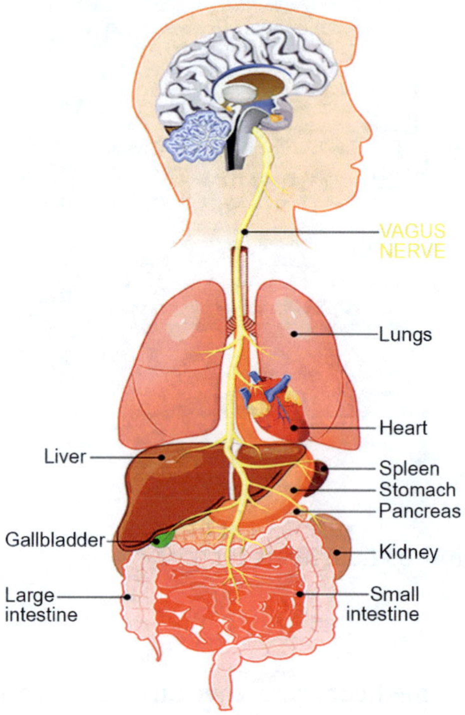

Figure 9.16. Vagus nerve.

Source: https://assets.lybrate.com/imgs/tic/enadp/image-of-the-vagus-nerve.jpg.

The breathing-cardiac rhythm interaction has been documented, and inspirations were seen to cause heart rate variation due to sympathetically generated variations. Respiratory influences highlight the importance of studies into how breathing states can influence cardiac responses. For instance, there can be an acute small hyperpolarization during inspiration that will serve to initiate heart rhythm variations related to neural signaling. Such mechanistic insight into the respiratory regulation of heart rate not only promises to open up new opportunities for improved understanding of physiological mechanisms but also prefigures therapeutic opportunities in treatment of disorders of both respiratory and cardiovascular systems, e.g., disorders of stress and arrhythmias (Jerath et al., 2015) (Figure 9.16).

9.5.2. Hormonal Influences on Heart Rate

The intricate interaction between hormones and regulation of heart rate is a fundamental concept of cardiac physiology that emphasizes the significance of neurohormonal systems. Hormones like adrenaline and norepinephrine, released by the adrenal medulla, profoundly affect heart rate, especially with stress or exercise. Such catecholamines activate beta-adrenergic receptors of the heart, which result in increased heart rate and myocardial contractility.

This system is significant in periods of increased demand, such as exercise, when increased cardiac output is required by the body to deliver oxygen and nutrients to tissues. In addition, hormonal signals conveyed in the blood may also modulate the heart's response to the autonomic nervous system, indicating that hormonal responses are not merely reactive but integrative processes that shape cardiovascular function under various physiological conditions. The role of other hormones, such as the renin-angiotensin-aldosterone system (RAAS), cannot be ruled out in this context of cardiac regulation. Activation of RAAS is essential for fluid regulation and blood pressure regulation and, secondarily, heart rate via regulation of vascular resistance. An increase in blood volume, for instance, results in an elevation of cardiac preload that typically leads to elevated heart rates to facilitate adequate circulation. Additionally, in elderly individuals, exercise has also been reported to have beneficial effects on catecholamine release and may significantly influence RAAS activity. Through exercise-induced maintenance of a healthy hormonal balance, patients can better adapt to age-related declines in cardiovascular effectiveness, thus making possible more optimal heart rate responses to various stressors (Allocca et al., 2013). This association highlights the importance of including exercise as a therapeutic intervention for maintaining optimal heart functioning. Furthermore, the influence of hormones is not confined to acute cardiovascular regulation but includes also longer-term adaptations responsible for cardiac well-being. Such chronic elevation in cortisol levels, for example, can lead to increased heart rates via catecholamine-mediated and inflammatory pathways. Elevated levels of cortisol are a common byproduct of stress and can ultimately contribute to the development of cardiovascular disease, illustrating how a lack of balance in hormones can set cardiac function up for pathological change. These dynamics are particularly significant in the study of space physiology, where fluid shifts and cardiovascular response alterations have been experienced in astronauts on microgravity (Hess et al., 1992). This dynamic hormonal environment demands an interdisciplinary research and clinical practice effort for elucidating the hormonal control of heart rate and ultimately promoting improved cardiovascular health and disease management outcomes (Figure 9.17).

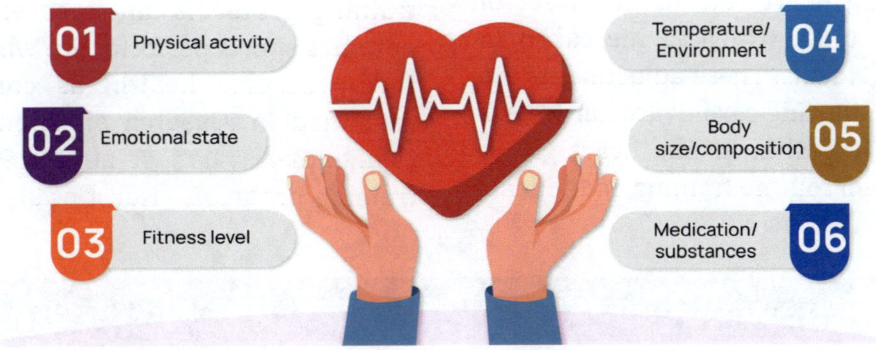

Figure 9.17. Factors affecting the pulse rate.

Source: https://sunfox.in/wp-content/uploads/2024/05/10.1-what-are-the-factors-affecting-the-Pulse-Rate_-scaled.webp.

9.5.3. Impact of Physical Activity on Heart Rate

The relationship between exercise and heart rate is an essential aspect of cardiac physiology that signifies the body's adaptive response to coping with increased metabolic demand. On presentation of physical exercise, the heart rate rises in order to deliver increased oxygen and nutrient supply to active muscles and removal of metabolic processes. This physiological response is mediated by autonomic regulation, namely by an increase in sympathetic nervous system activity that releases catecholamines that enhance cardiac output. Different intensities of exercise have been reported to generate varying degrees of heart rate elevation per study, demonstrating the resourcefulness and responsiveness of the body as well as its cardiovascular response. Longitudinal exercise programs not only improve the efficacy of muscles but also cardiovascular health by producing a more robust heart response both during and after exercise, with the consequent reduction in baseline resting heart rates in regularly active subjects.

Evidence confirms that specific types of training, e.g., sprint interval training (SIT) and endurance training (ET), can have drastic impacts on physiological values, including resting heart rate. In a single study, those who participated as volunteers in SIT experienced notable reductions in resting heart rate compared to control groups after an 8-week training regimen, confirming the efficacy of high-intensity training to enhance cardiac efficiency. Furthermore, long-term endurance exercise has been observed to reduce resting heart rate as an effect of enhanced vagal tone, which is increased in well-trained individuals. These adjustments are important to maximizing cardiovascular fitness and overall heart health. As the heart grows more efficient from routine training, individuals can have a reduction in resting heart rates in correlation with reduced cardiovascular risk and improved exercise function throughout life. The influence of exercise on heart rate is more than performance during exercise; it's critical during recovery and readiness to perform at a higher level.

Following high-intensity endeavors , such as ultra-endurance races, markers of cardiac stress, e.g., NT-proBNP and hs-TNT, have been found to increase significantly, reflecting the hearts reaction to prolonged exertion. Moreover, decreased heart rate variability post-exercise indicates temporary shifting towards sympathetic dominance, which mirrors the need for adequate recuperation time. The quicker athletes have larger increases in these markers of cardiac injury, which underscores the relationship between the intensity of training and cardiac health. Insights obtained through heart rate and recovery markers can then inform training protocols and recovery regimens to optimize sports performance while maintaining cardiovascular health, as comprehensively examined in research on endurance athletes (Martínez-Navarro et al., 2019) and interval training protocols (Hurst et al., 2014).

Test Your Knowledge

1. What part of the autonomic nervous system increases heart rate?
2. How does the parasympathetic nervous system affect heart rate?

9.6. Common Cardiac Disorders

Learning Outcome

1. Describe the overview of arrhythmias;
2. Define heart failure and its physiological implication;
3. Describe the coronary artery disease and its effects on cardiac function.

Under the broad category of common cardiac disorders, atrial fibrillation (AF) is the most prevalent arrhythmia encountered in everyday practice. AF is a syndrome when there is an irregular as well as accelerated rate of the heart, and this can lead to various complications , such as stroke as well as heart failure. Major risk factors for the development of AF include systemic arterial hypertension, diabetes, obesity, heart failure, and valvular heart disease. Recent literature has also highlighted the potential association between AF and anxiety disorders, pointing towards anxiety not only being a comorbidity of the condition but also possibly having a causative role in its development. This connection emphasizes the significance of holistic strategies in addressing psychological components as a component of comprehensive cardiac care, aiming to encourage health professionals to adopt whole measures that not only address the physiological status of AF but also its psychological underpinnings (Ceccacci et al., 2019).

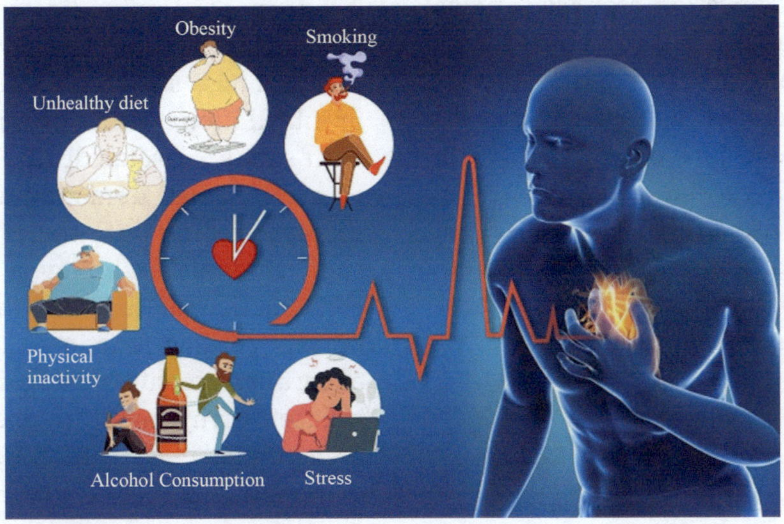

Figure 9.18. Prevent-cardiovascular-diseases.

Source: https://blog.thyrocare.com/wp-content/uploads/2021/11/prevent-cardiovascular-diseases.jpg.

Heart failure is another significant category of cardiac disease, characterized by the heart's inability to pump to meet the metabolic needs of the body. This condition is often caused by many underlying disorders , such as coronary artery disease, hypertension, and previous myocardial infarction. Heart failure complexity is caused by its multifactorial etiology and resultant pathophysiology, including ventricular remodeling and neurohormonal activation. Cardiac resynchronization therapy (CRT) has been identified as a key intervention in heart failure patients with ventricular desynchrony. Large clinical trials have established CRT to significantly enhance patient outcomes, reducing hospitalization and mortality and increasing functional capacity. At 70% positive response in the selected patients, CRT is a classic example of the evolution in heart failure therapy responsive to contemporary cardiac physiology and therapeutic dogma (Bătăiosu et al., 2018). Further, diagnosis and treatment of prevalent cardiac ailments solely depend upon the dynamic nature of cardiovascular health. Advancements in technology and strategies of patient care have transformed the processes of diagnosis and treatment of these ailments. For instance, advances in imaging techniques have improved the diagnostic effectiveness for heart diseases , such as coronary artery disease and cardiomyopathies. In addition, a greater emphasis on lifestyle modification, including dietary modification, exercise regimen, and smoking cessation, has played a central role in reducing cardiac disorder risk factors. Integration of prevention and education with patient management not only negates the acute expression of cardiac disease but also provides for long-term heart health. Lastly, an in-depth understanding of the physiological and behavioral aspects of cardiac disorders optimizes intervention success, enabling improved patient outcomes and quality of life (Figure 9.18).

9.6.1. Overview of Arrhythmias

Arrhythmias are defects in the heart's electrical conduction system with the ability to significantly disrupt normal cardiac function. These are characterized by the distortion of the heart rhythm, and can manifest as bursts of atrial fibrillation, ventricular fibrillation, or indeed bradycardia and tachycardia. This change affects the performance of the heart to pump blood efficiently, with clinical presentations ranging from benign to life-threatening. The mechanisms behind them are typically multifactorial, with some component of genetic susceptibility, structural heart disease, and ischemic substrates that interfere with the electrical conduction pathways of the heart. Awareness of the complexity of arrhythmias is crucial because they are one of the major determinants of morbidity and mortality among patients with cardiovascular disease, and hence, they are the cornerstone of cardiac physiology and therapeutic strategy studies. Pathogenesis of arrhythmias is due to many factors including myocardial structural changes, electrical remodeling, and metabolic alterations.

Ailments, such as heart failure and ischemic heart disease offer the background for arrhythmogenesis, in which abnormal ion channel operation and non-functional calcium handling become the rule. Ischemia, for instance, can result in hypoxia, which suppresses cardiac myocyte contractile performance and triggers abnormal electrical activity. Such modifications can trigger potentially fatal arrhythmias, such as ventricular tachycardia or fibrillation, which are strongly associated with sudden cardiac death. Effective treatment of arrhythmias demands a well-documented understanding of their mechanisms, as such an understanding is necessary for the construction of targeted therapies to restore normal cardiac function and rhythm. The use of cardioprotective strategies for treating drug-induced arrhythmias is one of the promising areas under investigation. Recent studies have demonstrated that certain compounds, among which is the pineal hormone melatonin, provide a protective effect against stress-induced cardiac arrhythmias and myocardial dysfunction. The capacity of melatonin to regulate certain signaling pathways of heart failure confirms its usefulness as an adjuvant therapy in patients treated with cardiotoxic drugs like doxorubicin. Moreover, refinement of animal disease models, including rabbit models, yields insight reflective of human physiology and leads the way for novel therapeutic opportunities. By acquiring a better understanding of arrhythmias and their pathophysiology, researchers can uncover new interventions that diminish the dangers of arrhythmias, enhancing patient results as a whole in cardiac physiology (Bers et al., 2008; Ganeshan, 2019) (Figure 9.19).

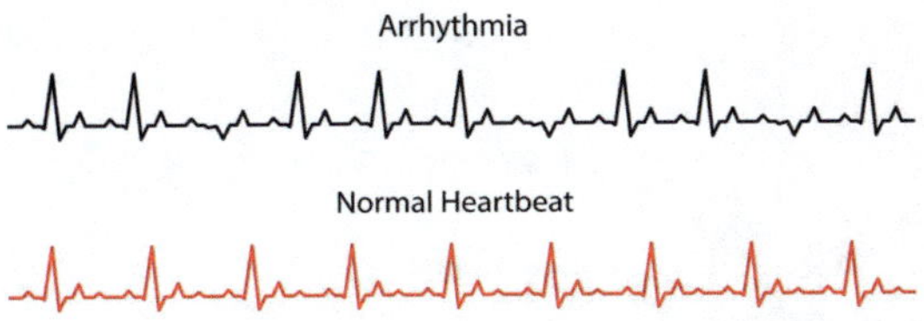

Figure 9.19. Arrhythmias: Causes, risk factors, symptoms, treatment.

Source: https://continentalhospitals.com/uploads/mceu_93856803611699523091260.png.

9.6.2. Heart Failure (HF) and Its Physiological Implications

HF is a significant problem of modern medicine in which the inefficiency of the heart to pump enough blood to meet the bodys metabolic needs reigns. The disease may be caused by many mechanisms of pathophysiology, including ischemic heart disease, hypertension, and diabetes. These lead to maladaptive remodeling of the heart and decreased efficiency of contractility. As the heart works to maintain production, adaptive mechanisms , such as increased heart rate and ventricular hypertrophy initially compensate for impairment but ultimately add to myocardial stress and lead to increased deterioration. This self-reinforcing spiral underscores the worth of HF not as a terminal illness, but as a chronic disorder that must be regulated repeatedly to alleviate symptoms and improve quality of life in afflicted patients. The intricate relationship between heart failure and metabolic dysregulation in diabetic patients is crucial to understanding the conditions physiological implications. Evidence indicates that diabetes negatively impacts cardiac inotropic response with patients exhibiting blunted β-adrenergic stimulation in response to apparently preserved contractile reserve. Moreover, recent evidence indicates that high-fat diets exacerbate insulin-adrenergic signaling pathways that result in amplified phosphorylation of the β2-adrenergic receptors and diminished cardiac contractile reserve. Notably, these changes can occur without remarkable structural alterations in the myocardium, and this indicates the benefits of early therapeutic interventions that target metabolic pathways to prevent subsequent cardiac sequelae.

The interplay between metabolic disease and heart failure highlights the benefits of multispecialty practice in managing cardiac care, as metabolic well-being assumes a central role in the optimization of cardiac function. In addition, the role of oxidative stress in pathogenesis in heart failure cannot be minimized. Myocardial redox disturbance is a pathogenic process in the development of heart failure, in which reactive oxygen species (ROS) and reactive nitrogen species (RNS) have both roles as toxic byproducts of cellular metabolism and essential signaling molecules. Excess accumulation of these species produces alterations in calcium handling, energy metabolism, and extracellular matrix deposition, all of which together create maladaptive cardiac remodeling. Recent advances in the elucidation of these signal transduction mechanisms have created pathways for therapeutic intervention to enhance antioxidant activity in myocardial tissue. Notably, however, the twelfth nature of both ROS and RNS must also be taken into account because abolition of both could compromise physiological myocardial homeostasis. Thus, the therapy development should strike a balance between preventing oxidative stress and not interfering with the protective roles played by these molecules in cardiac physiology (Angelini et al., 2016; Chiamvimonvat et al., 2017) (Figure 9.20).

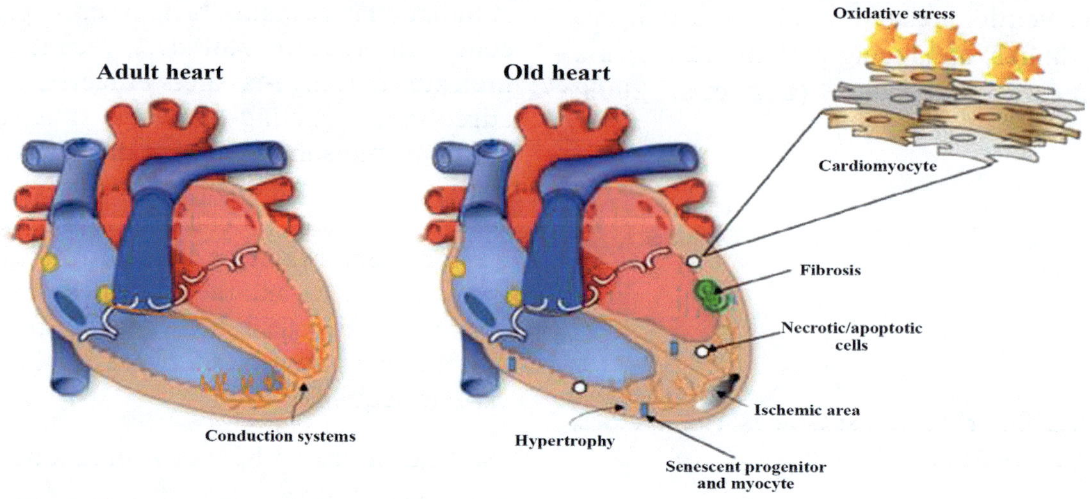

Figure 9.20. Heart failure (HF).

Source: https://www.physio-pedia.com/images/thumb/2/2d/Fig-2-Changes-in-the-myocardium-during-aging-Heart-and-vasculature-undergo-alterations.png/583px-Fig-2-Changes-in-the-myocardium-during-aging-Heart-and-vasculature-undergo-alterations.png.

9.6.3. Coronary Artery Disease (CAD) and Its Effects on Cardiac Function

CAD significantly impacts cardiac function through the narrowing of the coronary arteries, eventually restricting blood supply to the myocardium. This impaired perfusion can result in myocardial ischemia, presenting as chest discomfort, arrhythmias, or even myocardial infarction. Adaptive mechanisms like increased heart rate and myocardial hypertrophy may arise as the heart attempts to compensate for the decreased supply of appropriate oxygen and nutrients. These adaptations are typically insufficient in the long term, especially in the context of worsening atherosclerosis. Though initial symptoms could be harmless, chronic hypoxia can cause irreparable tissue damage to the heart, and hence the urgency for early intervention and lifestyle modification to oppose risk factors in CAD. The hemodynamic alteration by CAD has very important implications for the cardiac output. With falling coronary flow, the heart attempts to ensure adequate perfusion by various mechanisms, like increased ventricular rate and contractility. But as hinted at by simulations that maintained different heart rates as constants, the relationship between coronary perfusion and heart rate also becomes more complex. For instance, higher heart rates, especially when it is atrial fibrillation, can further exacerbate coronary perfusion deficits by warping pressure and flow behavior in coronary arteries. These dynamic changes underscore the imperative of critical understanding of hemodynamic responses in CAD patients for the best treatment strategy and improved cardiac outcomes (Anselmino et al., 2019). Explorations of the interaction between the epicardial adipose tissue and cardiac myocytes are necessary to understand the influence on cardiac performance. This adipose tissue contributes to local inflammation and exacerbates CAD pathophysiology through the release of pro-inflammatory cytokines, capable of further impairing myocardial function. Three-dimensional co-culture model experiments have elucidated the interactions of epicardial adipocytes with cardiac tissue, demonstrating how obesity- and lifestyle-related metabolic derangements are capable of exacerbating cardiac dysfunction. This cellular dynamics puts us in touch with CAD more effectively and brings out the need for multi-faceted management plans incorporating lifestyle modifications, drug therapy, and novel therapies aimed at the metabolism of adipose tissue (Agra et al., 2017).

Test Your Knowledge

1. What is coronary artery disease (CAD), and why does it occur?
2. How does high blood pressure affect the heart in the long term?

SUMMARY

The physiology of the heart reveals the high sensitivity to the varied forms of exercise, thus favoring the importance of personalized training protocols. A comparison of studies verifies that different modalities of training, such as SIT and ET, can yield significant improvements in cardiovascular indices, including resting heart rate and aerobic capacity. Specifically, there is evidence that the combination of these two types of training can further enhance overall physiological adaptations, yielding higher results in power performance. Based on recent studies, a structured organization can maximize work capacity for the body under both sports performance and overall well-being (Hurst et al., 2014). Secondly, understanding the body's physiological reactions to prolonged endurance efforts, i.e., ultramarathons, accounts for the sudden stress on the cardiac tissues. Biomarker determination post-event indicates a sharp elevation in markers of cardiac injury as a consequence of intense efforts, emphasizing the necessity of proper recovery procedures. Evidence has proven that considerate recovery periods are crucial, particularly among athletes who perform optimally, as such involved participants have been found to be marked by heightened responses in cardiac stress biomarkers. This connection has proven that the intensity of cardiovascular exertion is a major determinant in the bodys physiology, demonstrating that detailed training and recovery frameworks are necessary in sport science (Martínez-Navarro et al., 2019). Lastly, an increased understanding of cardiac physiology not only serves to improve the development of successful training programs but also benefits performance and helps cardiovascular health. As illustrated through the integration of various training modalities and investigation regarding endurance challenges, the adaptability of the heart can be harnessed for improved health benefits. As significant as the heart is in the capability to do athletics and overall health, further study in this field is necessary. Further research that continues to study the interaction of training schedules and cardiac adaptation will provide informative data, driving improvements in exercise science and ultimately leading to a better understanding of cardiac physiology.

Cardiac physiology is the process of mechanisms of all processes which regulate the heart's function, such as the proper circulation of blood within the body. Central to this understanding is the concept of the cardiac cycle, composed of phases of diastole and systole. During diastole, the cardiac chambers are filled with blood with the assistance of the atrioventricular valves opening rapidly. Conversely, systole is the phase of contraction, in which ventricles eject blood into the systemic and pulmonary circulations. It is important to be familiar with these phases since any dysfunction can lead to cardiovascular disease. Furthermore, the actions of specialized cardiac cells, such as pacemaker cells in the Sinoatrial node, reflect the way intrinsic electrical activity regulates heart rhythm and rate, adjusting dynamically from rest to exercise to physiological demand. Endurance sports , such as marathon running are common and have raised alarm about their impact on cardiac physiology. Among first-time marathon runners, there was significant cardiovascular remodeling without considerable improvement in cardiorespiratory function following intense training. These exercises have been originally associated with eccentric remodeling of the heart as reflected by both left and right ventricular cavity dilatations, suggesting an adaptation for blood volume and pressure changes to long-term exercise. Surprisingly, while decreases in blood pressure as well as enhancement of VO2 max were observed, only 11% of runners exhibited clinically relevant enhancements in VO2 max, suggesting a complex interaction between the magnitude of exercise and cardiovascular adaptation. These findings are significant in the assessment of long-term effects of endurance exercise on heart performance and health, and so the need for balanced training practices taking into consideration individual physiological responses (D'Silva et al., 2020).

The cardiac conductance system, responsible for the rhythmic contraction of the hearts, is the key to understanding cardiac physiology. Comprised of specialized tracts of conduction, this system guides the heart's electrical impulses through a highly coordinated chain that begins at the Sinoatrial node and quickly converges on the Atrioventricular node and bundle of His. Such conduction produces synchrony between atrial and ventricular contractions, optimizing the efficiency of the heart in terms of blood pumping. Disease within this system can lead to arrhythmias, demonstrating the delicate balance that these electrical pathways maintain. With advancements in new disease therapeutic models , such as Duchenne muscular dystrophy that targets muscular and cardiac function, cardiac physiology knowledge remains essential for the development of effective therapy. Comparing model analysis provides evidence for the necessity of comprehending underlying mechanisms for optimizing treatment protocol for cardiac-related disorders (Aartsma-Rus et al., 2018).

KEY TERMS FROM THIS CHAPTER

- Action Potential
- Atrioventricular (AV) Node
- Autonomic Regulation
- Baroreceptors
- Bundle of His
- Cardiac Cycle
- Cardiac Muscle
- Cardiac Output
- Coronary Circulation
- Diastole
- Electrocardiogram (ECG/EKG)
- Frank-Starling Law
- Heart Rate
- Heartbeat
- Myocardial Contractility
- Pacemaker Potential
- Purkinje Fibers
- Sinoatrial (SA) Node

CRITICAL THINKING QUESTIONS

1. **Which part of the heart is the body's natural pacemaker?**
   a. AV node
   b. SA node
   c. Purkinje fibers
   d. Bundle of His
2. **At what time of the cardiac cycle does the heart fill with blood?**
   a. Systole
   b. Diastole
   c. Isovolumetric contraction
   d. Ventricular ejection
3. **What is the normal resting heart rate for an adult?**
   a. 30–50 beats per minute
   b. 60–100 beats per minute
   c. 110–130 beats per minute
   d. 40–60 beats per minute
4. **Which ion is accountable for depolarization in cardiac muscle cells?**
   a. Chloride (Cl^-)
   b. Calcium (Ca^{2+})
   c. Potassium (K^+)
   d. Sodium (Na^+)
5. **Which one of the following best defines stroke volume?**
   a. Volume of blood ejected per minute
   b. Volume of blood ejected per beat
   c. Total blood volume in the body
   d. Volume of blood in the atria

Short Answer Questions

1. What is the function of the sinoatrial (SA) node?
2. Define cardiac output.
3. Name the two stages of the cardiac cycle.
4. Define stroke volume.
5. Define normal heart rate range in adults.
6. Discuss the function of the autonomic nervous system in the regulation of heart rate.
7. Describe excitation-contraction coupling in cardiac muscle.
8. Describe how an electrocardiogram (ECG) is utilized to assess cardiac function.
9. Compare and contrast the action potentials of pacemaker cells and ventricular muscle cells.
10. Describe the changes in heart sounds and pressure throughout the cardiac cycle.

Answers to Critical Thinking Questions

1. (b); 2. (b); 3. (b); 4. (d); 5. (b)

REFERENCES

1. Elizabeth L. Hess, Janice Wallace-Robinson, Katherine J. Dickson, and Janet V. Powers The George Washington University Washington, D.C (1992). NASA Contractor Report 4468*Publications of the Space Physiology and Countermeasures Program, Regulatory Physiology Discipline: 1980–1990*. Prepared for NASA Office of Space Science and Applications under Contract NASW-432.
2. D'Silva, A., Bhuva, A. N., van Zalen, J., Bastiaenen, R., Abdel-Gadir, A., Jones, S., Nadarajan, N., Menacho Medina, K. D., Ye, Y., Augusto, J., Treibel, T. A., Rosmini, S., Ramlall, M., Scully, P. R., Torlasco, C., Willis, J., Finocchiaro, G., Papatheodorou, E., Dhutia, H., Cole, D., ... Sharma, S. (2020). Cardiovascular Remodeling Experienced by Real-World, Unsupervised, Young Novice Marathon Runners. *Frontiers in physiology*, *11*, 232. https://doi.org/10.3389/fphys.2020.00232 (accessed on 16th June 2025).
3. Abid, A., Afonso, M., Ahmed, S., Alexander, G., Algranati, D., Altman, D., et al. (2017). Regulation of coronary blood flow. https://core.ac.uk/download/161627447.pdf (accessed on 16th June 2025).
4. Adjedj, J., Barbato, E., Esposito, G., Fearon, W. F., et al. (2017). Diabetes does not impact the diagnostic performance of contrast-based fractional flow reserve: Insights from the CONTRAST study. https://core.ac.uk/download/80696880.pdf (accessed on 16th June 2025).
5. Agmon, Y., Beach, R. E., Biondi, M., Burnstock, G., Casellas, D., Cohen, H. J., Edwards, R. M., et al. (2012). Renal pericytes: Regulators of medullary blood flow. https://core.ac.uk/download/30712009.pdf (accessed on 16th June 2025).
6. Ahmadian, N., Akiyama, T., Areosa, S., Attems, J., Babcock, D., Bailey, K., Baker, M., et al. (2019). A novel model of mixed vascular dementia incorporating hypertension in a rat model of Alzheimer's disease. https://core.ac.uk/download/323077251.pdf (accessed on 16th June 2025).
7. Alexander, D., Bergel, A., Boas, D. A., Burnham, B., Buxton, R., Deneux, T., et al. (2009). A time-invariant Visco-elastic wind Kessel model relating blood flow and blood volume. https://core.ac.uk/download/50544.pdf (accessed on 16th June 2025).
8. Allocca, E., Bonaduce, D., D'Amico, L., De Lucia, C., et al. (2013). Neuro-hormonal effects of physical activity in the elderly. https://core.ac.uk/download/76991216.pdf (accessed on 16th June 2025).
9. Alves-Lopes, R., Anagnostopoulou, A., Arner, A., De Lucca Camargo, L., et al. (2018). Vascular smooth muscle contraction in hypertension. https://core.ac.uk/download/150600176.pdf (accessed on 16th June 2025).
10. Attwell, D., Hall, C. N., & Hamilton, N. B. (2010). Pericyte-mediated regulation of capillary diameter: A component of neurovascular coupling in health and disease. https://core.ac.uk/download/1688588.pdf (accessed on 16th June 2025).
11. Jerath, R., Crawford, M. W., Barnes, V. A., & Harden, K. (2015). Widespread depolarization during expiration: a source of respiratory drive?. *Medical hypotheses*, *84*(1), 31–37. https://doi.org/10.1016/j.mehy.2014.11.010Bertolini, E., Buckley, H., Carlhoff, S., Feldman, M., et al. (2022). Female bone physiology resilience in a past Polynesian Outlier community. https://core.ac.uk/download/544385243.pdf (accessed on 16th June 2025).

12. Bertolini, E., Buckley, H., Carlhoff, S., Feldman, M., et al. (2022). Female bone physiology resilience in 750–300 BP 'Polynesian Outlier' community. https://core.ac.uk/download/516201971.pdf (accessed on 16th June 2025).

13. Bich, L., Moreau, J. F., & Pradeu, T. (2019). Understanding multicellularity: The functional organization of the intercellular space. https://core.ac.uk/download/228134961.pdf (accessed on 16th June 2025).

14. Birch, R. E., Peppiatt-Wildman, C. M., Schwiebert, E. M., Wildman, S. S., et al. (2013). Emerging key roles for P2X receptors in the kidney. https://core.ac.uk/download/30711999.pdf (accessed on 16th June 2025).

15. Blamire, A. M., Ford, G. A., Hallsworth, K., He, J., et al. (2014). Effects of community exercise therapy on metabolic, brain, physical, and cognitive function following stroke: A randomized controlled pilot trial. https://core.ac.uk/download/42130503.pdf (accessed on 16th June 2025).

16. Bonny, O., Gumz, M. L., Mazzoccoli, G., Vinciguerra, M., et al. (2017). Molecular bases of circadian rhythmicity in renal physiology and pathology. https://core.ac.uk/download/85210329.pdf (accessed on 16th June 2025).

17. Calhoun, V. D., Colenbier, N., Marinazzo, D., Poldrack, R. A., et al. (2019). Disambiguating the role of blood flow and global signal with partial information decomposition. https://core.ac.uk/download/287942331.pdf (accessed on 16th June 2025).

18. Casteleyn, C., Cornillie, P., Debbaut, C., Dierick, M., et al. (2014). Analyzing the human liver vascular architecture by combining vascular corrosion casting and micro-CT scanning: A feasibility study. https://core.ac.uk/download/55806749.pdf (accessed on 16th June 2025).

19. Cavarretta, E., Dal Sasso, E., Forte, M., Frati, G., et al. (2017). The light and shadow of senescence and inflammation in cardiovascular pathology and regenerative medicine. https://core.ac.uk/download/141694265.pdf (accessed on 16th June 2025).

20. Harwood, A. E., Cayton, T., Sarvanandan, R., Lane, R., & Chetter, I. (2016). A Review of the Potential Local Mechanisms by Which Exercise Improves Functional Outcomes in Intermittent Claudication. *Annals of vascular surgery*, *30*, 312–320. https://doi.org/10.1016/j.avsg.2015.05.043Cifarelli, V., & Eichmann, A. (2019). The intestinal lymphatic system: Functions and metabolic implications. https://core.ac.uk/download/212868551.pdf (accessed on 16th June 2025).

21. Crisafulli, A., Marongiu, E., Nobrega, A. C. L., O'Leary, D. S., et al. (2014). Neural regulation of cardiovascular response to exercise: Role of central command and peripheral afferents. https://core.ac.uk/download/pdf/54599119.pdf (accessed on 16th June 2025).

22. Martínez-Navarro, I., Sánchez-Gómez, J. M., Collado-Boira, E. J., Hernando, B., Panizo, N., & Hernando, C. (2019). Cardiac Damage Biomarkers and Heart Rate Variability Following a 118-Km Mountain Race: Relationship with Performance and Recovery. *Journal of sports science & medicine*, *18*(4), 615–622.(accessed on 16th June 2025).

23. Detmar, M., Di Nardo, A., Docherty, J. R., Holmes, C., et al. (2016). Multidisciplinary consideration of potential pathophysiologic mechanisms of paradoxical erythema with topical brimonidine therapy. https://core.ac.uk/download/323064570.pdf (accessed on 16th June 2025).

24. Di Giovanni, G., Muscat, R., Pierucci, M., Valentino, R. J., et al. (2011). Two-photon microscopy: Sequential imaging studies *in vivo*. https://core.ac.uk/download/46602303.pdf (accessed on 16th June 2025).

25. Dickson, K. J., Hess, E., Powers, J. V., Wallace-Robinson, S., et al. (2025). *Publications of the Space Physiology and Countermeasures Program, Regulatory Physiology Discipline: 1980–1990.* https://core.ac.uk/download/pdf/42811395.pdf (accessed on 16th June 2025).

26. Dignan, C. J. (2016). *The Benefits of a Plant-Based Diet for The Prevention and Treatment of Heart Disease.* https://open.bu.edu/bitstream/2144/14685/1/Dignan_bu_0017N_10517.pdf (accessed on 16th June 2025).

27. Zherebtsova, A. I., Dremin, V. V., Makovik, I. N., Zherebtsov, E. A., Dunaev, A. V., Goltsov, A., Sokolovski, S. G., & Rafailov, E. U. (2019). Multimodal Optical Diagnostics of the Microhaemodynamics in Upper and Lower Limbs. *Frontiers in physiology, 10,* 416. https://doi.org/10.3389/fphys.2019.00416(accessed on 16th June 2025).

28. Drinkhill, M. J., Hainsworth, R., & Wright, C. I. (2001). Responses to stimulation of coronary and carotid baroreceptors and the coronary chemoreflex at different ventricular distending pressures in anaesthetized dogs. https://core.ac.uk/download/57453.pdf (accessed on 16th June 2025).

29. Drinkhill, M. J., Hainsworth, R., McMahon, N. C., Myers, D., et al. (2000). Absence of reflex vascular responses from the intrapulmonary circulation in anaesthetized dogs. https://core.ac.uk/download/57443.pdf (accessed on 16th June 2025).

30. Drinkhill, M. J., Hainsworth, R., Myers, D. S., Noble, M., et al. (1998). Blood mobilization from the liver of the anaesthetized dog. https://core.ac.uk/download/57450.pdf (accessed on 16th June 2025).

31. Ekström, T. J., Nordfors, L., Shiels, P. G., Stenvinkel, P., et al. (2017). Current epigenetic aspects the clinical kidney researcher should embrace. https://core.ac.uk/download/84340482.pdf (accessed on 16th June 2025).

32. Fang, L., Haft-Javaherian, M., Muse, V., Nishimura, N., et al. (2019). Deep convolutional neural networks for segmenting 3D *in vivo* multiphoton images of vasculature in Alzheimer disease mouse models. http://arxiv.org/abs/1801.00880 (accessed on 16th June 2025).

33. Pierelli, G., Stanzione, R., Forte, M., Migliarino, S., Perelli, M., Volpe, M., & Rubattu, S. (2017). Uncoupling Protein 2: A Key Player and a Potential Therapeutic Target in Vascular Diseases. *Oxidative medicine and cellular longevity, 2017,* 7348372. https://doi.org/10.1155/2017/7348372(accessed on 16th June 2025).

34. Gerbes, A. L., Laggner, A., Arendt, C., Barratt-Boyes, G., Barry, M., Bauch, C., Brenner, T., et al. (1991). Ornipressin in the treatment of functional renal failure in decompensated liver cirrhosis. https://core.ac.uk/download/12166774.pdf (accessed on 16th June 2025).

35. Guzik, T. J., & Nosalski, R. (2017). Perivascular adipose tissue inflammation in vascular disease. https://core.ac.uk/download/77600990.pdf (accessed on 16th June 2025).

36. Haak, T., Jungmann, E., Kullmer, T., Meier-Sydow, J., et al. (1996). Hormonal modifications in patients admitted to an internal intensive care unit for acute hypoxemic respiratory failure. https://core.ac.uk/download/pdf/82065854.pdf (accessed on 16th June 2025).

37. Hills, G., Kuppusamy, H., Naing, P., Playford, D., et al. (2017). Non-invasive assessment of pulmonary vascular resistance in pulmonary hypertension: Current knowledge and future direction. https://core.ac.uk/download/213607322.pdf (accessed on 16th June 2025).

38. Holt, A. W., & Tulis, D. A. (2015). Vascular smooth muscle as a therapeutic target in disease pathology. https://core.ac.uk/download/322425090.pdf (accessed on 16th June 2025).

39. Kim, S. R., Lee, S. K., Jang, S. H., Choi, Y., et al. (2011). Expression of keratin 10 in rat organ surface primo-vascular tissues. https://core.ac.uk/download/pdf/82044703.pdf (accessed on 16th June 2025).

40. Kuchar, N. R. (2025). *Fluid Dynamics in Flexible Tubes: An Application to The Study of The Pulmonary Circulation*. https://core.ac.uk/download/pdf/85232914.pdf (accessed on 16th June 2025).

41. Lakin, W. D., Penar, P. L., Stevens, S. A., Tranmer, B. I., et al. (2007). Whole-body mathematical model for simulating intracranial pressure dynamics. https://core.ac.uk/download/pdf/10542011.pdf (accessed on 16th June 2025).

42. Leonard, J. I. (2025). *Description, Validation, And Modification of The Guyton Model for Space-Flight Applications. Part A. Guyton Model of Circulatory, Fluid and Electrolyte Control. Part B. Modification of the Guyton Model for Circulatory, Fluid and Electrolyte Control*. https://core.ac.uk/download/pdf/42845535.pdf (accessed on 16th June 2025).

43. Luck, J. C. (2019). *Effects of Peripheral Revascularization on Blood Pressure and Calf Muscle Oxygen Saturation in Peripheral Artery Disease*. https://core.ac.uk/download/345088588.pdf (accessed on 16th June 2025).

44. Machado, R. (2012). *The Molecular Genetics and Cellular Mechanisms Underlying Pulmonary Arterial Hypertension*. https://core.ac.uk/download/20320889.pdf (accessed on 16th June 2025).

45. Man, A. W. C., & Wang, Y. (2017). Age-associated arterial remodeling and cardiovascular diseases. https://core.ac.uk/download/84930825.pdf (accessed on 16th June 2025).

46. Mauroy, B., & Moreau, B. (2014). Functional optimization of the arterial network. http://arxiv.org/abs/1405.1281 (accessed on 16th June 2025).

47. Mauroy, B., & Moreau, B. (2015). Murray's law revisited: Quémada's fluid model and fractal trees. https://core.ac.uk/download/47087169.pdf (accessed on 16th June 2025).

48. Moskalenko, Y. Y. (2025). *Functional Stability of Cerebral Circulatory System*. https://core.ac.uk/download/pdf/42860883.pdf (accessed on 16th June 2025).

49. Mourot, L., Rakobowchuk, M., & Wilhelm, E. N. (2018). Exercise-derived macrovesicles: A review of the literature. https://core.ac.uk/download/288430488.pdf (accessed on 16th June 2025).

50. San, O., & Staples, A. E. (2012). An improved model for reduced-order physiological fluid flows. http://arxiv.org/abs/1212.0188 (accessed on 16th June 2025).

51. Solovyev, A., Stefanovska, A., Jackson, A. B., Solovyev, A., Bailey, A. M., Onigbinde, A. T., Brienza, D., et al. (2013). Hybrid equation/agent-based model of ischemia-induced hyperemia and pressure ulcer formation predicts greater propensity to ulcerate in subjects with spinal cord injury. https://core.ac.uk/download/12215249.pdf (accessed on 16th June 2025).

VASCULAR PHYSIOLOGY

10

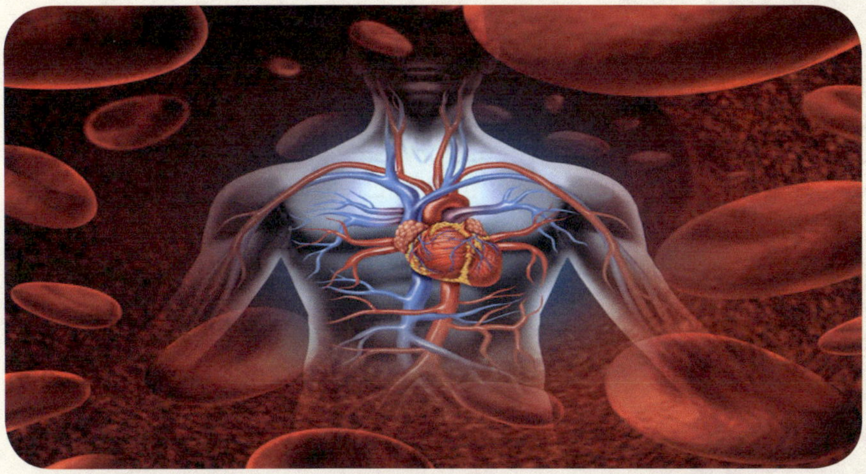

LEARNING OBJECTIVES

After studying this chapter, you will be able to:

1. Discuss the blood vessel structure;
2. Describe the dynamics of blood flow;
3. Discuss the vascular resistance;
4. Highlight regulation of blood pressure;
5. Study vascular pathophysiology;
6. Assess the therapeutic strategies in vascular health.

Introduction

The field of vascular physiology is at the core of understanding the complex network that facilitates blood circulation in the body. The complex network is comprised of a network of vessels, including arteries, veins, and capillaries, that have specific roles in delivering blood, nutrients, and oxygen to tissues. The elastic and muscular structure of the arterial system is essential for withstanding and regulating the blood pressure created by the contraction of the heart. Venous operation is of lower pressure and utilizes valves to ensure one-way blood return towards the heart. All these components create a dynamic equilibrium of blood flow that responds to the body's physiological requirements, revealing the essential mechanisms behind maintaining homeostasis and general health. To better delve into this vital topic, one must consider how vascular physiology is under the influence of countless variables, including neural, hormonal, and local tissue regulation. For instance, the autonomic nervous system plays a pivotal role in the control of vascular tone, affecting the dilation and constriction of blood vessels in regard to external stimuli. Norepinephrine and epinephrine hormones also facilitate these responses to develop rapid adaptations against physiologic stressors like exercise or changes in posture. In addition, local mechanisms , such as metabolic activity induce vasodilation through the release of substances like nitric oxide, allowing enhanced perfusion to active tissues. Such a multifaceted interaction poses the completeness of vascular response mechanisms that enable several organ systems to be perfused in proportion to their metabolic requirements. Greater insight into vascular physiology is crucial for research and also clinical practice. Techniques , such as advanced imaging techniques have enabled unprecedented visualization and quantification of vascular tissue at different scales, providing improved insight into microcirculation and its impact on pathology. For instance, recent hepatic circulatory research has employed vascular corrosion casting combined with micro-computer tomography to shed light on the hepatic vasculature at both macro and micro levels, showing exquisite detail of anatomical structure and blood dynamic parameters within the liver. These findings not only assist in surgical planning but also put into perspective investigating conditions involving improper blood circulation, like cirrhosis, where it can significantly influence liver functionality (Casteleyn et al., 2014). Furthermore, the breadth of research into vascular physiology, and how it can relate to regulatory physiology, continues to guide treatment of bodily reaction to a broad spectrum of adversities, such as space flight (Hess et al., 1992) (Figure 10.1).

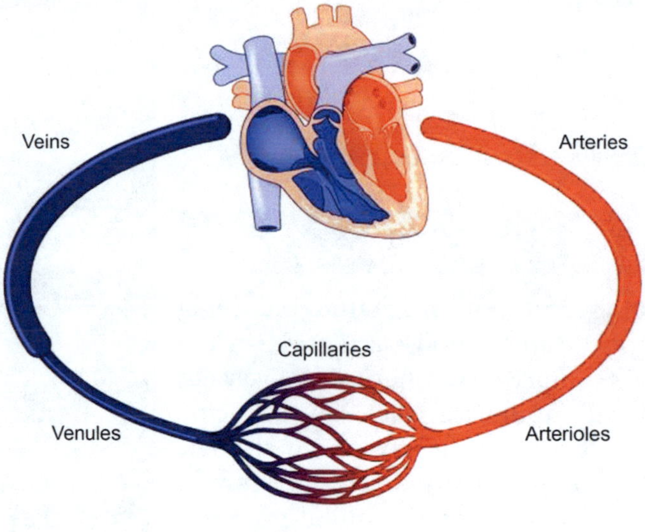

Figure 10.1. Vascular physiology.

Source: https://cdn.ps.emap.com/wp-content/uploads/sites/3/2018/03/Fig-1-The-five-types-of-blood-vessels_660.jpg.

Definition of Vascular Physiology

To really comprehend the intricacies of vascular physiology, one has to first take a glance at its definition, which entails the observation of the dynamics of blood flow in the vascular system. This understanding not only observes the structural components of blood vessels but also the mechanical properties of blood and how they interact. Vascular physiology plays a crucial role in the description of the delivery of nutrients, the elimination of waste, and hormonal signaling throughout the body. By integrating concepts from fluid mechanics and biophysics, the field describes how flow mechanics cross-talks with physiological needs and exposes how alterations in vascular function can lead to systemic disease. As the vascular system accommodates shifting physiological requirements, understanding these principles is crucial for the development of medical interventions designed to remedy dysregulation in blood pressure or flow. Mathematical modeling of blood flow dynamics is central to vascular physiology. Improved in recent years have established more advanced one-dimensional models containing numerous physiological parameters such that sophisticated comprehension of flow through the arterial network is achievable. For instance, a study suggests the inclusion of pulsed flow equations, where the dynamics of momentum variation in blood while flowing through the complex network of arteries are dynamically taken into account. This modeling helps researchers model the real-life physiological conditions, and it provides a platform for analyzing how changes in velocity and pressure of blood might dictate overall vascular health. These models should be effective in refining classical theories with profound steady-state conditions and be capable of incorporating nonlinear influences into the design, which are instrumental in occurrences like blood vessel bifurcations and varying outflow conditions, indicating the imperative requirement for accurate simulations in vascular research (San et al., 2012). Besides modeling techniques, technological innovations have also played a substantial role in vascular physiology analysis. The use of detailed system analysis to physiological tests in circumstances of normal gravity (1-g) and weightlessness is an example of the universality of this field. Through the utilization of powerful biomedical computer systems for simulation and analysis, researchers are able to develop detailed models of the entire vascular system. These consist of interactive software facilities that allow manipulation and observation of numerous parameters that affect vascular health. These advances enable enhanced understanding of short and long-term physiological responses to environmental changes, providing informative information on systemic adjustment and probable pathological processes. Therefore, the union of technology and vascular physiology has continued to open up opportunities for groundbreaking research and clinical use, eventually enabling us to gain a deeper understanding of human physiology.

Importance in the Circulatory System

The circulatory system serves as the foundation on which homeostasis is ensured in the body to ensure the delivery of essential nutrients, gases, and waste products. Such a sophisticated system comprising the heart, blood vessels, and blood is indispensable for effective oxygenation and nutrient delivery to the tissues while facilitating the elimination of metabolic waste. The significance of smooth blood flow is further realized with the interrelationship between vascular performance and the overall physiological integrity. Improvements in our understanding of vascular physiology, encompassing mechanisms controlling blood vessel reactivity, are at the forefront of the revelation of therapies for cardiovascular disease, which remains a predominant cause of morbidity and mortality globally. Maximizing circulatory function is self-evidently crucial to sustaining life and thus there is a pressing need for state-of-the-art therapeutic interventions targeting vascular pathways pivotal to homeostasis. There are advanced mechanisms in the circulatory system, and the cerebral region in particular, that ensure functional stability against varying physiological conditions. The intricate interaction between chemical and neurogenic stimuli controls the dilatation and constriction of cerebral vessels to ensure brain tissues receive an adequate blood supply regardless of systemic blood pressure changes. This versatility makes the brain's vascular response critical in the preservation of cognitive and motor function, as cerebral blood flow has a direct effect on the modulation of neuronal activity. Central nervous structure regulates this response that demonstrates the complexities that underlie vascular physiology and emphasizes the significance of more research. Consequently, cerebral circulation is an indication of the broader significance of vascular health, and assumes that failure in this system will lead to deleterious consequences like stroke and neurodegenerative illness (Moskalenko et al., 2025). Refinement of mathematical modeling techniques are advanced methods of understanding circulatory patterns of blood movement.

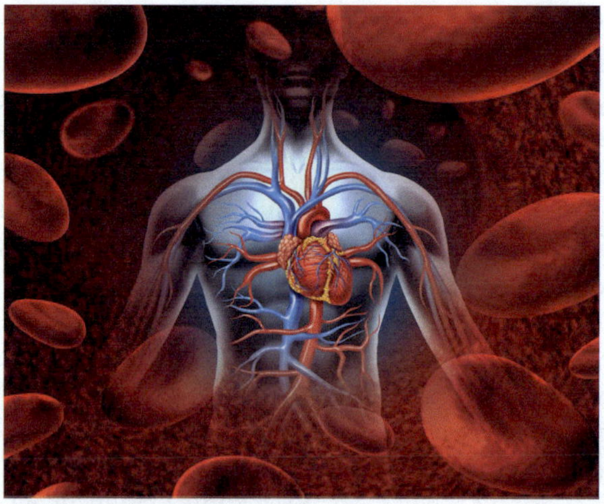

Figure 10.2. Circulatory system.

Source: https://cdn.mos.cms.futurecdn.net/pYF5YURHV2xggu6L2Dnjfb.jpg.

For instance, in the derivation of one-dimensional pulsatile flow equations, it is possible to analyze hemodynamics in various vascular geometries more effectively, particularly in complex arterial trees. Nonlinear equations typical of the dynamics of blood flow, as characterized in various studies, enable one to determine the behavior of blood under varying conditions, e.g., varying vessel diameter and pressure gradients. Using advanced numerical methods, such models provide an approach that clarifies the intricacies of vascular physiology. Through the better understanding of these fluid dynamics, potential intervention and treatment options for vascular disease can be conceived, underlining the importance of healthy vascular networks in guaranteeing physiological integrity (San et al., 2012) (Figure 10.2).

10.1. Structure of Blood Vessels

Learning Outcome

1. Describe the types of blood vessels: arteries, veins, and capillaries;
2. Note blood vessel wall layers: tunica intima, tunica media, tunica externa;
3. Investigate the structural and functional differences between types of vessels.

The structure of blood vessels is responsible for their role in helping sustain the circulatory system. The three primary layers of blood vessels are the tunica intima, tunica media, and tunica externa. The innermost one, tunica intima, is composed of endothelial cells, which create a smooth lining to produce the least amount of friction for blood flow. This is a significant role in vascular tone and permeability regulation. The intima is followed by the tunica media, which varies in thickness from vessel to vessel. This middle layer consists predominantly of smooth muscle cells and elastic fibers, which permit the vessel to contract or dilate in response to physiological demand. Last, the tunica externa, or adventitia, consists of connective tissue that provides structural support and flexibility such that blood vessels remain fixed in the larger vascular structure. Widespread structural differences between arteries, veins, and capillaries indicate their various functions in the circulatory system. Arteries possess stronger walls with more elastic tissue than veins and are capable of managing and regulating the high blood pressure that occurs in the heart pumping. The circular arrangement of smooth muscle in the tunica media makes vasoconstriction and vasodilation possible, required to maintain blood pressure and regulate the flow of blood. Conversely, veins are structured with thinner walls and larger lumen diameters that accommodate the lower pressure of returning blood. Valves within veins prevent the backflow of blood, ensuring unidirectional flow towards the heart.

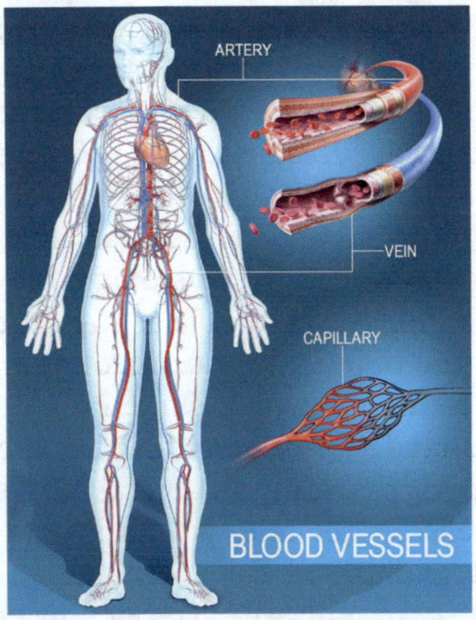

Figure 10.3. Blood vessels.

Source: https://www.visiblebody.com/hubfs/Learn_Articles/Circulatory_System/01B-Blood-Vessels.jpg.

Capillaries, the smallest and most numerous blood vessels, have walls that are only one cell thick. Such an organization is of prime importance for gas, nutrient, and waste product exchange between blood and tissue fluids, and thus serves to emphasize the importance of vessel organization in physiological processes. Advances in imaging technology, particularly in the use of volumetric imaging techniques , such as multiphoton microscopy, have enhanced our understanding of vascular architecture. These methods allow scientists to visualize 3D blood vessels with greater resolution than before, allowing the study of both normal physiology and disease pathology. For instance, applying convolutional neural networks to segment 3D vascular images has significantly improved vessel analysis accuracy, providing greater insight into vascular structure and function. Experiments with these tools have also demonstrated subtle structural remodeling of capillary beds associated with aging and neurodegenerative diseases like Alzheimer's. With the illumination of the intricate structure of blood vessels, these techniques tell us more about vascular physiology and what is in store for future research in health and disease (Kim et al., 2011; Fang et al., 2019) (Figure 10.3).

10.1.1. Types of Blood Vessels: Arteries, Veins, and Capillaries

The cardiovascular system relies on three main classes of blood vessels: arteries, veins, and capillaries, with each performing a specific function necessary for homeostasis. Arteries supply oxygenated blood to the rest of the tissues and organs from the heart. Thick and elastic walls on arteries enable them to withstand and regulate the high pressures generated by the contraction of the heart. This structural feature is significant because arteries must provide the required pressure to deliver enough blood flow, ensuring oxygen and nutrients are being distributed to the body's tissues effectively. Moreover, as arteries branch into smaller arterioles, they are tasked with regulating systemic blood pressure as well as dispersing blood flow to regions that require more oxygen supply during physical activity. Veins are the vessels that carry deoxygenated blood to the heart, completing the circulatory loop. Veins have thinner walls and larger lumens than arteries, to accommodate the lower pressure of blood return. The presence of valves in veins is a significant feature in that they oppose retrograde blood flow and promote unidirectional flow towards the heart, particularly in the peripheral circulation. The efficiency of venous return is also aided by the skeletal muscles around it that help propel blood in the veins as the individual moves. The muscle pump is significant, especially in the lower limbs, where blood must be pumped upwards against gravity. The combination of venous structure and muscle motion highlights the significant adaptations necessary to allow efficient circulation and play a notable part in overall cardiovascular health.

Capillaries are the body's smallest and largest number of blood vessels, creating the site of exchange with tissues and blood. Their thin walls, made up of a single layer of endothelial cells, allow rapid diffusion of gases, nutrients, and waste products. By having an extensive network of capillaries, all cells can be brought near to a blood supply, thereby allowing maximum metabolic activity. This intricate organization is particularly important in organs of high metabolic rate, e.g., muscles and the brain. Furthermore, advances in imaging techniques, as highlighted in the literature, depict the necessity of understanding capillary dynamics. The ability to image blood flow and cell-cell communication in real time has implications for clinical research and understanding of pathophysiological conditions, e.g., cerebrovascular disease (Valentino et al., 2011; Lakin et al., 2007) (Figure 10.4).

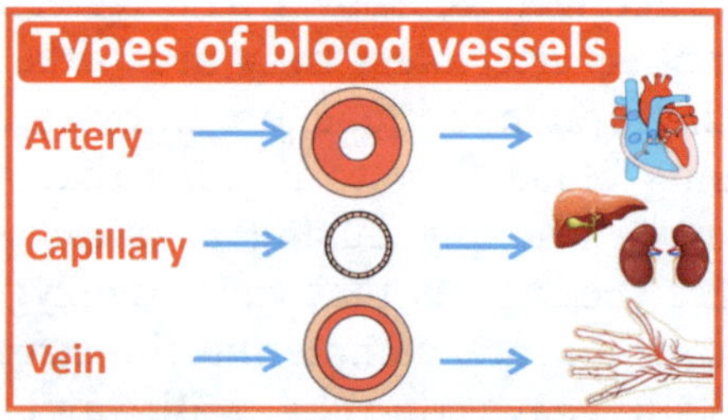

Figure 10.4. Types of blood vessels.

Source: https://i.ytimg.com/vi/Oq3SbxO8RBO/maxresdefault.jpg.

10.1.2. Layers of Blood Vessel Walls: Tunica Intima, Tunica Media, and Tunica Externa

The intricate blood vessel structure is made up of three simple layers, each crucial to vascular physiology. The innermost layer is the tunica intima, a smooth endothelial lining that minimizes resistance to blood flow and facilitates efficient gas and nutrient exchange. This layer is necessary for hemodynamic stability since it also regulates vascular tone and permeability by releasing various biochemical mediators. Injury to the endothelial structure can lead to vascular hyperpermeability and inflammation, increasing the risk of atherosclerosis and other cardiovascular diseases. Recognition of the functions of the tunica intima discloses not only its significance in vascular homeostasis but also in the pathophysiology of vascular disease, highlighting its role as the first contact between the blood and the surrounding tissue. The tunica media, which surrounds the tunica intima, is made up of smooth muscle cells and elastic fibers, providing structural reinforcement to the vessel wall and the ability to control pressure and blood flow. This layer enables arteries to carry pulsatile arterial flow efficiently and enables pressure variations resulting from cardiac contraction. During the aging process of the blood vessels, the architecture and function of the tunica media may be compromised and resulting in loss of elasticity along with an increase in stiffness. These alterations not only impact central artery health but also compromise peripheral vascular function and subsequently, give rise to microcirculatory complications. By understanding the pivotal role of the tunica media, researchers can better understand how its remodeling affects vascular health and investigate therapeutic approaches that can restore normal function in diseases like hypertension and atherosclerosis, which are significantly affected by vascular smooth muscle activity (Holt et al., 2015). The most external layer of blood vessels, the tunica externa, or adventitia, not only shields and supports the vessel but also houses the vascular network serving larger blood vessels. This outermost layer, composed mainly of connective tissue, gives structural support, meeting the requirements of nearby tissue by a very intricate interaction between blood vessels, nerves, and lymphatics. Since the tunica externa is crucial for overall vessel integrity and function, any pathological alteration of this layer has the potential to negatively impact the health of the vessels. Changes in the extracellular matrix elements may be involved in vulnerabilities of the vascular wall, predisposing to conditions , such as aneurysm or dissection. Stress on the function of the tunica externa enhances our understanding of vascular physiology and demands holistic answers to neutralize age-related vascular alterations as suggested by recent evidence linking structural arterial wall remodeling with cardiovascular health (Man et al., 2017) (Figure 10.5).

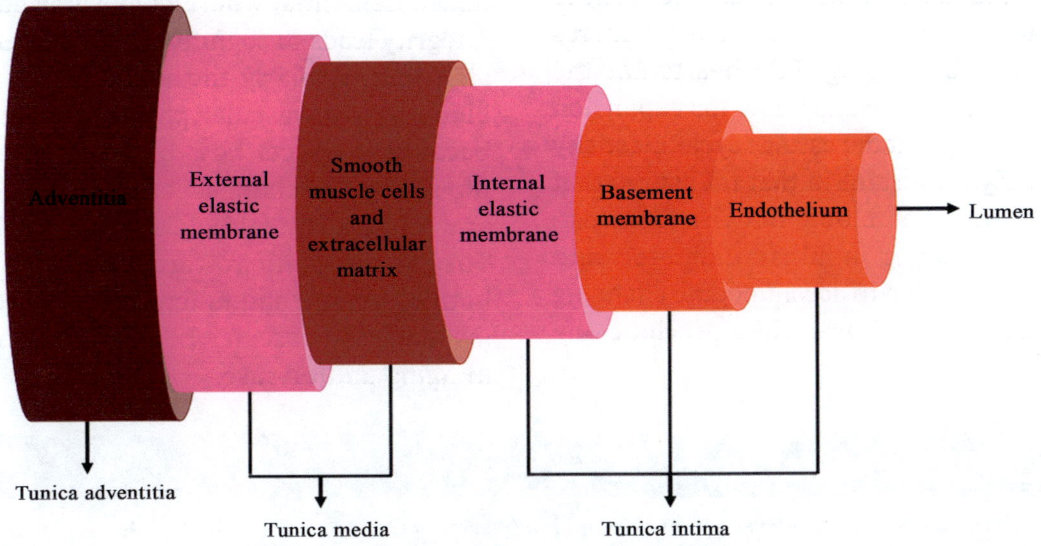

Figure 10.5. Layers of blood vessel walls.

Source: https://www.researchgate.net/publication/373753319/figure/fig1/AS:11431281205105911@1700103964303/Layers-of-the-arterial-wall-tunica-intima-tunica-media-and-tunica-adventitia-layer.png.

10.1.3. Differences in Structure and Function Among Vessel Types

The circulatory system consists of a network of vessel types, each with specific structural and functional objectives in the body. There are three primary blood vessels that differ significantly in constitution and function: arteries, veins, and capillaries. Arteries, which carry oxygenated blood away from the heart, possess strong, elastic walls made up mainly of smooth muscle and connective tissue. This type of structure allows them to resist and regulate the pressure of blood flow being high, so that they can distribute it effectively to tissues. On the other hand, veins have thinner walls, a larger lumen, and a backflow-preventing valve, which reflects their role of returning deoxygenated blood to the heart at lower pressure. The smallest of the vessels are the capillaries, which consist of a single layer of endothelial cells that facilitate exchange with the surrounding tissues, showing specialized adaptations that facilitate their own special functions in gas and nutrient exchange. Their structural differences are complemented by their own specific features. Capillaries, for instance, are structured for the exchange of nutrients since they possess a high surface area and thin walls, thus gases, nutrients, and waste products are able to diffuse rapidly. This is crucial where there is a high metabolic requirement, such as in muscles and organs. On the other hand, the firm walls of arteries render them robust enough to support the pressures generated by the pumping of the hearts, and the elastic fibers in their walls allow for expansion and recoil throughout the cardiac cycle. Elasticity is particularly important in that it ensures that there is permanent blood flow. In contrast, veins, whose larger luminal diameter and thinner walls function to accommodate changing blood volumes and whose valves preclude any backflow as the blood efficiently returns to the heart, especially in gravity-dependent areas , such as the legs. It is more than rudimentary physiology to comprehend differences in structure and function among vessel types because it calls forth their significance in pathophysiologic situations. For example, structural changes in the vasculature, such as in hypertension or atherosclerosis, can lead to deleterious effects on function and, ultimately, cardiovascular health. Vessel-type relationship is also significant in various conditions, such as mixed dementia, where compromised vascular integrity leads to cognitive decline (Ahmadian et al., 2019). Similarly, the addition of dynamics of blood flow to vascular physiology is important because it affects how blood vessels react to physiological changes and overall cognitive and systemic health (Calhoun et al., 2019). The results point towards the need to study both structural and functional properties when investigating vascular health and its relevance in aging and disease.

Test Your Knowledge

1. What are the three principal layers (tunics) of a blood vessel wall?
2. How structurally are arteries different from veins?

10.2. Blood Flow Dynamics

Learning Outcome

1. Explain the physiology of blood pressure and flow;
2. Define the determinants of blood flow: resistance and viscosity;
3. Study the role played by the heart in maintaining blood circulation;

Understanding blood flow dynamics forms the foundation of the science of vascular physiology since it accounts for the intricate mechanisms of hemodynamics within the body. Blood circulation is not a one-way process; it is, however, regulated by various factors , such as vessel diameter, blood viscosity, and resistance in the vascular system. Of interest, fluid dynamics principles regulate the circulatory system so that arteries and veins exhibit complicated behavior due to viscoelastic properties. A lumped-parameter model developed to characterize blood flow in the pulmonary vascular bed is especially representative of the nonlinear nature of resistance to flow, which is a function of transmural pressure. Besides aiding in the prediction of blood pressures and flow rates, this modeling helps in explaining pathological conditions influencing vascular health, enhancing the knowledge on blood flow dynamics within the context of vascular physiology (Kuchar et al., 2025). In addition, emerging models , such as the visco-elastic windkessel (VW) model, are significant to enhance our comprehension of cerebral blood volume (CBV) and cerebral blood flow (CBF). The model can account for the unique dynamics occurring following stimulation, capturing the effects of circumferential stress relaxation of veins on blood flow.

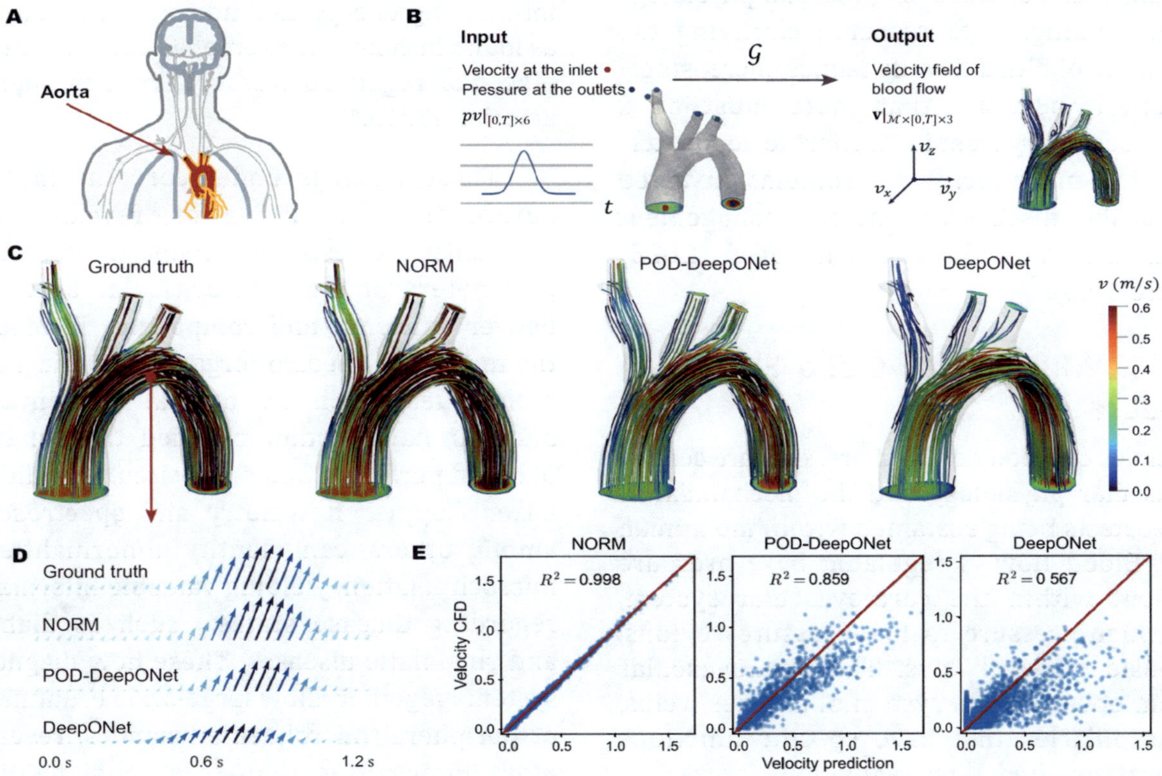

Figure 10.6. Blood flow dynamics prediction case.

Source: https://www.researchgate.net/publication/379780636/figure/fig4/AS:11431281236021200@1712974166819/Blood-flow-dynamics-prediction-case-Case-5-a-Illustration-of-the-human-thoracic.png.

By modeling the pressure-volume relationship of vessels as a state variable that is a function of the rate of change of CBV, the VW model accounts for vessel hysteresis during dilation and contraction. This information is significant, particularly in BOLD signal interpretation in fMRI experiments. The ability to predict flow dynamics following neural activity changes bolsters our understanding of blood flow regulation in the cerebral vasculature, validating the massive significance of blood flow dynamics in vascular physiology (Alexander et al., 2009). Blood flow dynamics is not only significant theoretically but also affects clinical practice and treatment of vascular disorders. A clear comprehension of these dynamics allows medical doctors to foresee and manage conditions , such as hypertension, atherosclerosis, and other cardiovascular illnesses more reliably. Scientists are able to model various pathological states with advanced modeling protocols and observe how variations in blood flow dynamics correlate with clinic manifestations. Also, continuous innovation in imaging technology continually enhances our capacity to image blood flow in real-time, further enhancing vascular physiology understanding. With research clarifying the intricacies of blood flow dynamics, increasingly evident it becomes that there must be a multidisciplinary front in an effort to adequately solve the multiplicity of problems involved in vascular disease and health management (Alexander et al., 2009; Kuchar et al., 2025) (Figure 10.6).

10.2.1. Principles of Blood Flow and Pressure

Principles of blood flow and pressure are central to vascular physiology and the mechanism of homeostasis being sustained within the human body. Blood flow is regulated by a pressure gradient within the cardiovascular system, from high-pressure to low-pressure regions, by basic physical laws. The cardiovascular system operates as a system of arteries, veins, and capillaries that have specific functions for pressure and flow regulation. Interactive dynamics keep tissues in the perfusion of cellular metabolism. Factors , such as vessel diameter, blood viscosity, and total vascular resistance all contribute to the modulation of blood flow, demonstrating the complexity of hemodynamics of the circulatory system. It is necessary to know these principles of diagnosis and treatment of many of the vascular diseases that can arise when these normal parameters are disrupted. The relationship between arterial pressure and blood flow is also significantly determined by evolutionary limitations built into the vascular architecture. Research shows that the morphology of the arterial tree has evolved to maximize tissue oxygenation at the cost of physiologic need, affecting pressure gradients and hematocrit within vessels. The evolution model postulates that arterial diameters must shrink proportionally to maintain sufficient shear stress and thereby affect red blood cell concentration. These physiological adaptation characteristics exhibit the compromise between maximizing the delivery of nutrients and minimizing energy expenditure on blood flow, as found in conclusions emphasizing the stresses placed on regulated pressure drops through the arterial network.

These findings underscore the intricate nature of blood circulation, revealing how mechanisms of evolution shape the functional parameters of the cardiovascular system to deliver efficiency and competency in meeting the metabolic needs of organs. New diagnostic techniques, such as optical non-invasive systems, have further clarified the dynamics of blood perfusion and microcirculatory health. Laser Doppler flowmetry and spectroscopy, among others, can identify abnormalities in microcirculation, yielding valuable information regarding disease states , such as diabetes and rheumatic diseases. These new diagnostic systems together allow large-scale examination of peripheral microhaemodynamics, revealing more information than traditional methods. The greater sensitivity and specificity of these techniques are of extreme relevance to early detection and intervention, particularly pertinent with the rising prevalence of vascular-related disease. By broadening our understanding of principles of blood flow and developing new diagnostic techniques, clinicians and researchers are able to promote improved patient outcomes, illustrating the continued progression of vascular physiology as a field of study committed to enhancing health and quality of life through rational medical intervention (Mauroy et al., 2014; Zherebtsova et al., 2019) (Figure 10.7).

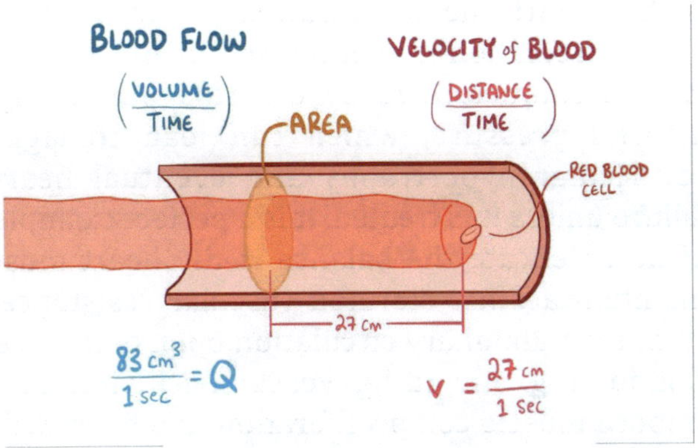

Figure 10.7. Principles of blood flow and pressure.

Source: https://d16qt3wv6xm098.cloudfront.net/2MzaxD9rSFqNZEcQb1cpgGS1Tx2BvyMP/_.jpg.

10.2.2. Factors Affecting Blood Flow: Resistance and Viscosity

In vascular physiology, those variables that influence the flow of blood must be explained. Of these variables, resistance and viscosity are significant in their role in how efficiently the blood circulates within the vascular system. Resistance, brought about by the friction of blood with the vessel walls, is based on the vessel size. According to Murrays law, which suggests fluid flow rate within a vessel to be directly proportional to the cube of vessel radius, dynamics of blood flow are significantly affected by variations in vessel diameter. The law is very applicable in macrocirculation, though it is somewhat discreet in microcirculation due to varying viscosity levels experienced in small vessels. Secondly, the Fåhræus-Lindqvist effect adds another level of complexity with the discovery that blood viscosity is not constant but rises with varying shear rates, hence influencing resistance and consequently blood flow. Viscosity itself, a measure of the resistance of fluids to flow, is inextricably linked with the transport characteristics of blood. The unique rheological properties of blood are not only its cellular constituents, i.e., red blood cells, but also the plasma in which they are suspended. The components can lead to non-Newtonian behavior in which viscosity is a function of the conditions of flow. As described in recent studies, the dependence of blood's viscosity on parameters like shear rate is crucial in vascular resistance and flow patterns assessment. For instance, at low shear rates, blood is thicker and can impede flow, especially in the smaller arteries where wall shear stress is significant. Such layered interaction of viscosity with shear rates is the basis of significant vascular health and disease, where various profiles of viscosity cause optimal flow or pathological conditions like thrombus formation and resistance in the vessels.

Clinical uses of these principles extend as far as clinical practice, particularly that of pulmonary hypertension (PHT) and its management. PHT is characterized by increased pulmonary vascular resistance, which causes alterations in the dynamics of blood flow in the pulmonary circulation. Measurement of pulmonary vascular resistance (PVR) is important in the determination of the etiology and type of PHT, whether pre-capillary or post-capillary in nature. Non-invasive assessments are aimed at differentiating among different underlying etiologies for the purpose of guiding appropriate therapeutic interventions. Understanding the role of viscosity and resistance in such clinical situations is paramount, since therapies aimed at increasing blood flow need to acknowledge both hemodynamic parameters as well as the complex rheological behavior of blood in states of varied physiological states. By synthesizing these concepts, clinicians can significantly enhance diagnosis and treatment protocols for conditions of vascular resistance and blood viscosity dependence, and reaffirm the importance of these factors in vascular physiology (Mauroy et al., 2015; Hills et al., 2017) (Figure 10.8).

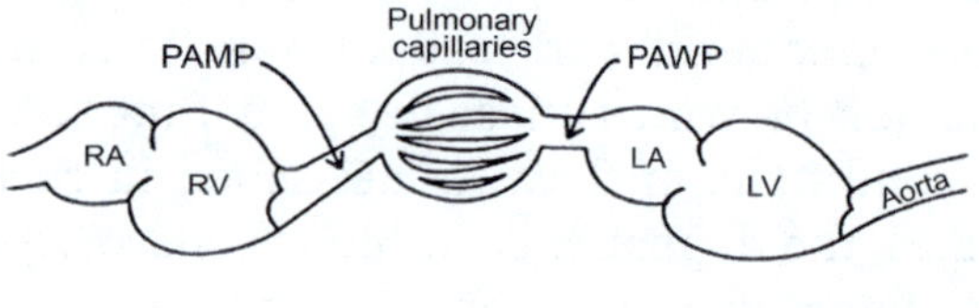

Figure 10.8. Normal pulmonary vascular resistance.

Source: https://external-content.duckduckgo.com/iu/?u=https%3A%2F%2Fwww.oakesacademy.com%2Fmembers%2Fimages%2F1591a.JPG&f=1&nofb=1&ipt=9b7d07236d1c337d65eb60c100361195fa3a047badb6e559c50483341f374b0a.

10.2.3. Role of the Heart in Maintaining Blood Circulation

The circulatory system's pump is the central heart, responsible for a continuous supply of blood to maintain homeostasis. The muscular organ consists of four chambers, two atria, and two ventricles that coordinate to regulate the flow of blood. The right side of the heart receives oxygen-depleted blood from the body and sends it to the lungs to be oxygenated, and the left side receives oxygenated blood from the lungs and sends it out to the body. The rhythmical contraction of the heart, in turn regulated by electrical impulses from intrinsic pacemaker cells, creates pressure differences that enable blood to flow throughout the complex network of arteries, veins, and capillaries efficiently. Understanding the mechanics of the heart and its electrical conducting system is required for an appreciation of how effective circulation preserves tissue perfusion and organ function in health and illness. During states of illness, such as PAH, the contribution of the heart to blood circulation is significantly compromised. PAH is characterized by elevated pulmonary arterial pressure, which can lead to right ventricular hypertrophy and eventual heart failure unless it is treated. It is a perfect example of how delicate the balance is the heart must maintain against elevated vascular resistance. With the pulmonary circulation open to intense remodeling, including vessel occlusion and smooth muscle cell proliferation, the heart will be forced to pump at increased pressure to effect proper blood flow into the lungs for oxygenation. The effects of such hemodynamic changes emphasize the heart's critical role in responding to varying vascular conditions and providing effective circulation for regular physiological function, a demonstration of how changes in one system can have extreme repercussions on the other (Machado et al., 2012). In addition, the heart is intricately coupled with other reflex mechanisms that regulate blood perfusion according to varying physiological requirements. Reflex cardiovascular reactions, for instance, may be provoked by localized intrapulmonary arterial and venous distension, demonstrating the adaptability of the heart. Investigative studies, such as those reporting responses to variations in intrapulmonary pressure, reveal that the heart and lungs collaborate to maintain vascular resistance and general stability in blood flow. Where intrapulmonary pressures significantly rise, the cardiovascular system tries to compensate through adjustment of vascular resistance. An understanding of these intricate mechanisms of feedback is critical to understanding how cardiovascular health is maintained and what the consequences of their failure are, for instance, in pulmonary hypertension (Drinkhill et al., 2000).

Test Your Knowledge

1. What controls the rate of blood flow through an artery?
2. How do blood pressure and flow vary with vessel diameter?

10.3. Vascular Resistance

Learning Outcome

1. Explain the function of vascular resistance;
2. Define the mechanisms of vasodilation and vasoconstriction;
3. Discuss the effect of vascular resistance on blood pressure.

Vascular resistance is a major determinant of blood flow in the cardiovascular system and is responsible for playing a central role in both physiological and pathological processes. It is typically characterized by pressure versus flow in the vessels, whereby increased resistance equates to decreased blood flow. This resistance is largely determined by blood vessel diameter, blood viscosity, and total vessel length. Importantly, small arterioles show large changes in diameter through contractions of smooth muscle, and these result in large changes in vascular resistance.

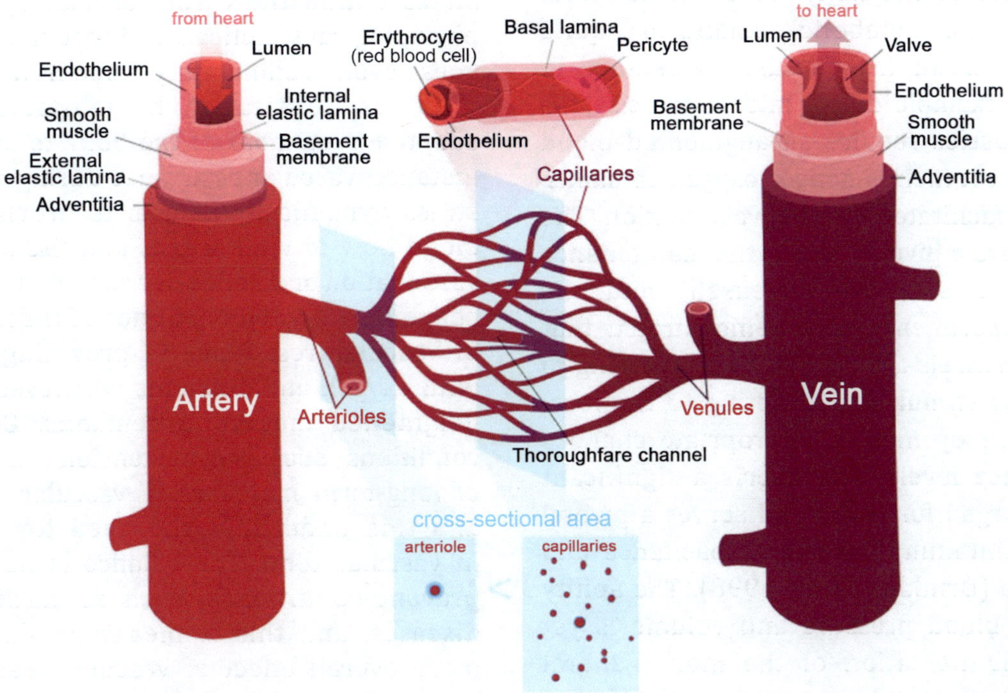

Figure 10.9. Vascular resistance.

Source: https://healthjade.net/wp-content/uploads/2019/11/vascular-resistance.jpg.

Understanding the causes of vascular resistance is important since vascular resistance is involved in disease states , such as hypertension and atherosclerosis, where abnormal or elevated vascular tone can exacerbate the disease process and enhance cardiovascular risk. Understanding the phenomenon of altered vascular resistance is not only intrinsic to the blood vessels but also dependent on neural and hormonal regulation. Specifically, the sympathetic nervous system releases norepinephrine and causes vasoconstriction and consequently, elevated resistance and ultimately, elevated blood pressure. On the other hand, vasodilators , such as nitric oxide play a significant role in reducing vascular resistance, resulting in increased blood flow and improved tissue perfusion. Exercise, particularly in conditions like intermittent claudication (IC), illustrates these effectively. During supervised exercise programs, as Harwood et al (2015) explain, the patients improve in terms of walking distances and cardiovascular fitness. All this is brought about by the complex interaction between reduced vascular resistance and improved endothelial function, which ultimately improves vascular health and quality of life. Besides, local conditions like metabolic demand are quite capable of modifying vascular resistance in tissues. For example, during intense exercise, the skeletal muscles require an augmented blood supply to meet their enhanced oxygen demands, and this is facilitated by local vasodilation. The process plays a pivotal role in the maintenance of homeostasis during increased metabolic activity. Experiments have demonstrated that resistance vessels are capable of responding to endogenous stimuli and adapting to the local environment by making appropriate changes in resistance levels. The liveris a significant reservoir organ for blood and serves a pivotal role in maintaining vascular capacitance and compliance (Drinkhill et al., 1998). The ability to control blood pressure and volume is yet another manifestation of the more general importance of vascular resistance to systemic circulation and overall physiological activity. Understanding these dynamic interactions is central to the development of effective targeted therapy for a variety of cardiovascular diseases (Figure 10.9).

10.3.1. Definition and Significance of Vascular Resistance

Vascular resistance is an important concept of vascular physiology describing the resistance to blood flow as it travels down the vascular system. Resistance varies with parameters like vessel diameter, length, and blood viscosity. Specifically, it is controlled by Poiseuilles Law, which explains how changes in the radius of the blood vessels are able to lead to significant variations in blood flow. Reduction in vessel size leads to exponential increase in resistance, highlighting the central role of vascular tone in the regulation of hemodynamics. Its significance is significant because vascular resistance directly influences blood pressure and circulatory effectiveness in general and establishes its significance in health and disease states within the cardiovascular system. The physiological significance of vascular resistance goes beyond rudimentary blood flow principles; it is very critical in homeostasis and the adaptive responses of the body to stimuli. For instance, vascular resistance during exercise or stress dynamically adjusts to provide greater blood flow to vital organs and tissues through vasodilation and hence decrease resistance. This adaptation is a demonstration of the importance of vascular resistance in providing the body with oxygen and nutrients whenever there are heightened metabolic demands. Conversely, conditions , such as hypertension can be a result of long-term increases in vascular resistance, and this underlines the need for a balance in vascular tone. The balance is necessary to prevent conditions , such as cardiovascular diseases, and this is meant to illustrate the more overall effect of vascular resistance on health. New research has revealed intriguing details on the role of vascular resistance in cellular communication, that is, in relation to microvesicles (MVs) released by cells upon physiological stress. Once simply viewed as cellular trash, MVs are now hailed for their role in intercellular communication and adaptation to stress, even in the form of mere exercise. Interestingly, systemic physiological need caused by physical training elicits the release of MVs into the circulation, which is capable of modulating vascular resistance through multifaceted mechanisms. The interaction between MVs and vascular physiology is an emerging field of study that has the potential to open up new therapeutic avenues for the regulation of conditions accompanying abnormal vascular resistance. With advancing research, gaining an insight into MVs and vascular resistance might become critical in the broader scheme of cardiovascular disease and management of health, as demonstrated by Drinkhill et al. (2001); Mourot et al. (2018) (Figure 10.10).

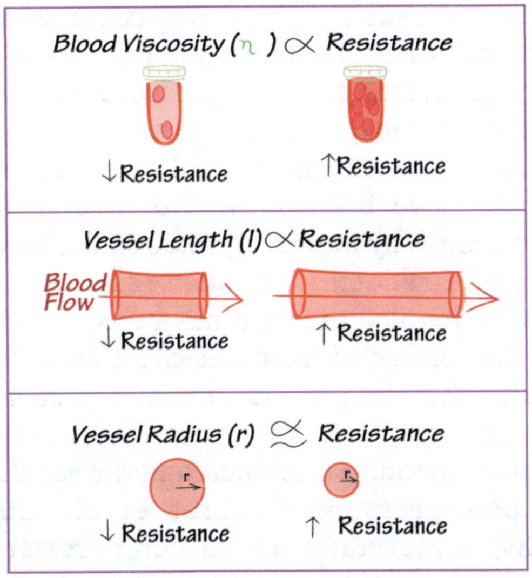

Figure 10.10. Significance of vascular resistance.

Source: https://d1j63owfs0b5j3.cloudfront.net/term/images/673-1494274890136.png.

10.3.2. Mechanisms of Vasodilation and Vasoconstriction

The vascular system regulates homeostasis through complex mechanisms of vasodilation and vasoconstriction control. Dilation of the blood vessels, or vasodilation, is mostly a reaction to a range of biochemical messengers , such as nitric oxide and prostaglandins. Relaxation of vascular smooth muscle results in increased blood flow and reduced vascular resistance. On the other hand, constriction of blood vessels, or vasoconstriction, is an operation largely mediated by the response of adrenergic receptors to catecholamines , such as norepinephrine. The interaction between these convergent processes is necessary for the regulation of blood pressure and adequate tissue perfusion. Understanding these processes is central to the correction of vascular pathologies, as dysregulation can lead to hypertension or peripheral artery disease, thus underscoring the significance of vascular tone to cardiovascular function as a whole. The modulating influence of the autonomic nervous system on vascular tone cannot be overemphasized. Under physiological stress, such as exercise, the sympathetic nervous system dominates and vasoconstriction of non-vital vascular beds takes place while vasodilation in contracting muscle is increased to address increased metabolic demand. Central command and reflex mechanisms coordinate this complex process by integrating sensory feedback from chemoreceptors and baroreceptors to gain control over blood pressure and flow. The mechanism is not uniform; different tissues respond in dissimilar ways to vasoconstrictive or vasodilatory stimuli, which can be explained by differential expression of adrenergic receptor subtypes. As oxygen demand rises with exercise, the proportion of vasodilation and vasoconstriction changes to prevent underperfusion, reflecting the dynamic nature of the vascular bed to maintain homeostasis with varying states of physical activity (Crisafulli et al., 2014). Recent developments in the mechanisms of vasodilation and vasoconstriction have illuminated their significance beyond classical cardiovascular physiology. For instance, the presence of local inflammation and perivascular inflammatory cells may result in aberrant vasodilation responses, such in rosacea. Some polymorphisms of certain receptors and genetic predispositions may also result in variations in vascular response between subjects, complicating treatment results. For instance, in some patients with rosacea managed with brimonidine, unexpected vasodilation is found due to these receptor function differences, causing erythema worsening after initial improvement. Elucidation of such intricacies not only explains vascular pathophysiology but also helps in the development of specific therapeutic strategies to manage vascular-associated disorders more effectively (Detmar et al., 2016) (Figure 10.11).

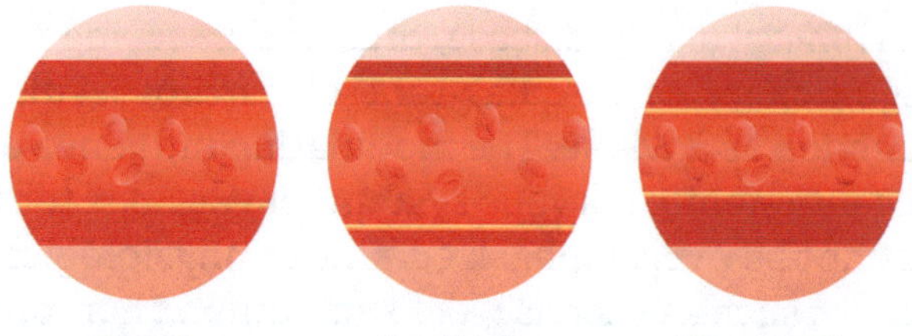

Figure 10.11. Vasodilation and vasoconstriction..

Source: https://external-content.duckduckgo.com/iu/?u=https%3A%2F%2Fstatic.vecteezy.com%2Fsystem%2Fresources%2Fpreviews%2F010%2F978%2F238%2Foriginal%2Fvasodilation-and-vasoconstriction-comparison-of-blood-vessels-vector.jpg&f=1&nofb=1&ipt=6aff5557b3350d32fc0c6ce9578982dfffc5ea1442700d0080ccdace3730f2ce.

10.3.3. Impact of Vascular Resistance on Blood Pressure

The interdependence of vascular resistance and blood pressure is a simple tenet of vascular physiology upon which the foundation of cardiovascular health rests. Vascular resistance, via regulation by blood vessel diameter, has a significant influence on hemodynamic parameters. As resistance increases, either by vasoconstriction or due to alterations in vascular wall structure, the blood pressure also has to rise so that adequate blood flow may be delivered. Such an interaction is consistent with the principles provided by Poiseuilles law, which provides the way in which smaller vessel diameters lead to resistance exponentially multiplied. Understanding this relationship is crucial as persistent elevation of blood pressure due to increased vascular resistance may lead to hypertension and its consequences, including heart disease and stroke. The importance of having appropriate vascular resistance thus provides a basis for therapeutic intervention for blood pressure control in clinical settings. Of perhaps even greater significance is the role of vascular resistance in disease states , such as atherosclerosis and diabetes. In such situations, endothelial dysfunction generally results in abnormal vasodilation and increased vascular resistance and therefore contributes to the effect on systemic blood pressure. The chronic elevation in vascular resistance is also capable of causing structural remodeling of the vasculature that in turn continues to feed back into elevated blood pressure as well as endothelial damage. Various interventions, from diet and lifestyle, pharmacologic therapy, to exercise, have been shown to reverse these abnormalities by improving endothelial function as well as reducing vascular resistance. For instance, regular exercise has been associated with the release of microvesicles that enhance vascular compliance and maintain good blood flow, highlighting a clear connection between vascular function, resistance, and the regulation of blood pressure (Mourot et al., 2018). Finally, understanding vascular resistance and blood pressure is essential to designing effective treatment strategies. The influence of pressure alterations on vascular resistance and consequent blood flow dynamics is best seen in specialized conditions, such as trauma or spinal cord injury, in which characteristics of blood flow can be markedly different from normal. Emerging modeling approaches, like the hybrid model combining ODEs for the blood flow with agent-based models for ulcer formation, reveal the complexities of these interactions in different populations (Solovyev et al., 2013). These new models emphasize overall strategies that consider both pathological and physiological status while addressing vascular resistance and its impact on blood pressure. These results pave the way for personalized clinical interventions, which in turn refine patient outcomes in various cardiovascular diseases.

Test Your Knowledge

1. What is vascular resistance, and how does it affect blood flow?
2. How does vasoconstriction affect vascular resistance and blood pressure?

10.4. Regulation of Blood Pressure

Learning Outcome

1. Identify the neural regulation: function of the autonomic nervous system;
2. Define the hormonal regulation: action of hormones like adrenaline and angiotensin;
3. Describe the local regulation: autoregulation within tissues.

Regulation of blood pressure is a critical topic in vascular physiology, as long as tissues and organs of the body are adequately perfused. Central to all of this are several mechanisms to sensitively regulate cardiac output and vascular resistance. Blood pressure is regulated by the cardiac cycle through its systolic and diastolic portions. During systole, blood is pumped from the heart into the arteries, generating pressure required for perfusion. During diastole, the heart relaxes and allows coronary blood flow that supplies oxygen to cardiac tissue. Such control is not a passive reaction but is directed by hormonal and neural mechanisms that respond to physiological demand, such that changes in blood flow are coordinated with tissue metabolic demand. Local metabolic factors are also of crucial importance in the control of blood pressure through adjustments in vascular tone. Oxygen supply-demand interaction governs this metabolic control such that metabolically active tissues release vasodilators , such as adenosine and nitric oxide. These induce vasodilation, thus lowering vascular resistance and hence lowering blood pressure. Furthermore, the role of the endothelium in regulating these responses cannot be overstressed, as it is one of the key regulators through secreting various signal molecules. The regulation of coronary blood flow shows these principles at work, revealing how metabolic needs influence endothelial function and vascular resistance. As indicated, "these mechanisms collectively modulate coronary vascular resistance" and represent a central aspect of delivering the hearts oxygen requirement without infringing systemic blood pressure (Abid et al., 2017). Circadian rhythm also plays a significant role in blood pressure regulation and demonstrates the complexity of vascular physiology. The kidneys play a central role in this regulation by adapting their function to the bodys circadian pattern. Kidney function involving fluid balance, electrolyte excretion, and hormone secretion varies depending on the time of day and impacts blood pressure fluctuation. For instance, increased sodium sensitivity and variability in autonomic function with changes in the time of day make contributions to these blood pressure level changes. This disruption of these circadian rhythms, or chronodisruption, has been associated with a variety of pathophysiological disorders, such as metabolic diseases and hypertension, thereby suggesting the widespread impact of biological timing on renal and vascular health. Such insight into the genetic and molecular mechanisms underlying such rhythms therefore anticipates new avenues for therapeutic interventions capable of reversing dysregulation of blood pressure and enhancing vascular health (Bonny et al., 2017) (Figure 10.12).

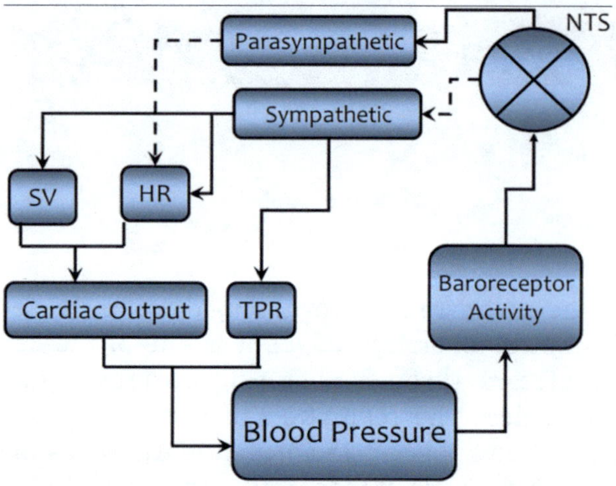

Figure 10.12. Regulation of arterial blood pressure physiology.

Source: https://www.researchgate.net/publication/339825352/figure/fig7/AS:11431281255839465@1719440490240/A-simplified-schematic-representation-of-the-regulation-of-arterial-blood-pressure-as-a.tif.

10.4.1. Neural Regulation: Role of the Autonomic Nervous System (ANS)

The ANS plays a central role in regulating vascular physiology through its dual components: the sympathetic and parasympathetic nervous systems. The sympathetic nervous system is primarily involved with the modulation of the tone of blood vessels, regulating the distribution of blood flow and systemic vascular resistance regulation. By releasing neurotransmitters , such as norepinephrine, the sympathetic division is responsible for vasoconstriction, increasing blood pressure to deal with physiological demands under stress or exercise. The parasympathetic nervous system acts on organs mostly through the action of the vagus nerve, which results in vasodilation and heart slowing. This delicate balance guarantees appropriate blood supply distribution according to the bodys varying demands, thereby placing the ANSs critical function in homeostasis of the vascular system into perspective. The autonomic nervous system and respiration are so integrated that they bring other features of vascular control into perspective. Changes in intrathoracic pressure during the respiratory cycle control venous return and consequently influence stroke volume and cardiac output. This respiration-mediated regulation of vascular dynamics is managed by neural processes implicated with respiration. For instance, inspiration causes minimal hyperpolarization in smooth muscle cells, leading to transient vasodilation, and expiration causes minimal depolarization that can lead to vasoconstriction. Identification of these physiological interactions, as detailed in studies on the Hering–Breuer reflex and respiratory sinus arrhythmia, provides the window to understand how breathing patterns can modulate cardiovascular responses in individual clinical conditions, providing new avenues for therapy. Increased appreciation of these mechanisms strengthens the ANSs involvement in the complicated interaction between vascular physiology and respiration (Jerath et al., 2015). The cardiovascular response to dynamic exercise is a quintessential example of the integrative function of the autonomic nervous system in vascular physiology. The body requires a heightened delivery of oxygen and nutrients to contracting muscles during exercise and thus requires a rapid and coordinated response from the ANS. It involves a withdrawal of parasympathetic tone and co-activation of the sympathetic system, leading to vasodilation of the skeletal muscles and sustaining blood pressure through vasoconstriction of non-vital vascular beds. Central command, baroreflexes, and chemoreflexes operate to ensure cardiovascular outputs are consistent with metabolic demands (Crisafulli et al., 2014). By ensuring optimal perfusion of the essential organs during the process of pressure fluctuation regulation, the ANS proves its pivotal role in the modulation of vascular responses to dynamic exercise physiological demands. These insights of neural regulation can inform cardiovascular wellness strategies, most importantly in the pathophysiology of exercise (Figure 10.13).

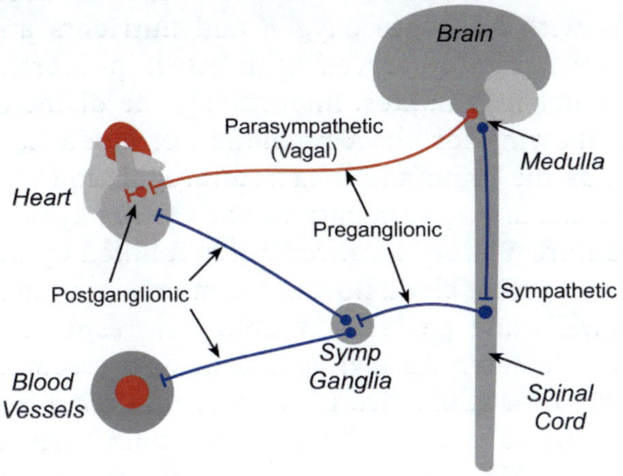

Figure 10.13. Neural regulation: role of the autonomic nervous system (ANS).

Source:

10.4.2. Hormonal Regulation: Influence of Hormones Like Adrenaline and Angiotensin

Hormonal regulation is the cornerstone of vascular physiology and plays an important role in cardiovascular response to stressors , such as hypoxia and circulatory instability. The two main hormones of the regulatory mechanism are adrenaline and angiotensin. Adrenaline secreted by the adrenal medulla in acute stress conditions results in increased heart rate and contractility and promotes augmented cardiac output. It plays a vital role in the sustenance of perfusion pressure and oxygen delivery to tissues during stress. Moreover, adrenaline induces vasodilation in skeletal muscle and vasoconstriction of non-vital vascular beds, reflecting its dual role in distributing blood supply. Modulation of vascular tone by adrenaline highlights the complex interaction between the sympathetic nervous system and endocrine mechanisms that act to keep vascular homeostasis in balance (Haak et al., 1996). Angiotensin, particularly angiotensin II, exerts powerful effects on vascular resistance and blood volume regulation. Being a strong vasoconstrictor, angiotensin II not only leads to arteriole narrowing, which produces increased systemic vascular resistance but also causes the secretion of aldosterone, leading to sodium and water reabsorption by the kidneys to be increased.

This combined action leads to an increase in blood volume and arterial blood pressure, important for the sake of keeping the perfusion adequate during states of decreased blood volume or renal hypoperfusion. The action of angiotensin is particularly important during critical illness or extreme loss of volume, where its action becomes vital to the restoration of hemodynamic stability. Angiotensin's role in pathophysiologic situations, such as acute renal failure, also underscores its role in the vascular response to hormonal stimuli (Gerbes et al., 1991). In a condition of extreme physiological stress, such as in severe physiological emergencies, the interaction between hormones , such as adrenaline and angiotensin takes on a certain importance. In patients with acute hypoxaemic respiratory failure, it has been observed that there is severe systemic modulation of these hormones, reflecting their elevated activity in states of stress (Haak et al., 1996). The above hormonal regulation is accountable for dynamic adjustments of vascular tone, blood flow distribution, and global hemodynamic stability. The ability of the vascular system to cater for varied physiological needs relies on effective hormonal regulation and implies that the underlying control mechanisms are of paramount importance in health as well as disease. The study of the interaction between hormones , such as adrenaline and angiotensin, therefore, enhances the current knowledge of vascular physiology and its implications for clinical practice and therapeutic interventions.

10.4.3. Local Regulation: Autoregulation in Tissues

Regulation of tissue blood flow locally, or autoregulation as it is commonly referred to, is crucial to maintain homeostasis irrespective of systemic circulatory changes. This physiological phenomenon allows tissues to adjust blood supply in response to variations in metabolic demand or local environmental stress in an attempt to supply cells with adequate oxygen and nutrients and facilitate removal of metabolic waste. The mechanism is mainly served by intrinsic properties of the concentration of carbon dioxide, oxygen, and other metabolites. Importantly, the diameter of blood vessels is able to change with high speed, allowing for strict regulation of blood flow, which is important in high-demanding tissues , such as the brain and heart. Autoregulation may differ from organ to organ, reflecting the unique functional requirements of each tissue type in the overall vascular physiology. An essential role in autoregulatory local control is fulfilled by the activity of pericytes in the form of specialized cells that regulate blood flow in the microcirculation. Pericytes are incorporated in capillary and venular walls and possess the ability to respond to several vasoactive stimuli, basically regulating vessel diameter. As highlighted in new research, these responses are not isolated events but are parts of a sophisticated web of autocrine and paracrine signaling involving nearby cells , such as endothelial and tubular epithelial cells. Pericyte function impacts the regulation of medullary blood flow (MBF), with important implications for renal function. Their responsiveness to changes in sodium chloride transport and oxygenation emphasizes their central function in autoregulatory processes within the renal system, emphasizing cellular communication as a fundamental feature of homeostasis (Agmon et al., 2012). In addition, understanding autoregulation goes beyond compartmentalized mechanisms, being founded on broader theoretical models , such as the Guyton model, an influential mathematical model within vascular physiology. This model shows how autoregulation interacts with systemic influences and adapts for physiological stressors like weightlessness in spaceflight. Through the integration of several physiological responses, the Guyton model enables researchers to model vascular responses under different scenarios, and our understanding of fluid and electrolyte regulation is improved as a result. This combined framework emphasizes the relationship between localized regulation within tissues and large-scale circulatory dynamics, demonstrating the complexity of autoregulatory processes in preserving effective organ function throughout varying environments (Leonard et al., 2025) (Figure 10.14).

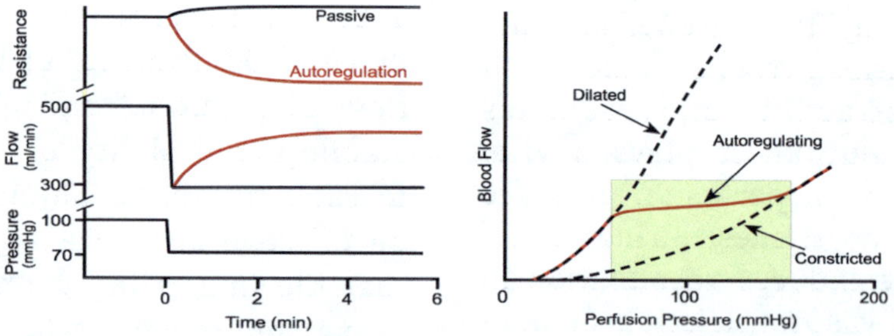

Figure 10.14. Autoregulation of organ blood flow.

Source: https://cvphysiology.com/s9v2f-3r4p7/share/bf004-autoregulation_c1519066067.png.

Test Your Knowledge

1. What role do baroreceptors play in the regulation of stable blood pressure?
2. What is the role of the renin-angiotensin-aldosterone system (RAAS) in regulating blood pressure?

10.5. Vascular Pathophysiology

Learning Outcome

1. Identify the common vascular diseases: hypertension and atherosclerosis;
2. Define the impact of lifestyle factors on vascular disease;
3. Describe the diagnostic methods for vascular disorders.

The study of vascular pathophysiology is significant because it describes how various diseases affect the blood vessels and cardiovascular health in general. Vascular pathophysiology typically consists of diseases , such as hypertension, atherosclerosis, and vascular endothelial dysfunction, all of which are critical to cardiovascular morbidity and mortality. The intricate interaction of vascular biology with systemic factors helps elucidate the way such conditions develop and progress. Atherosclerosis, characterized by the buildup of plaques within arterial walls, disrupts normal blood circulation and facilitates acute cardiovascular events. Hypertension, on the other hand, places excessive stress upon vascular tissues, triggering changes in structural and functional alterations that complicate related disease processes. Through extensive research, the mechanisms by which such conditions emerge can better be understood, thereby pointing toward more effective intervention strategies. Physical exercise has emerged as an essential factor in the prevention and management of vascular pathophysiology. It has been found through studies that regular physical exercise significantly reduces the risk of a series of cardiovascular diseases, including those associated with aging. Exercise, in particular, has been found to exert a beneficial effect on cardiovascular regulation and neuro-hormonal pathways. According to new data, physical activity influences catecholamine release and biosynthesis, exerts a positive action on the renin-angiotensin-aldosterone system, and reduces plasma concentrations of brain natriuretic peptides, all of which are important factors to take into consideration within vascular health. The role of exercise in enhancing endothelial function and the induction of vascular remodeling is particularly relevant in the older adult with increasing age-related chronic diseases. The use of optimal exercise protocols can hence be a foundation for preventing the detrimental effects of vascular pathophysiology in older adults (Allocca et al., 2013). Besides, the interaction of pharmacological therapies for the neuro-hormonal systems with exercise provides a multiple strategy for the treatment of vascular pathophysiology. In elderly individuals, pharmacologic agents that target such systems have been shown to enhance physical function and overall cardiovascular health. This combination strategy, exercise combined with pharmacotherapy, has the capacity not only to heal established disease but to prevent the development of cardiovascular diseases. The intersection of pharmacologic treatments with lifestyle interventions emphasizes the necessity of an integrated strategy in the care of vascular health. With the aging population, recognition and promotion of activities that enhance vascular function remain of primary significance. Upcoming studies must progress knowledge about how exercise and pharmacologic drugs interact synergistically on vascular pathophysiology for optimal patient response (Thierry et al., 2013) (Figure 10.15).

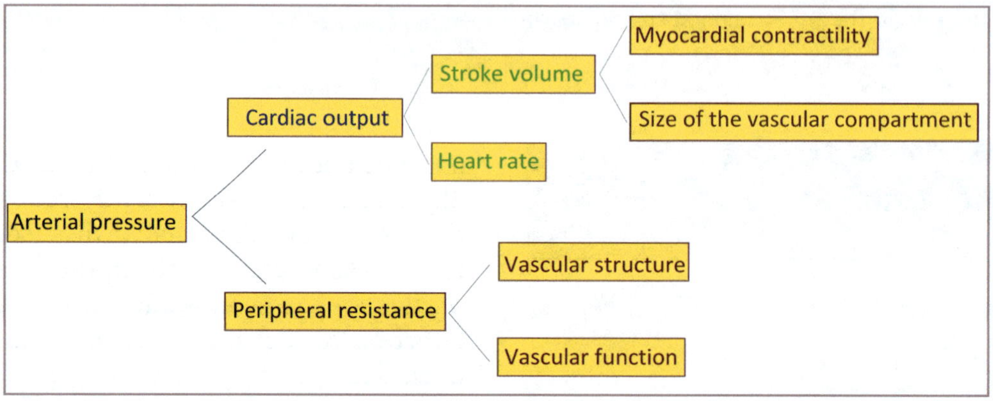

Figure 10.15. Pathophysiology of hypertension

Source: https://upload.wikimedia.org/wikipedia/commons/9/92/Arterial_pressure_diagram.png.

10.5.1. Common Vascular Diseases: Atherosclerosis and Hypertension

Atherosclerosis is the most common vascular disease, characterized by the accumulation of fatty plaques in the arterial wall. Atherosclerosis gradually narrows the arteries and reduces blood and oxygen supply to organs. The disease begins with endothelial injury, often caused by risk factors for hypertension, smoking, and hyperlipidemia. With progressive disease, there occurs chronic inflammation where immune cells emigrate into the arterial wall to phagocytose oxidized lipids. (Pierelli et al., 2017) highlights the role of uncoupling protein 2 (UCP2) in the causation of vascular disease with implications of reduced downregulation of the protein in heightened susceptibility to atherosclerosis and lesion formation. Furthermore, the presence of atherogenic factors can complicate pre-existing conditions like diabetes and obesity, aggravate vascular injuries, and accelerate the process of atherosclerosis itself. Hypertension, or high blood pressure, is another significant causative factor in vascular disease, which often occurs in conjunction with atherosclerosis. This condition can lead to the hardening of arteries as an aftereffect, which in turn promotes the deposition of atherosclerotic plaques and increases cardiovascular events , such as heart attack and stroke. There exists an intricate dynamic interplay of factors between hypertension and vascular health, with arterial stiffness and endothelial dysfunction. New research indicates that perivascular adipose tissue (PVAT) plays a key role in this respect because PVAT dysfunction is associated with inflammatory processes underlying hypertension and other cardiovascular diseases. (Guzik et al., 2017) provides some information on molecular mechanisms that take place in PVAT, where any imbalance of protective adipocyte-derived factors and pro-inflammatory factors disrupts normal vascular function, increasing both hypertension and atherosclerosis risk. Both hypertension and atherosclerosis highlight the importance of initial treatment and lifestyle modification, considering their interrelated status and thus compounded risk of serious cardiovascular complications. The management strategy should include dietary modification, physical exercise, and drug therapy for blood pressure as well as lipid levels. Furthermore, the identification of the pathophysiology behind these vascular diseases, such as the role of UCP2 in atherosclerosis and the inflammatory character of PVAT in hypertension, creates therapeutic possibilities. Considering that vascular health underlies overall welfare, continued study of these mechanisms will be critical to the formation of new treatment paradigms for the prevention of the burden of atherosclerosis and hypertension and, by implication, improving cardiovascular outcomes and patient quality of life (Figure 10.16).

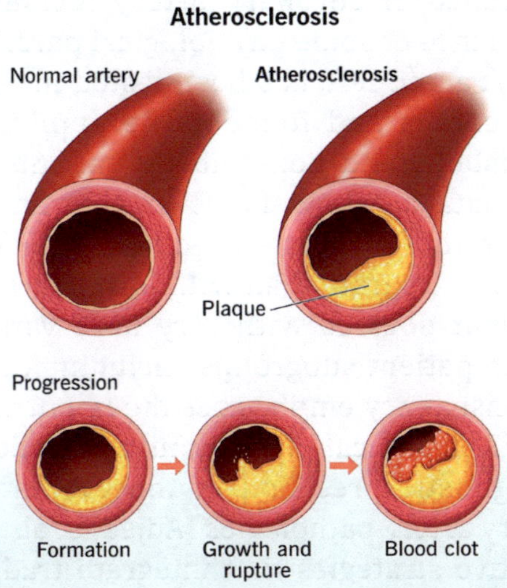

Figure 10.16. Atherosclerosis: Symptoms, causes and treatment.

Source: https://my.clevelandclinic.org/-/scassets/images/org/health/articles/16753-atherosclerosis-illustration?io=transform:fit,width:780.

10.5.2. Impact of Lifestyle Factors on Vascular Health

Lifestyle factors play a very crucial role in the health of the vascular system, having a great impact on the structure and function of blood vessels. Sedentary behavior, consumption of unhealthy foods, and smoking are some of the prime reasons for vascular dysfunction, which lead to atherosclerosis and hypertension. Exercise promotes endothelial health through the improvement of the production of nitric oxide and an increase in vascular permeability. Conversely, a diet rich in saturated fats and sugar not only results in obesity but also provokes inflammatory pathways that can be endothelium-destroying. It is the additive effect that places lifestyle modification at the forefront as a tool for maximizing vascular physiology and, potentially, reversing vascular damage. An analysis of these correlations is essential, as they form the basis for preventive health policies to reduce the incidence of lifestyle-related vascular diseases. Additionally, the interplay between lifestyle and genetic susceptibility must be addressed to better combat vascular health. For instance, while a genetic predisposition towards certain cardiovascular diseases may be hereditary, lifestyle may moderate these risks in significant ways. Studies indicate that regular cardiovascular exercise and a healthy balanced diet can prevent such hereditary risk factors, maintaining healthy vascular function and a reduced risk of developing hypertension or coronary artery disease. Along with this, stress reduction using behavioral interventions like mindfulness and adequate sleep has also been proven to positively impact vascular health by reducing cortisol levels, which otherwise cause endothelial dysfunction. Thus, understanding the dynamic interaction between lifestyle and genetic factors gives a comprehensive picture of vascular integrity, which can lead to individualized prevention. In addition to diet and exercise, psychosocial elements , such as stress and social support networks also play crucial roles in maintaining vascular integrity. Chronic stress is linked with high vascular inflammation and endothelial dysfunction, while supportive relationships promote healthier lifestyle habits and can act as a buffer against stress. Engaging in neighborhood-based health programs can reinforce social networks, leading ultimately to healthier behavior and reduced vascular risk. Moreover, findings emphasize that holistic approaches, such as physical, nutritional, and emotional status, are essential to optimal vascular health. Thus, intervention among lifestyle variables in a holistic framework is beneficial in terms of achieving better interventions that improve resilience for vascular disease and best outcomes for health in multiethnic populations under the scenario of vascular physiology (Figure 10.17).

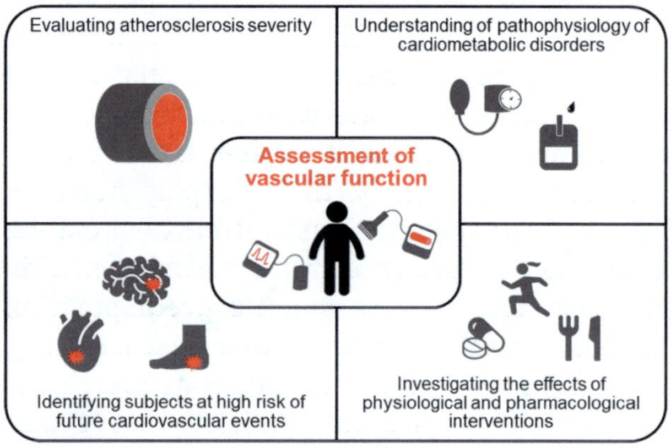

Figure 10.17. Vascular function in hypertension.

Source: https://media.springernature.com/full/springer-static/image/art%3A10.1038%2Fs41440-022-01147-0/MediaObjects/41440_2022_1147_Figa_HTML.png.

10.5.3. Diagnostic Methods for Vascular Conditions

Diagnosis of vascular disease highly depends on progress in a number of diagnostic methods that enable the exact assessment of vascular health. Of them, optical non-invasive techniques have turned out to be useful equipment in practical clinical work for early detection of microcirculatory pathology. These devices utilize laser Doppler flowmetry, absorption spectroscopy, and fluorescence spectroscopy, which are combined with functional tests, to provide full information on peripheral microhaemodynamics. Hybridization of such technologies has demonstrated excellent sensitivity and specificity in revealing alterations in microcirculation, particularly in rheumatic and diabetic patients. Being non-invasive, these optical methods not only enhance diagnostics but also minimize discomfort to patients, paving the way for expanded use in vascular physiology testing (Dremin et al., 2019). Aside from optical means, previous techniques , such as fractional flow reserve (FFR) measurements, continue to have an important role in coronary artery disease diagnosis. Studies have established the usefulness of adenosine-free coronary pressure wire measurements in evaluating the functional significance of coronary artery lesions. The performance of some physiological parameters, like Pd/Pa and iFR, has been tested in a multi-ethnic cohort and found to be applicable in both diabetic and non-diabetic patients. More recent data do show, however, that an all-or-none cutoff of contrast-based FFR (cFFR) is not only more accurate than with lower thresholds but that it does so with very little variability between patient subgroups, including diabetic. This consistency emphasizes the importance of the cFFR in clinical practice, further solidifying its diagnostic precision in the evaluation of coronary artery pathologies (Adjedj et al., 2017). Innovative strategies that integrate traditional and innovative technologies offer a holistic system for diagnosing vascular conditions, unleashing the dynamic nature of vascular physiology. Although established measures provide vital information for the evaluation of coronary health, the introduction of new non-invasive methods adds to the diagnostic potential in different patient populations. With the increasing knowledge of intricate vascular interactions, the diagnostic methods used in their detection will change. It is this intersection of conventional and advanced diagnostic methodologies that holds the key to better precision in vascular evaluation and, by extension, better patient outcomes. Consequently, continuing research and development in diagnostic technology remain imperative in the field of vascular physiology that drives the proficiency of health practitioners in the management of vascular diseases.

Test Your Knowledge

1. What are the primary etiologies of atherosclerosis, and what does it do to arteries?
2. How does hypertension contribute to vascular damage in the long term?

10.6. Therapeutic Approaches in Vascular Health

Learning Outcome

1. Describe the pharmacological treatment of vascular disease;
2. Define and describe lifestyle modification and its impact on vascular health;
3. Describe the surgical interventions: angioplasty and bypass surgery.

The therapeutic strategy environment in vascular health is rapidly evolving, with the utmost priority being given to the treatment of disease conditions involved in vascular dysfunction. At the center of such controversies is the role of UCP2, a mitochondrial protein that has fallen under the spotlight for its antioxidant activities against oxidative injury and vascular damage. The study suggests that UCP2 not only contributes to the regulation of mitochondrial function but also significantly contributes to the predisposition of individuals to numerous vascular diseases, especially in the conditions of obesity, diabetes, and hypertension. Experiments show that silencing the UCP2 gene worsens atherosclerosis and related vascular complications and that the overexpression of UCP2 can alleviate endothelial dysfunction. UCP2 is thus recognized as a pharmacological treatment target candidate, and drugs , such as fenofibrate and sitagliptin were found to be effective in inducing UCP2 expression and thereby providing vascular protection (Pierelli et al., 2017). Another highly innovative area for the enhancement of vascular health is understanding the lymphatic system and its role in lipid transport and immune capacity in the gut. The lymphatic system, previously an underemphasized part, has been recognized to have complex roles in homeostasis and metabolic control. Recent advances in molecular biology have put the workings of intestinal lymphatic function in the limelight, such as regulation of chylomicron entry into lymphatics by various signaling pathways involving vascular endothelial growth factors (VEGFs) and transcription factors. This new finding puts intestinal lymphatics at center stage in processes like metabolic syndrome, with the added possibility of them serving as therapeutic targets in vascular health regulation (Cifarelli et al., 2019). This information can lead to novel strategies aimed at optimizing vascular-related diseases caused by dysregulated lipid metabolism.

Therapeutic agents directed against endothelial function and vascular remodeling have also been of interest to most. The knowledge that endothelial cells play a pivotal role in vascular health induces the development of drugs aimed at enhancing endothelial function. These pharmacologic drugs significantly aim to modulate increasing the supply of nitric oxide, which is crucial for vasorelaxation and control of blood flow overall. Lifestyle modification, alongside pharmacotherapy, is a complementary approach to lowering vascular disease risk. Dietary modification rich in antioxidants and anti-inflammatory compounds supplement drug treatment by targeting root lifestyle causes that promote vascular disease. Both of these therapeutic strategies share a multiple-faceted agenda for vascular health where drug therapies, lifestyle change, and understanding molecular mechanisms are integrated to enhance patient outcomes for prevention and treatment of vascular disease (Figure 10.18).

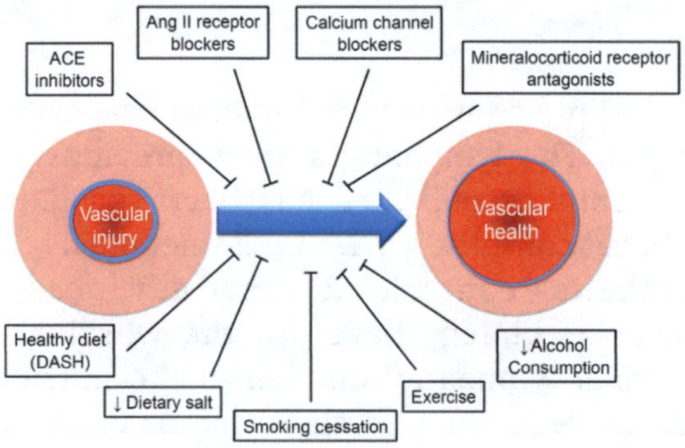

Figure 10.18. Drug treatment of hypertension: focus on vascular health.

Source: https://media.springernature.com/lw685/springer-static/image/art%3A10.1007%2Fs40265-016-0642-8/MediaObjects/40265_2016_642_Fig4_HTML.gif.

10.6.1. Pharmacological Treatments for Vascular Diseases

Pharmacological treatment of vascular disease represents a wide range of therapeutic agents aimed at diminishing the effect of disease on vascular physiology. Among the most widely applied medications are anticoagulants and antiplatelet drugs, which are essential drugs used to prevent thrombotic complications , such as myocardial infarction and stroke. These agents function by inhibiting platelet aggregation and the coagulation cascade, thereby reducing the risk of vascular perfusion and lessening the chances of vascular occlusions. Moreover, the introduction of newer anticoagulants with improved predictable pharmacokinetics and reduced monitoring requirements has reformed treatment in atrial fibrillation and venous thromboembolism patients. With improved patient compliance and outcomes, these advances in pharmacotherapy directly address the challenges posed by vascular health, supporting the vital link between drug and vascular physiology. In addition to antiplatelet and anticoagulant drugs, lipid-lowering drugs, particularly statins, are central to the pharmacological management of vascular disease. Statins competitively inhibit the enzyme HMG-CoA reductase, a key enzyme of cholesterol synthesis, and subsequently decrease the blood levels of low-density lipoprotein (LDL) cholesterol. This not only forestalls the progression of atherosclerosis but also has many pleiotropic actions, among which are improving endothelial function and affecting markers of inflammation. These pleiotropic effects attest to the role of statins beyond cholesterol reduction. Besides, with the increase in population age globally, control of cholesterol as a causative factor in the prevention of age-related vascular disease becomes more and more crucial, bearing in mind that aging and cardiovascular diseases like atherosclerosis and heart failure are interconnected (Cavarretta et al., 2017). Other interventions involving drugs target underlying mechanisms of vascular disease, such as hypertension, which is a significant risk factor for most cardiovascular events. Anti-hypertensive therapy, including angiotensin-converting enzyme (ACE) inhibitors and calcium channel blockers, not only facilitates the control of blood pressure but also plays a role in vascular remodeling and anti-arterial stiffness. The efficacy of these medications in promoting vascular compliance and endothelial function is well documented and reflects their central role in the comprehensive management of vascular disease. Furthermore, combination treatments using several drug classes can accomplish improved outcomes by addressing the nature of hypertension and its effects on vascular physiology. All these drug treatments are crucial in preparing therapeutic options for the treatment of patients with vascular disease, enabling an active style of approaching the role of aging and associated cardiovascular pathologies (Thierry et al., 2013) (Figure 10.19).

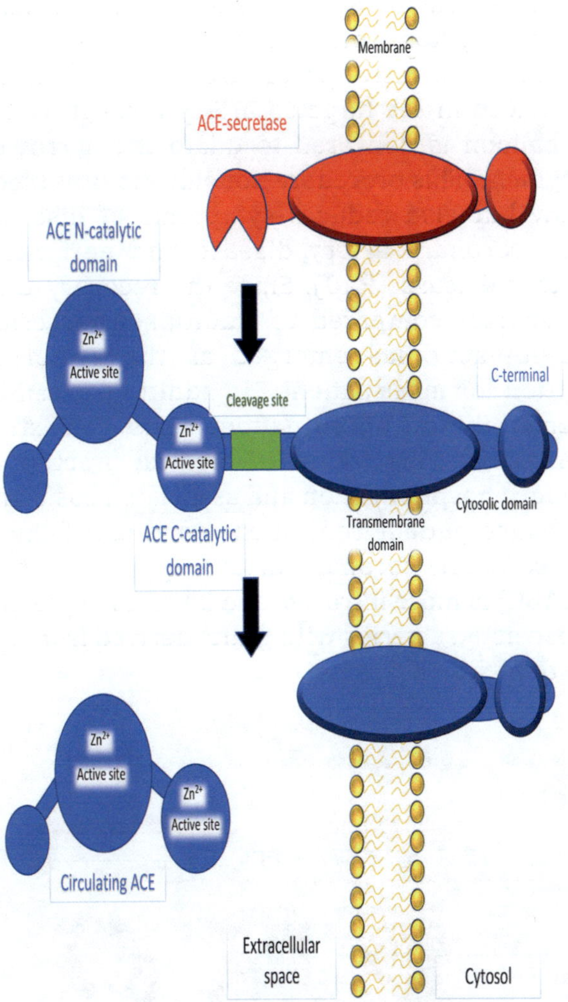

Figure 10.19. Two opposing functions of angiotensin-converting enzyme (ACE) that link hypertension, dementia, and aging.

Source: Le D, Brown L, Malik K, Murakami S. Two Opposing Functions of Angiotensin-Converting Enzyme (ACE) That Links Hypertension, Dementia, and Aging. International Journal of Molecular Sciences. 2021; 22(24):13178. https://doi.org/10.3390/ijms222413178

10.6.2. Lifestyle Modifications and Their Effects on Vascular Health

Lifestyle change plays a key role in enhancing vascular health, impacting a number of factors that are responsible for overall cardiovascular function. One of the key changes individuals can implement involves dietary change. A heart-healthy diet of high levels of fruits, vegetables, whole grains, and lean meats can reduce blood pressure, lower cholesterol, and improve blood vessel function. The evidence suggests that these diets, such as the Mediterranean diet, rich in healthy fats, especially those found in olive oil and nuts, have reduced the risk of vascular disease dramatically. Furthermore, reduced sodium intake has been advocated as a way to aid in the management of hypertension, which is a key risk factor for vascular health. When consumed together, these dietary modifications can create a setting that enhances healthier endothelial function and vascular reactivity, thereby minimizing risks of atherosclerosis and other cardiovascular conditions. In conjunction with diet, physical exercise is also imperative to a person's vascular well-being. Moderate aerobic exercise, such as walking, cycling, or swimming, has been shown to strengthen the heart and the circulation of blood, for instance. Vasodilation is promoted by frequent exercise so that increased blood supply is facilitated without increased blood pressure in the vessels. Physical exercise also keeps weight, reduces stress, and adjusts blood lipid profiles, and all these combined contribute to lowering cardiovascular risk. Studies confirm that even short bursts of exercise can yield profound enhancements in vascular function, and the importance of incorporating motion into ordinary daily activities cannot be overstated. Overall, compliance with habitual physical exercise not only improves vascular efficiency but serves as a protective modality against degenerative conditions , such as chronic kidney disease, which is linked to vascular complications (Ekström et al., 2017). Apart from diet and physical exercise, lifestyle modifications encompass management of stress levels, smoking status, and sleep habits. Stress has been implicated in exerting a negative influence on the vascular system in terms of inflammation and endothelial dysfunction, thus predisposing to vascular disease. Interventions , such as mindfulness, yoga, and meditation can attenuate such stress levels and lead to significant improvement in overall vascular function. Smoking, also an established risk factor for cardiovascular disease, adds numerous toxins to the body that degrade endothelial function and enhance atherosclerosis. Abstinence from smoking can reverse some of these negative effects, enhancing vascular hardness. Furthermore, quality, sufficient sleep is also essential to allow optimal vascular function; sleep loss is linked to dysregulated cardiovascular responses. Cumulatively, these lifestyle changes induce an overall plan of vascular health, blending several physiological systems to greater outcomes (Blamire et al., 2014).

10.6.3. Surgical Interventions: Angioplasty and Bypass Surgery

Surgical interventions , such as angioplasty and bypass surgery play a significant role in the management of vascular disease, particularly that of artery blockages. Angioplasty is a minimally invasive procedure where a catheter is placed in the targeted artery through which a balloon is delivered to dilate the narrowed segment. This procedure not only restores blood flow but also reduces symptoms of diseases like coronary artery disease and peripheral artery disease (PAD). Since the recovery time is shorter compared to traditional surgeries, angioplasty has emerged as the preferred option for most patients. In addition, it can be performed on an outpatient basis, consistent with prevailing trends in medical practice to reduce hospitalization and associated costs and enhance patient convenience and satisfaction. In contrast, coronary artery bypass grafting (CABG) is more intrusive and involves bypassing obstructed arteries with grafts derived from the patient's own tissue.

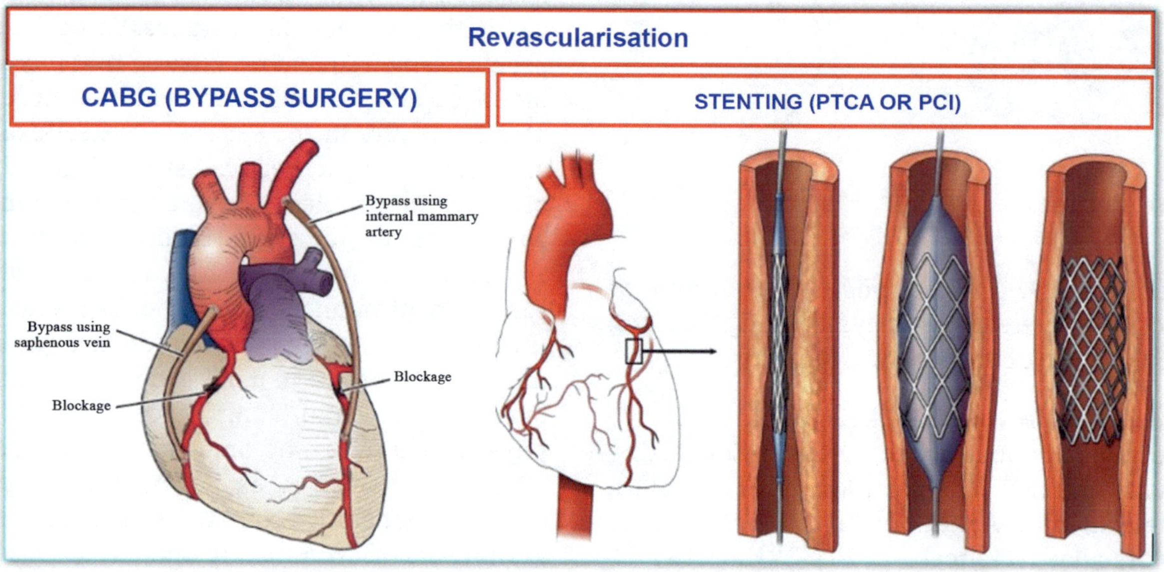

Figure 10.20. Bypass surgery versus angioplasty.

Source: https://www.cardiacwellnessinstitute.com/heart-disease-treatment-prevention/wp-content/uploads/2020/10/PTCA-BYPASS.jpg.

This operation is particularly valuable in the case of severe coronary artery disease, where multiple arteries are occluded. CABG will significantly increase blood flow to the heart muscle, thereby eradicating ischemic symptoms, reducing the potential for heart attack, and enhancing cardiovascular status. But this surgery is longer to recover from and risks complications more than with angioplasty. The choice between the two treatments generally depends on the patient's specific state, extent of arterial obstructions, and overall health profile, therefore necessitating a tailored approach to clinical practice. Current evidence indicates that both surgical methods can lead to significant improvements in exercise tolerance and hemodynamic adaptation in PAD patients. Specifically, revascularization therapies like angioplasty have been demonstrated to reduce the hyperkinetic blood pressure response to exercise, as observed in studies that report an improvement in skeletal muscle oxygen desaturation following these therapies. Those who underwent surgery not only experienced increased oxygen delivery to peripheral vasculature but also a significant decrease in mean arterial blood pressure during exercise (Luck et al., 2019). Also, since surgical procedures address the anatomical locations of occlusive disease, complementary lifestyle modifications, i.e., a plant-based diet, are mentioned as adjunct treatments for optimal cardiovascular health (Dignan et al., 2016). This multi-modality approach emphasizes the importance of integrating surgical interventions with overall health programs to enhance patient outcomes (Figure 10.20).

Test Your Knowledge

1. How do antihypertensive drugs contribute to the management of vascular disease?
2. What is the role of lifestyle modification in the promotion of vascular health?

SUMMARY

In vascular physiology as a field of study, one must recognize the dynamic interface between neural activity and blood flow regulation, particularly through the mechanisms of neurovascular coupling. As stressed, the assumption that heightened regional blood flow is coupled with heightened neural activity underscores the significance of being familiar with this interface. The pericyte function of regulating capillary diameter is a nuanced perspective of the neurovascular interaction, which postulates that blood flow regulation does not occur merely at the level of arterioles but also at the level of capillaries. Such an understanding is critical in the interpretation of findings from functional imaging investigations, especially in pathological conditions , such as ischemic stroke, where changes in neurovascular regulation lead to misattribution of underlying neural activity (Attwell et al., 2010). Additionally, the role of vascular smooth muscle dynamics in overall vascular physiology cannot be overemphasized. The pathophysiology of hypertension is a prime example of how sophisticated regulatory mechanisms can influence vascular reactivity and tone. Enhanced vascular resistance, which is caused by pathophysiological alterations in vascular smooth muscle cells, underscores the sophistication of blood pressure regulation. The convergence of several signaling pathways, such as the RhoA-Rho kinase and immune-mediated pathways, is the multiform character of vascular function and sensitivity to internal and external stress. Addressing these matters is important as we look for therapeutic avenues in chronic illness like hypertension because such conditions have wider implications for disease and health management (Alves-Lopes et al., 2018). Lastly, the significance of vascular physiology is not limited to the realm of basic science and transcends its clinical significance. Both dysfunction in neurovascular regulation and vascular smooth muscle signaling lead to a host of cardiovascular diseases, which is the testament to the importance of such information in developing proper treatment strategies. As research continues to advance, it will be essential to incorporate information from both vascular reactivity and neurovascular coupling to address conditions , such as vascular dementia and heart failure. Ultimately, a sophisticated comprehension of vascular physiology not only shines light on the underlying biology but also gives researchers and clinicians the tools to tackle the growing burden of related disease. The pursuit of novel therapies founded on such knowledge will be critical to furthering patient management and improving health in the decades ahead.

Vascular physiology is a multifaceted field that examines blood vessel function and structure, yielding vital information regarding the maintenance of hemodynamics and cardiovascular integrity. A fundamental aspect of vascular physiology is the understanding of mechanisms that regulate vascular tone. Mechanism involves several factors, like endothelial-derived signaling molecules like nitric oxide that play a vital role in vasodilation. These mechanisms are essential to regulate blood flow according to the demands of different organs and tissues. Furthermore, the particular cellular anatomy of arteries, veins, and capillaries ensures that blood flow is regulated in the correct manner, facilitating the delivery of nutrients and clearance of waste through the mechanism of an efficient integrated system of contraction and relaxation within vascular smooth muscle. Furthermore, specialized receptors and ion channels contribute significantly to the vascular responsiveness. Of these, P2X receptors (P2XR) are unique in vascular function, particularly in the kidney. Previous work has been primarily centered on P2X1R and its role in the autoregulation of renal blood flow. Recent research now suggests, though, that P2XR might have more generalized functions within the renal system and vascular system, influencing both health and illness. Activation and regulation of these receptors are key to maintaining balance in vascular responses, as they ensure the promotion of physiological responses to various stimuli. This refers to the complexity and interrelatedness of vascular physiology, where many regulatory pathways interact to maintain homeostasis of the cardiovascular system (Birch et al., 2013). In addition to overall vascular reactions, the impact of physical exercises like marathon running on vascular physiology reflects the influence of exercise on cardiovascular remodeling. Experiments have validated that novice marathon runners exhibit an eccentric remodeling of the heart, with increased ventricular cavity dimensions and reductions in blood pressure. These alterations highlight physiological mechanisms to enhance cardiac output and overall vascular efficiency. Despite the limited increase in peak oxygen uptake in this group, certain significant health benefits , such as reduced arterial stiffness, were recorded. These results form the foundation for an even deeper insight into how long-term physical activity can induce beneficial alterations in the vessels and the augmentation of the elaborate relationship between cardiovascular physiology and environmental determinants (D'Silva et al., 2020).

KEY TERMS FROM THIS CHAPTER

- Arteries
- Blood Pressure
- Capillary Exchange
- Hydrostatic Pressure
- Osmotic Pressure
- Pulse Pressure
- Tunica Intima
- Vascular Compliance
- Vasoconstriction
- Baroreceptors
- Capillaries
- Endothelium
- Mean Arterial Pressure (MAP)
- Peripheral Resistance
- Tunica Externa
- Tunica Media
- Vascular Resistance
- Vasodilation

CRITICAL THINKING QUESTIONS

1. **Which of the following blood vessels have the highest blood pressure?**
   a. Capillaries
   b. Veins
   c. Venules
   d. Arteries
2. **Which type of vessel is primarily responsible for creating peripheral resistance?**
   a. Arteries
   b. Capillaries
   c. Arterioles
   d. Veins
3. **Which of the following layer of blood vessels contains smooth muscle?**
   a. Tunica intima
   b. Tunica media
   c. Tunica externa
   d. Endothelium
4. **What is the main function of the capillaries?**
   a. Pump blood
   b. Transport hormones
   c. Exchange gases and nutrients
   d. Store blood
5. **Baroreceptors that regulate blood pressure are primarily located in the:**
   a. Renal arteries
   b. Coronary arteries
   c. Aortic arch and carotid sinus
   d. Pulmonary veins

Short Answer Questions

1. Name the three layers of a typical blood vessel wall.
2. Which vessel has the thickest smooth muscle layer?
3. What is the role of the endothelium within the blood vessel?
4. Define systolic and diastolic pressure.
5. Explain the structure and function of the artery, vein, and capillary.
6. Explain the regulation mechanisms of blood pressure.
7. Explain the role of the autonomic nervous system in vascular tone.
8. Compare and contrast pulmonary and systemic circulation in terms of pressure and resistance.

Answers to Critical Thinking Questions

1. (d); 2. (c); 3. (b); 4. (c); 5. (c)

REFERENCES

1. Abid, A., Afonso, M., Ahmed, S., Alexander, G., Algranati, D., Altman, D., et al. (2017). Regulation of coronary blood flow. https://core.ac.uk/download/161627447.pdf (accessed on 16th June 2025).
2. Adjedj, J., Barbato, E., Esposito, G., Fearon, W. F., et al. (2017). Diabetes does not impact the diagnostic performance of contrast-based fractional flow reserve: Insights from the CONTRAST study. https://core.ac.uk/download/80696880.pdf (accessed on 16th June 2025).
3. D'Silva, A., Bhuva, A. N., van Zalen, J., Bastiaenen, R., Abdel-Gadir, A., Jones, S., Nadarajan, N., Menacho Medina, K. D., Ye, Y., Augusto, J., Treibel, T. A., Rosmini, S., Ramlall, M., Scully, P. R., Torlasco, C., Willis, J., Finocchiaro, G., Papatheodorou, E., Dhutia, H., Cole, D., ... Sharma, S. (2020). Cardiovascular Remodeling Experienced by Real-World, Unsupervised, Young Novice Marathon Runners. *Frontiers in physiology*, *11*, 232. https://doi.org/10.3389/fphys.2020.00232(accessed on 16th June 2025).
4. Agmon, Y., Beach, R. E., Biondi, M., Burnstock, G., Casellas, D., Cohen, H. J., Edwards, R. M., et al. (2012). Renal pericytes: Regulators of medullary blood flow. https://core.ac.uk/download/30712009.pdf (accessed on 16th June 2025).
5. Ahmadian, N., Akiyama, T., Areosa, S., Attems, J., Babcock, D., Bailey, K., Baker, M., et al. (2019). A novel model of mixed vascular dementia incorporating hypertension in a rat model of Alzheimer's disease. https://core.ac.uk/download/323077251.pdf (accessed on 16th June 2025).
6. Alexander, D., Bergel, A., Boas, D. A., Burnham, B., Buxton, R., Deneux, T., et al. (2009). A time-invariant Visco-elastic wind Kessel model relating blood flow and blood volume. https://core.ac.uk/download/50544.pdf (accessed on 16th June 2025).
7. Allocca, E., Bonaduce, D., D'Amico, L., De Lucia, C., et al. (2013). Neuro-hormonal effects of physical activity in the elderly. https://core.ac.uk/download/76991216.pdf (accessed on 16th June 2025).
8. Alves-Lopes, R., Anagnostopoulou, A., Arner, A., De Lucca Camargo, L., et al. (2018). Vascular smooth muscle contraction in hypertension. https://core.ac.uk/download/150600176.pdf (accessed on 16th June 2025).
9. Attwell, D., Hall, C. N., & Hamilton, N. B. (2010). Pericyte-mediated regulation of capillary diameter: A component of neurovascular coupling in health and disease. https://core.ac.uk/download/1688588.pdf (accessed on 16th June 2025).
10. Jerath, R., Crawford, M. W., Barnes, V. A., & Harden, K. (2015). Widespread depolarization during expiration: a source of respiratory drive?. *Medical hypotheses*, *84*(1), 31–37. https://doi.org/10.1016/j.mehy.2014.11.010Bertolini, E., Buckley, H., Carlhoff, S., Feldman, M., et al. (2022). Female bone physiology resilience in a past Polynesian Outlier community. https://core.ac.uk/download/544385243.pdf (accessed on 16th June 2025).
11. Bertolini, E., Buckley, H., Carlhoff, S., Feldman, M., et al. (2022). Female bone physiology resilience in 750–300 BP 'Polynesian Outlier' community. https://core.ac.uk/download/516201971.pdf (accessed on 16th June 2025).
12. Bich, L., Moreau, J. F., & Pradeu, T. (2019). Understanding multicellularity: The functional organization of the intercellular space. https://core.ac.uk/download/228134961.pdf (accessed on 16th June 2025).

13. Birch, R. E., Peppiatt-Wildman, C. M., Schwiebert, E. M., Wildman, S. S., et al. (2013). Emerging key roles for P2X receptors in the kidney. https://core.ac.uk/download/30711999.pdf (accessed on 16th June 2025).

14. Blamire, A. M., Ford, G. A., Hallsworth, K., He, J., et al. (2014). Effects of community exercise therapy on metabolic, brain, physical, and cognitive function following stroke: A randomized controlled pilot trial. https://core.ac.uk/download/42130503.pdf (accessed on 16th June 2025).

15. Bonny, O., Gumz, M. L., Mazzoccoli, G., Vinciguerra, M., et al. (2017). Molecular bases of circadian rhythmicity in renal physiology and pathology. https://core.ac.uk/download/85210329.pdf (accessed on 16th June 2025).

16. Calhoun, V. D., Colenbier, N., Marinazzo, D., Poldrack, R. A., et al. (2019). Disambiguating the role of blood flow and global signal with partial information decomposition. https://core.ac.uk/download/287942331.pdf (accessed on 16th June 2025).

17. Casteleyn, C., Cornillie, P., Debbaut, C., Dierick, M., et al. (2014). Analyzing the human liver vascular architecture by combining vascular corrosion casting and micro-CT scanning: A feasibility study. https://core.ac.uk/download/55806749.pdf (accessed on 16th June 2025).

18. Cavarretta, E., Dal Sasso, E., Forte, M., Frati, G., et al. (2017). The light and shadow of senescence and inflammation in cardiovascular pathology and regenerative medicine. https://core.ac.uk/download/141694265.pdf (accessed on 16th June 2025).

19. Harwood, A. E., Cayton, T., Sarvanandan, R., Lane, R., & Chetter, I. (2016). A Review of the Potential Local Mechanisms by Which Exercise Improves Functional Outcomes in Intermittent Claudication. *Annals of vascular surgery*, *30*, 312–320. https://doi.org/10.1016/j.avsg.2015.05.043 (accessed on 16th June 2025).

20. Cifarelli, V., & Eichmann, A. (2019). The intestinal lymphatic system: Functions and metabolic implications. https://core.ac.uk/download/212868551.pdf (accessed on 16th June 2025).

21. Crisafulli, A., Marongiu, E., Nobrega, A. C. L., O'Leary, D. S., et al. (2014). Neural regulation of cardiovascular response to exercise: Role of central command and peripheral afferents. https://core.ac.uk/download/pdf/54599119.pdf (accessed on 16th June 2025).

22. Detmar, M., Di Nardo, A., Docherty, J. R., Holmes, C., et al. (2016). Multidisciplinary consideration of potential pathophysiologic mechanisms of paradoxical erythema with topical brimonidine therapy. https://core.ac.uk/download/323064570.pdf (accessed on 16th June 2025).

23. Mario Valentino, Christian Zammit, Giuseppe Di Giovanni, Massimo Pierucci, R. Muscat. Two-photon microscopy- sequential imaging studies in vivo. Malta Medical Journal Volume 23 Issue 03 2011(accessed on 16th June 2025).

24. Elizabeth L. Hess, Janice Wallace-Robinson, Katherine J. Dickson, and Janet V. Powers The George Washington University Washington, D.C (1992). NASA Contractor Report 4468*Publications of the Space Physiology and Countermeasures Program, Regulatory Physiology Discipline: 1980–1990.* Prepared for NASA Office of Space Science and Applications under Contract NASW-432(accessed on 16th June 2025).

25. Dignan, C. J. (2016). *The Benefits of a Plant-Based Diet for The Prevention and Treatment of Heart Disease.* https://open.bu.edu/bitstream/2144/14685/1/Dignan_bu_0017N_10517.pdf (accessed on 16th June 2025).

26. Zherebtsova AI, Dremin VV, Makovik IN, Zherebtsov EA, Dunaev AV, Goltsov A, Sokolovski SG and Rafailov EU (2019) Multimodal Optical Diagnostics of the Microhaemodynamics in Upper and Lower Limbs. Front. Physiol. 10:416. doi: 10.3389/fphys.2019.00416(accessed on 16th June 2025).

27. Drinkhill, M. J., Hainsworth, R., & Wright, C. I. (2001). Responses to stimulation of coronary and carotid baroreceptors and the coronary chemoreflex at different ventricular distending pressures in anaesthetized dogs. https://core.ac.uk/download/57453.pdf (accessed on 16th June 2025).

28. Drinkhill, M. J., Hainsworth, R., McMahon, N. C., Myers, D., et al. (2000). Absence of reflex vascular responses from the intrapulmonary circulation in anaesthetized dogs. https://core.ac.uk/download/57443.pdf (accessed on 16th June 2025).

29. Drinkhill, M. J., Hainsworth, R., Myers, D. S., Noble, M., et al. (1998). Blood mobilization from the liver of the anaesthetized dog. https://core.ac.uk/download/57450.pdf (accessed on 16th June 2025).

30. Ekström, T. J., Nordfors, L., Shiels, P. G., Stenvinkel, P., et al. (2017). Current epigenetic aspects the clinical kidney researcher should embrace. https://core.ac.uk/download/84340482.pdf (accessed on 16th June 2025).

31. Fang, L., Haft-Javaherian, M., Muse, V., Nishimura, N., et al. (2019). Deep convolutional neural networks for segmenting 3D *in vivo* multiphoton images of vasculature in Alzheimer disease mouse models. http://arxiv.org/abs/1801.00880 (accessed on 16th June 2025).

32. Pierelli, G., Stanzione, R., Forte, M., Migliarino, S., Perelli, M., Volpe, M., & Rubattu, S. (2017). Uncoupling Protein 2: A Key Player and a Potential Therapeutic Target in Vascular Diseases. *Oxidative medicine and cellular longevity, 2017*, 7348372. https://doi.org/10.1155/2017/7348372(accessed on 16th June 2025).

33. Gerbes, A. L., Laggner, A., Arendt, C., Barratt-Boyes, G., Barry, M., Bauch, C., Brenner, T., et al. (1991). Ornipressin in the treatment of functional renal failure in decompensated liver cirrhosis. https://core.ac.uk/download/12166774.pdf (accessed on 16th June 2025).

34. Guzik, T. J., & Nosalski, R. (2017). Perivascular adipose tissue inflammation in vascular disease. https://core.ac.uk/download/77600990.pdf (accessed on 16th June 2025).

35. Haak, T., Jungmann, E., Kullmer, T., Meier-Sydow, J., et al. (1996). Hormonal modifications in patients admitted to an internal intensive care unit for acute hypoxemic respiratory failure. https://core.ac.uk/download/pdf/82065854.pdf (accessed on 16th June 2025).

36. Hills, G., Kuppusamy, H., Naing, P., Playford, D., et al. (2017). Non-invasive assessment of pulmonary vascular resistance in pulmonary hypertension: Current knowledge and future direction. https://core.ac.uk/download/213607322.pdf (accessed on 16th June 2025).

37. Holt, A. W., & Tulis, D. A. (2015). Vascular smooth muscle as a therapeutic target in disease pathology. https://core.ac.uk/download/322425090.pdf (accessed on 16th June 2025).

38. Kim, S. R., Lee, S. K., Jang, S. H., Choi, Y., et al. (2011). Expression of keratin 10 in rat organ surface primo-vascular tissues. https://core.ac.uk/download/pdf/82044703.pdf (accessed on 16th June 2025).

39. Kuchar, N. R. (2025). *Fluid Dynamics in Flexible Tubes: An Application to The Study of The Pulmonary Circulation*. https://core.ac.uk/download/pdf/85232914.pdf (accessed on 16th June 2025).

40. Lakin, W. D., Penar, P. L., Stevens, S. A., Tranmer, B. I., et al. (2007). Whole-body mathematical model for simulating intracranial pressure dynamics. https://core.ac.uk/download/pdf/10542011.pdf (accessed on 16th June 2025).

41. Leonard, J. I. (2025). *Description, Validation, And Modification of The Guyton Model for Space-Flight Applications. Part A. Guyton Model of Circulatory, Fluid and Electrolyte Control. Part B. Modification of the Guyton Model for Circulatory, Fluid and Electrolyte Control.* https://core.ac.uk/download/pdf/42845535.pdf (accessed on 16th June 2025).

42. Luck, J. C. (2019). *Effects of Peripheral Revascularization on Blood Pressure and Calf Muscle Oxygen Saturation in Peripheral Artery Disease.* https://core.ac.uk/download/345088588.pdf (accessed on 16th June 2025).

43. Machado, R. (2012). *The Molecular Genetics and Cellular Mechanisms Underlying Pulmonary Arterial Hypertension.* https://core.ac.uk/download/20320889.pdf (accessed on 16th June 2025).

44. Man, A. W. C., & Wang, Y. (2017). Age-associated arterial remodeling and cardiovascular diseases. https://core.ac.uk/download/84930825.pdf (accessed on 16th June 2025).

45. Mauroy, B., & Moreau, B. (2014). Functional optimization of the arterial network. http://arxiv.org/abs/1405.1281 (accessed on 16th June 2025).

46. Mauroy, B., & Moreau, B. (2015). Murray's law revisited: Quémada's fluid model and fractal trees. https://core.ac.uk/download/47087169.pdf (accessed on 16th June 2025).

47. Moskalenko, Y. Y. (2025). *Functional Stability of Cerebral Circulatory System.* https://core.ac.uk/download/pdf/42860883.pdf (accessed on 16th June 2025).

48. Mourot, L., Rakobowchuk, M., & Wilhelm, E. N. (2018). Exercise-derived macrovesicles: A review of the literature. https://core.ac.uk/download/288430488.pdf (accessed on 16th June 2025).

49. San, O., & Staples, A. E. (2012). An improved model for reduced-order physiological fluid flows. http://arxiv.org/abs/1212.0188 (accessed on 16th June 2025).

50. Solovyev, A., Mi, Q., Tzen, Y. T., Brienza, D., & Vodovotz, Y. (2013). Hybrid equation/agent-based model of ischemia-induced hyperemia and pressure ulcer formation predicts greater propensity to ulcerate in subjects with spinal cord injury. *PLoS computational biology*, *9*(5), e1003070. https://doi.org/10.1371/journal.pcbi.1003070(accessed on 16th June 2025).

PULMONARY PHYSIOLOGY

11

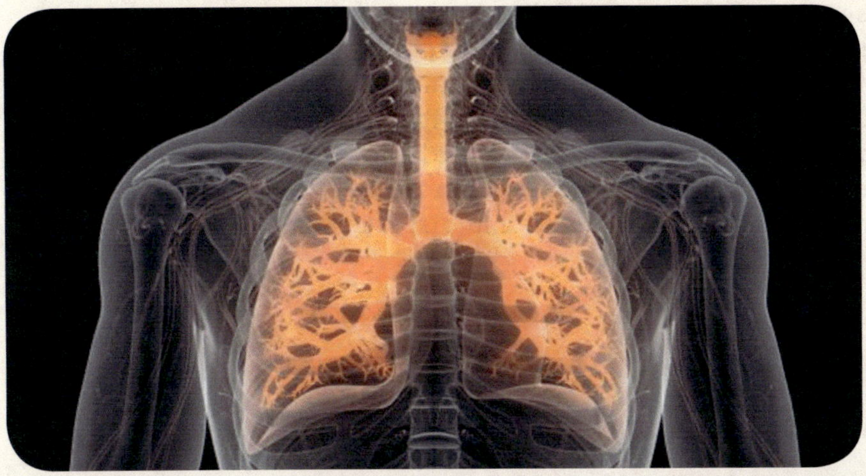

LEARNING OBJECTIVES

After studying this chapter, you will be able to:

1. Describe the respiratory system anatomy;
2. Discuss breathing mechanisms;
3. Describe gas exchange and transport;
4. Emphasize regulation of breathing for pulmonary physiology;
5. Learn pulmonary function tests;
6. Evaluate common pulmonary disorders.

Introduction

A study of pulmonary physiology is a prerequisite to a comprehension of the mechanics of respiration and gas exchange in the human body. Pulmonary physiology looks at how oxygen and carbon dioxide are exchanged through the lungs, essential for upholding homeostasis. Essential elements involve the respiratory system's anatomy, ventilation's mechanics, and the function of alveoli in gas exchange. The respiratory system consists of conducting airways, lungs, and pleura, each playing a vital role in respiration. The tracheobronchial tree, for example, is responsible for conducting air, whereas the alveoli, tiny air sacs within the lungs, facilitate gas exchange. Understanding these components is important to illustrate how respiratory disease can destabilize this tenuous balance and result in physiological complications. Ventilation is a significant pulmonary physiology process involving the passage of air in and out of the lungs. Air movement is reliant on the cooperative effort of the diaphragm and intercostal muscles responsible for inspiration and expiration. The mechanical process of ventilation relies on the law of pressure gradients governing the dynamics of air flow. When the person inhales, the diaphragm relaxes to increase the volume of the thorax and decrease the intrapulmonary pressure, thereby allowing air to fill the lungs. Exhalation is caused by the passive recoil of lung tissue. Moreover, understanding the finer details of ventilation can provide useful insight into important clinical implications since obstructive and restrictive lung diseases have serious effects on airflow and functional efficiency of gas exchange, and consequently emphasize the importance of precise test methods in research and clinical practice. CPET is a valuable tool in assessing functional pulmonary system capacity, particularly among patients with chronic pulmonary disease. Standardization of CPET protocols has optimized the efficacy of interpretation of results, guiding clinical decisions and research. Systematic literature reviews provide evidence for optimum testing parameters, with emphasis on a strict design involving a resting time, unloaded time, and increasing exercise time, with a subsequent recovery. CPET has been noted to impact patients greatly, demonstrating its usefulness in improving diagnostic testing and treatment planning. These developments highlight the contribution of patient input to the evaluation process, underscoring the interdisciplinary nature of research in pulmonary physiology and its translation into ensuring individualized patient care (Diller et al., 2009; Radtke et al., 2019). Understanding these protocols provides the framework for evaluating respiratory function across a variety of clinical scenarios, confirming the contribution of pulmonary physiology to health and disease (Figure 11.1).

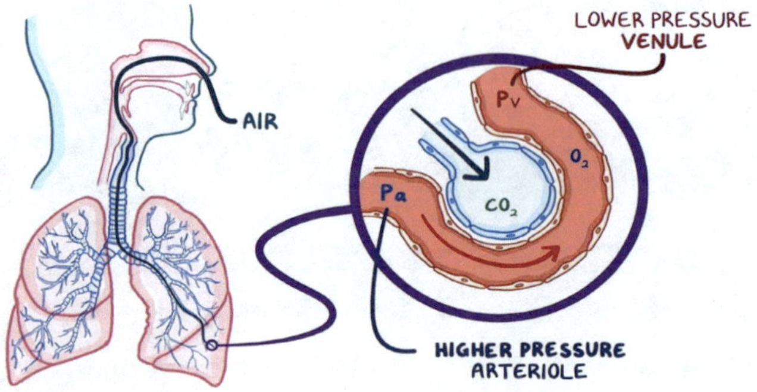

Figure 11.1. Pulmonary blood flow.

Source: https://www.osmosis.org/_next/image?url=https%3A%2F%2Fd16qt3wv6xm098.cloudfront.net%2Fro1Y0KtOTsGsy17lSyP86o6cQhewmdKT%2F_.jpg&w=3840&q=75.

Definition and Importance of Pulmonary Physiology

Pulmonary physiology is a critical discipline of medicine concerning the physiology of the breathing apparatus, or more precisely, the mechanics of breathing as well as gas exchange. It encompasses a number of processes, including ventilation, diffusion, and perfusion, which together make possible the crucial transfer of oxygen and carbon dioxide from the alveoli of the lung to the bloodstream. Understanding these physiological processes is critical not just for diagnosis and the management of respiratory disease but also for comprehending how external influences and lifestyle contribute to respiratory disease. Without first having an understanding of pulmonary physiology, health professionals would find it impossible to treat the complexities of diseases , such as asthma, COPD, and pulmonary fibrosis, requiring expertise to be managed appropriately. The relevance of pulmonary physiology extends beyond its medical applications because it is vital in the interpretation of body responses to various stressors like alterations in altitude, exercise, and disease. During exercise, the breathing system reacts by having higher ventilation rates and efficiency of gas exchange to meet the additional oxygen demand. This dynamic adjustment illustrates the body's remarkable ability for homeostasis and optimal performance under the threat of coping with changing environments. Research into pulmonary physiology also uncovers mechanisms of respiratory adaptation, allowing researchers to design interventions to enhance sporting performance or recovery in respiratory disease patients. Therefore, pulmonary physiology concepts are invaluable, not only in the clinical environment but also in exercise physiology and sports medicine. Additionally, the interdependence of systemic health and pulmonary physiology cannot be overstated, given the respiratory system's role in determining overall physiological well-being. Pulmonary hypertension and sleep apnea underscore pulmonary health with cardiovascular and metabolic health. Epidemiologic studies suggest that impaired lung function could be a precursor of broader health impairments, including heart disease and diabetes, and require a sweeping understanding and monitoring of pulmonary health. Further, progress in research on pulmonary physiology directs public health policy to reduce the prevalence of respiratory disease resulting from environmental toxins or occupational exposures. Therefore, the study of pulmonary physiology is essential to coming up with an anticipatory intervention for respiratory health and enhancing the quality of life in populations, because of its significant contribution to modern medicine and public health practice (Figure 11.2).

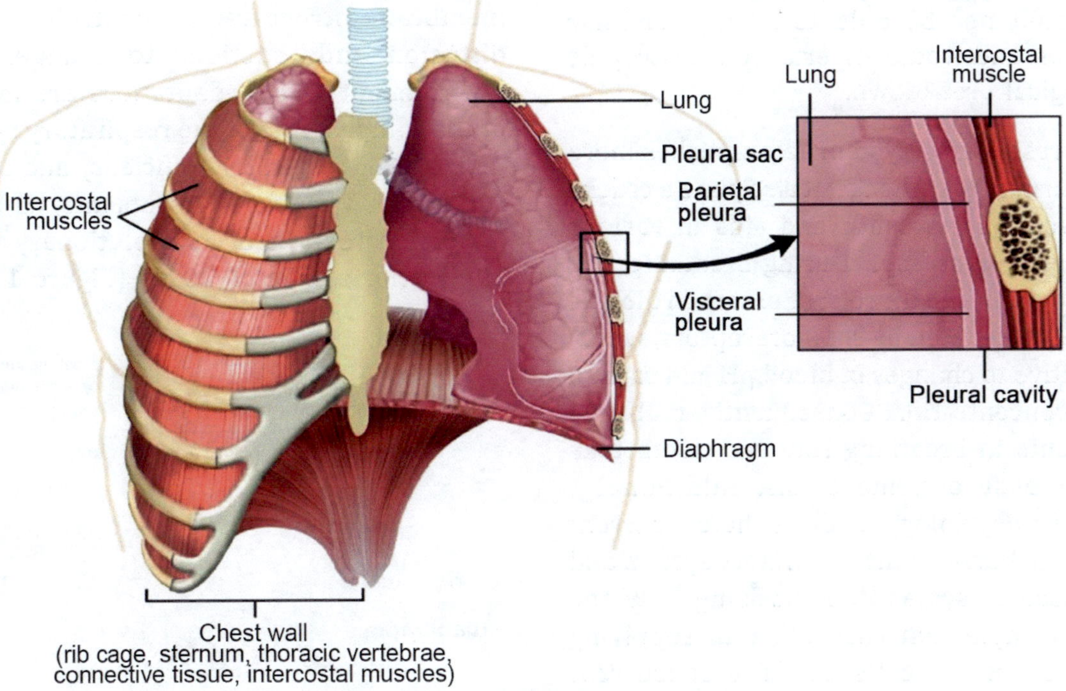

Figure 11.2. Pulmonary physiology.

Source: https://i.ytimg.com/vi/yzKWGIvqZWY/maxresdefault.jpg.

Overview of the Respiratory System

The respiratory system forms a critical component of homeostasis in the human organism and is primarily tasked with oxygen and carbon dioxide exchange. Consisting of passages , such as the nasal passage, trachea, bronchi, and lungs, this is a complex system that has the function of supplying oxygen to the blood while eliminating carbon dioxide, a body waste product of the metabolic process. The process begins with air being inhaled through the nasal passages, which is then warmed, humidified, and filtered. As the air enters the lungs, it is in contact with the alveoli, small, balloon-shaped sacs that enhance gas exchange because they have a huge surface area and thin walls. The preliminary gas exchange is through diffusion, a mechanism that utilizes concentration differences to facilitate effective transport of oxygen into the bloodstream and carbon dioxide out. Without such complex orchestration, the body would not be able to sustain cellular respiration and would experience catastrophic physiological breakdown.

The respiratory system accomplishes more than ensuring gas exchange; it also plays a crucial role in acid-base balance and aids in various physiological processes. During breathing, the need for oxygen and the release of carbon dioxide are closely regulated by chemoreceptors, which are sensitive to changes in blood pH and carbon dioxide concentration. Consequently, real-time adjustments in breathing rate and depth take place to ensure homeostasis. Additionally, pulmonary physiology involves the concurrent relationship between the respiratory system and cardiovascular system, emphasizing how the systems complement each other in supplying oxygenated blood to tissues. The concurrent relationship of these systems not only supports basic functions , such as metabolic support, but also supports the amount of physical performance ability. Knowledge of the respiratory system is thus required to comprehend how it supports human health and activity. Recent research has shown that some breathing techniques, such as pranayama, can likely have a profound impact on the physiological activity of the body. Pranayamic respiration, where there is voluntary control over breathing motions, has been discovered to create beneficial effects , such as lowered oxygen consumption, decreased heart rate, and reduced blood pressure. These effects point toward a likely reset of the autonomic nervous system, demonstrating the wide-ranging impact that breathing can have on overall health. These behaviors can be obtained by stretch receptor-mediated mechanisms, which provide inhibitory inputs upon inspiration and cause a parasympathetic state in the face of body requirements. Moreover, evolutionary stabilization of cellular structure , such as cholesterol-rich caveolae, demonstrates the relationship of respiratory function to membrane structure. By controlling oxygen diffusion and reactions to changes in the environment, these adaptations are indicative of the complex role of the respiratory system in maintaining respiratory efficiency and organism survival in variable environments, as outlined in current reviews of its evolutionary function Zuniga-Hertz & Patel, 2019) (Figure 11.3).

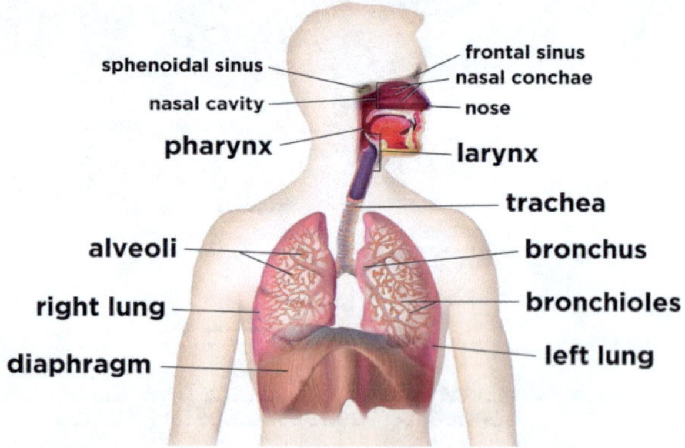

Figure 11.3. The respiratory system.

Source: https://i.ytimg.com/vi/ZB7uA5o0mS4/maxresdefault.jpg.

Historical Context and Key Discoveries

The history of pulmonary physiology is strongly embedded in the history of respiratory medicine, which stretches back to antiquity. The early medical men had naive ideas about breathing, most commonly equating it with a mere process of air exchange. Decisive discoveries over the centuries have flipped this idea on its head. Notably, the invention of the microscope in the 17th century made it possible for scientists to explore the microscopic lung structures, revealing the alveoli necessary for gas exchange. The 17th century also bore significant developments, particularly with William Harvey's discovery of blood circulation, illustrating the complex interaction between the circulatory and respiratory systems. This initial comprehension not only transformed pulmonary physiology but led to the development of increasingly complex theories and medical interventions on breathing and gas exchange within the body, ultimately birthing modern notions of respiratory well-being (Kosolosky et al., 2012). As scientific inquiry continued in the 18th and 19th centuries, the field of pulmonary physiology was transformed by revolutionary revelations in the chemical composition of respiration. The isolation of oxygen and the subsequent discovery of its status as a vital element for life transformed the understanding of respiratory functions. Doctors began to explore the implications of oxygen in the treatment of respiratory disorders, a shift still relevant today. Despite the advancements, there were then prevailing myths about oxygen therapy that had been around for decades. A study of early clinical practice reveals a reliance on empirical observation and inference, with the result of misleading assumptions regarding oxygen prescribing. For instance, certain practices were established in the absence of a uniform understanding of the potential dangers of over-liberal oxygen administration, exemplifying a complicated heritage that has influenced modern therapeutic practice (Kelly, 2014). Furthermore, the late 19th and early 20th centuries marked the formalization of pulmonary physiology as an academic discipline, responding to the need for systematic study in the burgeoning field of respiratory medicine. Research during this period catalyzed the formulation of key theories surrounding ventilatory mechanics and gas exchange dynamics. Advances , such as the development of spirometry enabled clinicians to measure lung function in a standard format, revealing patterns associated with various pulmonary diseases. The era also established environmental determinants , such as altitude and pollution as crucial factors shaping respiratory health. Through awareness of these determinants, practitioners began to individualize interventions for individuals suffering from acute and chronic pulmonary disease. The union of these discoveries utterly transformed the discipline, the forerunner to modern pulmonary medicine and ongoing research into the complexities of the respiratory system, thus providing a fertile background for modern clinical practice.

11.1. Anatomy of the Respiratory System

Learning Outcome

1. Describe the main structures: lungs, trachea, and bronchi;
2. Highlight the function of alveoli in gas exchange;
3. Appreciate supportive structures: diaphragm and intercostal muscles.

The anatomy of the respiratory system makes a significant contribution towards pulmonary physiology, guiding the intricate operations of gas exchange. The upper respiratory system, which comprises the nasal cavity and pharynx, begins the system and serves to filter the air, humidify the air, and regulate heat. Further down, air passes through the larynx and into the trachea, dividing into the bronchi and into the lungs. Its branching structure facilitates efficient distribution of air within the alveoli, the site where carbon dioxide's crucial exchange with oxygen occurs. The highly branched nature of this respiratory system maximizes surface area to an extreme degree, creating the best respiratory efficiency. Understanding the anatomical arrangement of the parts is necessary for an appreciation of the way alterations in structure can influence respiratory function and health, with a greater focus on disease states , such as asthma or chronic obstructive lung disease. Alveoli, tiny air bubbles within the lungs, are essential to pulmonary physiology due to their ability to allow for gas exchange. At the terminal ends of the bronchioles, the alveoli are covered by a thin layer of epithelium, forming the air-blood barrier that consists of the alveolar epithelium, interstitium, and capillary endothelium. Pulmonary surfactant, which is a lipoprotein complex secreted by type II alveolar cells, helps reduce surface tension and stabilize the alveoli during breathing. This surfactant layer not only sustains patency of the alveoli but also optimizes efficiency in gas exchange by facilitating the flow of gases across the barrier. The understanding of the structure and operation of the alveolar wall emphasizes its importance; failure of this system may lead to inefficient gas exchange, as in the case of most respiratory diseases (Hegermann et al., 2020). Additional investigation of pulmonary physiology uncovers the delicate balance provided by the respiratory system through both anatomical structures and physiological mechanisms. The thoracic cavity is central to this, with the diaphragm and intercostal muscles working together to generate pressure gradients responsible for ventilation. Added to this dynamic relationship is the neural control of breathing, modifying respiratory rates according to metabolic demand. Moreover, the systemic effects of respiratory function cannot be overlooked; proper gas exchange is essential to cellular respiration and energy production. Thus, the anatomy and physiology of the respiratory system are more than mere structure and encompass systemic health and the body's homeostatic mechanisms. The integrative methodology is called for, as evidenced in the controversy regarding the extendability of system-level thinking to physiological explanation, in response to reductionist methodologies focused primarily on separate details like the mechanics of gas exchange (Hutchins et al., 2015).

11.1.1. Major Structures: Lungs, Trachea, and Bronchi

Trachea, bronchi, and lungs are important pulmonary structures that are tasked with facilitating the all-important process of respiration in avian and mammalian life. The trachea, being the major airway, divides into the bronchi, which distribute inhaled air to the lungs. This division occurs at the carina, an anatomical characteristic in which the trachea divides into the right and left main bronchi. The structure of such airways, lined by ciliated epithelium and mucus-secreting glands, not only provides access for air but also traps particulate material and pathogens and eliminates them, and is hence a determinant of respiratory health. Regular maintenance of a clear airway is critical as obstructions or inflammation can lead to compromised gas exchange and increased susceptibility to respiratory disease, a consideration of specific relevance given that chronic respiratory disease is a primary global health concern (Dalamani et al., 2006). The lungs themselves consist of an intricate network of very small sacs known as alveoli, where true oxygen-carbon dioxide exchange occurs. Both lungs are also divided into lobes; the right lung has three lobes and the left one has two, making way for the anatomical positioning of the heart. This unique configuration increases the surface area for gas exchange needed to meet the metabolic demands. Observe that the pulmonary vasculature is closely associated with the alveoli to facilitate easy transportation of gases between the blood and air. Further, the functional characteristics of the lungs, including compliance and elasticity, are essential for proper ventilation. The lungs in avian species show an extremely organized architecture that includes bronchus-associated lymphoid tissue (BALT), reflecting the significance of immune defense in lung homeostasis (Dalamani et al., 2006). Further, the tracheobronchial tree is not only essential for its physiological functions but also for its participation in immune defense.

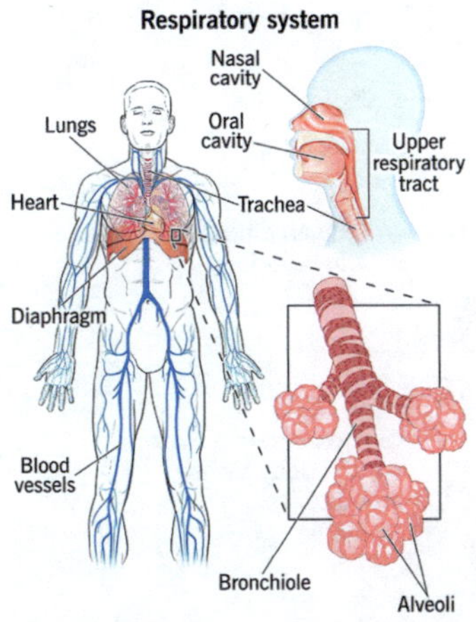

Figure 11.4. Respiratory system: Organs, facts, anatomy and function.

Source: https://my.clevelandclinic.org/-/scassets/images/org/health/articles/respiratory-system.

The bifurcating bronchi subdivide into progressively finer bronchioles, which terminate in the respiratory bronchioles that lead to alveolar sacs. The dynamic interaction of the respiratory tract with environmental exposures is a substantial contributor to the pathogenesis of respiratory disease. Notably, nonhuman primate models have been shown through research to reveal similarities between lung structure and immune mechanisms of nonhuman primates and humans. It is critical to appreciate these interactions because they demonstrate mechanisms whereby inhaled pathogens and pollutants cause inflammatory responses that contribute to chronic respiratory illness. These findings underscore the intricacy of pulmonary physiology and the necessity for continued investigation into its constituents and their roles in health and disease (Miller et al., 2017) (Figure 11.4).

11.1.2. Role of Alveoli in Gas Exchange

The functional units of the respiratory system are the alveoli that play a vital role in exchanging gases. An alveolus is a tiny balloon with an enormous surface area to exchange oxygen, carbon dioxide with air and blood. This is made possible by the thin architecture of alveolar walls, made up of a thin layer of epithelial cells, which provides a thin barrier for gas molecules to pass through. Collapsing of alveoli is prevented and breathing is made easier by surfactant, a lipoprotein secretion of type II alveolar cells, which reduces surface tension. This biophysical characteristic is essential for increasing the efficiency of gas exchange so that enough oxygen is absorbed into the bloodstream and carbon dioxide, a waste product of cellular metabolism, is expelled (Hegermann et al., 2020). The alveolar function is not just limited to the facilitation of gas diffusion but also plays a role in maintaining structural support to the air-blood barrier. Integrity of such a barrier is essential to normal respiratory function and is established by the alveolar epithelium and the capillary endothelium surrounding it. For maximal gas exchange, the air-blood barrier must be intact and thin so that gases may diffuse rapidly. A glycocalyx, or glycoprotein layer on the alveolar epithelial cells, has also been identified to exert significant interactions with the surfactant system. It helps in alveolar homeostasis by regulating the thickness and viscosity of the alveolar lining layer, which is required for optimal gas exchange and defense against inhaled pathogens (Hegermann et al., 2020). Moreover, variations in the efficiency of gas exchange can also be caused by pathologic conditions that affect the function of alveoli. For instance, while physiological adaptations within the alveoli facilitate gas exchange during normal respiratory status, they are compromised in scenarios , such as general anesthesia in horses, a condition whereby hypoxemia can arise. Although gas exchange is normally robust, during recumbency of animals, the gas exchange is compromised with altered ventilation-perfusion relationships in the lungs. This emphasizes the relevance of understanding and measurement of alveolar function during various states of disease and health, including in special populations , such as anaesthetized horses. Investigation into the management of deranged alveolar function remains relevant for improving patient outcomes, emphasizing the need for further study within this field of pulmonary physiology (Figure 11.5).

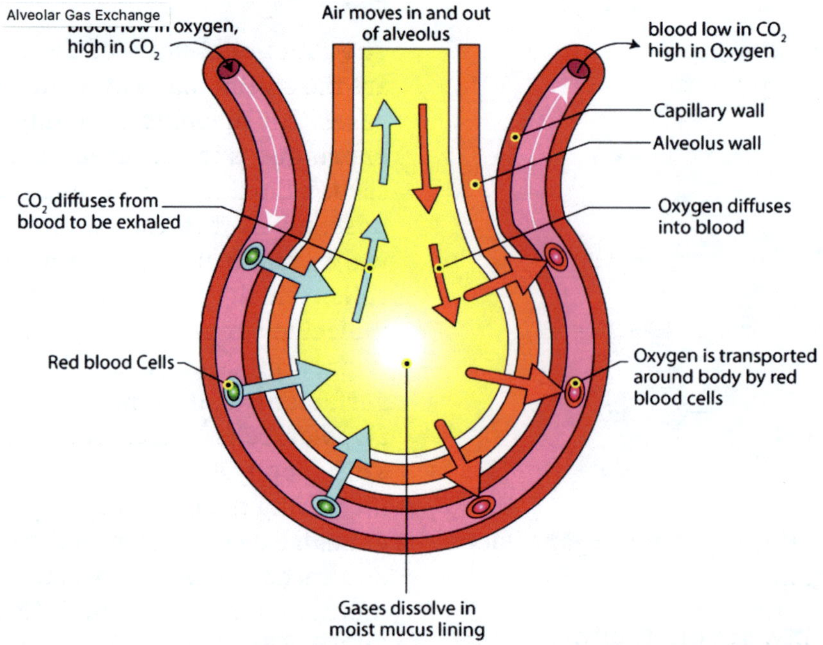

Figure 11.5. Role of alveoli in gas exchange.

Source: https://biologynotesonline.com/wp-content/uploads/2024/10/image-93.png.

11.1.3. Supporting Structures: Diaphragm and Intercostal Muscles

Diaphragm and intercostal muscles are significant components of the respiratory system and serve a significant role in pulmonary physiology. The diaphragm is a dome-shaped muscle at the base of the thoracic cavity and is involved in the process of taking in air during inhalation, mainly. The diaphragm flattens upon contraction, which expands the vertical dimensions of the thorax and creates a negative pressure that pulls air into the lungs. Intercostal muscles, which are positioned between the ribs, assist diaphragmatic action in that they stabilize and amplify the thoracic cage with respiration. When used together, these structures facilitate effective ventilation in that they provide adequate oxygen to alveoli while at the same time allowing for the removal of carbon dioxide. Their combined function represents their importance not only for normal respiration but also for assisting in the alteration of respiratory mechanics when physical exertion is increased. Understanding the biomechanics of the intercostal muscles and diaphragm is important while assessing respiratory function under varying physiological conditions. The activity of the diaphragm, for instance, is normally measured with invasive and non-invasive measures. Recent studies have highlighted that neuromechanical coupling (NMC) of the diaphragm is an important index of respiratory muscle function, particularly in neuromuscular conditions and cardiorespiratory diseases. The merging of non-invasive methods, including surface mechanomyography and electromyography, has proved to be an optimal substitute for conventional invasive measurement of transdiaphragmatic pressure. These are capable of providing a less restricted way of assessing diaphragm function, critical to early diagnosis and care for respiratory diseases (Petrocelli et al., 2019). Thus, refinements in measurement techniques not only enrich our understanding of respiratory mechanics but also promote clinical application. Intercostal muscles are crucial in aiding diaphragmatic function. During forceful or deep breathing, intercostal muscles contract to raise the rib cage and thereby enlarge lung volume and maximize air entry. This answer is particularly relevant under conditions of increased respiratory demand, exercise, or respiratory distress. Recent findings indicate strong relationships between measurements of non-invasive intercostal muscle activity and established invasive methods, reinforcing the notion that these muscles are essential for effective ventilation (Campos et al., 2018). By using intercostal muscle dynamics recording methods, the clinician can acquire valuable information on patient respiratory mechanics. Thus, the coordination between the diaphragm and intercostal muscles is an ideal example of complex mechanics of pulmonary physiology (Figure 11.6).

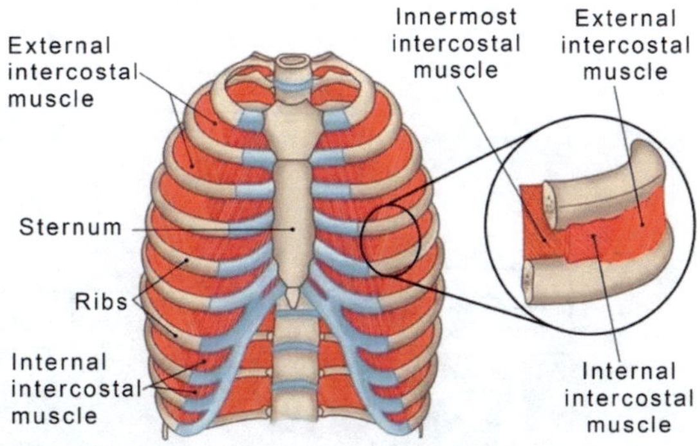

Figure 11.6. Intercostal muscles.

Source: https://samarpanphysioclinic.com/wp-content/uploads/2023/03/intercostal-muscles-1200x900.webp

Test Your Knowledge

1. What are the primary structures of the upper and lower respiratory tract?
2. Which structure links the bronchi and the larynx?

11.2. Mechanics of Breathing

Learning Outcome

1. Explain the process of expiration and inspiration;
2. Define pressure changes during respiration;
3. Explain factors affecting lung volume and capacity.

The breathing mechanics required for efficient gas exchange in the lungs involve complex interactions among multiple physiological structures. The fundamental process begins with intermuscular diaphragm and intercostal muscle contraction, creating negative thoracic cavity pressure. This negative pressure draws air into the lungs, while alveoli permit gas diffusion between the blood and air. In recent research, newer techniques , such as Forced Oscillation Technique (FOT) have been used in lung mechanics assessment without injuring patients via invasive examinations. The method allows for the assessment of respiratory function across different populations, for example, children and adults, in order to determine lung tissue mechanics differences caused by age and differences in body composition (Copot et al., 2019).

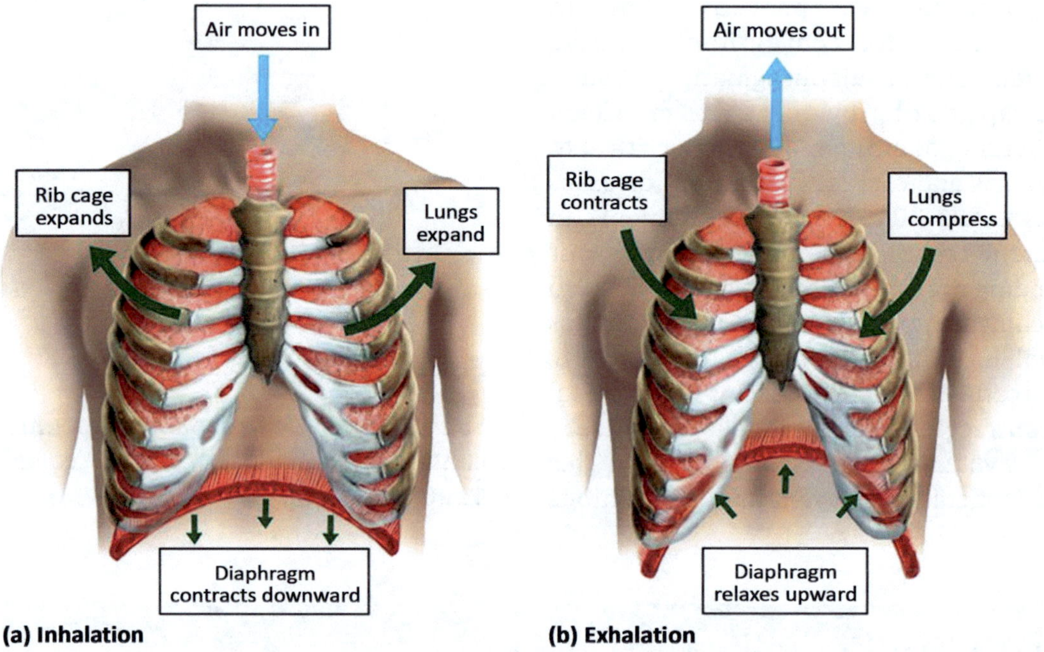

Figure 11.7. Mechanics of breathing.

Source: https://external-content.duckduckgo.com/iu/?u=https%3A%2F%2Fwww.online-sciences.com%2Fwp-content%2Fuploads%2F2021%2F06%2FMechanics-of-Pulmonary-Ventilation-4.jpg&f=1&nofb=1&ipt=c44d3ea1505d761def43d09fb6a37f1fcd48a8b0a932d886512496ab078553ac.

Such knowledge is critical in understanding the physiological differences in respiratory mechanics and, thus, the optimization of pulmonary health clinical strategies. The mechanics of exhalation and inhalation are not only passive events but also dependent upon chest wall compliance and lung tissue compliance. Low chest wall compliance, more particularly, presents certain breathing mechanics problems. For instance, very preterm infants have high respiratory compliance for the chest wall, which weakens the structural support necessary for effective inhalation. This disorder has the capacity to induce inappropriately generated pressures during breathing, posing a direct danger to their respiratory health. Recent advances in the modeling of respiratory mechanics have provided greater understanding of the problems in this susceptible population using nonlinear models that account for the unique biomechanical parameters involved (Brandes et al., 2018). By replicating mechanisms , such as laryngeal braking and compensatory alveolar pressure increments, researchers seek to develop more successful treatments in order to improve lung function in such infants. Beyond that, the applicability of pulmonary mechanics also reaches past the microscopic level of gas exchange within the alveoli to a more universal concern for respiratory therapy. The continued development of non-invasive ventilation techniques underscores the importance of investigating respiratory mechanics in medicine. For instance, figuring out the optimal balance of chest wall compliance and lung pressure can inform therapies like Continuous Positive Airway Pressure (CPAP) in infants and adults. By taking a personalized medicine approach to therapy, the effectiveness of breathing treatments can be enhanced and complications arising from different lung pathologies reduced. The integration of complex respiratory models with non-invasive testing procedures not only advances our understanding of mechanical breathing mechanisms but also paves the way towards novel applications in pulmonary therapy and management (Figure 11.7).

11.2.1. Inhalation and Exhalation Processes

The processes of inhalation and exhalation are at the heart of pulmonary physiology, enabling the exchange of gases needed in sustenance of life. In inhalation, intercostal muscles and the diaphragm contract, increasing the thoracic cavity volume. This inflation results in a reduction in intrapulmonary pressure, hence allowing atmospheric air into the lungs. The mechanism is complicated because it involves a number of physiological signals that ensure ventilation to the required degree. The major factors, including lung stretch receptors and chemoreceptors, affect the surveillance and response towards alterations in lung volume and blood gases. The integrated action in the respiratory center is a demonstration of the intricacy of such control mechanisms, further attested to by mathematical and computational models that faithfully capture the dynamics of such biological systems. Such integration generates insight into how inhalation maximally matches metabolic demand. Exhalation, on the other hand, is the essence of eliminating carbon dioxide, a byproduct of metabolism, from the body.

Unlike inhalation, it is passive or active, relative to the respiratory demand. During passive exhalation, the diaphragm is relaxed and the elastic properties of the lung tissues result in a natural tendency for recoiling, compressing air from the lungs as intrapulmonary pressure rises. Active exhalation, typically demanded during more vigorous activities, demands extra muscular contractions, primarily of the abdominal muscles and internal intercostals. This process is critical during exercise when the body must get rid of carbon dioxide quickly in a bid to maintain acid-base balance. The relationship between ventilation and perfusion is increasingly significant with exhalation, as effective gas exchange relies on maximally coordinated blood flow through the lungs and alveolar architecture (King et al., 2003). Thus, studying exhalation is crucial to measure pulmonary function and respiratory efficacy. The physiological function of respiration extends beyond the mere exchange of gases; it is the centerpiece of many metabolic and physiological processes. For instance, the regulation of inhaled substances, e.g., volatile organic compounds (VOCs), provides information on overall physiological states of the system. Breath analysis has been shown to expose the underlying metabolic processes, showing ventilation's interaction with blood composition under dynamic conditions , such as exercise (King et al., 2003).

Also, gases exhaled in much larger volumes during exercise can reveal something about tissue perfusion and the reactivity of the blood vessels to an increase in metabolic requirements. Information of this sort emphasizes the significance of studying such respiratory mechanisms not only for their mechanics but also for their potential application in a diagnostic function in clinical medicine. Lastly, the adjustment to a precise degree between exhalation and inhalation demonstrates the body's remarkable capacity to adjust and respond to an enormous number of physiological issues that are inherent in daily living (Figure 11.8).

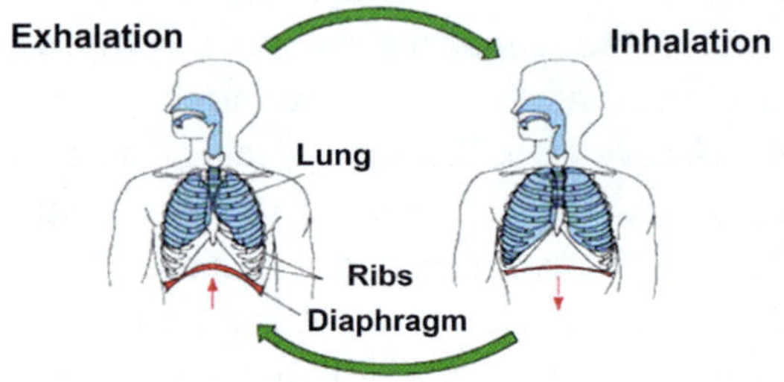

Figure 11.8. Difference between inhalation and exhalation.

Source: https://external-content.duckduckgo.com/iu/?u=http%3A%2F%2Ffiles.differencebetween.com%2Fwp-content%2Fuploads%2F2013%2F11%2FProcesses-of-Inhalation-and-Exhalation.png&f=1&nofb=1&ipt=414c88fe7a51786ad61d8c795128e6a64bd50f7fe4721446dd1f726a2c70a07e.

11.2.2. Role of Pressure Changes in Breathing

The role of pressure changes in breathing plays a pivotal role in pulmonary physiology mechanics. When breathing in and out, pressure gradients between the atmosphere and the thoracic cavity push ventilation. The diaphragm is relaxed on inspiration, expanding thoracic volume and consequently lowering intrapulmonary pressure relative to atmospheric pressure. The pressure gradient brings air into the lungs, demonstrating the significance of negative pressure mechanics. The reverse occurs upon expiration; the diaphragm falls, resulting in a reduction of thoracic volume and intrapulmonary pressure, thereby expelling air. This repetitive process of alternating pressure is not only critical for gas exchange but is also related to more advanced physiological processes, thus making it inevitable to understand the mechanics of breathing in terms of health and disease. In addition to increasing airflow, pressure changes in respiration influence other physiologic systems beyond the respiratory tract. Pressure changes have been shown to control heart rhythms, blood pressure, as well as neural activity throughout the phase of respiration. Respiratory sinus arrhythmia is one example of this, where heart rate fluctuates in synchrony with phases of respiration. On inspiration, the cardiac rate typically rises with reduced intrathoracic pressure that enhances venous return to the heart. At expiration, the cardiac rate typically falls. These relationships indicate the extent to which integrative respiratory functions shape overall homeostasis and can elucidate conditions like anxiety and stress disorders, further justifying the need for greater expertise in pulmonary physiology (Jerath et al., 2015). Also, ventilation control during exercise illustrates the complexities of pressure change during breathing. During exercise, the body transitions from the use of negative feedback systems used during resting conditions to an open-loop control system that facilitates greater ventilatory demand. This adjustment reflects compensations to maintain adequate oxygenation and carbon dioxide elimination with heightened metabolic activity. Specifically, respiration control is sensitive to adjustments in pulmonary CO2 production and acidosis of the blood since required to ensure effective gas exchange under conditions created by augmented exercise intensity (Thamrin & Murray-Smith, 2009). The adaptive processes pinpoint the dynamic interplay between pressure control and respiration and the need for continued research into the underlying respiratory physiology of treatment interventions within respiratory disease and enhanced performance (Figure 11.9).

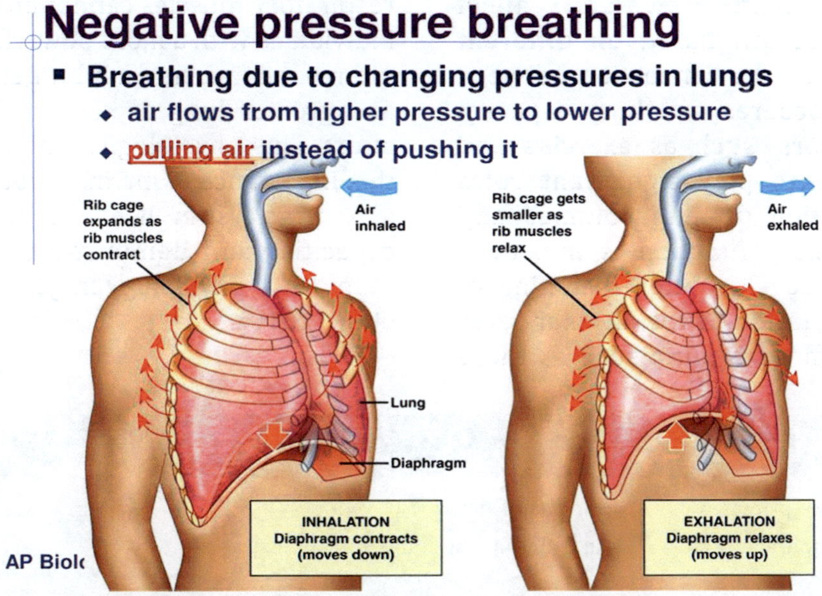

Figure 11.9. Role of pressure changes in breathing.

Source: https://image3.slideserve.com/7067155/negative-pressure-breathing-l.jpg.

11.2.3. Factors Affecting Lung Volumes and Capacities

Lung volumes and capacities are affected by a large number of factors, one of which is physiological state and overall health status. Age is of importance here, since lung function tends to decline with advancing years due to loss of elastic recoil and narrowing of airway diameter. This physiological decline results in reduced vital capacity and total lung capacity, which is also contributed to by long-term illnesses , such as emphysema or asthma. Body posture and composition also have a direct influence on lung volume; so, for instance, individuals with a higher body percentage of fat will have lower lung volumes than their thin counterparts. Furthermore, the mechanics of respiration can be undermined by illnesses involving obesity or restrictive pulmonary conditions, in which lung and chest wall compliance is adversely affected, which can lead to restriction of airflow and thereby change total lung capacity. Environmental factors have strong effects on lung volumes and capacities, particularly in regards to exposure to allergens and pollutants. Air quality is also most critical to pulmonary health due to the fact that exposure to chronic pollution can lead to long-term alterations of lung volumes and mechanics. For example, individuals who live in urban settings often have decreased lung function compared to individuals who live in rural areas due to being exposed to particulates and noxious gases that can lead to inflammatory responses of the lung. Furthermore, occupational exposure , such as inhalation of silica dust or asbestos, can result in restrictive lung disease that dichotomizes lung capacities. Furthermore, seasonal allergens trigger asthma or chronic obstructive pulmonary disease (COPD) exacerbation, affecting the variability of lung function since responses to increased inflammatory mediators affect the dynamics of breath based on different seasons, emphasizing the connection between environmental exposures and lung capacity. Physiological factors, such as exercise and physical fitness, also play significant roles in the determination of lung volumes and capacities. Pulmonary function is improved by physical exercise via better matching of ventilation and perfusion at the alveolar level. As has been shown by studies, such as those with real-time measurements of exhaled volatile organic compounds, factors like exercise-related ventilation and perfusion exhibit significant changes, having significant impacts on respiratory parameters (King et al., 2003). Greater perfusion during exercise provides optimal gas exchange, showing the interactive dynamic between the function of metabolism and lung capacity. Moreover, the power of respiratory muscles cannot be overemphasized; individuals with a more powerful diaphragm and intercostal muscles exhibit better lung function and greater lung capacities during maximum effort. This physiological interaction highlights the importance of intrinsic body welfare as well as extrinsic stimuli for regulating respiratory capacities and demonstrates the intricacy of pulmonary physiology in general (Kupferthaler et al., 2010).

Test Your Knowledge

1. Which muscles are primarily involved in inspiration?
2. How does the diaphragm play a role in inflating the lungs during inspiration?

11.3. Gas Exchange and Transport

Learning Outcome

1. Explain oxygen and carbon dioxide exchange mechanisms;
2. Define the role of hemoglobin in the transport of oxygen;
3. Describe the determinants of gas diffusion.

The intricate process of gas exchange within the lungs is core to the maintenance of homeostasis of the body. Oxygenation and elimination of carbon dioxide occur within the alveoli, where numerous small sacs of air permit diffusion of gases due to the vast surface area as well as thin walls. This process is supported by partial pressure gradients between blood and the alveoli. Oxygen will spontaneously move from the more concentrated setting of the alveoli to the less concentrated setting of deoxygenated pulmonary capillary blood. Concurrently, carbon dioxide, a waste product of cellular metabolism, moves from the blood where its concentration is more concentrated into alveoli, where it will be expelled during exhalation. This bidirectional interaction illustrates the effectiveness and the need for coordinated respiratory mechanics in maintaining effective gas transport and general pulmonary physiology. In evaluating the physiological processes of gas transport, it becomes necessary to consider how ventilation correlates with metabolic needs when the body is in activity. The body adapts to breathing rates and volumes responsively in order to maintain optimal oxygen delivery and carbon dioxide removal. As physical activity increases, the respiratory control shifts from negative feedback control to open-loop control mode as defined in research literature. Under this open-loop mode, the ventilation can be quickly adjusted according to increased pulmonary CO2 output and more blood acidity, which indicate increased metabolic function. These adaptations are credited with providing optimal oxygen requirements of the body's requirements while preventing the excessive accumulation of carbon dioxide, a critical component in the acid-base balance.

The fine adjustment between these systems underscores the importance of regulation of gas transport under various physiological conditions, particularly in the realm of exertion (Thamrin & Murray-Smith, 2009). In addition, evolutionary theories of gas exchange explain the adaptations by which complex organisms have been able to survive under varied environmental conditions. The earliest forms of life had to contend with specific challenges presented by increasing levels of atmospheric oxygen, resulting in profound biological adaptation to control intracellular oxygen levels. Cholesterol became an important biomolecule during this evolution and played the role of organizing cellular membranes as well as restricting the unregulated diffusion of oxygen. In contemporary systems, the specialized membrane structures known as caveolae have been identified as important mediators of gas exchange, serving as hubs of signaling pathways controlling cellular response to changing oxygen levels. These HIF processes are the pinnacle of complex membrane structure and respiratory function interplay, backing up the notion that gas exchange mechanism development has a close relationship with evolutionary forces and climatic changes (Zuniga-Hertz & Patel, 2019) (Figure 11.10).

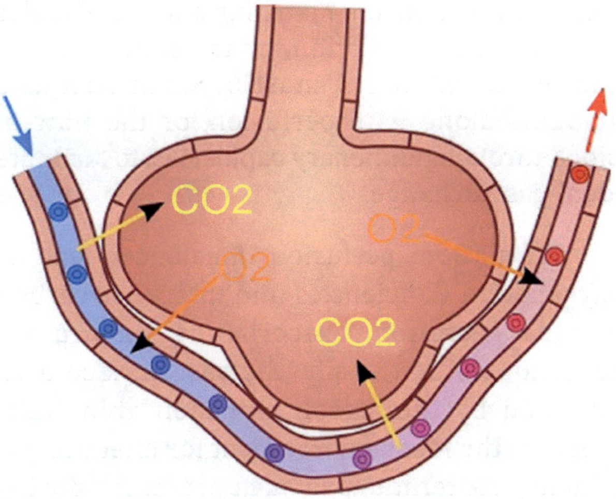

Figure 11.10. Factors that affect the human gas exchange system.

Source: https://study.com/cimages/multimages/16/gas_exchange_in_the_aveolus.jpg.

11.3.1. Mechanisms of Oxygen and Carbon Dioxide Exchange

The mechanisms of oxygen and carbon dioxide exchange are fundamental to pulmonary physiology and are chiefly performed in the alveoli of the lungs. The mechanism for the gas exchange is diffusion, as gases have a natural tendency to move from areas of higher partial pressure to areas of lower partial pressure. In the alveolar compartment, oxygen will tend to have a higher partial pressure than the deoxygenated blood entering from the body and thus will be transferred into the blood. Carbon dioxide, which is a metabolic waste in the body tissues, will have a higher partial pressure in the blood than in the alveoli and thus will be diffused into the air being exhaled from the lungs. This effective exchange is most crucial in facilitating homeostasis of the body, whereby cellular respiration involves oxygen and the effective elimination of carbon dioxide to prevent respiratory acidosis. Exchange efficiency of the carbon dioxide and oxygen is influenced by several factors, including ventilation-perfusion matching and the alveolar surface area. Ventilation, or the flow of air in and out of the lungs, must occur in adequate amounts along with perfusion, or the flow of blood through pulmonary capillaries, to facilitate ideal gas exchange.

Ventilation: perfusion imbalances lead to oxygenation deficiencies and improper carbon dioxide excretion, exacerbating respiratory conditions. Additionally, the vast surface area provided by the alveoli and their thin walls presents the ideal environment for effective gas exchange. Alterations in such processes during exercise, for instance, can have a tremendous effect on the body's ability to meet metabolic demands, which points out the dynamic nature of the pulmonary system in the states of physiology (Thamrin & Murray-Smith, 2009). Also, it is necessary to consider the role of carbon dioxide in ventilatory control, particularly in the case of exercise.

If there is an increase in metabolic activity, there is more production of carbon dioxide and, therefore, it will raise the acidity (lower the pH) of blood. This physiological response stimulates peripheral and central chemoreceptors that transmit signals to brain respiratory centers, which enhance ventilation so that carbon dioxide is eliminated efficiently while oxygen consumption is maximized.

This complexity is brought out by research indicating the range of reactions by different individuals to elevated carbon dioxide concentrations, particularly during exercise in a small enclosed space, such as space suits (Thamrin & Murray-Smith, 2009). Identification of these dynamics not only clarifies crude pulmonary physiology but also informs the development of strategies for the maintenance of respiratory health in a range of situations (Figure 11.11).

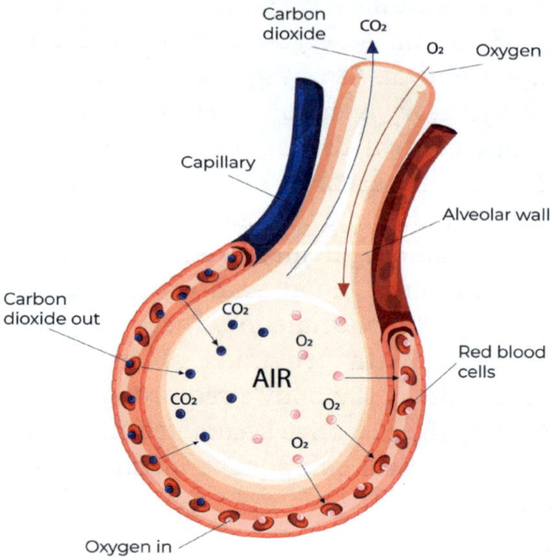

Figure 11.11. Oxygen-carbon-dioxide-exchange-alveolus-with-erythrocytes.

Source: https://img.freepik.com/premium-vector/oxygen-carbon-dioxide-exchange-alveolus-with-erythrocytes_458779-1135.jpg?w=2000.

11.3.2. Role of Hemoglobin in Oxygen Transport

Oxygen transport across the human body is greatly dependent on hemoglobin, an intricate protein component of red blood cells. This biomolecule also plays a vital role in binding oxygen in the lungs and delivering it to tissues throughout the body. Once oxygen is inhaled, which diffuses through alveolar spaces, it is delivered to the blood, where oxygen has a high affinity for hemoglobin under pulmonary capillary conditions. As it binds to oxygen, hemoglobin undergoes a conformational change that increases its affinity for binding additional oxygen molecules, a phenomenon known as cooperative binding. This feature significantly increases oxygen transport efficiency so that tissues can be maintained with an adequate oxygen supply even during varying metabolic demands. This adaptive control of oxygen affinity enables hemoglobin to maximize oxygen delivery, which is critical for the maintenance of cellular function and overall metabolic health. In hypoxic states, the physiological role of hemoglobin remains important for oxygen homeostasis. The adaptive ability of the body to low oxygen levels is often necessitated by increased hemoglobin production, as evidenced by observations that indicate significant alterations in hemoglobin levels in response to chronic hypoxia (Floros et al., 2014). The increase allows for increased oxygen transport capability despite lowered environmental oxygen concentrations. Moreover, since blood flow compensates against hypoxic stimuli, regulatory pathways , such as hypoxic vasodilation are triggered. Such a rise in local blood flow not only supplies more oxygen to tissues but also relies on the interaction of nitric oxide and hemoglobin, which is pivotal for vascular regulation under such stressors (Dyson et al., 2013).

Therefore, the key interaction between hemoglobin and vascular responses demonstrates how the body continuously compensates to uphold normal oxygen supply in adverse conditions. Furthermore, the role of hemoglobin extends beyond the mere transport of oxygen; it is instrumental in controlling the acid-base state of blood. Hemoglobin acts as a buffer by binding hydrogen ions and carbon dioxide, the end products of cell metabolism. This binding enables carbon dioxide to be carried back to the lungs, where it can be excreted from the body. During conditions of increased cellular activity, such as during exercise, hemoglobin's efficiency in both carrying oxygen and clearing carbon dioxide is essential. Advances in our understanding of hemoglobin dynamics have come to underscore its adaptability, particularly with respect to adjustment to variations in altitude or hypoxia, and the ability to regulate affinity according to pH and carbon dioxide status. By and large, these activities attest to its pivotal role in pulmonary physiology whereby oxygen delivery and respiratory gas exchange can be made effective under a range of physiological conditions (Figure 11.12).

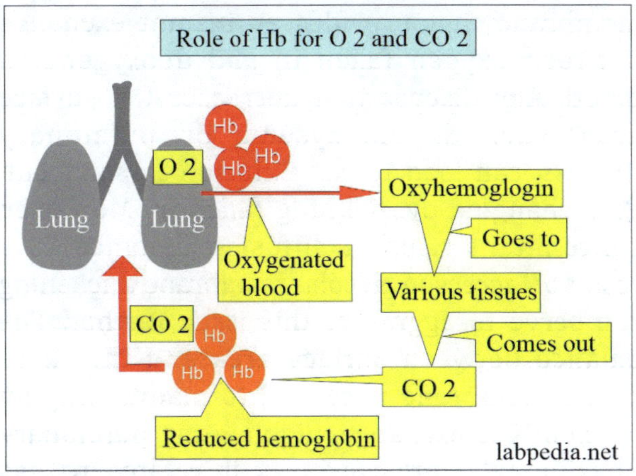

Figure 11.12. Role of hemoglobin in oxygen transport.

Source: https://labpedia.net/wp-content/uploads/2020/01/Hb-role-in-Oxygen-and-CO2.jpg.

11.3.3. Factors Influencing Gas Diffusion

Gas diffusion is largely influenced by several physiological factors, which have distinct roles in the efficiency of oxygen and carbon dioxide exchange in pulmonary circulation. Concentration gradient is one of the determining factors and is responsible for forcing gases from high partial pressure to low partial pressure areas. Oxygen partial pressure in the alveoli is typically greater than that of deoxygenated blood upon entry into the lungs to allow effective diffusion into the bloodstream. Carbon dioxide, on the other hand, diffuses from the blood, whose partial pressure is greater, into the alveolar air for exhalation. Thus, a perfect concentration gradient is essential to effective gas exchange, and this emphasizes the importance of factors , such as ventilatory rate and the overall health of the pulmonary system in achieving effective diffusion. Exposed surface area for gas exchange is crucial to gas diffusion efficiency. The lungs are gigantic organs providing a big surface area created by the vast number of alveoli, small air sacs inside the lungs. An alveolus is made up of a thin membrane that provides an instant exchange between oxygen taken in and deoxygenated blood. Any disease that decreases the surface area, such as emphysema or pulmonary fibrosis, can lead to gas diffusion impairment, thus changing overall lung function. Moreover, concomitant rises in diffusion distance as a result of increased alveolar membrane thickening can serve to aggravate this issue further. The balance between surface area and thickness of the membrane is central to maintaining an efficient gas exchange, highlighting pulmonary physiology's intricacies as it relates to gas diffusion. Environmental conditions also have a profound effect on gas diffusion in the lungs. Other properties like humidity, temperature, and pressure of the atmosphere can also alter the partial pressures of gases within the mixture. For instance, at higher altitudes where the pressure of the atmosphere is less, oxygen partial pressure is reduced, leading to decreased diffusion into the bloodstream and possibly causing hypoxia. In contrast, increased humidity may enable gas diffusion by preventing alveolar drying, maintaining the necessary concentration gradients. In addition, the role of cholesterol in cell membranes, especially in maintaining membrane order and integrity, is crucial under various environmental pressures. Cholesterol-enriched domains known as caveolae have been identified as significant sites for oxygen diffusion-related signaling and have shown another biological response to the outside gaseous environment, indicating the complexity of factors implicated in gas diffusion in pulmonary physiology (Zuniga-Hertz & Patel, 2019).

Test Your Knowledge

1. Where is gas exchange located in the respiratory system?
2. How is oxygen transported in the blood?

11.4. Regulation of Breathing

Learning Outcome

1. Describe the neural regulation of respiration;
2. Define the chemical regulation: CO2 and O2 levels' role;
3. Describe the reflexes and their impact on breathing patterns.

Breathing regulation is a complex interplay of neural, chemical, and mechanical elements converging to provide the optimal operation of pulmonary physiology. Respiration is regulated primarily by the respiratory centers within the brainstem, the medulla oblongata and the pons, which regulate the rhythm and depth of respiration. During inspiration, neurons fire to stimulate the contraction of the diaphragm and intercostal muscles to facilitate airflow into the lungs. During expiration, the neurons cease firing, enabling passive relaxation and airflow out. This rhythmic process is not only vital for gas exchange but also for the maintenance of homeostasis in the body, such as the maintenance of proper blood levels of oxygen and carbon dioxide. Understanding these regulatory processes is insightful regarding the physiological response to varied conditions, like stress and exercise, showing the dynamic nature of the respiratory system. The control of the respiratory system is also subject to considerable peripheral chemoreceptor control in the carotid and aortic arteries. The chemoreceptors in these arteries monitor arterial blood carbon dioxide, oxygen tension, and pH levels and send feedback to the brain to control the rate of breathing accordingly. For instance, an increase in carbon dioxide or a decrease in blood pH results in increased ventilation, while a decrease in oxygen levels invokes the same type of response to restore balance. Aside from the physiological, this homeostatic process is essential in treating conditions , such as sleep apnea and COPD, wherein mechanisms of feedback typically found are typically lost.

The intricate interplay between respiratory regulation and overall homeostasis highlights the importance of forceful patterns of respiration to healthy maintenance and prevention of disease, and the need for clinical intervention aimed at promoting respiratory efficiency and responsiveness. Another layer of breathing regulation is the autonomic nervous system, which modifies respiratory patterns as a response to emotional and somatic stimulation. The synchronization of breathing with autonomic nervous response offers a quick adaptation to changing situations, for example, exercise or stress. The sympathetic nervous system, among others, can augment respiratory drive during heightened activity or anxiety, while the parasympathetic system can promote slower, more tranquil breathing patterns. The relationship between these systems is used to underscore the importance of respiratory drive not only as a mechanical process but as a critical element in the physiological control of psychosomatic states. Continued research into the mechanisms, specifically their influence on cellular function, can potentially lead to new treatments for many medical conditions, and thus the value of knowing about breathing regulation within the scope of pulmonary physiology in general (Jerath et al., 2015; Torday, 2015) (Figure 11.13).

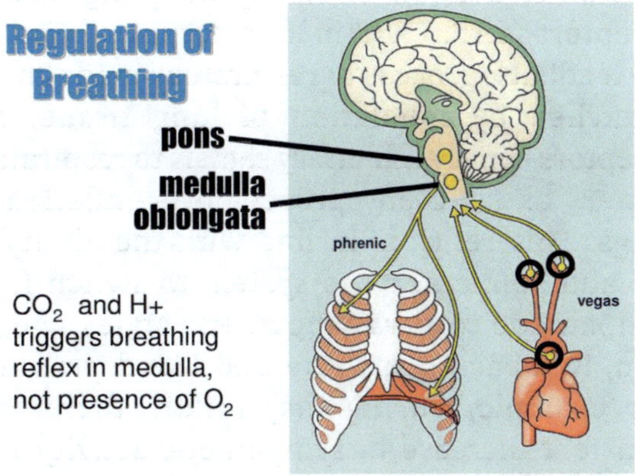

Figure 11.13. Regulation-of-breathing.

Source: https://image1.slideserve.com/1779231/regulation-of-breathing-l.jpg.

11.4.1. Neural Control of Respiration

Regulation of respiration is a complex coordination of nervous mechanisms to provide sufficient gas exchange under various physiological conditions. Central to this regulation is the brainstem respiratory center, which integrates into its inputs from peripheral and central chemoreceptors that inform about blood gases. Pons and medulla oblongata play a crucial role, where the center of medullary rhythmicity decides the basic rhythm of breathing. This rhythm pattern is also altered by higher brain center signals and by mechanical feedback from the lungs. Surprisingly, inspiration creates distinct neural pathways that result in the activation of respiratory muscles, while expiration is largely passive and driven by lung recoil and by a number of neuromuscular interactions. Over time, the intricate interaction of excitatory and inhibitory inputs is such that ventilation is controlled in terms of metabolic requirement and conditions of the environment, emphasizing the central role of the nervous system in pulmonary physiology. Mechanics of breathing are influenced by reflex actions and the autonomic nervous system, and these reveal the dynamic nature of respiratory control. Activation of slowly adapting stretch receptors (SARs) within lung tissue exemplifies the feedback process of respiratory modulation. Stretched by inhalation of lung tissue, the receptors convey inhibitory signals to respiratory centers and thereby prevent over-inflation of lungs. This reflex is in line with the ability of the autonomic nervous system to switch from sympathetic to parasympathetic states and, in turn, influence heart rate and blood pressure. For example, during inspiration, there is a transient increase in sympathetic activity that often happens to impact cardiac rhythm and vascular tone. This bidirectional communication between respiratory mechanics and autonomic modulation underscores the significance of having proper knowledge of neural control in connection with the regulation of breathing and generalized physiological response in the body (Jerath et al., 2015).

Furthermore, sophisticated techniques , such as pranayamic breathing show the striking interdependence between neural control and controlled breathing. Such respiration manipulation can trigger adaptive physiological responses, e.g., a decrease in heart rate and increased parasympathetic tone. Pranayamic exercises stimulate neural processes presumably responsible for the reset of the autonomic nervous system, illustrating how voluntary control of breathing dictates involuntary physiological processes. The fact that deep respiration leads to hyperpolarization currents through stretch receptors and fibroblast activity points towards a cellular-level mechanism that orchestrates various neural elements. These interactions are revealing the therapeutic potential of breathing techniques in the treatment of a range of disorders, from anxiety to chronic respiratory illness. Therefore, studies on pranayama and its effects resonate an even greater story on the importance of neural regulation of respiratory physiology, and there is a call for studies in this new field (Austin et al., 2006) (Figure 11.14).

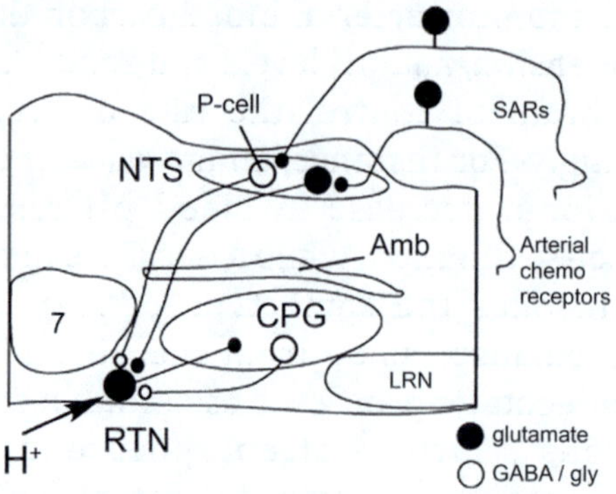

Figure 11.14. Inhibitory input from slowly adapting lung stretch receptors to retrotrapezoid nucleus chemoreceptors.

Source: https://external-content.duckduckgo.com/iu/?u=https%3A%2F%2Fphysoc.onlinelibrary.wiley.com%2Fcms%2Fasset%2F8d01075d-a2b8-44d2-a3fd-a8033816eb80%2Ftjp_2064_f8.gif&f=1&nofb=1&ipt=66f4124e53f041997f5d3f08f672e1dc57d4e5396b6676858ab175031286ed27.

11.4.2. Chemical Regulation: Role of CO_2 and O_2 Levels

Pulmonary physiology regulation is directly related to carbon dioxide (CO_2) and oxygen (O_2) content in the blood, and these are critical cues to respiratory control. Hypercapnia, or elevated CO_2, significantly affects ventilatory responses. The respiratory control system employs an open-loop system under exercise as opposed to the negative feedback system under resting conditions. This model demonstrates how the body maintains homeostasis through the regulation of ventilation in response to CO_2 production and the acidity of blood. With an increase in oxygen demand during exercise comes a corresponding increase in demand for adequate CO_2 clearance, highlighting the delicate relationship between these gases in the management of respiratory dynamics (Thamrin & Murray-Smith, 2009). This physiological reaction is required to sustain energy metabolism and prevent acidosis, actions that would jeopardize muscular function and performance. Besides CO_2, oxygen too is monitored closely by peripheral and central chemoreceptors, reporting to the brainstem respiratory centers the body's status of oxygenation. Hypoxia, as a condition of decreased oxygen supply, invokes a reflexive increase in ventilation to enhance the removal of CO_2, in addition to maximizing O2 uptake. Both these modulating mechanisms are utilized not only to satisfy the current demands of metabolism but also to avoid the risk of tissue oxygen deficit and its resultant cataclysmic physiological consequences.

This control mechanism ensures that the body can dynamically adapt to varying levels of oxygen demands, particularly with exercise. Moreover, the presence of CO_2 influences the sensitivity of the chemoreceptors, binds with hemoglobin to ensure O_2 delivery in tissues, hence showing the interdependency of the gases in maintaining aerobic metabolism with exercise and lifestyle activities (Abercromby et al., 2025). The level of interaction between O_2 and CO_2 becomes more pertinent in certain environments, such as microgravity or closed spaces where oxygen levels dip and CO_2 builds up, as during extravehicular activities (EVA) for astronauts. In such conditions, understanding the threshold of CO_2 exposure is imperative to ensure cognitive and physiological function. Research has shown that responses to hypercapnia are extremely variable among different individuals, and variability renders it difficult to define standardized CO_2 exposure levels in EVA. The lack of definitive guidelines for acceptable levels also serves to emphasize the need for real-time monitoring and regulation of respiration response under such unique circumstances. Thus, gas exchange chemistry not only regulates physiological function but also determines operational procedure within environments where normal atmospheric pressure is at risk, demonstrating the pre-eminent position that chemical control has in pulmonary physiology (Abercromby et al., 2025; Thamrin & Murray-Smith, 2009) (Figure 11.15).

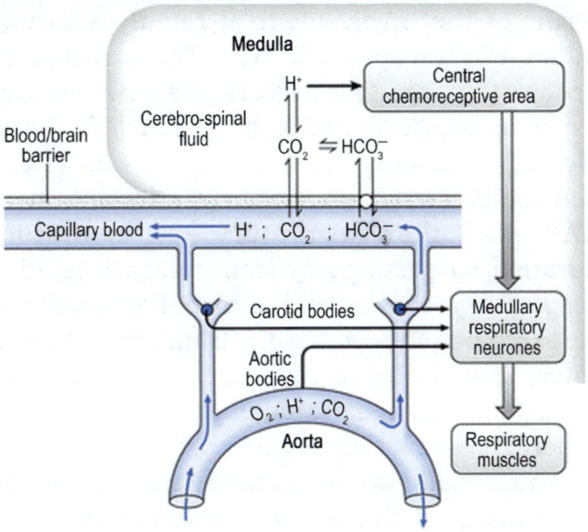

Figure 11.15. Chemical control of breathing.

Source: https://thoracickey.com/wp-content/uploads/2016/06/B9780702033704000098_gr1.jpg.

11.4.3. Reflexes and Their Impact on Breathing Patterns

Reflexes are also a key characteristic of the regulation of breathing patterns, acting as important mediators of respiration. The human respiratory system is finely tuned to react to a large number of stimuli via a network of neural pathways, including receptors in the lungs, airways, and chest wall. For instance, pulmonary stretch receptors (PSRs) monitor the degree of inflation of the lungs and give feedback to the brainstem, modulating the timing and extent of breathing. Such a feedback mechanism is important not only to maintain adequate gas exchange but also to alter respiratory patterns in different physiological states, e.g., exercise or stressors. Greater understanding of such reflex responses explains why certain modifications of respiratory patterns are feasible, particularly in pathophysiologic states when such reflexes may be deranged and thereby affect pulmonary function overall. Relationships among reflexes and respiratory patterns have been the subject of considerable investigation, particularly in terms of the involvement of rapidly adapting pulmonary receptors (RARs). These receptors are also important for triggering reflex responses , such as coughing and sighing, which facilitate airway clearance and maintain enhanced ventilation. Most importantly, stimulation of RARs can alter inspiratory and expiratory duration, suggesting a dynamic role in regulating respiratory timing and effort. For example, research has shown that RARs influence breath rates, specifically in response to irritation or during periods of elevated physical activity. The repetitive activation of these reflex pathways can potentially induce great alterations in the respiratory rhythm overall, demonstrating the significance of sensory and neural response integration to adaptive breathing mechanics (Davies et al., 2000). Understanding of the contribution of reflexes to the control of respiratory patterns extends to all areas of clinical and experimental practice, providing insight into therapeutic potential. Reflexive control impairments can cause decreased respiratory efficiency, for example, in COPD or asthma, where bronchial hyperreactivity warps the normal reflexive response. Recent research has also examined the implications of different ventilation strategies upon reflex activity to provide data on the treatment of patients with compromised pulmonary function. Besides, new techniques in the form of high-frequency ventilation illustrate the complex interaction between mechanical stimulation of the lung and the neural reflexes governing respiration. This multi-faceted approach underscores the necessity of further research in the integration of reflexes since it will certainly deliver revolutionary advancements in pulmonary rehabilitation and respiratory therapy.

Test Your Knowledge

1. Which part of the brain controls primarily the rate and depth of respiration?
2. How do chemoreceptors respond to changes in CO_2 and O_2 blood levels?

11.5. Pulmonary Function Tests (PFTs)

Learning Outcome

1. Describe the types of tests: spirometry, diffusion gas tests;
2. Define pulmonary physiology interpretation;
3. Discuss the clinical significance of pulmonary function tests.

Assessment of pulmonary function is significant in understanding respiratory physiology and in diagnosing pulmonary disorders. PFTs are a broad group of tests designed to evaluate lung volume, airflow, and gas exchange. Spirometry is a common test that measures how much air one can take in and out of their lungs. Diffusion capacity tests determine the ability of the lungs to exchange gases from inhaled air into the bloodstream.

These parameters furnish data on both obstructive and restrictive lung disease so that physicians can prepare individual treatment regimens. Lastly, PFTs not only serve as diagnostic tools but also as indicators of the severity of disease, patient responsiveness to therapy, and pulmonary function and therefore play a central role in patient management. Abnormal PFT results in children and adults can be symptomatic of an underlying disease that merits further investigation. For instance, research has indicated that children following coarctation repair exhibit considerably divergent oxygenation response compared to healthy controls, which affects exercise tolerance. It was observed in one study that peak power and oxygen uptake were substantially lower in the patients, but cerebral and muscle oxygenation response differences during incremental exercise underscore the complexity of pulmonary function tests (Vandekerckhove et al., 2019).

These findings confirm the importance of meticulous comprehension of patient physiology when applying the results of PFT. In the absence of contextualization to the health status of individual patients, it is simple for such tests to be misapplied, and treatment protocols are undermined. Furthermore, the addition of advanced imaging modalities is transforming pulmonary function testing by providing more enhanced insight into vascular and lung mechanics.

For example, investigations of pulmonary arterial tree mechanical behavior incorporate high-resolution volumetric imaging with physiological variations in arterial pressure. Such a method not only allows vessel mechanics to be characterized in a nondestructive manner but also relates these characteristics to anatomical regions of the pulmonary hierarchy (Dawson et al., 1999). These developments enhance the potential for the early detection of pathological change in pulmonary status, emphasizing the need for continuous development of PFT methods. Lastly, these developments highlight the value of pulmonary function testing, not only broadening its application to research studies in pulmonary physiology but also to clinical practice (Figure 11.16).

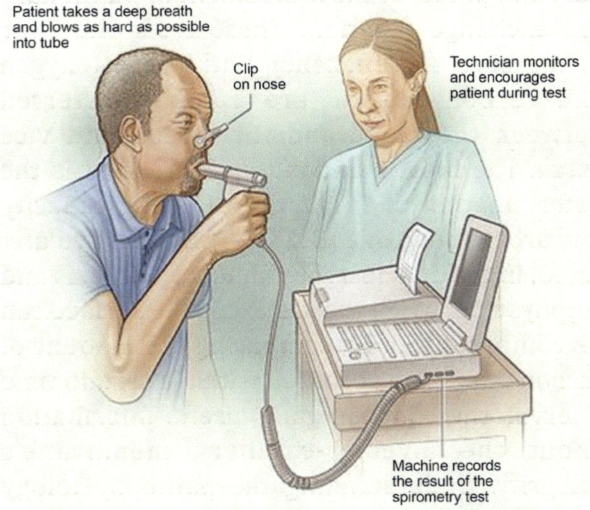

Figure 11.16. Pulmonary function test. (PFT)

Source: https://www.physio-pedia.com/images/thumb/a/a6/Spirometry1.jpg/399px-Spirometry1.jpg.

11.5.1. Types of Tests: Spirometry, Gas Diffusion Tests

Pulmonary function measurement involves a variety of tests, with one of the most frequent being spirometry. The test records forced vital capacity (FVC) and forced expiratory volume (FEV1) and provides useful information regarding lung volume and airflow obstruction. By measuring the volume of air forced out when breathing maximally, doctors can identify the existence of such conditions as COPD, asthma, COPD, and restrictive lung disease. The results are beneficial in the measurement and diagnosis of the disease process. Moreover, spirometry is quickly, easily performed and therefore is now an integral component of routine pulmonary evaluation, especially for application in outpatient settings. Comparison with normal standards by analysis of FEV1/FVC ratios allows clinicians to ascertain the severity of airway obstruction, and thus to correctly advise treatment and care for the patient. Apart from these spirometries, tests of gas diffusion are part and parcel of the assessment of pulmonary gas exchange function. These tests endeavor to measure the efficiency with which oxygen and carbon dioxide are being transferred between the blood and the alveoli and vice versa. The most mundane measurement is the determination of the lungs' diffusing capacity for carbon monoxide (DLCO). This is particularly useful in the diagnosis of pulmonary fibrosis and emphysema, when the gas exchange surface can be compromised. By comparing the amount of carbon monoxide absorbed within a certain time interval, the clinician gains useful information about the alveolar-capillary membrane's integrity. Understanding the pathophysiology of gas diffusion impairment facilitates individualized therapeutic management and ongoing evaluation of the patient, ultimately resulting in improved outcomes for patients with chronic respiratory disorders. Coupling spirometry and gas diffusion testing in clinical practice encapsulates the spectrum of pulmonary assessment. Comparison of spirometry values and gas diffusion parameters, for instance, can provide a more comprehensive overall assessment of a patient's respiratory condition. Such an approach is exemplified in the clinical setting with the use of cardiopulmonary exercise testing (CPEX), wherein ventilatory and gas exchange capacity are both assessed together with effort. This combined, multi-dimensional assessment serves not only for diagnosis of hidden pulmonary disease but for functional monitoring and pre-operative assessment in established cardiovascular patients. The mounting evidence in support of the application of these tests highlights the need for intensifying education in pulmonary physiology and its associated diagnostic techniques among medical practitioners, as they are central to providing the best possible patient care and personalized therapeutic strategies (Frenneaux et al., 2015). In addition, treatments , such as non-invasive ventilation can enhance maximal exercise capacity in patients with COPD, again emphasizing the importance of proper pulmonary assessment (Doggett et al., 2006) (Figure 11.17).

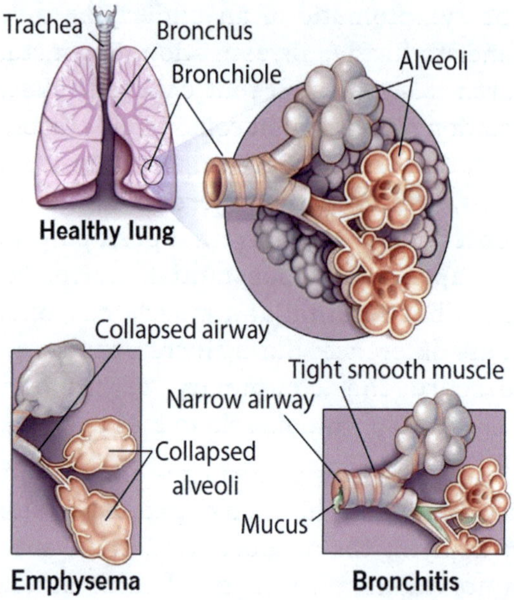

Figure 11.17. Chronic obstructive pulmonary disease (COPD): Causes, symptoms, diagnosis, treatment and prevention.

Source: https://my.clevelandclinic.org/-/scassets/images/org/health/articles/8709-copd.jpg.

11.5.2. Interpretation of Results

In pulmonary physiology, interpretation of diagnostic testing results is crucial to decipher respiratory health and disease processes. One of the key techniques employed in this field is cardiopulmonary exercise testing (CPET). With a standardized approach to CPET, clinicians are able to accurately quantify a patient's exercise tolerance and functional status, which is a key function in the diagnosis of chronic lung disease. A few studies have established that some exercise protocols yield consistent and reproducible results, particularly if they are composed of resting time and incremental work rates. In addition, the patient's perception of the usefulness of these tests underscores their potential to inform clinical practice and maximize therapeutic interventions. The concordance achieved by systematic reviews supports the premise that formalized protocols can automate the interpretive processes involved in CPET and other tests, with consequent advantages to patients (Radtke et al., 2019). In addition to exercise testing, exercise tolerance measurement and its implications in children also pose a unique aspect of interpreting results in pulmonary physiology. In a study of children following repair of coarctation, it was found that differences in oxygenation response were significant compared to normal controls and had a direct impact on exercise tolerance and capacity. The authors emphasized that decreased peak power outputs and altered oxygenated and deoxygenated hemoglobin responses signify a significant relationship between functional impairments and the physiological mechanisms involved in oxygen supply and utilization during exercise. Through a close analysis of these results, clinicians can derive crucial information about the pulmonary and systemic ramifications of congenital cardiac disease. Such a meticulous comprehension offers the intervention and monitoring strategies required for the optimization of health in the patients involved, thereby proving the importance of proper result interpretation in the clinical environment (Vandekerckhove et al., 2019). Lastly, result interpretation in pulmonary physiology is not just data analysis; it's combining clinical evidence to formulate comprehensive management plans for the patient. Both standardization of testing protocols and investigation in specific patient groups, such as children with major medical illnesses, point to a general phenomenon of pulmonary health. Its close attention to test result interpretation and understanding not only directs clinical practice but also stimulates research development. Ongoing development of methodology means that future horizons promise to include individualized test parameters tailored to each patient's profile. These advances will interpret outcomes increasingly accurate, promising improved health care outcomes for populations (Radtke et al., 2019; Vandekerckhove et al., 2019) (Figure 11.18).

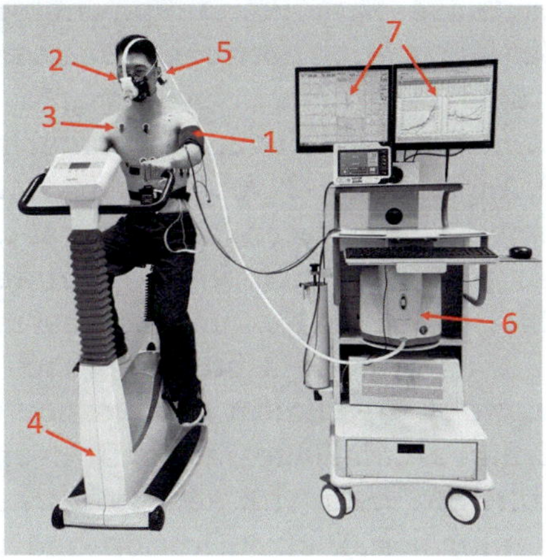

Figure 11.18. Cardiopulmonary exercise testing (CPET).

Source: https://www.researchgate.net/publication/356238804/figure/fig3/AS:1092564585324547@1637499104815/Standard-CPET-equipment-CPET-cardiopulmonary-exercise-testing-1-blood-pressure.jpg.

11.5.3. Clinical Significance of Pulmonary Function Tests (PFTs)

The clinical significance of PFTs in determining pulmonary physiology is important, as the tests perform essential assessments of lung function and the respiratory capacity. PFTs measure various pulmonary parameters, including lung volumes, rates of airflow, and effectiveness of gas exchange. Pulmonary disease diagnosis, including COPD and asthma, and determination of disease progression relies heavily on PFT data. Clinicians can create individualized treatment plans and enhance patient outcomes by monitoring parameters , such as forced expiratory volume and total lung capacity. Moreover, PFTs are also essential parts of preoperative evaluation, quantifying the risk of surgery in patients with pre-existing pulmonary disorders. In addition to diagnosis and treatment, the prognostic role of certain biomarkers of pulmonary diseases has been increasingly prominent. For example, research among patients with specific cardiovascular diseases, such as those with Fontan physiology, has shown an association between specific proteins and cardiac conditions , such as arrhythmias and pulmonary arteriovenous malformations (PAVM). Angiopoietin-2 (Ang-2) levels have been highly implicated in recent arrhythmias in these kinds of patients. Such findings underscore the utility of pairing biomarker assessment with PFTs as a multi-faceted approach to the assessment of the clinical significance of lung and cardiovascular interactions. Eventually, integrating PFT data with new biomarkers will further inform risk stratification and patient management in pulmonary medicine. Moreover, PFTs serve more than a diagnostic purpose; they are very important to assess the effectiveness of therapeutic interventions. Following lung function changes longitudinally allows the clinician to evaluate response to medication, therapeutic exercise, or lifestyle modification aimed at improving respiratory status. For example, in the reactive airway disease patient, serial PFTs can offer assurance that a treatment regimen is controlling symptoms. Regular monitoring of lung function tests can also detect reductions in respiratory status that need immediate attention. This continuous feedback system is essential not just for the management of existing pulmonary disease but also for preventing potential complications associated with respiratory worsening. Therefore, PFTs are essential in providing complete care and quality of life restoration for patients with various pulmonary diseases.

Test Your Knowledge

1. Which parameter measures the capacity of air that can be forcefully exhaled in one second (FEV1)?
2. How can PFTs make a differentiation between obstructive and restrictive lung diseases?

11.6. Common Pulmonary Disorders

Learning Outcome

1. Describe the asthma: pathophysiology and symptoms;
2. Define the chronic obstructive pulmonary disease (COPD);
3. Describe the interstitial lung diseases and their implications.

An understanding of the underlying mechanisms of common pulmonary diseases is essential in order to advance treatment methodologies and improve patient outcomes. COPD is a serious disease with persistent airflow limitation, most commonly caused by long-term exposure to harmful particles or gases, notably cigarette smoke. COPD accelerates the inflammatory response in the lung, leading to gradual deterioration of respiratory function. The patients typically develop disabling symptoms , such as chronic cough, sputum production, and dyspnea that may significantly impact their quality of life. Furthermore, new studies indicate a connection between COPD and circadian rhythm disturbance, affecting the secretion of hormones like corticosterone and serotonin—crucial for stress regulation and overall health. These endocrine disorders may further enhance the severity of mood disorders and insomnia in COPD patients, illustrating the complex relationship between pulmonary and overall wellness (Sundar et al., 2014). Asthma is another prevalent pulmonary condition, characterized by reversible airflow limitation and augmented airway responsiveness. Asthma pathophysiology involves the interplay of environmental stimuli and genetic factors, for instance, allergens, smoke, or pollution. It is characterized by repeated wheezing, shortness of breath, and chest tightness, generally exacerbated by precipitating factors. Recent studies have highlighted the role of respiratory physiology in asthma management, emphasizing the need for effective inhalation techniques and medication adherence. Additionally, respiratory pattern modulating interventions can improve balance within the autonomic nervous system, which influences heart rate rhythm and overall health (Jerath et al., 2015).

With these measures, the health professionals can enhance asthma control and significantly reduce the severity and frequency of acute exacerbations, thereby resulting in enhanced patient outcome and quality of life. Pulmonary diseases , such as pneumonia and pulmonary fibrosis are leading causes of morbidity and mortality globally. Pneumonia, an inflammation of the lung, is caused most often by infection (bacterial, viral, or fungal) and can have dire health effects if left untreated. Pneumonia presents with cough, fever, and difficulty in breathing, consistent with the impaired gas exchange due to the consolidation of the lung. In contrast, pulmonary fibrosis, resulting from the chronic scarring of lung tissue, causes permanent lung damage and limits airflow. Both conditions emphasize the importance of early diagnosis and intervention. An understanding of the associated physiological changes in the diseases, like changes in lung biomechanics and gas exchange efficiency, can assist clinicians in making targeted therapeutic regimens. By controlling such pulmonary conditions through early diagnosis and new treatment technologies, healthcare systems can remove a large percentage of individual burden and improve overall community general health (Sundar et al., 2014; Jerath et al., 2015) (Figure 11.19).

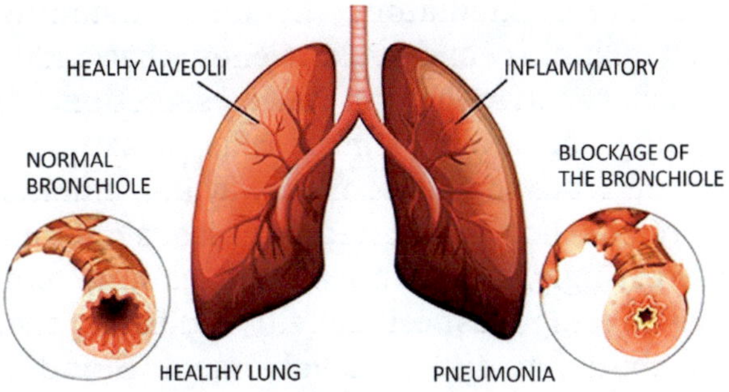

Figure 11.19. Pulmonary disorders.

Source: https://tx-hospital-blog-images.s3.ap-south-2.amazonaws.com/blogs/1743825513460-Image-showing-symptoms-of-lung-diseases.jpg.

11.6.1. Asthma: Pathophysiology and Symptoms

Asthma pathophysiology is complex, with predominantly chronic inflammation and airway hyperreactivity. Structural and functional changes in the airways result from an exaggerated immune response to environmental stimuli in this disease. Various symptoms can manifest with asthma, like wheezing, coughing, chest tightness, and dyspnea, typically exacerbated by allergens or irritants. One of the most important features of asthma is impaired cough reflex sensitivity that can lead to chronic cough as a usual symptom. Research indicates that chronic cough lasts in a high proportion of patients with asthma, from 8%–58% (Hirons et al., 2023). This highlights the importance of comprehending the multifaceted nature of the disease, as it helps identify patterns of symptoms for tailoring therapeutic interventions towards optimal patient outcomes. Identification of these symptoms is essential in evaluating asthma severity and providing effective management strategies. Mast cells play a central role in asthma pathophysiology and are powerful agents in immune modulation and inflammation of the airway. These cells, present in great numbers in the submucosa of the airway, release a broad spectrum of mediators, including histamine, prostaglandins, and leukotrienes, that induce bronchoconstriction and mucus secretion. The ongoing activation of mast cells in asthmatic patients leads to long-term airway inflammation and remodeling, manifested as disease symptoms. Interestingly, mild and severe asthma both have ongoing mast cell activity, indicating their contribution to disease development (Bradding, 2021). Understanding the mechanistic pathways of mast cell activation and the stimuli leading to their degranulation, is essential to designing targeted therapies. Exploration of such cellular behaviors has the promise to unveil new treatments that minimize symptoms through modulating the function of mast cells, basically enhancing patient quality of life. The interaction between various immune cells and inflammatory mediators makes asthma complex. In addition to mast cells, eosinophils and T-helper cells are also responsible for the inflammatory cascade that forms the basis of asthma pathology. Beyond influencing symptom severity, this dysregulation of the immune response is further involved in heterogeneity between patients, particularly when comparing different phenotypes of asthma. The divergence of T2-high and T2-low asthma also indicates the heterogeneity of the disease, with T2-high having heightened inflammatory response and eosinophil counts. Additionally, the chronicity of cough as an asthma symptom further emphasizes the need to explore chronic cough reflex hypersensitivity mechanisms more and whether or not they are associated with asthma exacerbations (Hirons et al., 2023). While sustained research unravels the intricate determinants of asthma pathophysiology, a more personalized treatment strategy is to be anticipated that will favor improved management programs based on patient-specific symptom profiles and underlying mechanisms (Figure 11.20).

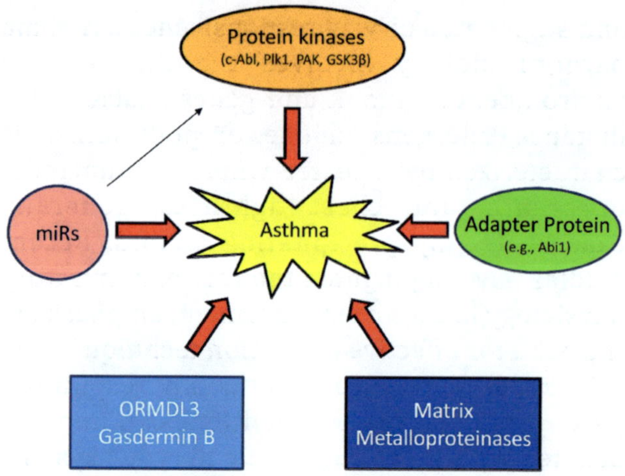

Figure 11.20. Asthma pathogenesis and biomarkers.

Source: Habib N, Pasha MA, Tang DD. Current Understanding of Asthma Pathogenesis and Biomarkers. *Cells*. 2022; 11(17):2764. https://doi.org/10.3390/cells11172764

11.6.2. Chronic Obstructive Pulmonary Disease (COPD)

COPD is a serious public health concern, characterized by chronic airway obstruction, which produces progressive respiratory disease. The pathogenesis of the condition is primarily caused by chronic exposure to toxic pollutants, with cigarette smoke being the greatest risk factor. With worsening of the disease, the condition develops classically in patients, with the presence of frequent episodes of acute exacerbations triggered by environmental triggers or infections. The physiological consequences of COPD are not confined to the lungs; it encroaches on other systemic processes, producing cardiovascular comorbidities and altering metabolic pathways. This chronic pulmonary disease tends to result in severe incapacitation of the quality of life, rendering complete management procedures that involve both the respiratory function and the systemic effects engendered by the disease absolutely essential. Ultimately, it is realizing the multifaceted character of COPD that becomes indispensable in developing personalized treatment procedures that reverse its extensive ramifications on patients' health. The pathophysiology of COPD relies on complex interactions between several systems of biology, namely the inflammatory mechanisms and airway remodeling. Noxious particle exposure triggers an abnormal inflammatory response, and this triggers immune cells and the secretion of pro-inflammatory cytokines. Persistent inflammation sets structural alterations in airways and lung parenchyma, including constricted airways, loss of alveolar elasticity, and gas exchange impairment. Along with this, COPD patients also have disrupted circadian rhythms that are further supplemented by the disease's physiological stress. Respiratory symptoms and lung function fluctuations daily illustrate the intimate relationship between respiratory health and circadian biology. As depicted by recent findings, both acute and chronic exposure to cigarette smoke has a strong impact on hormone secretion rhythms and ultimately affects sleep patterns and mood disorders in COPD patients (Sundar et al., 2014). This highlights the significance of systemic understanding of COPD in appreciating its implications beyond classical respiratory management. Exercise intolerance is a fundamental issue facing individuals with COPD, which has a great influence on their well-being and quality of life. Decreased oxygen availability to peripheral organs and muscles during exercise constitutes a central mechanism behind this constraint of exercise. Research has found that diseases , such as COPD and CHF share pathophysiological features typical of each other, which account for neuromuscular fatigue during exertion (Hirai et al., 2015). As the cardiopulmonary system is unable to match the brain and exercising skeletal muscles' metabolic requirements, patients will experience shortened physical exertion. This is particularly relevant since almost one-third of elderly patients have coexistent COPD-CHF, which is a predisposing condition for exertional symptoms. Thus, therapies that enhance oxygen delivery, such as by non-invasive ventilation with low-density gas mixtures, may be of critical significance in optimizing exercise capacity and alleviating symptoms of fatigability in this vulnerable group. Efforts to define and reverse such limitations are paramount to the enhancement of therapeutic interventions in managing COPD (Figure 11.21).

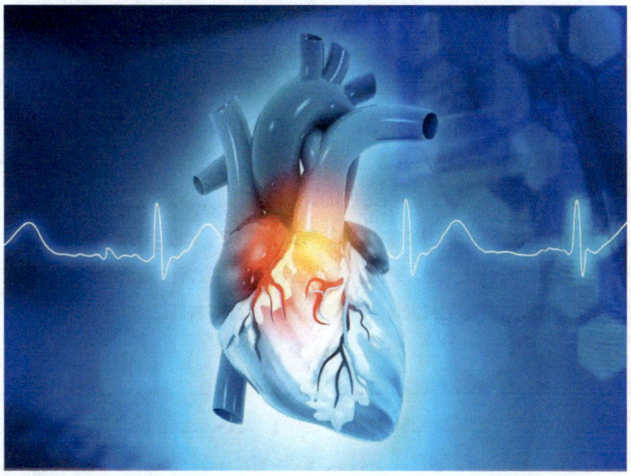

Figure 11.21. Chronic heart failure (CHF).

Source: https://etimg.etb2bimg.com/photo/94530943.cms.

11.6.3. Interstitial Lung Diseases (ILDs) and Their Impact

ILDs are a diverse group of pulmonary conditions that are characterized by inflammation and fibrosis of the lung interstitium, ultimately impairing gas exchange. The pathophysiology of such illnesses can vary, but they usually lead to increased lung stiffness and reduced lung compliance, with a major impact on pulmonary function. Due to the heterogeneity of ILDs, patients present with varying symptoms ranging from mild cough and dyspnea to end-stage respiratory failure. This variability hinders diagnosis and management as many patients present with overlapping clinical presentations and comorbidities. The progression of ILDs is more likely to result in high morbidity and mortality, and there is an acute necessity to learn about their physiological correlates and long-term effects on lung function and overall well-being. Interstitial lung disease diagnosis is often a multidisciplinary endeavor involving clinical evaluation, imaging, and in certain situations, lung biopsy to determine the underlying pathology. Clinicians are faced with the task of discriminating between various subtypes of ILDs, for example, idiopathic pulmonary fibrosis and connective tissue disease-associated ILDs. Based on recent research, the design of clinical trials must be enhanced to improve treatment modalities in ILD patients. For instance, a work group focused on connective tissue disease-associated ILD has established a consensus set of outcome measures that include lung physiology, imaging, and symptom-based patient-reported outcomes, including dyspnea and quality of life. These measurement scores have been standardized to enhance the validity and reliability of further studies on the effectiveness of ILD treatment, hence enabling enhanced patient management and care (Antoniou et al., 2013). The impact of interstitial lung diseases also extends beyond pulmonary function to the quality of life of patients. Severe psychological distress, including depression and anxiety, occurs in most ILD patients, with added chronic dyspnea and fatigue. The progressive nature of these diseases may also lead to activity and social interaction restrictions, adding to the psychological burden. Successful management of ILDs, therefore, should not only encompass pharmacotherapies but also supportive care aimed at mental health and psychosocial well-being. Interventions , such as pulmonary rehabilitation have been shown to be effective in improving physical and emotional health outcomes for ILD patients. With continuous research advancement, it remains important to consider the cumulative impact of interstitial lung disease in the framework of pulmonary physiology for better patient-focused therapy (Assaad et al., 2018).

Test Your Knowledge

1. What are the key characteristics of chronic obstructive pulmonary disease (COPD)?
2. How does asthma affect the airways and breathing?

SUMMARY

In assessing the complexity of pulmonary physiology, it is realized that the intricate interplay of structure and function is intrinsic to an understanding of a multitude of pulmonary diseases. The culmination of research gives one an understanding of how alterations in pulmonary vessel architecture might have significant pathophysiological ramifications. An understanding of this interplay enables one to develop an overall picture of disease states like pulmonary hypertension, wherein vascular remodeling has direct effects on hemodynamics. Additionally, technological advancements, as described in various studies, in imaging techniques permit profound observation of such changes at a microstructural level, permitting a better understanding of the underlying mechanisms. With pulmonary physiology as an ever-evolving field, the integration of novel technologies into traditional paradigms promises to contribute to our knowledge of dysfunctional deficits of the pulmonary system, thus allowing for the development of precision therapies. The culmination of research findings provides a guide for future research into pulmonary physiology, particularly in the context of genetic influence on vascular remodeling and hemodynamics. Varying animal model studies, including Fawn-Hooded, Sprague-Dawley, and Brown Norway rat strains, reveal significant findings regarding the genetic determinants for pulmonary disease. The suggestion that genetic heterogeneity is responsible for vascular alteration is essential for considering potential therapeutic avenues. As investigation increasingly illuminates the interplay between genetic coding and lung function, symptomatic improvement can not only be the aim of specific treatment, but also intervention on the responsible genetic basis for vascular dysregulation. This is a framework of thought that aligns with new paradigms that are moving toward individualized therapy in pulmonary disease management, incorporating genetics into standard treatment regimens. Lastly, the intersection of new imaging modalities and genetic research foretells an innovative future for pulmonary physiology, enhancing laboratory and clinical research. Certainly, there is a very strong rationale for wanting to know about the mechanical properties of remodelled pulmonary arteries because they so heavily influence therapeutic interventions in diseases , such as pulmonary hypertension. With new technologies, researchers can potentially gain a better appreciation of how structural alterations lead to functional deficits in the pulmonary circuit. As described in the recent study, such awareness can yield valuable information regarding clinical presentation of hypoxic damage and the subsequent hemodynamic alterations observed in the involved patients. Such data consolidates the rationale for interdisciplinary pulmonary healthcare founded on a sincere integration of innovative research and clinical expertise that can yield patient advantages in respiratory disease (Dawson et al., 2004; Diller et al., 2009).

To advance medical science and improve the lives of patients, an understanding of pulmonary physiology is critical. The pinnacle of this science is to conquer the challenge of imaging lungs *in vivo* during the entire respiratory cycle. The dynamic motion of lungs requires innovative techniques to minimize motion artifacts that will compromise data quality. Traditional methods , such as real-time gating through ventilation, are not the best, particularly with small animal models, in which fast rates of ventilation make image acquisition challenging. To tackle such shortfalls, researchers have looked for post-acquisition gating techniques using automated algorithms to track ventilatory phases from a series of projection images. The method of improved signal-to-noise ratio and finally produces clearer images for both the qualitative and quantitative analysis of pulmonary structures and functions, and thus supports critical physiological investigations within the discipline (Dawson et al., 2004). The evolution of protein and genomic research over the past few decades has been an essential background to the progress in pulmonary physiology. Historically, there has been a dramatic association between basic science and clinical application. There is evidence from research in the area of neonatal intensive care, for instance, that scientific study has shifted from purely clinical procedures to fundamental research that informs clinical procedures. This shift is brought to attention by the work of Comroe and Dripps, who assumed that most clinically relevant articles are the result of basic research. However, subsequent studies have cast doubt on the replicability of their findings, inferring that fewer breakthroughs are indeed the result of basic research strategies. Such dialogue is essential because it brings to the fore the necessity of reassessing funding priorities for biomedical research (Grant et al., 2010). The application of pulmonary physiology research results to clinical practice is very important for enhancing healthcare. It is important to understand how findings from basic research are converted into effective treatments and interventions. By measuring progress from early research to application within the clinical universe, stakeholders can better allocate resources to places that demonstrate clear, meaningful returns. Establishing sound methodologies by which follow-up on the value added by early research can be fairly and accurately measured lends legitimacy to the debate within the scientific community. Emphasizing an integrative approach with fundamental science knowledge in clinical practice ensures that medical progress is not only based on retrospective efficacy but also in relation to a full understanding of underlying mechanisms at the physiological level (Grant et al., 2010).

KEY TERMS FROM THIS CHAPTER

- Alveoli
- Chemoreceptors
- Diaphragm
- Hemoglobin
- Oxygen Diffusion
- Partial Pressure
- Pulmonary disorders
- Pulmonary Ventilation
- Respiratory Membrane
- Carbon Dioxide Diffusion
- Dead Space
- Gas Exchange
- Intercostal Muscles
- Oxyhemoglobin
- Pulmonary Circulation
- Pulmonary function tests
- Respiratory Control Center
- Respiratory Rate

CRITICAL THINKING QUESTIONS

1. Which muscle is primarily responsible for inspiration?

a. Internal intercostals
b. Diaphragm
c. External oblique
d. Rectus abdominis

2. Which of the following volumes is the volume of air remaining in the lungs after forced expiration?

a. Tidal volume
b. Inspiratory reserve volume
c. Residual volume
d. Expiratory reserve volume

3. The partial pressure of oxygen is highest in:

a. Pulmonary arteries
b. Alveolar air
c. Venous blood
d. Systemic veins

4. Which structure prevents food from entering the trachea during swallowing?

a. Epiglottis
b. Vocal cords
c. Bronchioles
d. Larynx

5. The process by which oxygen binds to hemoglobin is called:

a. Diffusion
b. Perfusion
c. Oxygenation
d. Oxygen saturation

Short Answer Questions

1. What is tidal volume?
2. What is residual volume in the lungs?
3. Specify the principal muscle of inspiration.
4. What is the role of alveoli?
5. Define vital capacity.
6. Explain how pulmonary circulation is different from systemic circulation.
7. Explain the effect of high altitude on pulmonary physiology.
8. Explain ventilation-perfusion matching within the lungs.

Answers to Critical Thinking Questions

1. (b); 2. (c); 3. (b); 4. (a); 5. (d)

REFERENCES

1. Abercromby, A. F. J., Bekdash, O. S., Conkin, J., Downs, J., et al. (2025). Evidence-based approach to establish space suit carbon dioxide limits. https://core.ac.uk/download/pdf/323104209.pdf (accessed on 16th June 2025).

2. Aboulhosn, J. A., Boström, K. I., Conrad, M. B., Guihard, G., et al. (2019). Angiopoietin-2 predicts morbidity in adults with Fontan physiology. https://core.ac.uk/download/323079832.pdf (accessed on 16th June 2025).

3. Radtke, T., Crook, S., Kaltsakas, G., Louvaris, Z., Berton, D., Urquhart, D. S., Kampouras, A., Rabinovich, R. A., Verges, S., Kontopidis, D., Boyd, J., Tonia, T., Langer, D., De Brandt, J., Goërtz, Y. M. J., Burtin, C., Spruit, M. A., Braeken, D. C. W., Dacha, S., Franssen, F. M. E., ... Hebestreit, H. (2019). ERS statement on standardisation of cardiopulmonary exercise testing in chronic lung diseases. *European respiratory review : an official journal of the European Respiratory Society*, *28*(154), 180101. https://doi.org/10.1183/16000617.0101-2018(accessed on 16th June 2025).

4. Sundar, I. K., Yao, H., Huang, Y., Lyda, E., Sime, P. J., Sellix, M. T., & Rahman, I. (2014). Serotonin and corticosterone rhythms in mice exposed to cigarette smoke and in patients with COPD: implication for COPD-associated neuropathogenesis. *PloS one*, *9*(2), e87999. https://doi.org/10.1371/journal.pone.0087999(accessed on 16th June 2025).

5. Antoniou, K., Baughman, R. P., Brown, K. K., Castelino, F., et al. (2013). Connective tissue disease related interstitial lung diseases and idiopathic pulmonary fibrosis: Provisional core sets of domains and instruments for use in clinical trials. https://core.ac.uk/download/77004246.pdf (accessed on 16th June 2025).

6. Assaad, S., Friedman, M. B., Kratzert, W. B., Perrino, A. C., et al. (2018). Assessment of pulmonary edema: Principles and practice. https://core.ac.uk/download/145643671.pdf (accessed on 16th June 2025).

7. Auckburally, A., & Nyman, G. (2017). Review of hypoxemia in the anaesthetized horse: Predisposing factors, consequences and management. https://core.ac.uk/download/46558350.pdf (accessed on 16th June 2025).

8. Austin, D., Benson, H., Bhargava, A., Bhattacharya, R., Bijlani, R., Brown, J., Busek, M., et al. (2006). Physiology of long pranayamic breathing: Neural respiratory elements may provide a mechanism that explains how slow deep breathing shifts the autonomic nervous system. https://core.ac.uk/download/131210060.pdf (accessed on 16th June 2025).

9. Jerath, R., Crawford, M. W., Barnes, V. A., & Harden, K. (2015). Widespread depolarization during expiration: a source of respiratory drive?. *Medical hypotheses*, *84*(1), 31–37. https://doi.org/10.1016/j.mehy.2014.11.010(accessed on 16th June 2025).

10. Vandekerckhove, K., Panzer, J., Coomans, I., Moerman, A., De Groote, K., De Wilde, H., Bové, T., François, K., De Wolf, D., & Boone, J. (2019). Different Patterns of Cerebral and Muscular Tissue Oxygenation 10 Years After Coarctation Repair. *Frontiers in physiology*, *10*, 1500. https://doi.org/10.3389/fphys.2019.01500(accessed on 16th June 2025).

11. Borrione, P., CECI GALANOS, R., Crescioli, C., Di Luigi, L., et al. (2017). Phosphodiesterase type 5 inhibitors, sport and doping. https://core.ac.uk/download/141695235.pdf (accessed on 16th June 2025).

12. Bou-Antoun, S., Cromwell, D. A., Gurol-Urganci, I., Lim, C., et al. (2013). Impact of Caesarean section on subsequent fertility: A systematic review and meta-analysis.

13. Bradding, P. (2021). Mechanisms of mast cell activation in severe asthma: Beyond IgE. *American Journal of Respiratory and Critical Care Medicine, 205*, 375–377. https://www.semanticscholar.org/paper/2c39fbcd479aefe476856ae642c42ce544a0e36d (accessed on 16th June 2025).

14. Brandes, M., Fix, L. E., Khoury, J., Linkous, J., et al. (2018). Theoretical open-loop model of respiratory mechanics in the extremely preterm infant. https://core.ac.uk/download/232207327.pdf (accessed on 16th June 2025).

15. Kelly C. (2014). Oxygen therapy: time to move on?. *Therapeutic advances in respiratory disease*, *8*(6), 191–199. https://doi.org/10.1177/1753465814549011(accessed on 16th June 2025).

16. Copot, D., Ghita, M., Ghita, M., Ionescu, C., et al. (2019). A medical information system for monitoring respiratory function and related nonlinear dynamics. https://core.ac.uk/download/322827882.pdf (accessed on 16th June 2025).

17. Dalamani, G., Kaspers, B., & Reese, S. (2006). The avian lung-associated immune system. https://core.ac.uk/download/12174987.pdf (accessed on 16th June 2025).

18. Davies, A. (2000). *Studies of Lung Function*. https://core.ac.uk/download/429712282.pdf (accessed on 16th June 2025).

19. Dawson, C. A., Haworth, S. T., Heinrich, A., Molthen, R., et al. (2004). Changes in pulmonary arterial wall mechanical properties and luminal architecture with induced vascular remodeling. https://core.ac.uk/download/213084606.pdf (accessed on 16th June 2025).

20. Dawson, C. A., Haworth, S. T., Hu, J., Molthen, R., et al. (2004). Post-acquisition small-animal respiratory gated imaging using micro cone-beam CT. https://core.ac.uk/download/213084633.pdf (accessed on 16th June 2025).

21. Dawson, C. A., Johnson, R. H., Karau, K. L., Molthen, R., et al. (1999). Quantification of pulmonary arterial wall distensibility using parameters extracted from volumetric micro-CT images. https://core.ac.uk/download/213084473.pdf (accessed on 16th June 2025).

22. Diller, G. P. (2009). Pathophysiologic correlates of exercise intolerance in adults with pulmonary hypertension and congenital heart disease. https://core.ac.uk/download/17294714.pdf (accessed on 16th June 2025).

23. Doggett, A. (2006). Effect of inspiratory pressure support on exercise performance in patients with chronic obstructive pulmonary disease. https://core.ac.uk/download/11310949.pdf (accessed on 16th June 2025).

24. Dyson, A., Audibert, G., Berne, R. M., Blitzer, M. L., Boutilier, R. G., Brown, I. P., Devlin, C., et al. (2013). The key role of nitric oxide in hypoxia: Hypoxic vasodilation and energy supply-demand matching.

25. Estrada Petrocelli, L. C., Jané Campos, R., Jolley, J., Lozano García, M., et al. (2019). Noninvasive assessment of inspiratory muscle neuromechanical coupling during inspiratory threshold loading. https://core.ac.uk/download/294829794.pdf (accessed on 16th June 2025).

26. Floros, J., López Barneo, J., Olmeda, B., Pascual Bravo, M., et al. (2014). Effect of hypoxia on lung gene expression and proteomic profile: Insights into the pulmonary surfactant response. https://core.ac.uk/download/161254450.pdf (accessed on 16th June 2025).

27. Frenneaux, M. P., Gollop, N. D., Loudon, B. L., Parasuraman, S., et al. (2015). Healthcare professional's guide to cardiopulmonary exercise testing. https://core.ac.uk/download/41992557.pdf (accessed on 16th June 2025).

28. Grant, J., Green, L., & Mason, B. (2010). From bedside to bench: Comroe and Dripps revisited. https://core.ac.uk/download/336628.pdf (accessed on 16th June 2025).

29. Hegermann, J., Kuebler, W. M., Lopez-Rodriguez, E., Matuszak, J., et al. (2020). On top of the alveolar epithelium: Surfactant and the glycocalyx. https://core.ac.uk/download/323256852.pdf (accessed on 16th June 2025).

30. Hirai, D. M., O'Donnell, D. E., Neder, J. A., Zelt, J. T. J., Jones, J. H., et al. (2015). Does impaired O_2 delivery during exercise accentuate central and peripheral fatigue in patients with coexistent COPD-CHF? https://core.ac.uk/download/37741944.pdf (accessed on 16th June 2025).

31. Hirons, B., Rhatigan, K., Kesavan, H., Turner, R., Birring, S., & Cho, P. (2023). Cough in chronic lung disease: A state-of-the-art review. *Journal of Thoracic Disease, 15*, 5823–5843. https://www.semanticscholar.org/paper/1316acf894b3a408db134b3ebf403587d39f5043 (accessed on 16th June 2025).

32. Hutchins, B. R., Brown, D., Buchwald, C., Clarke, D., et al. (2015). Descartes, corpuscles and reductionism: Mechanism and systems in Descartes' physiology. https://core.ac.uk/download/147061302.pdf (accessed on 16th June 2025).

33. Jané Campos, R., Jolley, J., Lozano, M., Moxham, J., et al. (2018). Surface mechanomyography and electromyography provide non-invasive indices of inspiratory muscle force and activation in healthy subjects. https://core.ac.uk/download/187265990.pdf (accessed on 16th June 2025).

34. King, J., Koc, H., Unterkofler, K., Mochalski, P., et al. (2003). Physiological modeling of isoprene dynamics in exhaled breath. http://arxiv.org/abs/1010.2145 (accessed on 16th June 2025).

35. Kosolosky, L., & Provijn, D. (2012). William Harvey's bloody motion: Creativity in science. https://core.ac.uk/download/11923424.pdf (accessed on 16th June 2025).

36. Miller, L., Pinkerton, K., Royer, C., Schelegle, E., et al. (2017). Nonhuman primate models of respiratory disease: Past, present, and future. https://core.ac.uk/download/323069778.pdf (accessed on 16th June 2025).

37. Thamrin, H. and Murray-Smith, D.J. (2009) A mathematical model of the human respiratory system during exercise. In: IASTED International Conference on Modelling, Simulation and Identification (MSI 2009), Beijing, China, 12-14 Oct 2009,(accessed on 16th June 2025).

38. Zuniga-Hertz, J. P., & Patel, H. H. (2019). The Evolution of Cholesterol-Rich Membrane in Oxygen Adaption: The Respiratory System as a Model. *Frontiers in physiology, 10*, 1340. https://doi.org/10.3389/fphys.2019.01340(accessed on 16th June 2025).

39. Torday J. S. (2015). Homeostasis as the Mechanism of Evolution. *Biology, 4*(3), 573–590. https://doi.org/10.3390/biology4030573(accessed on 16th June 2025).

RENAL PHYSIOLOGY: STRUCTURE AND FILTRATION

12

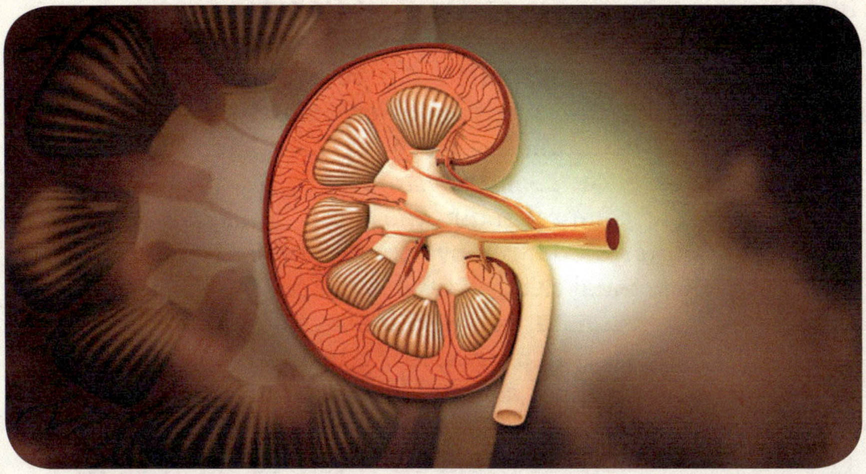

Introduction

A good understanding of renal physiology is required to explain the intricacy of kidney structure and function, particularly in relation to the filtration process. The kidneys play a key role in homeostasis through the regulation of fluid status, electrolytes, and the elimination of waste through urine secretion. This intricate process is enabled through specific structures of the nephron, the functional unit of the kidney, consisting of glomeruli, tubules, and collecting ducts. Each part of the nephron is specialized to carry out certain functions that are collectively responsible for the process of filtration and reabsorption. Additionally, the mechanism of these structures is also important for comprehending different kidney diseases and their causative mechanisms, so work needs to be done in research and discovery in the field of renal physiology. Current studies have put a focus on deciphering the mechanisms of renal pathologies, such as cystic kidney disease (CKD) and acute kidney injury. CKD affects millions of people globally and is characterized by fluid-filled cysts that develop from nephric

LEARNING OBJECTIVES

After studying this chapter, you will be able to:

1. Explain the anatomy of the kidneys;
2. Describe nephron structure;
3. Discuss glomerular filtration;
4. Emphasize tubular reabsorption;
5. Learn tubular secretion;
6. Evaluate the regulation of renal function.

tubules, highlighting cellular responses to flow and proliferation. Studies have shown that the molecular mechanisms of CKDs are not well understood, and innovative experimental models are needed to explore further. Specifically, findings suggest that the planarian excretory system demonstrates remarkable conservation with vertebrate nephrons and offers a promising model with which to study the etiology of CKDs and elucidate the evolution of kidney function. Using such models, we can deepen our knowledge of kidney structure and mechanisms of filtration in disease and health and translate this ultimately into the development of therapeutic approaches. In addition to CKDs, etiologies of acute kidney injury also demonstrate the intricate interrelationship between cell function and renal structure.

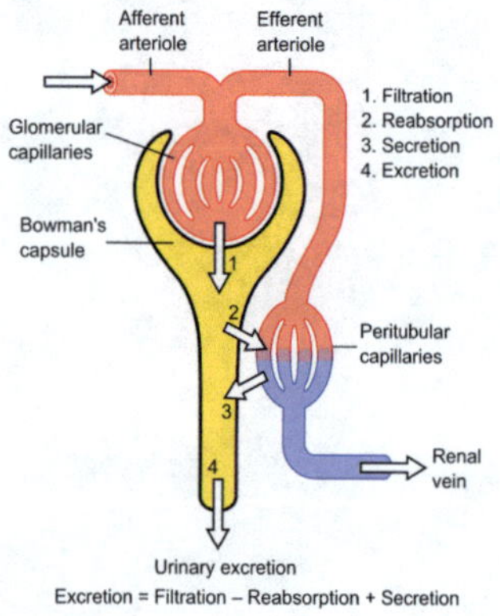

Figure 12.1. Renal physiology.

Source: https://almostadoctor.co.uk/wp-content/uploads/2017/06/Physiology_of_Nephron.png.

For example, TMIGD1 (Transmembrane immunoglobulin domain 1) has been recognized as a critical receptor that controls cell morphology and adhesion in renal epithelial cells. Its regulation is assigned significant importance when renal stress is taken into consideration because reduced expression of TMIGD1 has been correlated with increased cell death in injury models. Their identification is critical for the development of effective treatments since treatments currently are predominantly transplantation due to unfavorable responses in the acute state. The inclusion of cellular mechanisms understanding in our awareness of renal filtration mechanisms brings us closer to the big picture of kidney physiology and opens doors to future research in combating renal disease (Figure 12.1).

Definition of Renal Physiology

Renal physiology is a vital branch of research that encapsulates the complex functions of the kidneys, a pair of organs that are critical to maintaining the body in homeostasis. In essence, renal physiology is the mechanism for comprehending how the kidneys work to filter blood, remove waste products, and keep essential electrolytes in balance, thereby playing an essential role in fluid status. This intricate interplay of processes is crucial not only to toxin removal but also to blood pressure control and overall body fluid balance. Because the kidneys are always responding to various physiological states, their role is not merely a matter of simple filtration; they also serve as a primary regulator of body homeostasis and therefore, emphasize the importance of renal function in more general physiological mechanisms. Within renal physiology, it is impossible to ignore the importance of nephron anatomy and its influence on filtration and absorption. Nephrons, or the working nephron structures of the kidney, have varying segments like the glomerulus, proximal convoluted tubule, loop of Henle, distal convoluted tubule, and the collecting duct. These segments play different functions to perform together, which cumulatively assist the kidneys in filtering blood and reabsorbing the essential nutrients along with expelling the wastes. For instance, glomerular filtration is heavily reliant on podocyte integrity because damage to the specialized cells will typically lead to severe renal impairment. Recent studies indicate that urinary biomarkers of podocyte injury may be employed as prospective indicators of kidney function, demonstrating the manner in which renal physiology commingles with pathophysiologic evolution to inform practice (Sekulic et al., 2013). Besides, renal physiology knowledge has come a long further in the realm of research into the acute kidney injury (AKI), which explains the abrupt failure of the kidney commonly seen in the clinical setting. AKI, being an acute loss of kidney function within hours to days, is plagued by difficulties in treatment, and the need for new therapeutic strategies highlights this imperative. Recent research has shown that sphingolipids, and in particular sphingosine-1-phosphate (S1P) and its receptors, may be a potential future direction for therapeutic intervention in the mitigation of kidney injury (Hoffman, 2021).

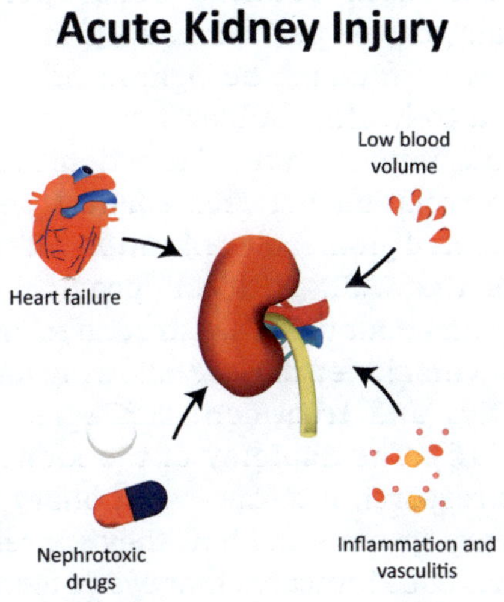

Figure 12.2. Acute-kidney-injury (AKI).

Source: https://wp04-media.cdn.ihealthspot.com/wp-content/uploads/sites/464/2024/08/Acute-Kidney-Injury-1.jpg.

The relationship between renal physiology and AKI is also used to highlight the dynamic nature of renal function, together with the requirement for increased knowledge of the attendant underlying biological processes that regulate renal health and disease. As continuous studies uncover the intricate interactions in renal physiology, it becomes increasingly evident that maintaining kidney function is pivotal in overall body function (Figure 12.2).

Importance of the Kidneys in Homeostasis

The kidneys contribute significantly to maintaining homeostasis in the body through various mechanisms, primarily by regulating the composition and volume of body fluids. They do this through the complex processes of filtration, reabsorption, and secretion that maintain the balance of electrolytes, salts, and waste products. The nephron, the functional unit of the kidney, is specifically engineered to facilitate this, consisting of a glomerulus for filtering and a variety of tubules for metabolizing the filtrate. This intricate architecture allows the kidneys to react appropriately to physiological changes, such as changes in hydration status or electrolyte status, and thus maintain a stable internal environment necessary for cell functioning. Without this renal homeostatic property, such imbalances may develop and lead to disorders , such as dehydration or electrolyte imbalance, underlining the kidneys' invaluable contribution to homeostasis. Apart from fluid and electrolyte balance, the kidneys also play a role in acid-base balance for maintaining normal physiological processes. The kidneys manage the blood pH range by reabsorbing bicarbonate and secreting hydrogen ions selectively, which is vital for enzymatic reactions and metabolic processes. This acid-base regulation of the kidneys has a direct impact on other organ systems, namely the respiratory and cardiovascular systems, necessitating an interdependent response to maintain overall homeostasis. Moreover, the kidneys dynamically regulate in response to fluctuations in dietary intake and metabolic demand, demonstrating flexibility and importance in physiological control. The outcome of renal impairment can thus be severe, inducing acidosis or alkalosis, in order to once again emphasize the role of the kidneys in ensuring metabolic balance and overall health. Continuous research continues to uncover the complexities of renal physiology, especially in the role of kidney impairment in systemic homeostasis. Recent advances highlight the need to find new ways to preserve renal viability and function, particularly in situations like organ transplantation. For instance, recent findings highlight the importance of the renal vasculature in maintaining homeostasis and the general well-being of the renal apparatus. Injury to the endothelium can initiate a series of interruptions in renal function and systemic balance. Therefore, enhancing pre-transplant evaluation methodologies and the pathophysiology of the renal vasculature are increasingly essential. These efforts highlight not only the kidney's central role in homeostasis but also the need for ongoing research to enhance understanding and the treatment of renal disease, eventually to be of utility to healthcare (Vu et al., 2015; Pamplona et al., 2023).

12.1. Anatomy of the Kidneys

Learning Outcome

1. Explain the location and size of the kidneys;
2. Point out outer structure: renal capsule and hilum;
3. Teach the inner structure: renal cortex and medulla.

The kidneys are critical organs with important functions , such as filtration, excretion of waste products, and maintenance of fluid balance. Structure-wise, one kidney is divided into three main areas: the cortex, the medulla, and the pelvis. The renal cortex, the outer portion, is where nephrons, the functional units of the kidney, responsible for blood filtration and urine production, are housed. A nephron has a glomerulus, where the blood is filtered, and a tubule, where reabsorption and secretion occur. The medulla, under the cortex, consists of renal pyramids that house collecting ducts and loop of Henle segments, which play a role in urine concentration. The renal pelvis is the urine drain funnel from the kidney to the ureter. Understanding this anatomy is essential in learning the complex mechanism of renal physiology and structure and their role in filtration processes. Another sophisticated technique utilized to ascertain kidney function and structure is Arterial Spin Labeling (ASL) MRI, which quantitates renal perfusion in the absence of contrast agents. ASL MRI studies have proved unique kidney physiology differences between healthy humans and patients with chronic kidney disease (CKD). Results have indicated that CKD patients possess increased T1 relaxation times, which indicate structural alterations with reduced renal perfusion. Specifically, cortex perfusion levels among CKD patients were found to be significantly reduced compared to healthy subjects, reflecting CKD's deleterious impact on renal function. Moreover, a high correlation between cortical perfusion and estimated glomerular filtration rate (eGFR) suggests that ASL MRI can provide critical information about the renal structures' health in patients with kidney disease, allowing for better diagnostics and treatment strategies (Delles et al., 2016). The anatomy of the kidneys also involves research into the evolutionary history of excretory systems and how they are related to CKDs. Evidence indicates that cystic formations arise due to nephric tubule developmental abnormalities, a sign of profound dysregulation of cellular processes, e.g., proliferation and perception of flow. Ironically, comparisons between vertebrate nephrons and planarian excretory systems reveal a conserved process with ultrafiltration and modification of flow. Moreover, genetic manipulation in planarians has created phenotypes that are similar to human CKDs, establishing them as novel models for the verification of underlying pathophysiological mechanisms. This evolutionary perspective highlights the importance of structural conservation between species, facilitating a better understanding of renal physiology and relevant studies in human kidney disease (Vu et al., 2015) (Figure 12.3).

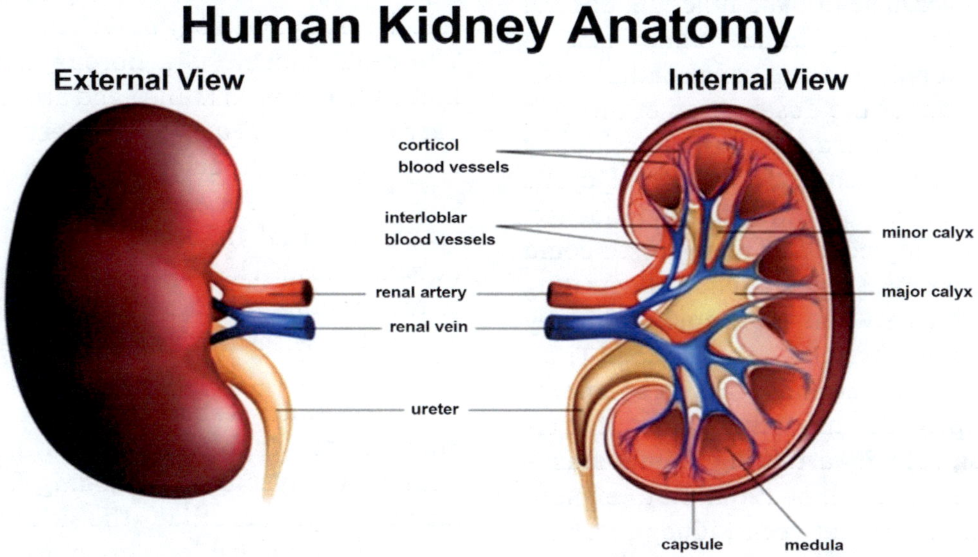

Figure 12.3. Anatomy of the kidneys.

Source: https://www.news-medical.net/image-handler/picture/2018/10/shutterstock_1027902178.jpg.

12.1.1. Location and Size of the Kidneys

The kidneys, the vital components of the renal apparatus, are located strategically in the posterior part of the abdominal cavity, i.e., retroperitoneal to peritoneum. This position allows for efficient filtering of the blood but is minimal in the way of injury from external forces. The left kidney is typically a bit higher than the right, a consequence of the liver mass occupying space on the right. The kidneys are about 11–14 cm in length, 6 cm in width, and about 4 cm in thickness, bean-shaped. Their size not only facilitates their function of filtering the blood but also sustains a balance necessary for nephron adjustment with changes in body needs or environmental conditions. This anatomical design accentuates the evolutionary specializations of the kidneys to achieve maximum function under varying physiological conditions (Natochin et al., 1996). Their comparative size to body weight reflects the significance of the kidneys in maintaining homeostasis. Each kidney contains around one million nephrons, functional units responsible for filtration as well as electrolyte, water, and waste product balance. Because the kidneys are so vital, their size ensures sufficient surface area for glomerular filtration according to the body's overall anatomy. The dense compactness of the kidney is important in ensuring proper blood supply, and it is supplied with about 20%–25% of cardiac output. This enhanced blood supply allows the kidneys to effectively filter enormous volumes of blood, maintain fluid balance, and regulate blood pressure through renin-angiotensin mechanisms. The renal flexibility to size and position also highlights its evolutionary adaptation so that organisms may respond better to a range of environmental stresses (Musacchia, 1972). In addition, kidney size also becomes an indicator of overall health and function. Clinical assessments frequently utilize kidney size as a parameter for diagnosing renal pathologies. For example, under the observation of imaging techniques like ultrasound, irregular kidney size could reflect diseases , such as polycystic kidney disease or chronic kidney disease. Both underdevelopment and overgrowth could severely compromise renal function, illustrating the connection between morphologic kidney appearance and physiological function. Thus, understanding the anatomical measurements of the kidneys provides us with a sense of their fundamental role in attaining homeostasis. Additional research will be required to explore the interrelatedness between kidney location, size, and evolutionary adjustment to fully detail how these account for renal physiology and wellbeing (Natochin et al., 1996) (Figure 12.4).

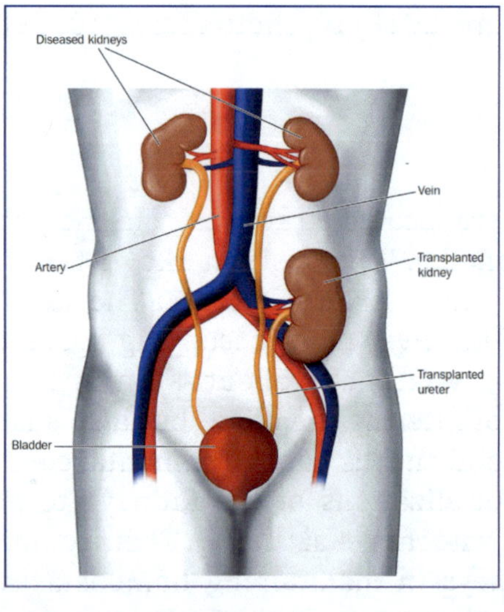

Figure 12.4. Location and size of the kidneys.

Source: https://www.researchgate.net/profile/Fiona-Murphy-7/publication/6260322/figure/fig1/AS:830239500406786@1574955930999/Location-of-the-trasplanted-kidney.png.

12.1.2. External Structure: Renal Capsule and Hilum

The external kidney anatomy is made up of functional components, which are the renal capsule and the hilum, and they both play a vital role in renal physiology as well as renal function. The renal capsule is a fibrous, hard covering that envelops each kidney and acts as a physical barrier to trauma as well as infection. This tight connective tissue structure is responsible not only for the preservation of the shape but also as an essential first defense line against the outside world. The capsule resilience is crucial to the kidneys' tolerance of pressure variations associated with urine production and storage, and thus the nephron's function is maintained constant under varying physiological states. Further, the involvement of renal capsules within the layer of surrounding fat and renal fascia helps stabilize the kidneys within the abdominal cavity and place themselves optimally for efficient filtration. Adjoining the renal capsule is the hilum, a significant kidney anatomical structure through which vital vessels and structures enter and exit. The hilum is the window through which the renal artery, renal vein, ureter, lymphatics, and nerve structures pass, signifying the course through which there is blood supply and drainage. The area is significant in that it serves to ensure that the kidney is adequately supplied with oxygen and nutrients and efficiently eliminates toxins and metabolic end-products. The complexity of structuring within the hilum serves to underscore the kidneys' multifunctional nature in physiological homeostasis because it orchestrates the mixing of urinary and vascular functions. The organization and structure of the hilum are vital because their disruption could initiate significant renal health and functionality complications. Appreciation of the interaction between the capsule and renal hilum is essential to understanding the broader concepts of renal physiology, particularly related to processes of filtration. In addition to securing the renal structure, the capsule also assists the kidneys in resisting and adapting to the variable pressures that come with filtration. With well-controlled renal blood flow and glomerular filtration rates, the hilum's role becomes essential in allowing these processes. Furthermore, the advancement in imaging techniques, like the ones explained in research comparing CT-based methods of assessing renal function, further justifies the importance of these extrinsic structures in clinical evaluation (Siddarth et al., 2014). A proper understanding of the renal hilum and capsule not only educates anatomic knowledge but also clinical practice in renal diseases and transplant planning, further justifying their importance in disease and health (Figure 12.5).

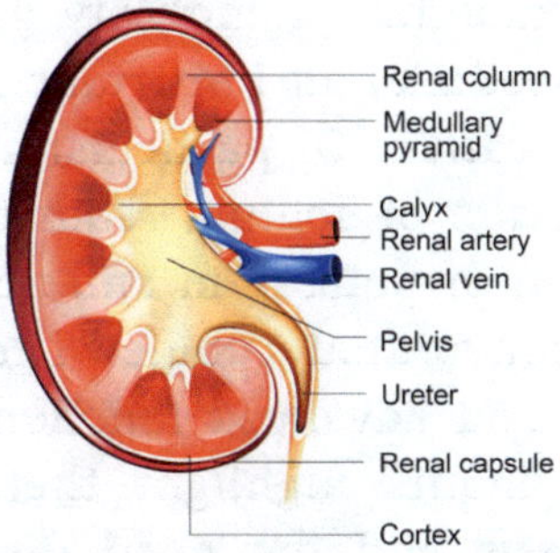

Figure 12.5. External and internal features of the kidney.

Source: https://cdn1.byjus.com/wp-content/uploads/2022/06/kidney-diagram.png.

12.1.3. Internal Structure: Renal Cortex and Medulla

The intricate internal architecture of the kidneys is divided into two broad categories: the renal cortex and the renal medulla, which both play significant roles in renal physiology and the filtration process. The renal cortex, being the outer layer of the kidney, is packed with numerous renal corpuscles, where blood filtration begins. These corpuscles contain glomeruli and Bowman's capsules. Their cortices are rich with nephrons, the kidney's functional units, through which the first filtration step and reabsorption of essential elements like glucose, ions, and water are facilitated. Importantly, the cortex also contains a significant number of peritubular capillaries that aid in solute and fluid transfer, thereby facilitating homeostasis in the body's internal environment. Understanding these features of the renal cortex is crucial to learning about how the kidneys drain blood and are part of other physiological functions. The renal medulla, however, is responsible for concentrating urine and regulating the body's fluid balance. It consists of renal pyramids, which contain the loops of Henle and collecting ducts. These renal structures are organized to attain peak concentration efficiency for urine concentration through a process called countercurrent multiplication in which the renal medulla-generated osmotic gradient facilitates water reabsorption from collecting ducts. This inner special anatomy allows the kidneys to produce urine several times more concentrated than plasma, an important function to maintain the body's hydration status. The interaction of the medullary structures with the endocrine control, such as the antidiuretic hormone (ADH), is essential for the kidney's ability to adapt to varying fluid intake situations. As stressed in studies, medullary lesions can result in severe pathophysiologic states of renal and overall health (Keith et al., 1994). The renal cortex-medulla interaction describes the kidneys' sophisticated filtration and regulatory processes. Abnormality in both regions can cause pathological processes like autosomal dominant polycystic kidney disease (ADPKD) or other renal dysfunctions that disrupt normal mechanisms of filtration. To make a point, in ADPKD, studies have found that impaired medullary trapping of ammonia aggravates acid-base disturbances, highlighting the renal medulla's contribution to the kidney's overall health (Keith et al., 1994). Furthermore, studies on renal physiology, e.g., the role of the cortex and the medulla, are utilized to further cement the necessity of sound educational materials within the field. This information is essential for both medical students and healthcare professionals as they prepare to handle complex renal diseases efficiently using evidence-based and knowledge-centered approaches.

Test Your Knowledge

1. What are the three major regions of the kidney?
2. Where are the renal cortex and renal medulla?

12.2. Nephron Structure

Learning Outcome

1. Outline the function of nephrons;
2. Outline nephron structure: glomerulus and tubules;
3. Understand nephron types: cortical and juxtamedullary.

The nephron, the kidney's fundamental structural and functional unit, is beautifully crafted to enable the vital processes of filtration, reabsorption, and secretion. A renal corpuscle and a renal tubule, each nephron consists of these two units, which together work to control blood composition and volume. The renal corpuscle is made up of the glomerulus, a tuft of capillaries that filters blood effectively, and the Bowman's capsule, which encloses the glomerulus and contains the resulting filtrate.

This initial filtration step is important because it will determine the composition of urine and enable the discharge of waste products. Nephron morphology is essential to understand when interpreting renal physiology, as modifications to any of these elements can have great effects on renal function and overall well-being, making it worth examining nephron pathology in disease states , such as chronic kidney disease and hypertension within the overall framework of renal filtration. As the filtrate goes on from the renal corpuscle to the renal tubule, it is heavily altered by three important segments: the proximal convoluted tubule (PCT), the loop of Henle, and the distal convoluted tubule (DCT). The PCT is tasked with reabsorbing the majority of the filtrate's sodium, chloride, and water, thereby preventing excessive loss of essential substances. Next, the loop of Henle is employed to concentrate urine further and maintain osmolarity gradients in the kidney medulla, an important function in water conservation. Of particular importance is the regulation of sodium reabsorption and the regulation of potassium and acid-base by the distal convoluted tubule. The intricate architecture and advanced functions of these nephron segments highlight their function in homeostasis and the need for extensive research on how their malfunction results in such conditions as hypertension, where aberrant sodium handling can be observed (Graham et al., 2017). Moreover, our advancing knowledge on nephron structure has provided significant information regarding varied kidney diseases, such as CKDs. It has been confirmed by science that the pathological characteristics of CKDs, in which water-filled cysts result from defective cellular mechanisms, share mechanistic properties with the nephron structure. Structural function conservation across species, illustrated by the comparison between vertebrate nephrons and less complex invertebrate systems, indicates a shared evolutionary origin that affirms our insight into nephron dysfunction in human disease (Vu et al., 2015). These findings identify the need for more research into the nephron structural integrity and how it relates to kidney well-being, identifying the need for cross-disciplinary investigation that crosses molecular biology, physiology, and clinical sciences in finding useful cures for kidney disease (Figure 12.6).

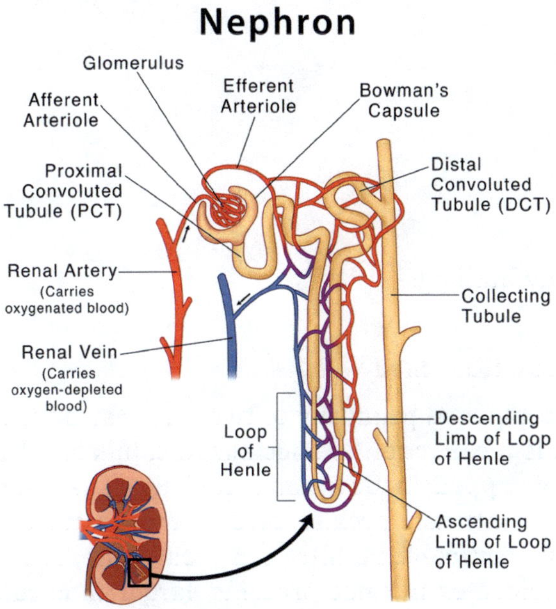

Figure 12.6. Nephron structure.

Source: https://classnotes123.com/wp-content/uploads/2022/06/Nephron-diagram-Class-10-983x1024.jpg.

12.2.1. Definition and Function of Nephrons

Nephrons, the functional units of the kidney, are tasked with attaining homeostasis by virtue of filtration, reabsorption, and secretion. The kidney contains a population of approximately one million nephrons, structured intricately to allow efficient filtration of blood and elimination of wastes. The nephron is structured into various segments like the glomerulus, proximal tubule, loop of Henle, distal tubule, and collecting duct, each playing unique roles in the composition of urine. The glomerulus accomplishes the initial filtration of the blood, during which water, ions, and small molecules are filtered and larger proteins and cells remain in the blood. The unique structure bears witness to the nephron's ingenious design for effective renal physiology regulation. Nephrons not only serve the function of simple filtration; they also ensure the electrolyte balance, fluid composition, and acid-base state of the body. Through reabsorption and secretion, nephrons control the concentration of various solutes, such as sodium, potassium, and bicarbonate, according to the body's needs. For instance, in the tubule of the proximal part, almost 65% of the sodium and water filtered are reabsorbed, essential to ensure blood pressure and overall fluid balance. When blood is traveling through the nephron, further changes occur in the loop of Henle and the distal tubule that more precisely regulate the composition of urine. This complex regulation shows how the nephrons are essential routes for the excretion of metabolic waste along with homeostatic equilibrium. Nephron function is also associated with renal autoregulation mechanisms that offer stable renal blood flow, required in maintaining their filtering capacity. Renal perfusion is regulated by myogenic responses and tubuloglomerular feedback, which are crucial to counteract varying systemic blood pressures. These mechanisms not only maintain the rate of filtration when there is a fluctuation in blood pressure levels but also detect the dynamic interaction between nephrons and their vascular supply. Mathematical models have been applied in recent studies to analyze these autoregulatory mechanisms and discovered them to be intricate and oscillatory under certain conditions in renal function, as published in Arciero et al. (2015). Knowledge of these mechanisms has clinical relevance, particularly in conditions like Acute Kidney Injury (AKI), where there is dysfunction of the nephrons, pointing to the significance of targeting some pathways for therapeutic development, as reported in Hoffman (2021) (Figure 12.7).

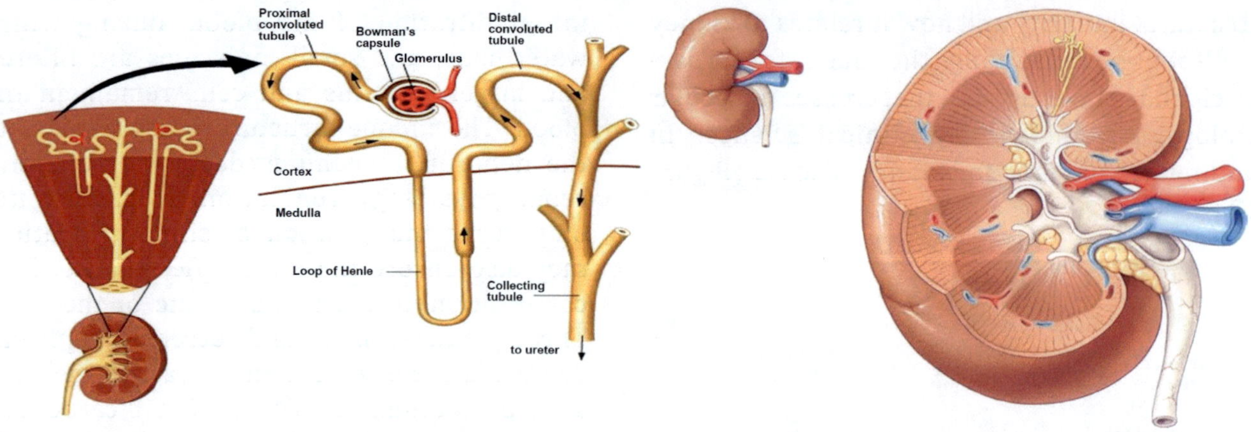

Figure 12.7. Functions of nephrons.

Source: https://i.ytimg.com/vi/fhRJmc4JHwU/maxresdefault.jpg.

12.2.2. Components of the Nephron: Glomerulus and Tubules

The nephron, or basic functional unit of the kidney, is composed primarily of two major structures: the renal tubules and the glomerulus. The glomerulus is a collection of specialized capillaries that carries out the initial process of filtration of blood. Wrapped in Bowman's capsule, it is where blood gets filtered from the body into the kidney. The intrinsic architecture of the glomerulus, which contains very permeable endothelial cells and a characteristic filtration membrane, is such that the selective passage of water, ions, and small molecules but not proteins, larger molecules into the filtrate is enabled. This efficient filtration process is crucial, as it regulates the balance of fluids and electrolytes in the body and removes waste and toxins from blood, ultimately influencing the homeostasis as a whole (Speck, 2020). The resultant fluid, now referred to as tubular fluid, moves into the renal tubules, which comprise the proximal convoluted tubule, the loop of Henle, and the distal convoluted tubule. Each segment of the tubule has a distinct role to play in the reabsorption and secretion of substances. The proximal convoluted tubule, for example, reabsorbs nearly 65% of filtered sodium, water, and other solutes, while the loop of Henle establishes a concentration gradient that is essential to the kidney's capacity to concentrate the urine. The distal convoluted tubule fine-tunes electrolyte balance even more and responds to hormonal signals , such as aldosterone. The form and function of the tubules are responsible for the kidneys' ability to respond to changed states of physiology and homeostasis (Andersson et al., 2014). In addition to each serving their distinct function, the renal tubules and glomerulus collaborate to serve as an integrated filtration system. The interface between filtration and reabsorption is regulated by several physiological mechanisms that respond to the body's need. The system more and more comes at center stage in the scenario of increasing numbers of chronic kidney diseases, where glomerular damage is the chief contributor to renal damage. Clarification of cellular and molecular processes of glomerular filtration and tubular reabsorption forms the foundation for the initiation of efficient therapeutic interventions in chronic kidney disease and other nephropathies. Hence, learning about the components of the nephron not only increases our understanding of kidney physiology but also brings into perspective the intricacy of kidney function and the significance of its contribution to overall health in the body (Andersson et al., 2014; Speck, 2020) (Figure 12.8).

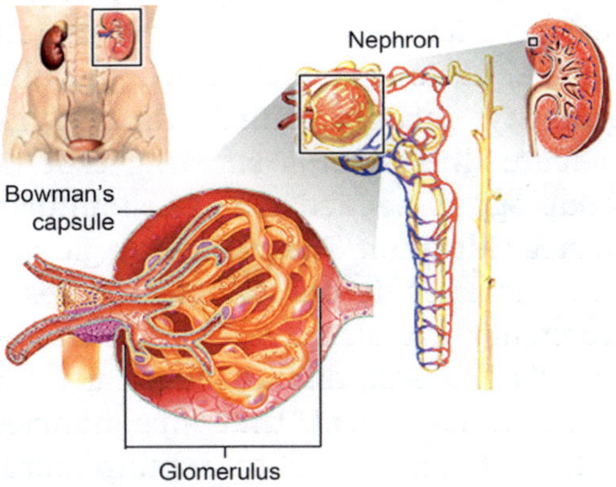

Figure 12.8. Glomerulus and nephron.

Source: https://medlineplus.gov/ency/images/ency/fullsize/24353.jpg.

12.2.3. Types of Nephrons: Cortical Versus Juxtamedullary

The human kidney has two primary types of nephrons: cortical nephrons and juxtamedullary nephrons, each with distinct structural and functional characteristics. Cortical nephrons, constituting approximately 85% of all nephrons, are found primarily in the renal cortex. These nephrons have short loops of Henle that extend only a limited distance into the medulla. Their primary role is to allow the filtering of blood and the removal of waste substances while also being involved in the regulation of body water and electrolyte balance. Although cortical nephrons are very critical to general renal function, they are less involved in urine concentration than the juxtamedullary ones that are crucial in more specialized renal function. On the other hand, juxtamedullary nephrons are for the kidney's ability to concentrate urine. These nephrons occur close to the renal medulla and contain longer loops of Henle that penetrate deep within the medulla. The unique structural pattern of the juxtamedullary nephrons facilitates them in creating a concentration gradient required for the reabsorption of water. The osmotic pressure generated in the medullary space, in which the Henle loops exist, enables effective recovery of water back into the circulation. This function testifies to their importance, especially in dehydration or during periods of limited fluid intake when the body must conserve water. As such, juxtamedullary nephrons are important in maintaining homeostasis, especially during unfavorable physiological conditions. The differences in functioning between cortical and juxtamedullary nephrons reveal their complementary role in the renal system. While cortical nephrons deal with ordinary day-to-day waste filtration and electrolyte balance, the juxtamedullary nephrons have an extremely vital role in concentrating urine through making use of the renal medulla's steep osmotic gradient. This complementarity between the two nephrons is essential for the best renal functioning, particularly in adapting to varying physiological demands. It is imperative to appreciate the variations because they inform us of nephron capability and the renal general efficacy in maintaining fluid and electrolyte homeostasis. Studying these adaptations may also help us learn about renal pathologies, hence the types of nephrons becoming a vital component of renal physiology and related medical sciences, and therefore how much more research is required in this area (Jamison et al., 1987; Stadt, 2022).

Test Your Knowledge

1. What are the two major parts of the nephron?
2. What nephron structure is given the task of filtration of blood?

12.3. Glomerular Filtration

Learning Outcome

1. Explain the mechanism of filtration of the glomerulus;
2. Define determinants of glomerular filtration rate (GFR);
3. Explain the role of the filtration barrier.

The mechanism of glomerular filtration is the cornerstone of renal physiology, enabling the kidneys to efficiently filter blood and maintain homeostasis. This is a process that takes place in the glomeruli, specialized nephron structures where blood plasma is filtered into the Bowman's capsule. The main determinants of GFR are blood pressure, the permeability of the glomerular membrane, and the filtration surface area. The peculiar structure of glomerular capillaries featuring fenestrations and a negatively charged basement membrane permits size and charge-selective filtration. It is crucial to recognize the regulatory processes and pathways of glomerular filtration for effective diagnosis and treatment of various renal diseases. More specifically, accurate measurement of GFR is central to assessing renal function and determining kidney disease progression, as the implication is that accurate eGFR equations are critical in clinical practice (Kirwan et al., 2013). In the critically ill patient, the estimation of glomerular filtration must be interpreted with caution because renal function varies significantly. Standard eGFR equations, for instance, those applied using serum creatinine, may not be the best measurement of acute changes in kidney function, particularly in cases of AKI. It has been demonstrated that although these equations carry some data regarding renal function, their accuracy is lower in such a group of patients. For instance, studies reveal that including such markers as cystatin C would refine the accuracy of estimated GFR, offering a potentially more precise measurement of renal function (Kirwan et al., 2013). However, current clinical practice demonstrates the limitations of such equations, which were initially set to quantify chronic kidney disease rather than acute illness, thus showing that better methodology is needed for live monitoring of glomerular filtration. The changes in glomerular filtration in specific physiological states, such as pregnancy, are also worthy of investigation to unravel the adaptability of renal function. Investigations reveal that pregnancies at term have been shown to exhibit increased glomerular filtration rates compared with those in non-pregnant women owing to systemic hemodynamic adaptations and plasma volume expansion. However, in preeclampsia, glomerular filtration is further impaired by glomerular and functional changes in the kidneys, such as glomerular endotheliosis. These observations underscore the value of employing cystatin C as a biomarker indicating both structural and functional changes in the kidneys in pregnancy. Such findings are important in the differentiation between physiological adaptive responses and pathological conditions, thereby informing clinical strategies towards monitoring and managing risks of renal complications during pregnancy (Figure 12.9).

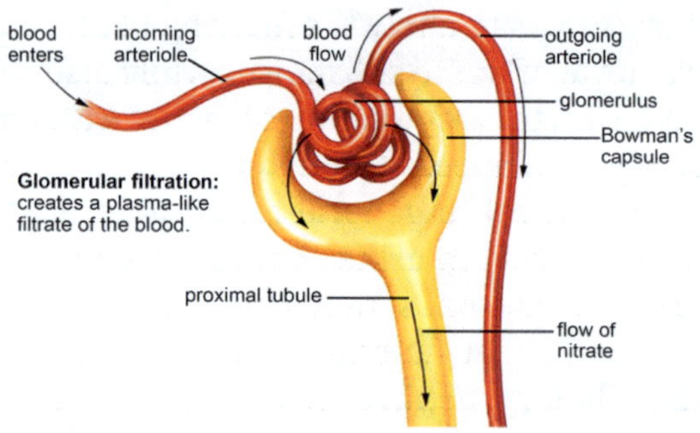

Figure 12.9. Glomerular filtration.

Source: https://4.bp.blogspot.com/-j_kDNHm-ZNQ/ULjhGK7XvXI/AAAAAAAAAOI/Z0VPb4zXJc4/s1600/path-of-urine-formation-i10.jpg.

12.3.1. Mechanism of Filtration in the Glomerulus

The glomerulus is the initial location of the process of filtration in the renal physiology system and is a critical component of the separation of blood constituents based on size and charge. Located within Bowman's capsule, the glomerulus is a network of capillaries which by nature are permeable to water, ions, and small solutes but not to larger molecules , such as proteins and blood cells. The three principal barriers to such selective filtration include the fenestrated endothelium of glomerular capillaries, the glomerular basement membrane, and the podocytes lining the capillaries. Each of these structures is crucial to the integrity of the filtration barrier and to permitting only the proper substances into the renal tubules for future processing. The dynamics of filtration pressure are critical to glomerular function, since it is sustained by hydrostatic and oncotic forces. This ultrafiltration is regulated primarily by hydrostatic blood pressure within the glomerular capillaries, which is resisted by osmotic blood pressure caused by plasma proteins. As the blood traverses the glomerulus, the elevated hydrostatic pressure drives water and solutes into the Bowman's capsule, where they are known as filtrate. GFR is a critical indicator of renal function and is typically preserved by mechanisms , such as autoregulation and hormonal regulation, e.g., the renin-angiotensin-aldosterone system. These regulatory pathways regulate response to changes in systemic blood pressure and volume, thus ensuring uniform filtration efficacy. The glomerulus itself is not merely a passive filter; it actively participates in renal homeostasis and metabolism. For instance, the presence of specialized transporters in the proximal tubule , such as sodium-glucose cotransporters SGLT1 and SGLT2, indicates the importance of reabsorption mechanisms in maintaining glucose homeostasis. Surprisingly, a study reveals that knockout mice lacking these transporters result in hyperglycemia due to excessive loss of glucose in urine, indicating their role in preventing glucose excretion (Ghezzi et al., 2018). Alongside, ongoing research on the understanding of glomerular function has identified several genes with specific mRNA expressions critical for structural stability and vulnerability to disease, shedding light on conditions like diabetic nephropathy (Anders et al., 2010). This knowledge sheds light on the complex interplay between mechanisms of filtration and renal integrity and provides an avenue to potential therapeutic advances (Figure 12.10).

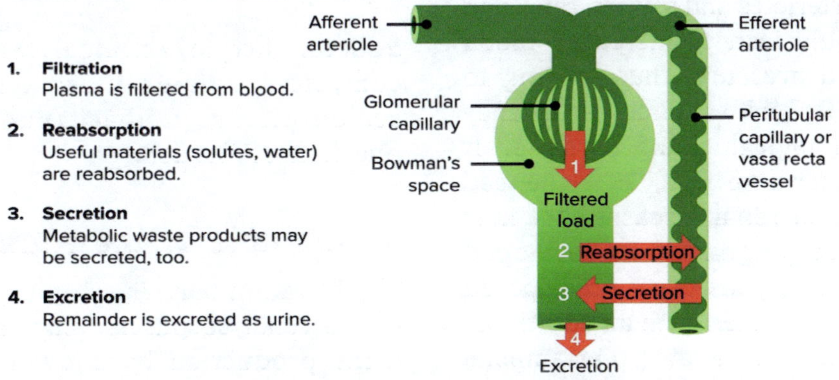

Figure 12.10. Primary-renal-functions.

Source: https://cdn.lecturio.com/assets/Primary-renal-functions.jpg.

12.3.2. Factors Affecting Glomerular Filtration Rate (GFR)

The GFR is a crucial measure of renal function, which is open to the influences of many physiological and pathological variables. One of the determining factors of GFR is renal blood flow, which is determined by the fine balance between efferent and afferent arteriolar resistance. Systemic blood pressure can also profoundly affect glomerular perfusion; for instance, elevated mean arterial pressure (MAP) tends to support increased GFR through more effective glomerular filtration. In other research, low birth weight was linked to hypertension and renal insufficiency, indicating that conditions in the womb also contribute to long-term regulation of the GFR. More specifically, individuals who have had low birth weight tend to have lower numbers of nephrons, which can lead to hypertension and lowered GFR in later life, indicating how early development affects kidney function (Daniels et al., 2015). Yet another important determinant of GFR is the hormonal regulation of renal activity, particularly by substances , such as renin, angiotensin, and aldosterone. These hormones play a considerable role in the control of renal blood flow as well as in the filtering process. For example, the renin-angiotensin system (RAS) is responsible for regulating both resistance in the arterioles and sodium retention and activation could lead to increased blood volume and blood pressure, thus leading to an increase in GFR. Besides, under pregnancy conditions, physiological changes render it challenging to determine GFR, as evidenced by the occurrence of renal diseases that may be dormant before pregnancy. In developed countries, chronic kidney disease is predisposed to occur in pregnant women with an additional layer of conditions , such as preeclampsia, which distorts renal physiology and should be managed by appropriate monitoring of GFR with reliable instruments (Noto, 2020). In addition to blood perfusion and hormonal regulation, native kidney function is essential in the regulation of an optimal GFR. Pathologies , such as glomerulonephritis or CKD can severely compromise renal filtration capacity. Structural integrity of the glomeruli, as the prime filter organ, is compromised directly by pathology, such that there is altered permeability and filtration capacity. For instance, in chronic or acute inflammation, glomerular structural change can manifest as proteinuria, clinically showing kidney stress and inflammation. Interestingly, physicians are challenged by the proper staging of CKD, particularly in pregnancy, where physiological hyperfiltration complicates the interpretation of GFR. Therefore, the use of serum creatinine and albuminuria assessment becomes important in making a diagnosis and observing the function of the kidneys over time, illustrating the multifaceted influences on GFR in renal health (Noto, 2020) (Figure 12.11).

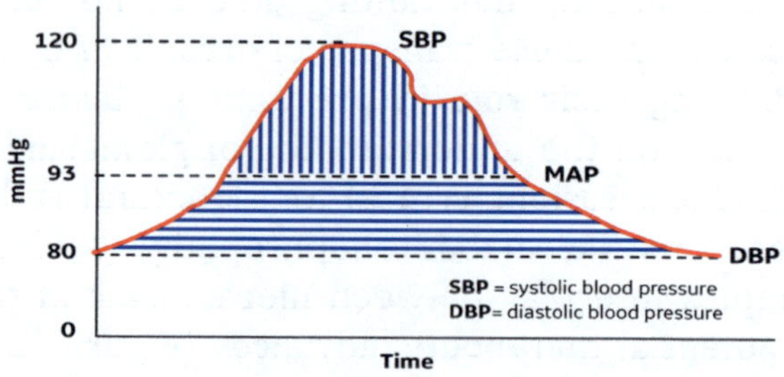

Figure 12.11. Measuring mean arterial pressure.

Source: https://clinicalview.gehealthcare.com/sites/default/files/styles/paragraph_scaled_picture_fallback/public/39_graph1.png?itok=rFFH9EeE.

12.3.3. Role of the Filtration Barrier

The filtration barrier, a sophisticated structure of the renal corpuscle, plays a crucial role in urine production by allowing only selective compounds to travel from the blood to the nephron. Composed of three distinct layers, glomerular endothelial cells, basement membrane, and podocytes, the barrier prevents the loss of essential solutes and water while preventing the passage of larger molecules and cells. The complex cell structure enhances permeability by a network of filtration slits formed by podocytes, such that small molecules like ions and glucose can be transmitted. Interestingly, barrier integrity is very important; dysfunction or damage will result in serious pathophysiological conditions, which suggests the intimate relationship between function and structure in renal physiology. In addition to selective permeability, the filtration barrier is also involved in the body's overall fluid balance and homeostasis. The endothelial glycocalyx layer, which lies on the luminal surface of the glomerular endothelium, is critical to protecting the underlying cells and regulating the passage of fluids through the barrier. This very sensitive layer can be compromised by various pathological conditions and thereby compromise the efficiency of filtration. Maintenance of the endothelial glycocalyx is critical in intravenous fluid treatments since improper management can complicate existing injuries of this layer and interfere with fluid homeostasis (Goswami et al., 2019). For this reason, identification of the function of the filtration barrier not only proves invaluable for understanding the structural requirements for optimal kidney function but also draws attention to its relevance in clinical environments. The disruption of the filtration barriers is most essential in CKDs, where the alterations could lead to proteinuria and other clinical manifestations. Structural integrity of the filtration barrier is lost in CKD, and there is inappropriate entry of proteins into the urine. This pathologic leak is a consequence of the podocyte structure changes and loss of the normal filtration barrier structure, essentially changing the dynamics of glomerular filtration. Current studies show that there is a conserved process that is accountable for cyst formation in CKDs, which connects the structural characteristics of excretory systems across species with human pathophysiology. By exploring such conserved mechanisms, researchers can make correlations that increase our understanding of CKD and develop targeted therapeutic interventions (Vu et al., 2015). Thus, the filtration barrier not only is central to renal physiology but also embodies avenues for emerging research into kidney disease and health management.

Test Your Knowledge

1. What are the substances usually filtered by the glomerulus?
2. Why is blood pressure essential to efficient glomerular filtration?

12.4. Tubular Reabsorption

Learning Outcome

1. Describe the tubule reabsorption mechanism within the proximal tubule;
2. Define reabsorption mechanisms: active or passive;
3. Explain the significance of reabsorption in the balance of fluids and electrolytes.

Tubular reabsorption is a major function of the nephron that helps to regulate the body fluids and electrolytes. It is the mechanism of selective reabsorption of water, ions, and other substances back into the bloodstream after their initial filtration in the glomeruli. It is a complex system that allows the kidneys to reabsorb critical compounds , such as glucose, amino acids, and bicarbonate that are crucial to the preservation of homeostasis. Apart from the process of simple reabsorption, the nephron is very sensitive to the changing needs of the body, such that waste is removed while necessary solutes are preserved. Consequently, the effectiveness of this process is of much concern, providing the foundation of general renal physiology and demonstrating the kidneys' vital role in blood filtration and the support of varied physiological parameters. The PCT, the first segment of the nephron to be involved with reabsorption in the tubules, is tasked mainly with the reclamation of an enormous proportion of the filtered substance. Approximately 65-70% of the produced filtrate is absorbed in this segment, including critical solutes like sodium, chloride, bicarbonate, and nearly all the glucose and amino acids. The mechanism, which makes this very high rate of reabsorption possible, involves passive and active transport mechanisms. Sodium ions are actively effluxed out of the tubular lumen, and this creates an osmotic gradient for water reabsorption. These activities, as demonstrated in compensatory hypertrophic responses, establish that increases in tubular surface area can maximize reabsorption efficiency, exhibiting the plasticity of renal adaptation to altered physiological demands (Beck et al., 1998).

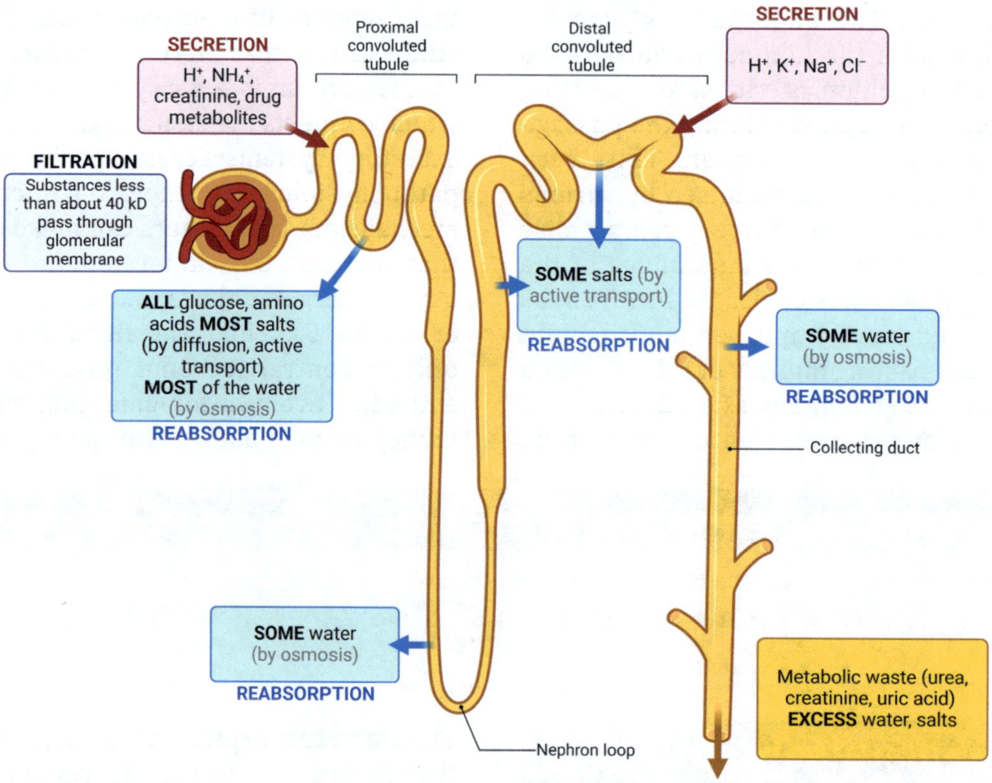

Figure 12.12. Reabsorption in the nephron.

Source: https://uen.pressbooks.pub/app/uploads/sites/462/2024/06/U19-011-Reabsorption-in-the-Nephron-v3.png.

In addition, the role of PCT in acid-base homeostasis through bicarbonate reabsorption is particularly critical in the prevention of metabolic acidosis, thus illustrating its importance in the entire process of kidney function. The collecting duct (CCD) and DCT subsequently refine the process of reabsorption initiated in the PCT, completing the body's meticulous fluid and electrolyte control. The DCT has a more specialized function, reabsorbing sodium and chloride under the influence of hormonal regulation, particularly aldosterone, resulting in sodium retention and potassium excretion. The ability of the DCT to control sodium reabsorption based on the body's demand is a testament to its significance in blood pressure regulation and electrolyte balance. Most notably, the thick ascending limb of the loop of Henle is also a significant determinant of sodium reabsorption, incriminating alterations within this segment in the etiology of hypertension, highlighting the highly coordinated interconnectedness of kidney physiology and total health (Graham et al., 2017). This highly coordinated integration highlights not only the importance of tubular reabsorption in renal physiology but also its devastating impact on broader physiological systems (Figure 12.12).

12.4.1. Process of Reabsorption in the Proximal Tubule

The proximal tubule is a key site for the renal physiological mechanisms of reabsorption, which enables the recovery of essential solutes and water from the glomerular filtrate. Microvilli line it to offer a larger surface area and utilize several forms of transport to recover valuable nutrients , such as glucose, amino acids, and bicarbonate. Proximal tubule reabsorption is largely an active transport process, relying on energy-driven sodium-potassium pumps to create electrochemical gradients. Such gradients permit sodium to carry other substances like glucose and amino acids across the tubular epithelium, thus preventing their excretion and ensuring their availability to systemic processes.

Thus, the proximal tubule plays a pivotal role not just in fluid balance but also in homeostasis of vital compounds that are needed for various functions in the body. At the heart of reabsorption are specialized membrane proteins that facilitate the movement of molecules through the apical and basolateral membranes of the proximal tubules. Sodium-glucose cotransporters SGLT1 and SGLT2 are especially responsible for glucose reabsorption by the kidneys to prevent the body from losing unnecessary amounts of glucose, something required for the process of energy metabolism.

The function of these transporters underscores the intersection of renal physiology and health at the metabolic level: when they are disrupted, as happens in diabetes, glucose spills into the urine because it is not reabsorbed properly. Clinically, these dysfunctions have informed the development of SGLT2 inhibitors to manage type 2 diabetes, and they highlight the importance of proximal tubule reabsorption in both health and disease (Ghezzi et al., 2018). The relationship between reabsorption processes and kidney pathologies is also implied with conditions , such as diabetic nephropathy, where changes in transport expression can detrimentally compromise tubular function. Experiments show that reductions in expression of major transporters, megalin and cubilin, correlate with increased tubular damage and reduced protein reabsorptive capacity. This is particularly relevant in diabetic models where alterations to intracellular trafficking of the receptors add to the compromise of their function (Bahamonde et al., 2017). The understanding of these processes reveals the complexity of renal physiology; the proximal tubule is not only a conduit for filtrate but an active participant in the preservation of renal and overall well-being. This underscores the importance of having transporter systems to enable the reabsorption of not only sodium and water, but also essential proteins, which marks the proximal tubule focal role in renal function (Figure 12.13).

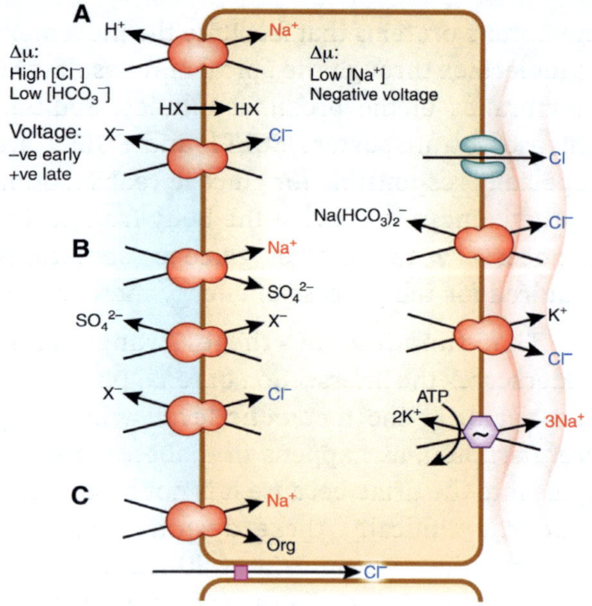

Figure 12.13. Process of reabsorption in the proximal tubule.

Source: https://www.researchgate.net/profile/Orson-Moe-2/publication/254280597/figure/fig1/AS:616389098364929@1523970021132/Proximal-tubule-NaCl-reabsorption-Unlike-the-thick-ascending-limb-or-distal-convoluted.png.

12.4.2. Mechanisms of Reabsorption: Active Versus Passive

In renal physiology, understanding solute reabsorption mechanisms is fundamental in the realization of how the kidneys achieve homeostasis. Active and passive reabsorption are two significant mechanisms through which recovery of essential compounds from the renal tubules to the blood system is made possible. Active transport mechanisms are energy-dependent, most often from adenosine triphosphate (ATP), to move solutes against their concentration gradient to reabsorb nutrients , such as glucose and amino acids efficiently. For instance, in the proximal tubule, sodium-glucose cotransporters (SGLTs) are significant by leveraging the sodium gradients established through the Na+/K+ ATPase pump for energizing the active reabsorption of glucose (Ghezzi et al., 2018). Passive reabsorption, on the other hand, occurs without energy expenditure but instead through electrochemical gradients and concentration gradients, directly affecting water and a few ions. Coordination between active and passive reabsorption is required to control urine composition and biochemical homeostasis. Of particular interest, the regulation of sodium (Na+) reabsorption provides clues on how the processes work synergistically. For example, the thick ascending limb of the loop of Henle is a segment in which active reabsorption is the norm, actively transporting sodium ions from the filtrate. This is a key segment in preventing excessive sodium loss, and alterations in reabsorption significantly impact blood pressure and fluid status (Graham et al., 2017). The complex renal structure, such as the special cell types and segmental tubular pattern, allows for coordination of these reabsorption strategies, thereby underscoring the fineness of renal function. Additionally, the consequences of deranged reabsorption mechanisms underscore the clinical significance of these mechanisms in health and disease states. The diseases , such as diabetes and hypertension elucidate the requirement of adequate management of solute within the nephron. In diabetes, for instance, reabsorptive inefficiencies of glucose can lead to glucosuria when transporter processes , such as SGLT2, are overburdened (Ghezzi et al., 2018). Similarly, in hypertension, sodium hyperreabsorption in the nephron, particularly in the thick ascending limb, leads to elevated blood pressure through fluid overload and vascular remodeling (Graham et al., 2017). Understanding these mechanisms is important not only to appreciate renal function but also to the development of targeted therapeutic interventions in the treatment of renal and cardiovascular disease, reflecting the subtle interplay between renal physiology and general health (Figure 12.14).

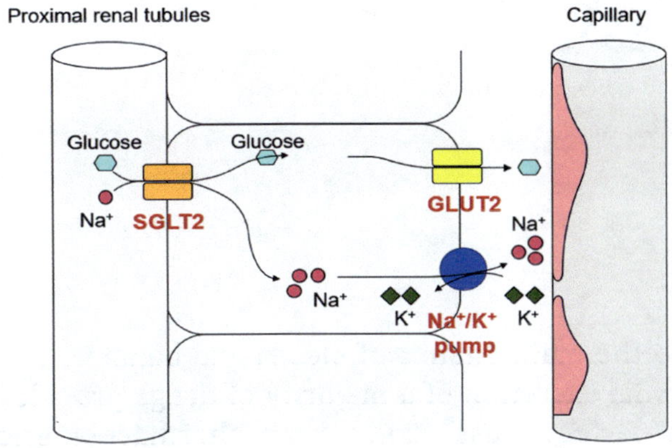

Figure 12.14. A role of sodium-glucose co-transporter 2 in cardiorenal anemia iron deficiency syndrome

Source: Sano M. A Role of Sodium-Glucose Co-Transporter 2 in Cardiorenal Anemia Iron Deficiency Syndrome. International Journal of Molecular Sciences. 2023; 24(6):5983. https://doi.org/10.3390/ijms24065983

12.4.3. Importance of Reabsorption for Fluid and Electrolyte Balance

Renal reabsorption is a critical fluid and electrolyte balance mechanism in the body and has direct implications for homeostasis. Reabsorptive renal tubular processes reclaim essential substances , such as sodium, chloride, glucose, and water following glomerular filtration, during which blood plasma is converted into filtrate. By selectively stripping these important components from the filtrate and returning them to the blood, the kidneys ensure that there is not too great a loss of essential electrolytes and fluids that would cause imbalances, posing a danger to overall health. Of note, this not only maintains normal physiologic function but also helps maintain the body's acid-base state. Thus, reabsorption of filtered substances is a contributing factor to the maintenance of cellular environments ideal for metabolism, ultimately affecting the systemic function of the body and its ability to resist stressors. The nephron, or kidney functional unit, is defined by distinctive regions that enable effective reabsorption, notably in the proximal tubule and collecting duct. In the proximal tubule, approximately 65-70% of filtered water and sodium are reabsorbed, along with nutrients , such as glucose and amino acids, further highlighting the tubule's fundamental role in the conservation of nutrients. Additional reabsorption occurs in the collecting duct and loop of Henle, where additional water and electrolytes are regulated based on the body's level of hydration. The mechanisms by which hormonal stimuli, such as ADH for water reabsorption and aldosterone for sodium, are a reflection of how responsive the kidneys are to hormonal requirements. It is significant because it ensures that fluid and electrolyte balances are regulated based on intake, activity, and hydration status, demonstrating the kidneys' function as homeostatic controllers. Besides, structural adaptations within the renal collecting ducts are required for modulating urinary composition and directly affect fluid and electrolyte balance. The tight epithelial barrier formed by specific proteins known as claudins allows for selective permeability of the collecting duct, thus playing a significant role in reabsorptive processes. As highlighted in studies, particular claudins , such as Cldn-3 and Cldn-4, contribute to the integrity, enabling the passage of coupled water and solutes while effectively isolating intraluminal urine from the interstitium. Such structural competence ensures that collecting ducts are capable of controlling water excretion based on the body's hydration status, an excellent example of the significant interaction between reabsorption and fluid homeostasis. Disturbances in this barrier can potentially result in major disruptions in blood pressure and homeostasis, making reabsorption so vital in renal physiology (Natochin et al., 1996; Leiz et al., 2019).

Test Your Knowledge

1. What substances are commonly reabsorbed in the proximal convoluted tubule?
2. How does the loop of Henle assist in water and salt reabsorption?
3. Why is tubular reabsorption so vital for homeostasis?

12.5. Tubular Secretion

Learning Outcome

1. Explain the importance of tubular secretion;
2. Identify the main substances secreted by the renal tubules;
3. Explain the role of secretion in acid-base balance.

The renal system plays a crucial role in maintaining homeostasis, primarily by processes , such as filtration, reabsorption, and tubular secretion. Tubular secretion is one of the major processes by which the kidneys can control the composition of the blood by secreting certain substances from the peritubular capillaries into the fluid of the tubules. This function occurs almost exclusively in the renal tubules, i.e., in the proximal convoluted tubule, distal convoluted tubule, and collecting duct, where various organic and inorganic substances , such as drugs, electrolytes, and metabolic waste, are secreted. Through such activities, tubular secretion not only helps to eliminate harmful substances from the body but is also a determinant mechanism in acid-base balance, controlling the pH of body fluids and the balance of the internal environment overall. Tubular secretion mechanisms are as diverse as the chemicals being subjected to the process. Facilitated diffusion and active transport are essential for the movement of solutes through the tubular epithelium. The secretion of hydrogen ions, for example, is essential in the regulation of blood pH, while active secretion of potassium ions contributes to the maintenance of electrolyte balance. The renal excretion of a majority of drugs provides a perfect illustration of the pharmacokinetic relevance of tubular secretion, as it plays a decisive role in drug efficacy and duration of action. The reabsorption of materials back into the tubules, often mediated by specialized transporters, illustrates the complexity of renal processes and the interaction between various transport mechanisms. Combined, these mechanisms demonstrate how tubular secretion enables the ability of kidneys to modulate body functions subtly and offer homeostasis. This discussion on the evolutionary significance of tubular secretion requires one to appreciate the conservation of renal processes across species. Surprisingly, studies have proven that those same mechanisms governing tubular secretion are highly conserved from ancient creatures to modern vertebrates, as evidenced by the similarity in vertebrate and planarian excretory systems.

This suggests an evolutionary origin for the renal adaptations. For example, glomerular nephron and tubular morphogenesis have been influenced to respond to specific pressures of the environment, such as freshwater adaptation in early vertebrates and the necessity for proper excretion of waste and osmoregulation. Awareness of these evolutionary milestones can provide a person with an appreciation of the underlying mechanisms of renal physiology, showing how such primitive processes still affect our modern understanding of kidney function and regulation that is involved in maintaining fluid and electrolyte balance throughout different life forms (Natochin et al., 1996; Vu et al., 2015) (Figure 12.15).

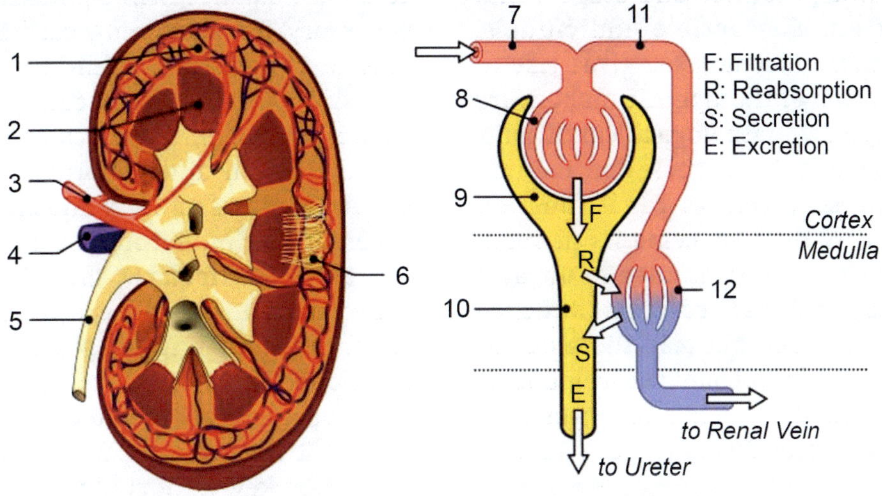

Figure 12.15. Tubular secretion.

Source: https://biologydictionary.net/wp-content/uploads/2017/05/Kidney-And-Nephron.jpg.

12.5.1. Definition and Significance of Tubular Secretion

Tubular secretion is an important renal physiological process necessary for the preservation of homeostasis. It is a mechanism by which selected substances—, such as ions, organic acids, and foreign substances—are actively secreted from peritubular capillaries into renal tubules. In contrast to the passive glomerular filtration, tubular secretion actively regulates blood chemical makeup and what ultimately excretes in urine. The efficiency of tubular secretion is essential in removing excess material and toxins from the blood in order not to cause likely imbalances that would adversely affect physiological processes. The intricacy among tubular secretion and other renal processes signifies its significant role in the overall process of renal physiology and homeostasis, which describes the kidney's adaptability under varying internal and external changes. The significance of tubular secretion extends beyond waste removal per se; it is crucially significant in acid-base balance and electrolyte homeostasis. By secreting hydrogen ions and reabsorbing bicarbonate, the kidneys can effectively regulate blood pH, a critical variable for numerous enzymatic and metabolic processes. Tubular secretion is also critically involved in potassium and sodium management, regulating systemic blood pressure and water balance. For instance, during times of hyperpotassemia from dietary excess, potassium tubular secretion is elevated in order to prevent hyperkalemia and thus dangerous cardiovascular effects. This is particularly meaningful given the increased frequency of electrolyte imbalance in numerous clinical illnesses and illustrating just how not only a normal renal function, but actually a vital determinant of overall well-being and physiologic stability, tubular secretion of potassium truly is. Current research highlights the complexity and multi-dimensionality of tubular secretion, and its relevance in disease conditions , such as primary hyperoxaluria. Evidence has established that increased oxalate secretion from the proximal tubule lays the ground for supersaturation and crystallization of calcium oxalate, leading to renal injuries and potential end-stage renal disease (ESRD) in susceptible individuals. Understanding these mechanisms gives rise to a further exploration of therapeutic maneuvers aimed at limiting such pathological conditions, as the regulation of tubular secretion may be crucial to the preservation of renal function in the long term. With advancements in renal physiology, research now continues to unravel how the nuances of tubular secretion influence not only renal pathology but also the broader metabolic and systemic mechanisms, cementing its significance in the study of human physiology (Coe et al., 2013; Shokr, 2016) (Figure 12.16).

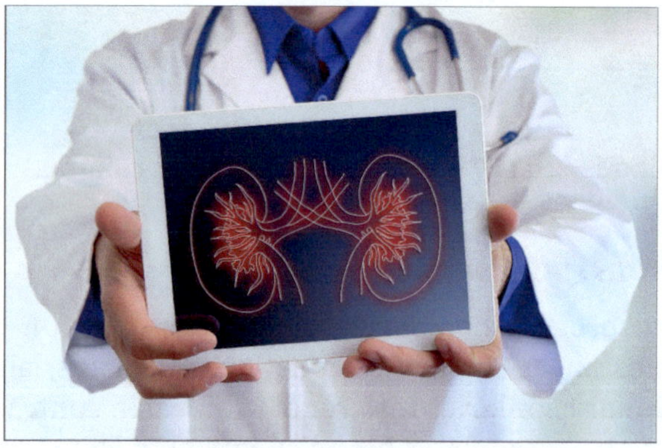

Figure 12.16. End-stage renal disease (ESRD).

Source: https://en.lepumedical.com/uploads/image/20210831/kidney.jpg.

12.5.2. Key Substances Secreted by the Renal Tubules

The renal tubules are responsible directly for the delicate balance of homeostasis, in great measure through the secretion of some substances that impact body functions. The tubules are located within the nephron and are tasked with such functions as acid-base balance, control of electrolytes, and excretion of waste products. Among the most significant substances secreted are hydrogen ions, potassium ions, and ammonia, all of which have a significant impact on the body's physiological balance. For instance, hydrogen ion secretion is necessary for acid-base balance, while potassium secretion is necessary for sustaining cardiac function and muscle contraction. Additionally, ammonia is necessary in the detoxification of nitrogenous waste products, specifically in maintaining renal function and general metabolic health. Renal tubules secretory mechanisms are thus necessary for numerous essential physiological processes. Particularly, the PCT is a major site of secretion and reabsorption and serves as the major interface between glomerular filtrate and the blood. There, numerous organic anions and cations are actively secreted, including drugs and metabolic waste products. It is selective secretion that is of key importance to renal clearance of drugs and, therefore, their therapeutic effect and toxic potential. Besides that, renal tubules are directly involved in the transport of organic compounds like bicarbonate, which is very important for acid-base homeostasis. The renal tubules also secrete other compounds like erythropoietin during hypoxia, thus regulating erythropoiesis. All these extensive functions give implications to the role of renal tubules in maintaining the body's health and underscore their necessity in renal physiology and pathology studies (Shokr, 2016; Ayati et al., 2018). In addition to maintaining ionic balance and eliminating metabolic waste, renal tubules have the function of controlling blood pressure via renin secretion. Renin is an important enzyme that initiates the renin-angiotensin-aldosterone system (RAAS) to maintain systemic vascular resistance and circulating volume. As blood pressure decreases, certain cells within the juxtaglomerular apparatus release renin, triggering a cascade of hormonal responses that cause sodium reabsorption and vasoconstriction. This function places greater emphasis upon the larger role in cardiovascular health and homeostasis. Secondly, malfunctioning secretion of these vital substances can also lead to severe health problems, such as high blood pressure and electrolyte imbalance, further accentuating the need for continued research into renal physiology. Hence, renal tubules' secretion of vital substances is not just a sophisticated process but also a determinant of overall physiological equilibrium (Shokr, 2016; Ayati et al., 2018) (Figure 12.17).

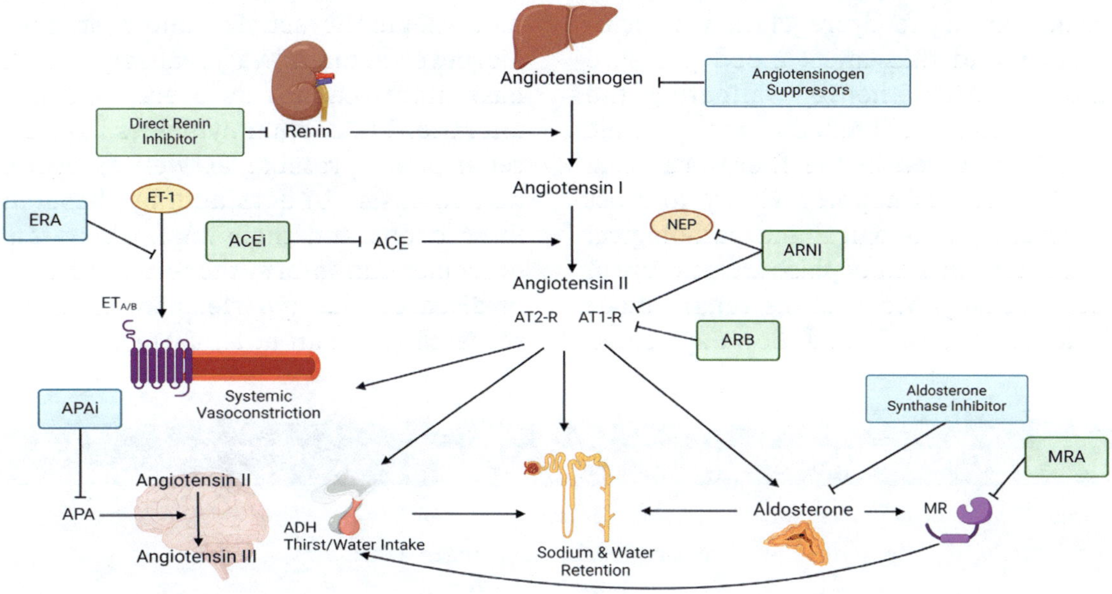

Figure 12.17. Renin-angiotensin-aldosterone system.

Source: Ksiazek SH, Hu L, Andò S, Pirklbauer M, Säemann MD, Ruotolo C, Zaza G, La Manna G, De Nicola L, Mayer G, et al. Renin–Angiotensin–Aldosterone System: From History to Practice of a Secular Topic. International Journal of Molecular Sciences. 2024; 25(7):4035. https://doi.org/10.3390/ijms25074035

12.5.3. Role of Secretion in Maintaining Acid-Base Balance

The role of maintenance of acid-base balance by secretion is pivotal to renal physiology, particularly in the case of the nephrons varied segments. As blood travels through the renal system, kidneys regularly filter and selectively secrete material to regulate pH levels. This process is ongoing in the proximal tubule and collecting duct, where hydrogen ions (H^+) and bicarbonate ($HCO3^-$) are secreted or reabsorbed based on the metabolic needs of the body. This balance avoids acidosis or alkalosis, which will become seriously disrupting to cellular function and homeostasis as a whole. Furthermore, the capacity of renal tubular epithelial cells to adaptively alter mechanisms of secretion in accord with systemic acid-base status just underscores their central role in metabolic regulation. Finally, adequate acid-base homeostasis is not simply a matter of excretion but an elegant ballet of secretion and reabsorption that preserves physiological equipoise. Secretion mechanisms in the renal collecting duct have a dual role, helping not only with electrolyte balance but also acid-base balance regulation at a fine level. Collecting duct epithelium contains tight junctions that control paracellular movement, which subsequently supports precise ion exchanges. There is the capability of cells in this segment to actively secrete H+ ions into the urine with the active reabsorption of bicarbonate and to create a counter-regulatory mechanism. The effectiveness of this process is decided by the expression of various claudins, which take care of the integrity and function of tight junctions. For instance, any functional impairment in claudins would compromise the barrier, leading to dysregulation of acid-base balance, and thus affect blood pressure and fluid retention, thereby validating the interdependence of renal function and systemic control as highlighted in the literature (Leiz et al., 2019). Further, nephron ability to react under different physiological and pathological conditions determines the sophisticated nature of its secretory activity. With acidosis, renal tubules increase the secretion of H^+ and allow augmented reabsorption of HCO_{3-}, thereby compensating for the pH abnormality. With alkalosis, H^+ secretion may be decreased to provide space for augmented excretion of bicarbonate to allow equilibration. This flexibility is paramount to the capacity to accommodate fluctuations in diet, metabolic activity, and systemic health. Moreover, sodium (Na^+) reabsorption and acid-base status cannot be overemphasized since alterations in sodium dynamics have effects on renal blood pressure as well as overall renal homeostasis. Understanding these intricate interactions and their implications on health outcomes can inform therapeutic management of diseases like hypertension, as discussed in research (Graham et al., 2017).

Test Your Knowledge

1. What is tubular secretion, and how is it distinct from reabsorption?
2. Which parts of the nephron are primarily accountable for tubular secretion?
3. How does tubular secretion regulate the body's pH?

12.6. Regulation of Renal Function

Learning Outcome

1. Describe the hormonal regulation: aldosterone and ADH role;
2. Describe the neural regulation: sympathetic nervous system effect;
3. Identify the blood pressure on renal function.

Regulation of renal function is a complex but necessary part of controlling total homeostasis within the body. The kidneys filter blood and remove waste products and preserve electrolytes, fluids, and acid-base balance. This precise regulation is sustained by a blend of intricate mechanisms , such as neural, hormonal, and local controls that influence renal blood flow and GFR. For example, the RAAS plays a significant role in blood pressure and fluid regulation through the alteration of the reabsorption of sodium and water in the nephron. In this, then, the kidneys can regulate filtration dynamics in keeping with physiological demand, as evidenced by blood pressure and volume changes that reflect overall metabolic status. Pregnancy demonstrates the flexibility of renal function further, since extensive morphological and functional adaptation takes place to preserve maternal and fetal health. It has been found via research that renal structural adaptations take place during pregnancy, in the form of increased renal blood flow and glomerular filtration rates above non-pregnant states. These adaptations play an important role in meeting the increased metabolic demands and body fluid volume changes. Surprisingly, however, evidence attests that renal effects during normal pregnancies can be the same as those seen under preeclampsia, with pathological alterations indicative of underlying diseases. This comparison of variation in renal function emphasizes the importance of renal regulation in normal physiology as well as the identification of possible complications during pregnancy, therefore shedding light into their importance as indices of fetal and maternal health (Strevens, 2002). In addition to determinants of renal filtration and function, understanding the evolutionary history of kidney disease also sheds light into the intrinsic mechanisms that govern renal regulation. CKDs, characterized by fluid-filled cysts derived from nephric tubules, have been linked to aberrant cellular processes. Of specific interest are comparative studies between vertebrate and invertebrate urinary systems, which reveal that certain processes of CKD pathogenesis are evolutionarily conserved. Findings indicate that planarian excretory systems and vertebrate nephrons both possess similar processes with regard to filtration and flow mechanics. This conservation means that new invertebrate models, such as planarians, are able to affect the understanding of human renal pathologies, telling us about the regulation of renal function and pathophysiology of kidney diseases (Vu et al., 2015) (Figure 12.18).

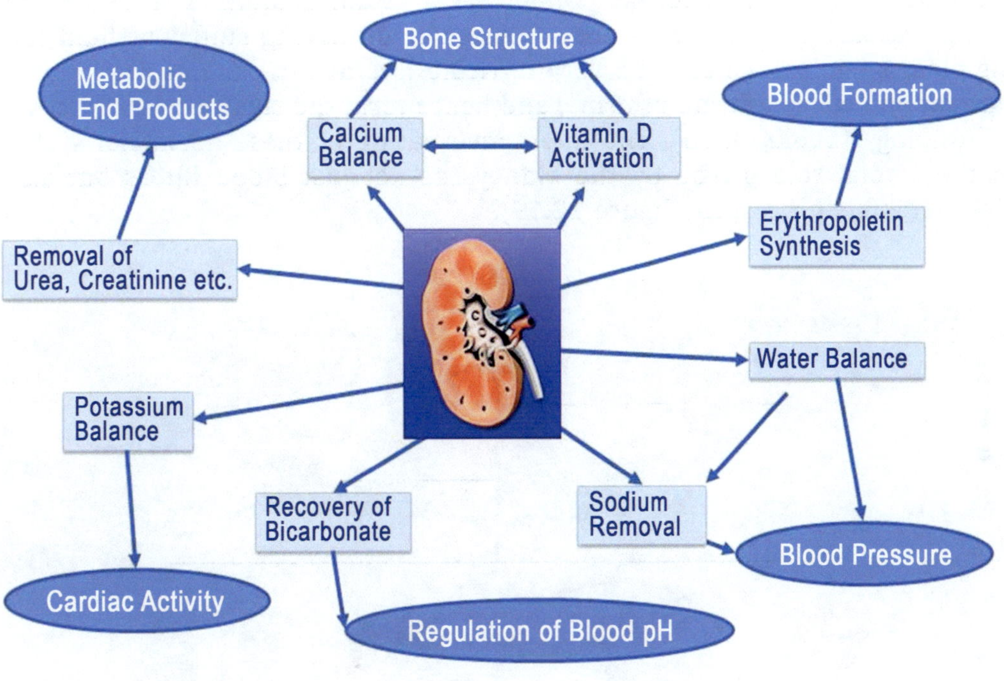

Figure 12.18. Kidney functions and regulation.

Source: https://slideplayer.com/13119203/79/images/slide_1.jpg.

12.6.1. Hormonal Regulation: Role of Aldosterone and Antidiuretic Hormone (ADH)

Fluid balance and electrolyte homeostasis in the human body largely rely on hormones, particularly on aldosterone and ADH. Aldosterone is a steroid hormone produced by the adrenal cortex with a very critical function of sodium and potassium regulation in the renal system. Through stimulation of sodium reabsorption from collecting ducts and the distal convoluted tubule of the nephron, aldosterone stimulates water retention that has direct effects on blood pressure and volume. The hormone is stimulated through various triggers like low blood pressure and increased potassium levels, underlining its function in maintaining cardiovascular activity and uniform electrolyte environment (Shokr, 2016). The interaction between aldosterone and renal anatomy drives the body to properly respond to fluctuating homeostatic demands. ADH, also known as vasopressin, acts primarily on the collecting ducts of the nephron to enhance water reabsorption. Released from the posterior pituitary gland in response to an increase in plasma osmolality or decreased blood volume, ADH stimulates the insertion of aquaporin-2 channels into renal epithelial cells. This mechanism enhances the concentrating ability of the kidneys, restricting water loss and osmotic equilibrium in the blood (Leonard et al., 2025). ADH functions not only control the body's hydration status but are also crucial to oppose dehydration from disparate forms of physiological stress. Aldosterone and ADH hence play pivotal roles to define renal physiology and fluid dynamics. Synergistic action of aldosterone and ADH has a fine control mechanism that maintains homeostasis in the renal system. During dehydration, when plasma osmolality is elevated, secretion of ADH is amplified, leading to enhanced reabsorption of water. Concurrently, diminished volume of circulating blood stimulates the secretion of aldosterone, which helps retain sodium. The two hormones work together to ensure that the body does not compromise on having sufficient fluid levels without endangering electrolyte imbalance. This very intricate interaction enables the kidneys to control both the amount and concentration of urine, and hence form the significance of hormonal control of kidney physiology (Shokr, 2016). The interactive nature of these hormonal systems helps to underscore the pivotal role played by the kidneys as not just blood filters but also as crucial regulators of metabolic processes (Figure 12.19).

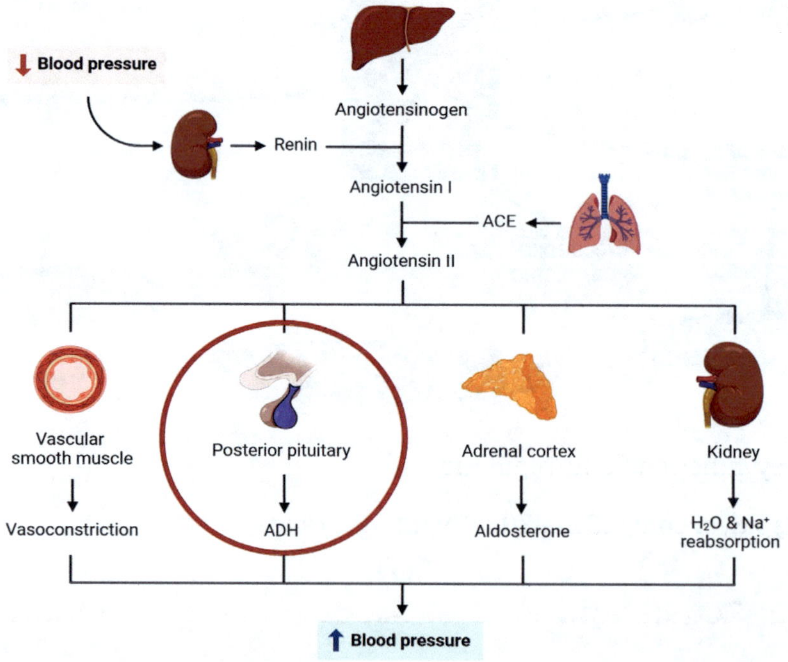

Figure 12.19. Renin-angiotensin-system.

Source: https://microbenotes.com/wp-content/uploads/2024/04/Renin-Angiotensin-System.jpeg.

12.6.2. Neural Regulation: Sympathetic Nervous System (SNS) Influence

The SNS is crucial in the control of renal function, particularly in controlling GFR and electrolyte homeostasis in the kidney. During stress or decreased blood volume, sympathetic nerve activity is increased with ensuing vasoconstriction of the renal blood vessels. Such a mechanism can shunt blood to the priority organs while simultaneously decreasing GFR by decreasing hydrostatic pressure in the glomerulus. Furthermore, the SNS controls the juxtaglomerular apparatus and influences the secretory apparatus of renin, the centerpiece of the RAAS. The ability of the SNS to synthesize these responses emphasizes its role not merely in the preservation of hemodynamic homeostasis but in the control of renal physiology during physiological stress (Peak et al., 2016). Apart from its vascular impact, the SNS affects nephron transport processes, particularly in the collecting duct and the proximal tubule. Sympathetic outflow increases brings about alterations in the reabsorption of sodium and water, which aids in the maintenance of body fluid when there are emergencies.

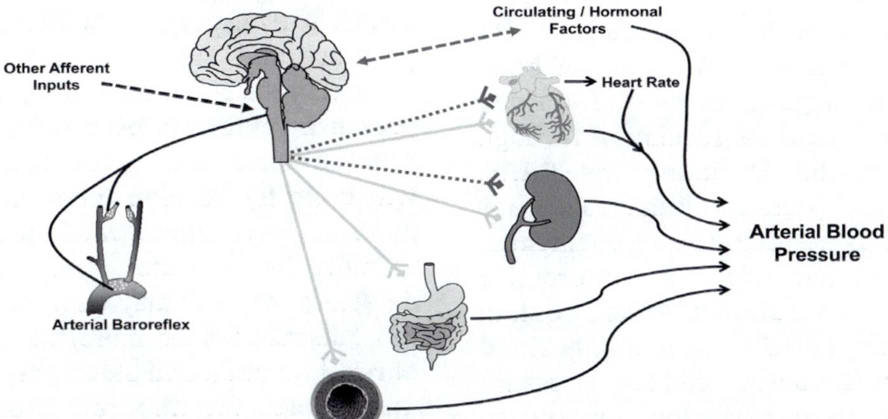

Figure 12.20. Neural regulation: sympathetic nervous system influence.

Source: https://www.researchgate.net/profile/Colin-Young-13/publication/51250285/figure/fig1/AS:277544470368270@1443183166859/Schematic-illustrating-neural-cardiovascular-control-Sympathetic-light-gray-lines-and.png.

Experimental data derived from studies imply sympathetic innervation to directly influence nephron function, increasing sodium reabsorption and modulating the osmotic regulation of urine production. This adaptation is most pertinent under conditions , such as dehydration or hypotension, where water and electrolyte conservation is essential for survival. Synergy among sympathetic nerves and renal tubular cells points to the multifaceted role of neural control of renal physiology, facilitating systemic action with regional renal responses (Burnstock et al., 2016). Furthermore, the impact of SNS on renal function has general applicability to a number of renal diseases, including diabetes and hypertension. Pathologically exaggerated sympathetic output is often observed in these diseases and is associated with structural and functional alterations in the kidney in accordance with disease pathology. For instance, prolonged elevation of sympathetic output can lead to renal ischemia, which in turn causes fibrosis as well as chronic kidney injury. Research has shown that modulation of sympathetic activity is therapeutic in value, with the potential targeting of neural pathways for the treatment of renal pathologies, emphasizing the potential of sympathetic modulation in addressing renal pathology. The interaction between renal dysfunction and sympathetic nerve activity speaks to the complex interaction between neural control and renal disease, which remains a continuing stimulus to research on the contribution of sympathetic modulation to clinical therapy (Figure 12.20).

12.6.3. Impact of Blood Pressure on Renal Function

The interrelation of blood pressure with renal function forms the foundation of body homeostasis. Kidneys possess the unique function of blood pressure regulation through various mechanisms, including the RAAS. During high blood pressure, renal ability for plasma filtration is elevated, causing augmented renal blood flow and GFR. This interactive process ensures elimination of excess sodium and water, which helps in controlling blood pressure. Conversely, decreased blood pressure can jeopardize renal perfusion, leading to compromised GFR and accumulation of waste products. Understanding how altered levels of blood pressure impact renal function is significant in preventing the development of kidney diseases, particularly in hypertensive individuals or diseases that compromise vascular integrity, i.e., atherosclerosis. Hypertension, or high blood pressure, causes tremendous stress on the intrarenal organs and renal vasculature. Chronic hypertension can induce nephrosclerosis, a diffuse thickening of arterial walls that further impairs renal blood supply and filtration ability. Subsequent capillary damage leads to nephron loss due to a vicious cycle of increasing hypertension and deteriorating renal insufficiency. This concept is supported in research that points out the role of the thick ascending limb of the loop of Henle (TAL) in the kidneys, which plays a crucial role in sodium reabsorption. If the segment is overactive due to excess intake of dietary salt, as has been reported in salt-sensitive hypertension literature, nephrons ability to maintain sodium and fluid homeostasis is lost, leading to increased worsening blood pressure rise and renal injury (Graham et al., 2017). The effects of such interactions of blood pressure and kidney function become most evident in the situation of CKD, where abnormal pressure relationships can induce a cycle of renal deterioration. The involved subjects will typically develop increasingly worsening nephron dysfunction, which in turn might lead to more hypertension, generating a cycle of deterioration that may culminate in end-stage renal disease. Furthermore, the interdependency of renal function and blood pressure variability underscores the importance of proper blood pressure control to avoid further aggravation of CKD. New approaches aimed at interrupting sodium reabsorption in the TAL may hold potential for new therapeutic maneuvers to break this vicious cycle. Research also established that shifting diet therapy or utilizing the application of pharmacologic agents to change renal sodium regulation has a spectacular influence on blood pressure management and on renal health, and this indicates that a multidimensional strategy is necessary for general patient management (Lu et al., 2010).

Test Your Knowledge

1. What hormone increases water reabsorption in the kidneys and from where is it secreted?
2. What role does the renin-angiotensin-aldosterone system (RAAS) play in blood pressure control and kidney function?
3. How does antidiuretic hormone (ADH) control urine concentration?

SUMMARY

Examination of renal physiology, with particular emphasis on the intricate relationship between kidney anatomy and the filtration process, reveals significant implications for knowledge of and therapy for CKD. Advanced imaging techniques, such as ASL MRI, have provided significant insight into renal perfusion patterns. Evidence indicates that T1 relaxation time alterations are correlated with decreased perfusion in CKD patients and emphasize the role of renal structural alterations towards functional deficits (Delles et al., 2016). Such findings emphasize combining functional with structural assessment to enhance diagnostic efficiency and treatment response. In addition, learning about the mechanisms involved in the resistance of various animal species to kidney disease can give new therapeutic strategies to manage CKD in humans. For example, certain animals, such as the naked mole rat, are highly long-lived and are highly resistant to oxidative stress-associated injury (Stenvinkel et al., 2018).

Such species, when analyzed, can provide important information regarding probable therapeutic strategies that can employ natural renal protective mechanisms. By tapping into information from diverse biological models, researchers are able to construct novel interventions that lower the onset of renal dysfunction. Last, a collaborative exchange among nephrologists, veterinarians, and biologists has the promise to lead to progress in the study of kidney disease. The application of a multisciplinary method allows a broader exploration of renal physiology, enabling the study of new forms of therapy and prevention. As the burden of disease associated with CKD increases globally, it is necessary that the scientific community embraces integrative strategies in order to combat the disease on an effective level. Ultimately, the intersection of structural and functional knowledge and knowledge gleaned from nature will be significant in advancing our knowledge and management of renal health.

A clear understanding of renal physiology calls for a deep exploration of the anatomy of the kidneys and the filtration mechanisms necessary for body homeostasis. The nephron, the kidney's functional unit, plays the central role in the process through blood filtration, reabsorption of essential substances, and waste product elimination. Various sections of the nephron, including the glomerulus, proximal tubule, loop of Henle, distal tubule, and collecting duct, have distinct roles to play in the filtration process as a whole. The intricate combination of these sections offers the mechanisms necessary for the control of electrolytes, water balance, and acid-base homeostasis, reflecting the kidneys' significant role in physiological regulation.

These complex architectures must be maintained since any disruption will lead to renal pathologies and loss. New research highlights the significance of evolutionary understanding in the interpretation of renal health and disease. Science has demonstrated how comparative analysis between vertebrate nephron architectures and others, i.e., planarians, reveals conserved mechanisms that constitute the core of kidney function and disease pathology. Specifically, the pathological manifestation of CKDs has been discovered to be similar between species, meaning that information on the diseases may be learned from evolutionary models. The ultraconservation of ultrafiltration as well as flow-associated filtrate modification mechanisms is proof of a long-standing evolutionary adaptation across animal excretory systems, suggesting an integrated concept of how the processes have evolved to specific ecological niches (Vu et al., 2015). This evolutionary outlook provides richness to the study of renal physiology, creating a fascinating background for existing research. Additionally, multi-disciplinary studies are more and more critical in working to understand complex kidney disease, as evident through comparative susceptibility of various species to diseases , such as CKD. For instance, whereas domestic cats are very prone to CKD due to diet, other animals like naked mole rats and hibernating bears possess protective mechanisms against chronic illness by nature (Stenvinkel et al., 2018). These findings suggest that resistance to oxidative stress and metabolic adaptation under stressful conditions can offer new insights for the prevention and treatment of CKD in humans. It may well happen that a synergistic interaction between nephrologists, ecologists, and veterinarians can result in new approaches using the inherent abilities observed in various animal models. Interdisciplinary gap bridging can potentially open new avenues towards enhancing renal function and surmounting pathological barriers in human beings.

KEY TERMS FROM THIS CHAPTER

- Afferent Arteriole
- Collecting Duct
- Efferent Arteriole
- Glomerular Filtration
- Glomerulus
- Kidney
- Nephron
- Proximal Convoluted Tubule (PCT)
- Renal Cortex
- Bowman's Capsule
- Distal Convoluted Tubule (DCT)
- Filtration Membrane
- Glomerular Filtration Rate (GFR)
- Juxtaglomerular Apparatus
- Loop of Henle
- Peritubular Capillaries
- Renal Blood Flow
- Renal Medulla

CRITICAL THINKING QUESTIONS

1. **What is the functional unit of the kidney?**
   a. Glomerulus
   b. Nephron
   c. Renal tubule
   d. Bowman's capsule
2. **Where is the primary site of filtration in the nephron?**
   a. Loop of Henle
   b. Distal tubule
   c. Proximal tubule
   d. Glomerulus
3. **What pressure plays the chief role in glomerular filtration?**
   a. Oncotic pressure
   b. Hydrostatic pressure in Bowman's capsule
   c. Tubular osmotic pressure
   d. Glomerular capillary hydrostatic pressure
4. **Which cells form the filtration slits in the glomerulus?**
   a. Mesangial cells
   b. Macula densa cells
   c. Endothelial cells
   d. Podocytes
5. **Which arteriole enters the glomerulus and controls blood supply to the nephron?**
   a. Afferent arteriole
   b. Efferent arteriole
   c. Peritubular capillaries
   d. Vasa recta

Short Answer Questions

1. What is the functional unit of the kidney?
2. Where is the major site of glomerular filtration?
3. Define glomerular filtration rate (GFR).
4. What is the role of the afferent arteriole in the nephron?
5. Describe the structure of the nephron and its functional components.
6. What is glomerular filtration and what forces are involved?
7. What are the determinants of glomerular filtration rate (GFR)?
8. How do afferent and efferent arterioles differ in maintaining glomerular pressure?

Answers to Critical Thinking Questions

1. (b); 2. (c); 3. (c); 4. (c); 5. (b)

REFERENCES

1. Thi-Kim Vu, H., Rink, J. C., McKinney, S. A., McClain, M., Lakshmanaperumal, N., Alexander, R., & Sánchez Alvarado, A. (2015). Stem cells and fluid flow drive cyst formation in an invertebrate excretory organ. *eLife*, *4*, e07405. https://doi.org/10.7554/eLife.07405 (accessed on 16th June 2025).
2. Anders, H. J., Cohen, C. D., Edenhofer, I., Eichinger, F., et al. (2010). Systematic analysis of a novel human renal glomerulus-enriched gene expression dataset. https://core.ac.uk/download/12175685.pdf (accessed on 16th June 2025).
3. Andersson, A. C. (2014). *Characterization of Novel Glomerular Proteins: Role in Physiology and Disease*. https://core.ac.uk/download/70341242.pdf (accessed on 16th June 2025).
4. Arafa, E. (2016). *Determining Cellular and Biochemical Function of a Novel Adhesion Molecule in Kidneys*. https://open.bu.edu/bitstream/2144/16062/1/Arafa_bu_0017N_11077.pdf (accessed on 16th June 2025).
5. Arciero, J. C., Ellwein, L., Ford Versypt, A. N., Layton, A. T., et al. (2015). Bifurcation study of blood flow control in the kidney. https://core.ac.uk/download/46962683.pdf (accessed on 16th June 2025).
6. Stenvinkel, P., Painer, J., Kuro-O, M., Lanaspa, M., Arnold, W., Ruf, T., Shiels, P. G., & Johnson, R. J. (2018). Novel treatment strategies for chronic kidney disease: insights from the animal kingdom. *Nature reviews. Nephrology*, *14*(4), 265–284. https://doi.org/10.1038/nrneph.2017.169(accessed on 16th June 2025).
7. Ayati, B. P., Holstein, S. A., & Walk, J. C. (2018). Modeling the effects of multiple myeloma on kidney function. http://arxiv.org/abs/1602.03214 (accessed on 16th June 2025).
8. Bahamonde, J., Ezquer, F., Ezquer, M., Giraud Billoud, M., et al. (2017). Tubulointerstitial injury and proximal tubule albumin transport in early diabetic nephropathy induced by type 1 diabetes mellitus. https://core.ac.uk/download/159301014.pdf (accessed on 16th June 2025).
9. Beck, F. X., Giebisch, G., Ohno, A., Pfaller, W., et al. (1998). Quantitative morphology of renal cortical structures during compensatory hypertrophy. https://core.ac.uk/download/16432494.pdf (accessed on 16th June 2025).
10. Beebe, L., Hesse, D., & Massey, A. (2019). *UGA Anatomy and Physiology 2 Lab Manual* (3rd ed.). https://core.ac.uk/download/217306575.pdf (accessed on 16th June 2025).
11. Bruno, R. M. (2025). *Sympathetic Regulation of Vascular Function in Health and Disease*. https://core.ac.uk/download/pdf/37830788.pdf (accessed on 16th June 2025).
12. Burnstock, G., & Loesch, A. (2016). Sympathetic innervation of the kidney in health and disease: Emphasis on the role of purinergic cotransmission. https://core.ac.uk/download/79521483.pdf (accessed on 16th June 2025).
13. Campos Pamplona, C., Leuvenink, H. G. D., Moers, C., van Leeuwen, T. T., et al. (2023). Expanding the horizons of pre-transplant renal vascular assessment using *ex vivo* perfusion. https://core.ac.uk/download/571868157.pdf (accessed on 16th June 2025).
14. Coe, F. L., Evan, A. P., Krambeck, A., Lingeman, J. E., et al. (2013). A test of the hypothesis that oxalate secretion produces proximal tubule crystallization in primary hyperoxaluria type I. https://core.ac.uk/download/46962645.pdf (accessed on 16th June 2025).

15. Daniels, M. (2015). *A Translational Study of The Correlation Between Low Birth Weight, Hypertension, And Kidney Function Using a Rat Model*. https://core.ac.uk/download/148695115.pdf (accessed on 16th June 2025).

16. Delles, C., Gillis, K. A., Mark, P. B., McComb, J. M., et al. (2016). Non-contrast renal magnetic resonance imaging to assess perfusion and corticomedullary differentiation in health and chronic kidney disease. https://core.ac.uk/download/42373079.pdf (accessed on 16th June 2025).

17. Graham, L. A., Dominiczak, A. F., & Ferreri, N. R. (2017). Role of renal transporters and novel regulatory interactions in the TAL that control blood pressure. *Physiological genomics*, *49*(5), 261–276. https://doi.org/10.1152/physiolgenomics.00017.2017(accessed on 16th June 2025).

18. Ghezzi, C., Loo, D. D. F., & Wright, E. M. (2018). Physiology of renal glucose handling via SGLT1, SGLT2 and GLUT2. https://core.ac.uk/download/323079917.pdf (accessed on 16th June 2025).

19. Goswami, S., & Kundra, P. (2019). Endothelial glycocalyx: Role in body fluid homeostasis and fluid management. https://core.ac.uk/download/212867445.pdf (accessed on 16th June 2025).

20. Hoffman, Nicholas A., "The role of sphingolipids in AKI and the progression to CKD: potential therapuetic targets." (2021). Electronic Theses and Dissertations. Paper 3746. https://doi.org/10.18297/etd/3746 (accessed on 16th June 2025).

21. Jamison, R. L. (1987). Short and long loop nephrons. https://core.ac.uk/download/pdf/82811392.pdf (accessed on 16th June 2025).

22. Keith, D. S., Kon, S. P., Offord, K. P., Torres, V. E., et al. (1994). Renal ammonia in autosomal dominant polycystic kidney disease. https://core.ac.uk/download/pdf/82698346.pdf (accessed on 16th June 2025).

23. Kirwan, C. J., Macphee, I. A., & Philips, B. J. (2013). Estimated glomerular filtration rate correlates poorly with four-hour creatinine clearance in critically ill patients with acute kidney injury. https://core.ac.uk/download/17298026.pdf (accessed on 16th June 2025).

24. Leiz, J., & Schmitt-Ott, K. M. (2019). Claudins in the renal collecting duct. https://core.ac.uk/download/286097290.pdf (accessed on 16th June 2025).

25. Leonard, J. I. (2025). Analysis of head-down tilt as an analog of weightlessness using a mathematical simulation model. https://core.ac.uk/download/pdf/42845539.pdf (accessed on 16th June 2025).

26. Lu, Y., & Wang, W. (2010). Multiscale modelling of fluid and solute transport in soft tissues and micro vessels. https://core.ac.uk/download/46170774.pdf (accessed on 16th June 2025).

27. Musacchia, X. J. (1972). The role of depressed metabolism in increased radio-resistance. Document ID

28. 19760013710, Acquisition Source Legacy CDMS; Report Number: NASA-CR-146512(accessed on 16th June 2025).

29. Natochin, Y. V. (1996). Evolutionary aspects of renal function. https://core.ac.uk/download/pdf/82128875.pdf (accessed on 16th June 2025).

30. Noto, A. (2020). *Renal Disorders in Pregnancy*. https://core.ac.uk/download/333568139.pdf (accessed on 16th June 2025).

31. Pichler Sekulic, S., & Sekulic, M. (2013). A compendium of urinary biomarkers indicative of glomerular podocytopathy. https://core.ac.uk/download/28947337.pdf (accessed on 16th June 2025).

32. Ragul Siddarth, K. (2014). Estimation of relative bilateral renal function of potential voluntary kidney donors using various computerized tomography methods. https://core.ac.uk/download/288216014.pdf (accessed on 16th June 2025).

33. Shokr, E. (2016). *Introduction to Human Physiology for Medical Students.* https://core.ac.uk/download/322470167.pdf (accessed on 16th June 2025).

34. Speck, P. L. (2020). *The Kidney: A Designed System for Plasma Homeostasis.* https://core.ac.uk/download/351114222.pdf (accessed on 16th June 2025).

35. Stadt, M. M. (2022). *Mathematical Modeling of Kidney Function During Pregnancy.* https://core.ac.uk/download/534414719.pdf (accessed on 16th June 2025).

36. Strevens, H. (2002). *Blood Pressure, Renal Functional and Structural Changes, In Normal and Preeclamptic Pregnancy.* https://core.ac.uk/download/83727645.pdf (accessed on 16th June 2025).

INDEX

C

N

O

P

R

S

T

U

V

W